DATE DUE

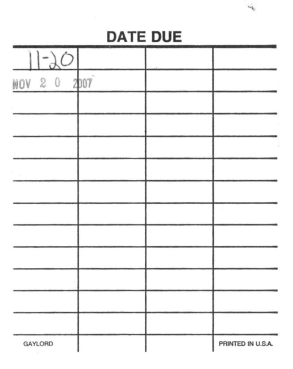

11-20			
NOV 2 0 2007			
GAYLORD			PRINTED IN U.S.A.

Mood Disorders

Mood Disorders

Clinical Management and Research Issues

Editors

Eric J. L. Griez

Department of Psychiatry and Neuropsychology
University of Maastricht, The Netherlands

Carlo Faravelli

Department of Neurology and Psychiatry
University of Florence, Italy

David J. Nutt

Psychopharmacology Unit
University of Bristol, UK

and

Joseph Zohar

Department of Psychiatry
University of Tel Aviv, Israel

John Wiley & Sons, Ltd

Other Wiley Editorial Offices

John Wiley & Sons Inc., 111 River Street, Hoboken, NJ 07030, USA

Jossey-Bass, 989 Market Street, San Francisco, CA 94103-1741, USA

Wiley-VCH Verlag GmbH, Boschstr. 12, D-69469 Weinheim, Germany

John Wiley & Sons Australia Ltd, 33 Park Road, Milton, Queensland 4064, Australia

John Wiley & Sons (Asia) Pte Ltd, 2 Clementi Loop #02-01, Jin Xing Distripark, Singapore 129809

John Wiley & Sons Canada Ltd, 22 Worcester Road, Etobicoke, Ontario, Canada M9W 1L1

Wiley also publishes its books in a variety of electronic formats. Some content that appears in print may
not be available in electronic books.

Library of Congress Cataloging-in-Publication Data

Mood disorders: clinical management and research issues/edited by Eric J.L. Griez. . . [et al.].
    p. ; cm.
  Includes bibliographical references and index.
  ISBN 0-470-09426-5 (alk. paper)
    1. Affective disorders. 2. Depression, Mental.   I. Griez, E. J. L.
  [DNLM: 1. Mood Disorders. WM 171 M8172 2005]
  RC537.M664 2005
  616.85'27–dc22

                                                                              2004053722

British Library Cataloguing in Publication Data

A catalogue record for this book is available from the British Library

ISBN 0 470 09426 5 (HB)

Typeset by Dobbie Typesetting Ltd, Tavistock, Devon
Printed and bound in Great Britain by TJ International Ltd, Padstow, Cornwall
This book is printed on acid-free paper responsibly manufactured from sustainable forestry in which at
least two trees are planted for each one used for paper production.

Contents

Contributors

Saena Arbabzadeh-Bouchez   *Hôpital Fernand Widal, 200, rue de Faubourg St. Denis, 75475 Paris Cedex 40, France*

Nicolò Baldini-Rossi   *University of Florence, Psychiatry Unit, Department of Neurology and Psychiatry, Viale Morgagni, 85, 50134 Florence, Italy*

Giovanni Battista Cassano   *University of Pisa, Facoltà di Medicina e Chirurgia, Dipartimento di Psichiatria, Clinica Psichiatrica II, Via Roma, 67, 56100 Pisa, Italy*

Fiammetta Cosci   *University of Florence, Department of Neurology and Psychiatry, Viale Morgagni, 85, 50134 Florence, Italy*

Phil J. Cowen   *University Department of Psychiatry, Warneford Hospital, Oxford OX3 7JX, UK*

Diego De Leo   *Australian Institute for Suicide Research and Prevention, Mt Gravatt Campus, Griffith University, 4111 Queensland, Australia*

Carlo Faravelli   *University of Florence, Department of Neurology and Psychiatry, Viale Morgagni, 85, 50134 Florence, Italy*

Renee Goodwin   *Department of Epidemiology, Mailman School of Public Health, Columbia University, 722 West 168th St, Rm 1706, New York, NY 10032, USA*

Eric J. L. Griez   *Department of Psychiatry and Neuropsychology, University of Maastricht, PO Box 616, 6200 MD Maastricht, The Netherlands*

Anthony S. Hale   *Kent Institute of Medicine and Health Sciences, University of Kent, Canterbury, Kent CT2 7PD, UK*

Frank Jacobi   *Dresden Technical University, AG Epidemiologie und Versorgungsforschung, Chemnitzerstrasse 46, 01187 Dresden, Germany*

Gunter Kenis   *Department of Psychiatry and Neuropsychology, University of Maastricht, PO Box 616, 6200 MD Maastricht, The Netherlands*

Markus Kosel   *Psychiatric Neuroimaging Group, Department of Psychiatry, University Hospital Bern, 3010 Bern, Switzerland*

Jean-Pierre Lépine   *Hôpital Fernand Widal, 200 rue de Faubourg St. Denis, 75475 Paris Cedex 40, France*

Michael Maes   *Department of Psychiatry and Neuropsychology, University of Maastricht, Hospital Vjverdal, Vijverdalseweg, 6200 AB Maastricht, The Netherlands*

Andrea L. Malizia   *University of Bristol, Psychopharmacology Unit, Dorothy Hodgkin Building, Whitson Street, Bristol BS1 3NY, UK*

Mario Miniati   *University of Pisa, Facoltà de Medicina e Chirurgia, Dipartimento di Psichiatria, Clinica Psichiatrica II, Via Roma, 67, 56100 Pisa, Italy*

Peter Muris   *Department of Medical, Clinical and Experimental Psychology, University of Maastricht, PO Box 616, 6200 MD Maastricht, The Netherlands*

David J. Nutt   *University of Bristol, Psychopharmacology Unit, Dorothy Hodgkin Building, Whiston Street, Bristol BS1 3NY, UK*

Pierre Oswald   *Erasmus Hospital, Department of Psychiatry, Free University of Brussels, 808, Route de Lennik, B-1070 Brussels, Belgium*

Thea Overbeek   *Department of Psychiatry and Neuropsychology, University of Maastricht, PO Box 616, 6200 MD Maastricht, The Netherlands*

Stefano Pini   *University of Pisa, Facoltà di Medicina e Chirurgia, Dipartimento di Psichiatria, Clinica Psichiatrica II, Via Roma, 67, 56100 Pisa, Italy*

Claudia Ravaldi   *University of Florence, Psychiatry Unit, Department of Neurological and Psychiatric Sciences, Viale Morgagni, 85, 50134 Florence, Italy*

Jeffrey Roelofs   *Department of Medical, Clinical and Experimental Psychology, University of Maastricht, PO Box 616, 6200 MD Maastricht, The Netherlands*

Hans M. Rollema   *Pfizer Global Research and Development, Groton Laboratories, MS 8220-4159, Department of Neuroscience, Eastern Point Road, Groton, CT 06340, USA*

Simone Rosi   *University of Florence, Psychiatry Unit, Department of Neurological and Psychiatric Sciences, Viale Morgagni 85, 50134 Florence, Italy*

Thomas E. Schlaepfer   *Department of Psychiatry, The Johns Hopkins University School of Medicine, Baltimore, MD, USA, and Psychiatric Neuroimaging Group, Department of Psychiatry, University Hospital Bern, 3010 Bern, Switzerland*

Alessandro Serretti   *H.S. Raffaele, Department of Psychiatry, University Vita-Salute, School of Medicine, Via Stamira D'Ancona 20, 20127 Milan, Italy*

Daniel Souery   *Department of Psychiatry, University Clinics of Brussels, Erasmus Hospital, Free University of Brussels, 808 Route de Lennik, 1070 Brussels, Belgium*

Kym Spathonis   *Australian Institute for Suicide Research and Prevention, Mt Gravatt Campus, Griffith University, 4111 Queensland, Australia*

Jeffrey Sprouse   *Pfizer Global Research and Development, Groton Laboratories, MS 8220-4159, Department of Neuroscience, Eastern Point Road, Groton, CT 06340, USA*

Leonard Tondo   *Centro Lucio Bini, Stanley Foundation Research Center, 28, Via Cavalcanti, 09128 Cagliari, Italy*

Elisabetta Truglia   *University of Florence, Psychiatry Unit, Department of Neurological and Psychiatric Sciences, Viale Morgagni, 85, 50134, Florence, Italy*

Herman M. van Praag   *Department of Psychiatry and Neuropsychology, Academic Hospital Maastricht, and The Brain and Behavior Research Institute, University of Maastricht, Maastricht, The Netherlands*

Dirk van West   *University Centre of Child and Adolescent Psychiatry Antwerp – AZM, University of Antwerp (UA), Lindendreef 1, 2020 Antwerp, Belgium*

Sue J. Wilson   *University of Bristol, Psychopharmacology Unit, Dorothy Hodgkin Building, Whitson Street, Bristol BS1 3NY, UK*

Joseph Zohar   *Ministry of Health, The State of Israel and Department of Psychiatry, Tel Aviv University, Sackler School of Medicine, Tel Hashomer 52621, Tel Aviv, Israel*

Preface

The present book complements *Anxiety Disorders: an Introduction to Clinical Management and Research* by the same editors.

These publications reflect the core materials of the European Program in Affective Neuroscience, formerly known as The European Certificate in Anxiety and Mood Disorders. Both volumes are linked to the dynamic process of an ongoing series of academic events, which has been repeated year after year since 1989. The present book on mood disorders, like its predecessor on anxiety disorders, relies on the essential contribution of a broad faculty of worldwide experts who have been involved in our teaching program. The book does not aim to be exhaustive. All basic issues on mania and depression are covered, but, as far as advanced topics are concerned, the volume concentrates on a limited number of selected key issues. The choice is intended as an introduction in critical thinking and research-mindedness applied to the field of bipolar and depressive disorders.

This book reflects an education program at a level of excellence, which favors scientific debate rather than the propagation of any particular view or doctrine-driven opinion on the origin and mechanisms of affective disorders. It will therefore come as no surprise that in the following chapters, authors at some point differ in the interpretations of existing data. More often than not, evidence, when looked at in a critical way, appears to be ambiguous. The acceptance of this limitation belongs to the essence of science, scientific activity itself being kept alive by the diversity of new hypotheses.

In the preface of our volume on anxiety disorders we defined the European Certificate in Anxiety and Mood Disorders as a pioneering transnational teaching initiative in the field of mental health. In the mean time, this initiative has evolved as a formal interuniversity consortium now awarding a joint academic degree in Affective Neuroscience. Scientific activity is a worldwide endeavor; likewise scientific education should become an international enterprise.

Eric J. L. Griez
Chairman of the Board of Directors

Introduction

Herman M. van Praag

Scientific Advisor Department of Psychiatry and Neuropsychology, Academic Hospital Maastricht, and The Brain and Behavior Research Institute, Maastricht University, The Netherlands

This is yet another book on depression. So many have been published about this subject over the past 40 years, that the question arises of possible redundancy. I do not believe this to be the case. First, the domain of mood disorders is in motion, and has been so for many years. Slowly but steadily our data base is, and has been enriched. One needs regular reviews and updates to keep abreast. Second, the field of mood disorders confronts us with fundamental and unresolved issues, pertaining not only to depression, but to psychiatry at large. Attention to them should not slacken.

How, for instance, can one mark the border between the still normal and the just pathological. In the case of depression, what differentiates so called 'case depression' from states of distress. Is it number of symptoms, their persistence, their seriousness, or the measure of social or professional impairment they cause? Is it whether they occur in isolation or are embedded in a syndrome? We do not yet know, and this state of affairs hampers research, for instance that into the biological determinants of depression and into the efficacy of antidepressant drugs. As an analogy: the cause and treatment of pneumonia would have remained in darkness if groups of pneumonia patients had been mixed with patients suffering from a common cold. This question is all the more urgent now that it has been well documented that phenomena we know from true psychopathological states also occur, and with considerable frequency, in the normal population (Johns and Van Os, 2001). Death ideation, for instance, was reported by 35% of those interviewed, death wish by 10.6%, suicide contemplation by 11.7%, suicide attempt by 2.8% (Neeleman et al., in press). In a cohort of school-aged youths the frequency of suicidal ideation was even higher: 30.8% in females, and 25.3% in males (Miotto et al., 2003).

What, furthermore, is the role of stress in depression? Stress so often precedes depression, but what is its pathogenic weight. Is it merely responsible for a measure of distress or can it truly cause (certain forms of) depression. We do not yet know, but the latter seems likely (Van Praag et al., 2004). If probability were to become certainty, the focus of biological depression research would be diverted from depression per se, to the neurobiology of stress (at least for certain types of depression), and proper treatment of (certain) depressions should become primarily stress-focused.

Another rather crucial point is the status of anxiety. Anxiety may be, and often is, prominent in depression, and mood and anxiety disorders often go hand in hand. Is anxiety a mere component of the depressive syndrome or should its status be upgraded. Could it be that anxiety is a precursor and pacemaker of (certain forms of) depression, as suggested by Van Praag (1996). Pacemaker symptoms I defined as symptoms that are primordial and may cause disturbances in other psychic domains (Van Praag, 2001).

Another pertinent question is whether anxiety and mood disorders are in fact discrete categories or to that degree intermingled that it is highly artificial to distinguish them categorically – does a dimensional characterization of mixed depression/anxiety states, therefore, seem more appropriate?

This, in its turn, raises a truly fundamental question. Is categorical classification the appropriate way to classify disordered mental states, or are categories rather man-made artefacts, and should the categorical way of diagnosing be replaced, or at least be complemented, by a functional/dimensional system (Van Praag, 1997). In such a system psychopathological syndromes are dissected into their basic constituents, i.e. psychic dysfunctions, such as disturbances in anxiety, mood, and aggression regulation, in cognitive functions, in emotional regulation and many others. Those dysfunctions will be assessed and measured as to presence and intensity. In this way a detailed map is obtained of dysfunctioning domains in the 'psychic apparatus'.

In a direct line with this reasoning arises the question whether biological treatment of mental pathology should remain categorically directed or should shift to a functional/dimensional focus; whether 'disorders' should be treated – such as major depression, dysthymia, mixed anxiety depression disorder etc. – or rather psychic dysfunctions such as disturbances in anxiety regulation, mood regulation and aggression regulation. For such functional orientation of psychopharmacology there are clear precedents in other branches of medicine. The cardiologist, for instance, does not treat myocardial infarction, he treats its functional consequences, and this with a variety of medications.

Since it would clearly be impossible to treat each and every psychic dysfunction in a given psychopathological state, the functional approach would become only feasible and adequate if the concept of pacemaker symptoms were to be validated. Functional psychopharmacology would require a strategic turnaround of research efforts within the pharmaceutical industry.

What, one may ask, is the potentiality of biology for treatment purposes. Is it possible to conceive of future antidepressant drugs that approach 100% efficacy in treating and preventing depression, or does that seem an illusion and will psychological interventions always be an indispensable complement to biological treatment. This is another of such fundamental issues. I believe the latter possibility is more likely than the former. In most cases depressive disorders are preceded by stressors, that produce undue stress, because of personality traits impeding coping abilities. To the extent that stress plays a role in the pathogenesis of depression, psychological methods, geared towards ego-strengthening and betterment of coping skills, will be an indispensable complement to biological treatments, in most cases.

Psychological treatments today are globally oriented, that is to say are geared towards personalities as a whole. One wonders whether a more functional orientation would be beneficial in this field as well. Which personality features one wants to address and what coping skills should be strengthened will then be the primary questions. Functional psychotherapy would be, I presume, a significant step forward.

And finally, then, to end this enumeration of some fundamental issues, the interest in which has been significantly enhanced by depression research, there is the question of what the pathogenetic significance is of the neurobiological disturbances gathered in psychiatric disorders. Biological studies, so far, have unearthed bits and pieces of information. In the study of depression, for instance, aberrations have been traced in all monoaminergic systems, the glutamate and CRH/cortisol systems, in that of some growth factors, and several others.

Is depression, biologically speaking, a multifaceted disorder in which various biological dysfunctions have the same pathogenic 'valence', or is there a common biological denominator to which the 'bits and pieces' are subordinate? This question remains of central concern to biological psychiatric research in general.

Depression research yields data literally every day. Yet many questions remain, some practical in nature, some touching the very foundations of psychiatry. Regular reporting is essential to keep the profession informed, researchers and clinicians alike.

Another book on depression, then, is no superfluity.

Johns LC, Van Os J (2001) The continuity of psychotic experiences in the general population. *Clin Psychol Rev* **21**: 1125–1141.

Miotto P, Coppi de M, Frezza M, Petretto D, Masala C, Preti A (2003) Suicidal ideation and aggressiveness in school-aged youths. *Psychiat Res* **120**: 247–255.

Neeleman J, de Graaf R, Volleberg W (in press) The suicidal process; prospective comparison between early and later stages. *J Affect Disor.*

Van Praag HM (1996) Faulty cortisol/serotonin interplay. Psychopathological and biological characterization of a new hypothetical depression subtype (SeCa depression). *Psychiat Res* **65**: 143–157.

Van Praag HM (1997) Over the mainstream: diagnostic requirements for biological psychiatric research. *Psychiat Res* **72**: 201–212.

Van Praag HM (2001) Historical and contemporary notes on the treatment of depression, or, How classification shaped therapeutic approaches. In den Boer JA, Westenberg HGM (eds) *Antidepressants: Selectivity or Multiplicity?* Amsterdam: Benecke.

Van Praag HM, De Kloet R, Van Os J (2004) *Stress, the Brain and Depression.* Cambridge, UK: Cambridge University Press.

PART I
Epidemiology/Genetics

The Epidemiology of Mood Disorders

**Frank Jacobi[1], Simone Rosi[2],
Carlo Faravelli[2], Renee Goodwin[3],
Saena Arbabzadeh- Bouchez[4] and Jean-Pierre Lépine[4]**

[1]*Dresden Technical University, Dresden, Germany*
[2]*University of Florence, Florence, Italy*
[3]*Columbia University, New York, USA*
[4]*Fernand Widal Hospital, Paris, France*

INTRODUCTION

Research in epidemiology is critical to understanding mood disorders for several reasons. First, on a societal level, health care planning can be assisted by assessing the magnitude of the burden of disease in the population. Mood disorders are among the major health problems world wide for two reasons: they are highly prevalent in the general population, and they cause significant loss of quality of life and social functioning in the affected individual. Further, mood disorders contribute to a poorer outcome of comorbid mental as well as somatic conditions. On the basis of epidemiological data and health economic measures based on clinical severity ratings it has been projected that major depression will be responsible for the largest burden of disease of any illness by the year 2020 (Murray and Lopez, 1996). With regard to health care planning, the assessment of the effectiveness of intervention programs in the community is important. Second, in addition to the mere reporting of prevalence or incidence rates in a circumscribed population (*descriptive epidemiology*), *analytical epidemiology* supplements clinical research in identifying vulnerabilities as well as factors that trigger the onset, and influence the course of the condition under study. This is particularly applicable to mental disorders. It is well known that subjects with mental disorders often do not seek psychiatric consultation (Goldberg and Huxley, 1980); therefore, cases that come under the observation of specialists cannot be considered fully representative of the characteristics of psychiatric disorders in the general population. Epidemiological community surveys consistently show that the number of cases referred to psychiatrists is relatively small and unlikely to be representative of psychiatric disorders as they occur in the

Mood Disorders: Clinical Management and Research Issues. Edited by E. J. L. Griez, C. Faravelli, D. J. Nutt and J. Zohar.
©2005 John Wiley & Sons Ltd. ISBN 0 470 09426 5.

general population (Bijl et al., 2003). Psychiatric samples, therefore, could be biased not only quantitatively but also qualitatively (Galbaud du Fort et al., 1993). Thus, studies conducted with non-clinical samples are necessary in order to complete our knowledge of psychiatric pathology – in basic research on mechanisms as well as in refining diagnostic criteria and nosology.

This chapter will focus on the following topics: (1) methodological issues in the epidemiological investigation of mood disorders; (2) distribution of mood disorders in the general adult population (prevalence, comorbidity, onset, course) and (3) risk factors and correlates of mood disorders.

METHODOLOGICAL ISSUES

Historical Development: First, Second and Third Generation Studies

In a classic review Dohrenwend and Dohrenwend (1982) identified three generations of psychiatric community epidemiological surveys. In the first generation of studies, which dates back to the mid-1800s, community residents were not directly interviewed and the identification of cases of psychiatric disorders relied essentially on agency records and key informants, such as general practitioners and clergymen. The second generation of studies began after World War II and its major advancement is represented by the fact that randomly selected community residents were directly contacted; in these surveys subjects either filled out forms which yielded global ratings of psychopathology (but not a diagnosis) or were assessed by interviewers (generally clinicians) who determined the diagnoses (Streiner, 1998). When diagnoses were obtained, the lack of clear operationalized diagnostic criteria and of standardized and reliable assessment instruments resulted in a poor reliability and represented a major shortcoming of these studies. Diagnostic categories of affective pathology in particular were quite different from current ones. Due to a unitary view of psychopathology, milder forms of mood disorders were generally grouped together with anxiety and other disorders and labelled as 'neuroses', while the category of 'affective psychosis' included both depressive and bipolar severe mood disorders. Neugebauer et al. (1980) reviewed 3 North American and 13 European (mostly Scandinavian) second generation studies and reported period prevalence rates for affective psychosis ranging from 0.0% to 1.9%.

In spite of their limitations, the first and second generation studies were fundamental for the development of psychiatric epidemiology since they clarified that mental illness was a major public health problem and that most subjects suffering from psychiatric disorders did not seem to have adequate access to treatment (Tohen et al., 2000).

During the 1970s concerns about the low reliability of psychiatric diagnoses led to the development of explicit, operationalized sets of diagnostic criteria such as the St.

Louis criteria (Feighner et al., 1972), the Research Diagnostic Criteria (RDC; Spitzer et al., 1978), the third edition of the American Psychiatric Association's Diagnostic and Statistical Manual (DSM-III and the subsequent editions DSM-III-R and DSM-IV; American Psychiatric Association, 1980, 1987, 1994/2000), the ninth and tenth revisions of the World Health Organization's International Classification of Diseases (ICD-9 and ICD-10; World Health Organization, 1978, 1993). Concurrently, standardized diagnostic interviews were developed in order to reduce potential sources of disagreement between different assessors (Box 1).

Utilization of operationalized diagnostic criteria and standardized interviews in community samples reflect the major advance of the *third and current generation* of psychiatric epidemiological surveys. These developments allowed researchers to obtain reliable information about the prevalence rates of specific disorders and as a result the past 20 years have been a highly productive period for psychiatric

---

Box 1: Selected Assessment Instruments

Along with the development of diagnostic systems based on explicit criteria, standardized diagnostic interviews were developed and refined in order to reduce potential sources of disagreement between different assessors. There are basically two types of instruments (Brugha et al., 1999a): semi-structured interviews (for use by interviewers with clinical experience) and fully standardized interviews (for use by lay interviewers). Note: in some recent studies mandatory standardized assessment is accompanied by clinical severity ratings, preferably administered by clinically trained interviewers; thus, the dichotomy of these approaches is not absolute.

   Prominent examples are:

(A) Semi-structured interviews

- Present State Examination (PSE; Wing et al., 1974)
- Schedule for Affective Disorders and Schizophrenia (SADS; Endicott and Spitzer, 1978)
- Schedules for Clinical Assessment in Neuropsychiatry (SCAN; Wing et al., 1990)
- Structured Clinical Interview for DSM-IV (SCID; First et al., 1997)

(B) Standardized interviews

- Diagnostic Interview Schedule (DIS; Robins et al., 1981)
- Composite International Diagnostic Interview (CIDI; Robins et al., 1988, and several modified/updated versions)
- Revised Clinical Interview Schedule (CIS-R; Lewis et al., 1992).

Another example for a widely used instrument is the Mini-International Neuropsychiatric Interview (Sheehan et al., 1998), a short structured diagnostic interview, developed jointly by psychiatrists and clinicians in the United States and France, for DSM-IV and ICD-10 psychiatric disorders. With an administration time of approximately 15 minutes, it was designed to meet the need for a short but accurate structured psychiatric interview for multicentre clinical trials and epidemiology studies and to be used as a first step in outcome tracking in nonresearch clinical settings.

epidemiology, with a large number of surveys conducted in several countries, although little evidence is still available from nations with low-income economies (de Girolamo and Bassi, 2003).

Assessment and Design Issues

Despite the remarkable advances of current semi-structured or standardized assessments, important methodological issues still remain unresolved. Most importantly, the validity of community diagnostic assessment remains controversial. This is a crucial issue since it has been repeatedly shown in community samples that even relatively small changes in diagnostic criteria and assessment methods may produce substantially different results (Brugha et al., 1999b; Regier et al., 1998; Narrow et al., 2002). Thus, it is important to investigate whether differences in prevalence rates between studies are attributable to real differences or to methodological factors (population/sampling, threshold definitions (see Box 2), modifications in the instrument, or use of clinically trained vs. lay interviewers).

In mood disorders, valid assessment is difficult for various reasons (see Box 3). The standardized approach of the assessment (e.g. M-CIDI; Wittchen et al., 1998) offers good reliability and validity, in particular in its current versions, for depressive disorders but to a lesser degree in bipolar disorders (Kessler et al., 1998, 2003; Wittchen, 1994). Considering the difficulties in assessing the whole spectrum of mood disorders the use of clinicians as interviewers might be of special importance, as well as in certain other domains (e.g. psychosis, mental disorder due to general

---

Box 2: Subthreshold Mood Disorders

Various studies suggest that a large proportion of subjects with clinically significant depression in the community fail to meet current diagnostic criteria for either major depressive disorder or dysthymia (Angst and Merikangas, 1997). For instance, in the NCS the lifetime prevalence of DSM-III-R 'minor depression' was 10.0% and its correlates were substantially similar to major depression (Kessler et al., 1997), while in a recent Italian survey the lifetime prevalence of DSM-IV 'depression not otherwise specified' was 7.8% (Faravelli et al., 2004b).

Recurrent brief depression is perhaps the most extensively studied subthreshold mood disorder since its first operationalized definition on the basis of epidemiological observations from the Zurich study (Angst and Dobler-Mikola, 1985). In a recent review of four community studies the lifetime prevalence of recurrent brief depression ranged between 2.6% and 21.3%; the disorder also seems associated with significant clinical impairment (Pezawas et al., 2003).

Data from the Zurich study also suggest the broadening of the boundaries of bipolarity; in this survey about 11% of community residents could be included in the expanded spectrum of bipolar disorders and 13% presented attenuate expressions of bipolarity intermediate between bipolar disorder and normality (Angst et al., 2003a,b); however, these findings, being derived from a single small-size study, need replication.

> **Box 3: Challenges in the Assessment of Mood Disorders in Epidemiological Studies**
>
> In mood disorders, valid assessment is difficult for various reasons:
>
> - Even chronic and recurrent mood disorders show an episodic and fluctuating course. This results in difficulties in assessing exact time frames where enough symptoms are present concurrently with sufficient severity to justify the diagnosis. Example: Results will differ if the 12-month time frame is completely assessed before further lifetime psychopathology (for the disorders where no 12-month symptoms were present) vs. lifetime episodes are inquired about first, followed by a recency question (When was the last time it happened?) and prescribing a 12-month diagnosis according to the answer to this recency question. The first interview version produces better 12-month prevalence estimates.
> - With regard to the unstable course it may be reasonable also to take subthreshold conditions into account (e.g., to identify prodromal states, partial remissions, or a new diagnosis in its own right, see Box 2), describing further potential complications.
> - Mood disorders require lifetime assessment especially with regard to (differential) diagnosis of bipolar disorders. Distinguishing normal mood swings and nonpathological exalted mood states from (hypo-) manic symptoms requires additional procedures to achieve reliability as well as clinical relevance of the diagnosis; the use of clinically trained interviewers may be necessary.

medical factor, somatoform disorders). This also refers to the validity of study designs (e.g. one cross-sectional interview in household vs. sequential assessment by the subject's primary care physicians; Faravelli et al., 2004a).

The debate about a 'gold standard' of the epidemiological assessment – semi-structured vs. standardized interviews (Brugha et al., 1999a) – may continue until the theoretical advantage of a clinical approach provides more promising psychometric properties than standardized interviews do. In some areas such as disclosure vs. bias due to social acceptability standardized methods can even achieve better results than a method that resembles clinical practice (Turner et al., 1998). Following Wittchen et al.'s (1999a) arguments, the use of semi-structured clinical interviews as the central approach to carrying out epidemiological surveys might be likely to create more problems than it solves. In any case, the results of CIDI and SCID diagnoses seem to converge, presumably due to the development of improving accuracy within the latest CIDI versions. Also Faravelli et al. (2004b) conclude that their results of a naturalistic study are comparable to previous studies: in spite of the broad methodological differences, the similarities seem much greater than the differences.

Among other current methodological developments in the assessment of mood and other mental disorders as well as in the design of epidemiological studies, are: the inclusion of severity measures and more comprehensive analyses of disability and help-seeking, enhanced probing and rating procedures, inclusion of variables suited for health economic analyses, and the increasing availability of longitudinal data, allowing more sophisticated analyses with regard to causes and courses of mental disorders.

THE DISTRIBUTION OF MOOD DISORDERS IN THE COMMUNITY: PREVALENCE, COMORBIDITY, AND THEIR CORRELATES

Lifetime and Current Prevalence Rates in the General Population

Major Depression and Dysthymia

Prevalence rates of Major Depression and Dysthymia in selected third generation epidemiological surveys are presented in Table 1.1. Note that in the total rates shown, male and female values are averaged: prevalence rates have been consistently found 1.5–2.5 times higher in women than in men; for example, in the German study (Jacobi et al., 2004) the prevalence of any depressive 12-month-diagnosis in women is 14% vs. 7.5% in men. Prevalence rates for major depression and dysthymia in these surveys vary widely across countries (for references see Table 1.1) and, in particular, very low rates of major depression have been reported in studies conducted in Eastern Asian nations. Sociodemographic differences (e.g. discrepancies in the distribution of marital status) or cross-cultural variations (e.g. different social acceptability of the expression of emotions) could explain the discrepancies between the results. Also variability of instruments and design used in these studies can account for differences. For example, the clinicians in the Sesto Fiorentino Study diagnosed 'depressive disorder NOS' significantly more frequently than is reported in studies based on a different methodology; this might explain lower rates of major depression (9.5% vs. 13–17% lifetime prevalence in other recent studies).

Roughly 20–40% of unipolar depressive cases are assigned dysthymia as a diagnosis (3–6% lifetime prevalence over most studies). Studies are generally concordant in pointing out that major depression and dysthymia frequently coexist, a disorder sometimes referred to as 'double depression'. The lifetime prevalence of double depression has been reported to range between 1.5% and 2.5% (Bland, 1997).

Data from most cross-sectional community surveys suggest that the prevalence of major depression is increasing in successive generations born after World War II (Cross-National Collaborative Group, 1992; Kessler et al., 1996, 2003). However, studies relying on single retrospective interviews may be biased by methodological factors such as recall bias increasing with age (Bland, 1997; Paykel, 2000). Long-term longitudinal follow-up surveys are a much more reliable source of information about this topic; however, available evidence from such studies is limited and inconsistent (Hagnell et al., 1982; Lehtinen et al., 1991; Murphy et al., 2000a,b) and therefore this issue remains open to debate. Selected findings about the prevalence in primary care are presented in Box 4.

Bipolar Disorders

Prevalence rates of bipolar disorders in selected third generation epidemiological surveys are presented in Table 1.2; here, rates in women and men are roughly the same (lifetime 1–2% in most studies). The differences between lifetime and current (12-month) rates are smaller than in unipolar depressions; this could indirectly indicate a higher chronicity. It has to be mentioned that in this overview bipolar I and bipolar II disorders are lumped together, but most by far of the epidemiological studies on bipolar illness have examined bipolar I disorder.

Younger and Older Age

This chapter focuses on the epidemiology of mood disorders in adults but some basic information for children and adolescents is given in Box 5. The results for depressive symptoms among the elderly population are quite variable across studies. These results are summarized in Table 1.3. By contrast with depressive symptoms, rates of major depression seem to be much lower. When the Diagnostic Interview Schedule (DIS) (Robins et al., 1981) is used, the 6-month prevalence of major depression in the community ranged from 1.7% (Weissman et al., 1985) to 4.85% (Potter et al., 1995). Other methods have been used in order to assess depressive disorders in the elderly (Uhlenhuth et al., 1983; Ben-Arie et al., 1987; Carpiniello et al., 1989; Forsell et al., 1995; Steffens et al., 2000). The prevalence rates found in theses studies vary from 5.1% (Uhlenhuth et al., 1983) to 15.8% (Steffens et al., 2000).

Box 4:   Depression in primary care

In addition to representative community studies it should be noted that the prevalence of depressive disorders has also been examined in primary care all over the world (e.g. WHO studies; Üstün and Sartorius, 1995). Point prevalence estimates of major depression have varied widely across 15 centres (Simon et al., 2002); from a low of 1.6% in Japan to a high of 26.3% in Chile. In Germany, recent studies in primary care with large samples ($N > 20\,000$) report point prevalence estimates of over 10% for depressive disorders (Jacobi et al., 2002a; Wittchen and Pittrow, 2002).

Although primary care physicians show better recognition rates than in former WHO studies, there is still much room for improvement. Case recognition (any mental disorder among the patients diagnosed by the physicians as depressive) is better than diagnostic recognition (correct depressive diagnosis) – but often primary care physicians tend to over-diagnose depression (compared to standardized study assessment; Höfler and Wittchen, 2000).

TABLE 1.1   Third generation prevalence studies of major depression and dysthymia

			Major depression			Dysthymia		
			Lifetime	6–12-month	1-month	Lifetime	6–12-month	1-month
Semi-structured interviews								
Weissman and Myers, 1978	New Haven, USA	SADS/RDC	18.0	–	3.7[a]	–	–	–
Faravelli et al., 1990	Florence, Italy	SADS/DSM-III	–	6.3	2.8[a]	–	3.0	1.0[a]
Angst, 1996	Zurich, Switzerland	SPIKE/DSM-III	16.1	7.3	1.5	–	–	–
Almeida-Filho et al., 1997	Brazil (3 samples)	Semi-structured interview/DSM-III	1.9–10.2[b]	–	–	–	–	–
Faravelli et al., 2004a,b	Florence, Italy	FPI/DSM-IV	9.5	3.4	2.7[a]	1.5	0.9	0.8[a]
Henderson et al., 1979, 1981	Canberra, Australia	PSE/ICD-9	–	–	4.8[b]	–	–	–
Bebbington et al., 1981	Camberwell, UK	PSE/ICD-9	–	–	7.0[b]	–	–	–
Mavreas et al., 1986	Athens, Greece	PSE/ICD-9	–	–	7.4[b]	–	–	–
Hodiamont et al., 1987	Nijmegen, the Netherlands	PSE/ICD-9	–	–	5.4[b]	–	–	–
Vazquez-Barquero et al., 1987	Santander, Spain	PSE/ICD-9	–	–	6.2[b]	–	–	–
Lehtinen et al., 1990	Finland (2 samples)	PSE/ICD-9	–	–	4.6[b]	–	–	–
Roca et al., 1999	Formentera, Spain	SCAN/ICD-10	–	–	1.6	–	–	3.1
Ayuso-Mateos et al., 2001	Finland (2 samples)		–	–	4.1–4.7	–	–	0.3–1.1
	Ireland (2 samples)		–	–	6.2–8.9	–	–	0.5–2.9
	Norway (2 samples)	SCAN/ICD-10	–	–	7.0–8.4	–	–	0.9–1.5
	Santander, Spain		–	–	1.8	–	–	0.5
	UK (2 samples)		–	–	4.8–15.0	–	–	0.2–0.3
Fully structured interviews								
Regier et al., 1988; Weissman et al., 1991	USA (ECA; 5 samples)	DIS/DSM-III	5.8	3.0	2.2	3.3	–	–
Canino et al., 1987	Puerto Rico	DIS/DSM-III	4.6	3.0	–	4.7	–	–
Bland et al., 1988a,b	Edmonton, Canada	DIS/DSM-III	8.6	3.2	2.3	3.7	–	–
Wells et al., 1989; Oakley-Browne et al., 1989	Christchurch, New Zealand	DIS/DSM-III	12.6	5.3	–	6.4	–	–

(continued)

Study	Location	Instrument/Criteria						
Hwu et al., 1989	Taiwan (3 samples)	DIS/DSM-III	0.9–1.7	0.6–1.1	—	0.9–1.5	—	—
Lee et al., 1990a,b	Korea (2 samples)	DIS/DSM-III	3.3–3.5	—	—	1.9–2.4	—	—
Wittchen et al., 1992	Former West Germany	DIS/DSM-III	9.0	3.0	—	3.9	—	—
Chen et al., 1993	Hong Kong	DIS/DSM-III	1.3 (M)–2.4 (F)	—	—	1.0 (M)–2.8 (F)	—	1.6
Szadoczky et al., 1998	Hungary	DIS/DSM-IIIR	15.1	7.1	2.6	4.5	—	—
Kessler et al., 1994b; Blazer et al., 1994	USA (NCS)	CIDI/DSM-IIIR	17.1	10.3	4.9	6.4	2.5	—
Offord et al., 1996	Ontario, Canada	CIDI/DSM-IIIR	—	4.1	—	—	0.8	—
Bijl et al., 1998	The Netherlands	CIDI/DSM-IIIR	15.4	5.8	2.7	6.3	2.3	—
Wang et al., 2000	USA (MIDUS)	CIDI/DSM-IIIR	—	14.1	—	—	—	—
Kringlen et al., 2001	Oslo (Norway)	CIDI/DSM-IIIR	17.8	7.3	—	10.0	3.8	—
Sandanger et al., 1999	Norway (2 samples)	CIDI/ICD-10	—	—	2.6[a,c]	—	—	—
Abou-Saleh et al., 2001	Al Ain, United Arab Emirates	CIDI/ICD-10	3.4	—	—	—	—	—
Andrade et al., 2002	S3o Paulo, Brazil	CIDI/ICD-10	16.8	7.1	4.5	4.3	1.4	1.1
Andrews et al., 2001	Australia	CIDI/DSM-IV	—	6.3	3.2	—	1.1	0.9
Kessler et al., 2003	USA (NCS-R)	CIDI/DSM-IV	16.2	6.6	—	—	—	—
Jenkins et al., 1997	Great Britain	CIS-R/ICD-10	—	—	2.3[a]	—	—	—
Araya et al., 2001	Santiago, Chile	CIS-R/ICD-10	—	—	5.5[a]	—	—	—
Jacobi et al., 2004	Germany	M-CIDI/DSM-IV	14.8	8.3	3.4	4.5	4.5	3.6
The ESEMeD-MHEDEA 2000 Investigators, 2004	Belgium, France, Germany, Italy, the Netherlands, Spain	WMH-CIDI/DSM-IV	12.8	3.9	—	4.1	1.1	—

ECA: Epidemiologic Catchment Area Study; NCS: National Comorbidity Survey; MIDUS: Midlife Development in the United States survey; SADS: Schedule for Affective Disorders and Schizophrenia (Endicott and Spitzer, 1978); SPIKE: Structured Psychopathological Interview and Rating of the Social Consequences for Epidemiology (Angst et al., 1984); FPI: Florence Psychiatric Interview (Faravelli et al., 2001); PSE: Present State Examination (Wing et al., 1974); SCAN: Schedules for Clinical Assessment in Neuropsychiatry (Wing et al., 1990); DIS: Diagnostic Interview Schedule (Robins et al., 1981); CIDI: Composite International Diagnostic Interview (Robins et al., 1988); CIS-R: Revised Clinical Interview Schedule (Lewis et al., 1992).

[a] 1–2-week prevalence.
[b] PSE/CATEGO/ICD-9 depressive disorders.
[c] Major depressive episode and dysthymia.

Among the specific difficulties in this area are: great variability according to age group (>55 vs. >65 vs. >70 vs. >80 in different studies), problems with diagnostic instruments developed for younger adults (Knäuper and Wittchen, 1994), interference/symptom overlap with comorbid somatic conditions, and the need for modified (but not yet established) diagnostic criteria for the elderly.

But independently of the assessment method used, prevalence rates of depressive symptoms and major depression are lower in elderly people in the community than in younger people. These results may be explained by a selective mortality bias, a recall bias of psychiatric symptoms, a more frequent denial of psychiatric symptoms by elderly, more prominence of physical symptoms of depression in aged people or a possible cohort effect.

Comorbidity, Onset, and Course

Comorbidity

Community studies are generally concordant in pointing out that major depression is a highly comorbid disorder. Figure 1.1 presents comorbidity data from a German study (Jacobi et al., 2002b, 2004) with percentages and odds ratios for anxiety, somatoform and substance disorders when a major depression or dysthymia is

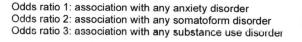

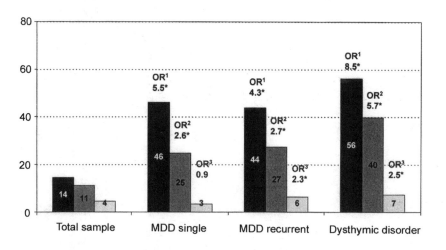

Figure 1.1 Comorbidity of 12-month depressive disorders: proportions and associations with anxiety, somatoform and substance use disorders in respondents with any disorder, MDD single, MDD recurrent and dysthymic disorder (GHS-MHS; N=4181)

TABLE 1.2   Third generation prevalence studies of bipolar disorder

			Lifetime	6/12 month	1 month
Semi-structured interviews					
Weissman and Myers, 1978	New Haven, USA	SADS/RDC	1.2	–	0.0[a]
Faravelli et al., 1990	Florence, Italy	SADS/DSM-III	–	1.5	0.5[a]
Almeida-Filho et al., 1997	Brazil (3 samples)	Semistructured interview/DSM-III	0.3–1.1	–	–
Angst and Gamma, 2002	Zurich, Switzerland	SPIKE/DSM-IV	2.3	–	–
Faravelli et al., 2004a,b	Florence, Italy	FPI/DSM-IV	0.8	0.3[a]	0.3[a]
Henderson et al., 1979, 1981	Canberra, Australia	PSE/ICD-9	–	–	0.2
Bebbington et al., 1981	Camberwell, UK	PSE/ICD-9	–	–	0.8
Hodiamont et al., 1987	Nijmegen, the Netherlands	PSE/ICD-9	–	–	0.1
Vázquez-Barquero et al., 1987	Santander, Spain	PSE/ICD-9	–	–	0.1
Lehtinen et al., 1990	Finland (2 samples)	PSE/ICD-9	–	–	0.4
Roca et al., 1999	Formentera, Spain	SCAN/ICD-10	–	–	0.9
Fully structured interviews					
Regier et al., 1988; Weissman et al., 1991	USA (ECA; 5 samples)	DIS/DSM-III	0.8	0.5	0.4
Canino et al., 1987	Puerto Rico	DIS/DSM-III	0.5	0.3	–
Bland et al., 1988a,b	Edmonton, Canada	DIS/DSM-III	0.6	0.1	0.1
Wells et al., 1989	Christchurch, New Zealand	DIS/DSM-III	0.7	–	–
Hwu et al., 1989	Taiwan (3 samples)	DIS/DSM-III	0.1–0.2	0.1	–
Lee et al., 1990a,b	Korea (2 samples)	DIS/DSM-III	0.4	–	–
Witchen et al., 1992	Former West Germany	DIS/DSM-III	0.2	0.2	–
Chen et al., 1993	Hong Kong	DIS/DSM-III	0.1 (M)–0.2 (F)	–	–
Szadoczky et al., 1998	Hungary	DIS/DSM-IIIR	1.5	0.9	0.5
Kessler et al., 1994	USA (NCS)	CIDI/DSM-IIIR	1.6	1.3	–
Offord et al., 1996	Ontario, Canada	CIDI/DSM-IIIR	–	0.6	–
Bijl et al., 1998	The Netherlands	CIDI/DSM-IIIR	1.6	0.9	–
Kringlen et al., 2001	Oslo (Norway)	CIDI/DSM-IIIR	1.8	1.1	0.6
Abou-Saleh et al., 2001	Al Ain, United Arab Emirates	CIDI/ICD-10	0.3	–	–
Andrade et al., 2002	São Paulo, Brazil	CIDI/ICD-10	1.0	0.5	0.4
Jacobi et al., 2004	Germany	M-CIDI/DSM-IV	1.0	0.8	0.6

ECA: Epidemiologic Catchment Area Study; NCS: National Comorbidity Survey. SADS: Schedule for Affective Disorders and Schizophrenia (Endicott and Spitzer, 1978); SPIKE: Structured Psychopathological Interview and Rating of the Social Consequences for Epidemiology (Angst et al., 1984); FPI: Florence Psychiatric Interview (Faravelli et al., 2001); PSE: Present State Examination (Wing et al., 1974); SCAN: Schedules for Clinical Assessment in Neuropsychiatry (Wing et al., 1990); DIS: Diagnostic Interview Schedule (Robins et al., 1981); CIDI: Composite International Diagnostic Interview (Robins et al., 1988).

[a]1-week prevalence.

Box 5:   Mood Disorders in Children and Adolescents

Empirical studies have documented that the phenomenology of depression is quite similar between adolescents and adults (Roberts et al., 1995; Ryan et al., 1987) even if differences exist in the expression of mood disorders between adults and children and adolescents. One of those differences is irritability, which is a symptom of depression in children and adolescents but not in adults.

Assessment of depression in children and adolescents encounters several methodological difficulties:

- Dimensional or diagnostic instruments assessing depression specifically in delimited age groups do not exist yet. So, clinicians and researchers use the same instrument to assess mood disorders in children and adolescents regardless of the fact that the reliability and validity of these instruments change with the age of the patient.
- When a diagnostic interview is used, the multiplicity of informants (parents, teachers or the patient) and the uncertainty as to how combine these data to yield a diagnosis constitute a methodological problem.
- Another difficulty with diagnostic interviews is the lack of explicit criteria assessing the impairment or the distress due to the mental disorder in children. In DSM-IV, this criterion is made more explicit.
- Dimensional self-report checklists assessing mood disorders in children and adolescents are numerous but there is a lack of specificity with most high-scoring youngsters failing to meet diagnostic criteria for depression.

Major Depression

In the community, the point prevalence of major depression ranges between 1% (McGee and Williams, 1988) to 6% (Kessler and Walters, 1998). Canino et al. (2004) assessed the prevalence of mental disorders in 1897 children and adolescents aged 4 to 17 years. The 12-month prevalence of major depression according to DSM-IV criteria was 3% in this population. The rates of lifetime prevalence of major depression in children and adolescents are higher, ranging from 4% (Whitaker et al., 1990) to 25% (Lewinsohn et al., 1998), which is comparable to the lifetime rate of major depression in adults. The gender ratio of major depression is 1:1 in children and increases to 2:1 female-to-male ratio in adolescents (Kessler et al., 1994b).

Bipolar Disorders

Between 20% and 40% of adolescents with major depressive disorder develop Bipolar I disorder within a period of 5 years after the beginning of the mood disorder (Rao et al., 1995; Geller et al., 1994; Strober et al., 1993). Risk factors of bipolar disorder in adolescents with depressive disorder include early-onset depression, mood disorder with psychotic features, family history of bipolar disorder and pharmacologically induced hypomania (Akiskal et al., 1995; Geller et al., 1994). It is important to recognize the existence of bipolar disorders in adolescents because this mood disorder may be misdiagnosed as conduct disorder or a personality disorder. Studies assessing the prevalence of bipolar disorder in children and adolescents are rare and reported estimates range from 0.0% to 1.0% (Kessler and Walters, 1998; Costello et al., 1996).

TABLE 1.3   Prevalence of depressive symptoms in the elderly

Site	Author	N	Age	Methods of assessment	Prevalence (%)
US community studies					
Durham County	Blazer and Williams, 1980	997	⩾65	OARS, Depression Scale	14.7
Los Angeles County	Frerichs et al., 1981	126	⩾65	CES-D⩾16	16.7
Kentucky	Murrell et al., 1983	2517	⩾55	CES-D⩾20	F: 18.2, M: 13.7
Washington	Goldberg et al., 1985	1144	65–75	CES-D⩾16	9.5
New Haven	Berkman et al., 1986	2806	⩾65	CES-D⩾16	F: 19.2, M: 11.3
New York	Copeland et al., 1987	445	⩾65	GMS-AGECAT	16.2
New York	Kennedy et al., 1989	2317	⩾65	CES-D⩾16	F: 19.9, M: 11.1
Duke-EPESE	Blazer et al., 1991	3998	65–74	Revised CES-D	8.1
			75–84		10.3
			⩾85		12.3
New York City	Potter et al., 1995	1140	⩾65	CES-D⩾16	11.4
Tennessee	Okwumabua et al., 1997	110	⩾60	CES-D⩾16	19.8
European community studies					
Liverpool	Copeland et al., 1987	1070	⩾65	GMS-AGECAT	11.5
London	Lindesay et al., 1989	890	⩾65	CARE Depression Scale	13.5
North London	Livingston et al., 1990	811	⩾65	Short CARE	15.9
France	Dufouil et al., 1995	2797	⩾65	M: CES-D⩾17, F: CES-D⩾23	15.9 15.9
London	Prince et al., 1997	654	⩾65	Short CARE	17
Dublin	Kirby et al., 1997	1232	⩾65	GMS-AGECAT	10.3

CES-D: Center for Epidemiologic Studies Depression Rating Scale. GMS-AGECAT: Automated Geriatric Examination for Computer Assisted Taxonomy Package. CARE: Comprehensive Assessment and Referral Evaluation.

present vs. the base rates of the disorders in the total sample. There are markedly elevated rates, reaching up to 56% anxiety disorders in dysthymia (vs. 14% in the general population); overall, roughly 60% of major depressions and 80% of dysthymia were accompanied by at least one additional diagnosis.

The strong association with anxiety has been consistently reported before (Weissman et al., 1996; Kessler et al., 1996; Angst, 1996). Regarding specific anxiety disorders, an examination of the findings of six epidemiological surveys (Merikangas et al., 1996) showed that panic disorder had a much stronger association with major depression than phobias. Of the phobic disorders, social phobia had a stronger association with major depression than either agoraphobia or simple phobia; a significant association with both generalized anxiety disorder and obsessive-compulsive disorder has also been reported. Generally anxiety disorders (possibly with the exception of panic disorder) appear temporally primary to major depression in the majority of subjects in both cross-sectional and prospective long-itudinal studies (Merikangas et al., 1996; Wittchen et al., 2000; Kessler et al., 2003).

In most studies substance use disorders are also associated with major depression, although findings are less consistent than those regarding anxiety disorders, and the association appears weaker.

Finally, data from the recent US National Comorbidity Survey Replication (Kessler et al., 2003) also suggest that about one-third of the subjects with major depression may have a lifetime comorbid impulse control disorder, although comorbid impulse control disorder is often thought to be more strongly related to bipolar than to unipolar depression (McElroy et al., 1996); according to the authors this could reflect broader factors of the existence of what has recently been called 'soft bipolar spectrum' in which comorbid impulse control disorder among patients with major depression represents a marker of bipolar susceptibility (Perugi et al., 1998).

Dysthymia also shows a high co-occurrence rate with anxiety disorders; of the specific anxiety disorders, dysthymia seems more strongly comorbid with general-ized anxiety disorder and panic disorder and less strongly comorbid with phobias and obsessive-compulsive disorder.

A comorbid anxiety disorder is diagnosed in 40% to 90% of subjects with bipolar disorder in community samples (Kessler et al., 1997; Szadoczky et al., 1998); the stronger associations appear to be with panic disorder, obsessive-compulsive disorder and generalized anxiety disorder, while the comorbidity with phobias seem weaker. It has also been suggested that subjects with bipolar II disorder may have a particularly high comorbidity rate with anxiety disorders when compared to subjects with bipolar I disorder (Rihmer et al., 2001).

Co-occurrence of bipolar and addictive disorders is also particularly frequent. A comorbid lifetime alcohol/substance use disorder is present in 20% to 70% of bipolar subjects (Regier et al., 1990; Fogarty et al., 1994; Kessler et al., 1997; Fara-velli et al., 2004b); in the ECA study the prevalence of alcoholism in bipolar disorder was three times higher than in major depression (Helzer and Pryzbeck, 1988).

Age of Onset

In the majority of studies, the mean age of onset is in the mid to late 20s for major depression while for bipolar disorder it ranges between the mid-teens and the mid-20s. More differentiated than the comparison of means is the comparison of the whole cumulative age of onset distributions (i.e. curves that show what proportion of all lifetime cases report the onset before a given age). These are presented in Figure 1.2 for several types of mood disorders. The differences between bipolar disorders, major depression and dysthymia are obvious: bipolar disorders begin very early (50% of the subjects with a lifetime diagnosis report an onset before 18 years), whereas the median age of onset in major depression is 30 years and in

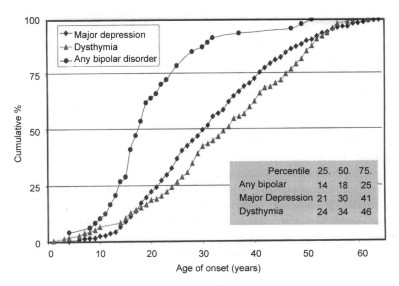

Figure 1.2 Age of onset distributions (source: GHS-MHS; Jacobi et al., 2004)

dysthymia 34 years. Only 25% develop a bipolar disorder after age of 25, whereas the 75th percentile in major depression is 41 and 46 years in dysthymia.

There are no marked effects on type of major depression (single vs. recurrent), type of bipolar disorder (bipolar I vs. bipolar II), when considering gender either. But age effects are very significant: younger cohorts consistently report an earlier onset. Age-related differential recall, differential willingness to disclose, or other methodologic factors could play important parts in this pattern, although a genuine increase in the prevalence in recent cohorts may have occurred (Kessler et al., 2003).

Course of Major Depression and Bipolar Disorders

As evidence to date suggests, the course of depression is likely to differ considerably depending on several factors, often considered subtype qualifiers, such as age of onset (early vs. late), subclinical vs. clinical criteria, vegetative vs. non-vegetative. The commensurate treatment implications of information about course are considerable. For instance, a seemingly increasingly important and timely, but difficult to study, emerging area appears to be the relationship between treatment use (both antidepressant and psychotherapy, as well as other treatments) and the course of major depression in the community. In addition, information gained from clinical follow-up studies showing that the majority of severe depression cases are recurrent have led to a re-focusing of much depression treatment to a prevention of recurrence, rather than being purely directed toward offset of current episode.

Yet, to date there is relatively little available epidemiologic information on the course of major depression in the community. Specifically, there are only a few prospective, long-term, community-based studies with multiple follow-ups of depression, which are needed in order to understand the natural course of the disorder. While bipolar disorder is thought to be a very chronic condition (Coryell and Winokur, 1992), most available information comes from clinical samples not representative of the course of bipolar disorder and bipolar spectrum disorder in the community. Little epidemiologic evidence is available on the course of bipolar disorder, largely due to the methodological challenges mentioned above, as well as some additional obstacles to accurate and reliable measurement needed to describe course. Additional challenges to measuring the course of bipolar disorder in the community include prospective measurement of onset, episodes and remission, as well as periods when subclinical symptoms may be present. Since there have been few prospective studies of bipolar disorder in the community, reliance on retrospective recall of first onset and past episodes has been much more common than in research on depression or other mental disorders.

Correlates and Risk Factors

Epidemiologic research is the key to the identification of risk factors for mental disorders. Cross-sectional epidemiologic studies can be used to describe associations or even *correlates* of major depression. Such associations between the investigated factors and major depression reflect that they are symptoms, maintaining factors or the consequences of having a major depression. The identification of *true risk factors* is not possible in cross-sectional studies due to reliance on retrospective recall with some exceptions for fixed factors such as race and gender. In most cases, longitudinal data are needed in order to identify potential risk factors and examine them prospectively. Given that most findings concerning major depression are based on cross-sectional epidemiologic data, according to Kraemer et al. (1997) we prefer to use the term 'correlate' rather than 'risk factor'.

Sociodemographic Variables: Gender, Marital and Socioeconomic Status

Specific demographic characteristics are differentially associated with the prevalence and risk of depression onset among adults in the community. Among the most striking is female gender. So, we will review first the associations between depression and gender.

The importance of gender differences in mental health is usually illustrated in significantly different prevalences and incidence rates of major depression, whereas the explanations for these findings remains poorly studied. Despite the wide variations in lifetime prevalence estimates of major depression across countries and studies, the roughly 2:1 sex ratio is consistent cross-culturally (Weissman et al., 1993; Kessler et al., 1994a; Meltzer et al., 1995; Bebbington, 1998; Gater et al., 1998; Jacobi et al., 2004). Conversely, most studies have found no gender difference in the prevalence of bipolar disorder (Tohen and Goodwin, 1995; Weissman et al., 1996).

In general, *biological, psychosocial* and *artefact* explanations have been proposed to explain the predominance of depressive disorders in women (for an extensive overview see Wilhelm and Parker, 1994; Bebbington, 1998; Piccinelli and Wilkinson, 2000; Kessler, 2003).

Artefact explanations assume that much of the observed differences in prevalence rates may be produced by gender-related bias or even artefacts such as differences in help-seeking behaviour and symptom-reporting patterns (Kessler et al., 1981; Nolen-Hoeksema, 1990; Loewenthal et al., 1995; Kessler, 1998), quality and quantity of symptoms (symptom profile; Young et al., 1990; Silverstein, 1999), recall bias (Ernst and Angst, 1992; Wilhelm and Parker, 1994), definitions of cases in epidemiological studies (threshold for caseness; Angst and Dobler-Mikola, 1985; Wilhelm and Parker, 1994; Piccinelli and Wilkinson, 2000), or even gender-biased case-finding measurements (Salokangas et al., 2002). It has been suggested that these artefactual factors may contribute to the female preponderance in depressive disorders to some extent, yet gender differences still seem to be genuine and can be shown even after these are accounted for (Nazroo et al., 1998; Piccinelli and Wilkinson, 2000).

Biological theories have proposed differences in brain structure and functioning between men and women, including neurotransmitter, neuroendocrine and circadian rhythms, as well as genetic factors and reproductive functioning (Joffe and Cohen, 1998; Kornstein, 1997; Paykel, 1991; Pajer, 1995; Leibenluft, 1999). Although attractive, explanations in biological terms face a number of difficulties. If higher rates in mental disorders, particularly in depressive disorders in women, are due to a universal biological vulnerability, the sex ratio ought to be unaffected by, for example, sociodemographic attributes. There is no convincing evidence for this, however (e.g. Bebbington, 1998). Therefore, biological explanations alone are not sufficient. This inevitably moves the focus of interest to psychosocial hypotheses for gender differences in depressive disorders.

From a *psychosocial* perspective, several possible explanations for gender differences have been suggested (Pajer, 1995; Kornstein, 1997; Bebbington, 1998; Piccinelli and Wilkinson, 2000), for example that women, in general, have a lower socioeconomic status. Surveys since the 1970–1980s have indicated a higher prevalence of mental disorders in the lower social classes, though perhaps only for women (Weissman and Myers, 1978; Kessler et al., 1994a). Higher rates of mood disorders for women may also reflect issues related to the fact that they may be subject to more significant, or more upsetting stressful life events or chronic difficulties (Brown and Moran, 1997; Bebbington, 1996; Nazroo et al., 1997, 1998), low social support (Brown and Andrews, 1986; Fuhrer et al., 1992), victimization and adverse experiences in childhood (e.g. sexual or physical abuse or parental separation/

divorce with resulting lack of child care in early years; Cutler and Nolen-Hoeksema, 1991; Rodgers, 1994; Bebbington, 1998), and maladaptive coping styles (Hobfoll et al., 1994; Nolen-Hoeksema et al., 1994). Other issues suggested to contribute to a higher risk of depressive disorders among women have been social roles, such as marital and employment status (unequal adult gender role stresses; Vazquez-Barquero et al., 1992; Cramer, 1993; Kessler et al., 1993; Loewenthal et al., 1995). Yet, in the light of contradictory findings, the reason for these differences remains unclear.

Overall, the emotional advantages or disadvantages of certain sociodemographic variables (marital status, employment status, number of children, parenthood and social class) apply *equally* to men and women (Klose and Jacobi, 2004). We cannot explain the female preponderance in most mental disorders by detecting specific unfavourable patterns of sociodemographic correlates, suggesting that determinants of gender differences in common mental disorders are still far from being understood.

Regarding marital status, the literature suggests that in general currently married persons had lower rates of both depressive and bipolar disorders than those who had never married or were currently separated, divorced or widowed (Kessler et al., 2003; Tohen and Goodwin, 1995; Weissman et al., 1996). Several studies have investigated the relationship between various measures of socioeconomic status and mood disorders but evidence is quite mixed, thus not allowing definitive conclusions (Kohn et al., 1998).

Familial Transmission

Family studies have shown that risk of depression onset and severity is associated with family history of depression (Bridge et al., 1997; Kendler et al., 1997; Klein et al., 2001; Warner et al., 1999; Wickramaratne et al., 2000). Yet, the majority of these data are drawn from clinical or other highly selected samples, and therefore it is not known whether findings are generalizable to the population. In one of very few community-based studies examining familial risk of depression, Lieb et al. (2002) showed that parental history of depression was associated with a significantly increased risk among offspring. Additionally, parental depression was associated with earlier onset and higher levels of morbidity (severity, impairment, recurrence). This study also showed that having two parents with depression was associated with higher risk than only one, though there did not appear to be any difference conferred by paternal or maternal risk. Of interest, this study also showed that parental depression was associated with increased risk of substance use disorders and anxiety disorders in offspring. Kendler et al. (1996) have also shown that familial history is associated with increased risk of depression, and that stressful life events are associated with an even higher risk of depression onset among those with familial or genetic vulnerability to depression. In particular, findings suggest that the increase in risk is pronounced during the first month following the event, and then is no longer evident. Another interesting question is whether major depression and anxiety disorders are transmitted independently within families. Some studies suggest that there is an independent transmission and that the comorbidity between depression and anxiety is caused by non-familial aetiologic factors (e.g. Klein et al., 2003; Weissman et al., 1993).

Early Adversity

Several factors reflecting adversity in early childhood have been shown to increase the risk of depression onset, severity, and recurrence in longitudinal studies (Brown and Harris, 1993). Investigators have repeatedly documented associations between childhood physical and sexual abuse and neglect and increased risk of depression in adulthood (e.g. Brown and Harris, 1993; Kessler et al., 1997). In terms of life events and early adverse exposures, loss-related events appear particularly potent and somewhat specific to depression, compared with anxiety, as research has shown that a severe threatening event involving loss was most often involved in the onset of depression (Brown, 1993). Parental loss during childhood, by death or separation, is also associated with increased risk of depression in adulthood. Childhood abuse is associated with increased risk of a wide range of mental disorders during adulthood, while loss events appear strongly and somewhat specifically depressogenic.

Psychiatric Symptoms and Other Mental Disorders

Studies have consistently shown that previous mental disorders strongly increase the risk of first onset of major depression as well as increasing the likelihood of persistence, severity, and recurrence of the disorder (e.g. Hettema, 2003). Specifically, anxiety disorders have been shown to precede and predict the onset of major depression.

Research has shown that the link between prior symptoms and risk of major depression spans all developmental stages. Canals et al. (2002) looked at predictors of depression onset at age 18 and found that 80% with depression onset at 18 had symptoms of major depression between the ages of 11 and 14. These findings support a continuity of depression from adolescence to young adulthood with subclinical scores on the Children's Depression Inventory (CDI; del Barrio, 1993) as an early indicator of long-term risk. This study also found early symptoms of anxiety to be a predictor of depression at 18, but only among boys.

Stressful Life Events

Major stressful life events are a well-known risk factor for major depression (Paykel, 2001). Research suggests that there is no gender or age difference in susceptibility to depression associated with stressful life events, but that women have a greater risk of depression related to distal losses (Maciejewski et al., 2001). Additionally, there are some data suggesting that different types of losses pose greater risks of depression between genders; for instance, familial conflict is associated with an increased risk of depression among females while financial strain is more strongly associated with depression among males. Brown and colleagues (Brown et al., 1995) have done extensive work on the aetiology of depression among women in the community. Their findings suggest that loss events are particularly depressogenic when combined with the experience of humiliation and entrapment. Such studies have also shown that loss is important in provoking depression and that positive events (i.e. fresh-start events) involving hope are particularly important in recovery from depression (Brown, 1993).

Other Factors

There are additional factors thought to be associated with risk of major depression. For instance, personality traits (e.g. neuroticism) (Kendler et al., 2003, 2004) and cognitive coping styles are associated with higher rates of depression.

ARE PREVALENCE ESTIMATES FOR MOOD DISORDERS TOO HIGH?

The high prevalence rates of mood disorders, especially in the recent CIDI surveys, has generated some scepticism about diagnostic validity (Parker, 1987; Frances, 1998; Bebbington, 2000; Henderson, 2000) and it has been proposed that a proportion of the syndromes identified in community surveys may represent transient homeostatic responses that are neither pathologic nor in need of treatment (Regier et al., 1998). Furthermore, it has been shown that cases identified in the community are not always consistently associated with social impairment (Bebbington, 1994; ten Have et al., 2002). For instance, Narrow et al. (2002) found that the application of a clinical significance criterion lowered the 1-year prevalence rates of mood disorders by 44% in the ECA study and by 32% in the NCS, while Henderson et al. (2001) showed that about 15% of subjects with a 1-month CIDI diagnosis of depressive disorder in an Australian sample reported no disability in daily life.

On the one hand, these findings suggest that the mere diagnosis cannot be equated with clinically relevant treatment need. In addition, it should be noted that no health care system in the world could ever provide (adequate) mental health care for roughly a third of the population. To estimate treatment need for public health reasons, prevalence rates must be supplemented by information on comorbidity, severity, treatment demand, social impact etc. But criticizing the absence of clinically significant disability or claiming irrelevance for clinical practice in a relevant proportion of the diagnosed subjects in epidemiological studies needs to be separated from the question of whether 'mild' disorders should be eliminated from the DSM or other diagnostic systems. Kessler et al. (2003) show, for example, that longitudinal analyses using severity strata indeed produce differences in the risk of clinically significant outcomes – but differences between mild cases and noncases are consistently larger than differences between mild and moderate cases. Considerations should be given not only to current distress and impairment but also to the risk of progression from a mild to a more severe disorder. Thus, treatment of mild disorders may be cost-effective (prevention of later need of intensive treatment and long-term cost of illness). Also it should be acknowledged that mental disorders (like physical disorders) vary in severity, and the investigation of pathways and outcomes of psychopathology should not depend on arbitrary societal views of treatment need and the naturally limited health care resources.

SUGGESTED READINGS

Since the reference list is quite exhaustive, some selected recent publications that can be easily accessed via internet from universities and other institutions are recommended here for first suggested readings. More 'classic' references on diagnosis and nosology can be found in Chapter 3 of this book by Faravelli, Ravaldi and Truglia.

A comprehensive paper on the epidemiology of major depression in the *JAMA* reports, besides recent prevalence rates data on correlates, role impairment and treatment issues (from the second National Comorbidity Survey in the USA, NCS-R; Kessler et al., 2003). A short overview on the important issue of comorbidity is given by Wittchen (1996), and Merikangas et al. (1996) present an exemplary analysis on the comorbidity of mood disorders with anxiety disorders and substance use disorders. The discussion about clinical semi-structured versus standardized approaches is exemplarily included in an editorial section of *Psychological Medicine* (Brugha et al., 1999a vs. Wittchen et al., 1999a). Interesting information on self-report methodology is summarized by Kessler et al. (2000). A benchmark paper on risk factors is the one by Kraemer et al. (1997). As an example of a modern CIDI-study using clinically trained interviewers and investigating a relatively broad spectrum of disorders, the German Health Interview and Examination Survey and its Mental Health Supplement (Jacobi et al., 2004) is also mentioned here because this data set is available as a public use file and can be ordered from F.J., as well as the data from the prospective Early Developmental Stages of Psychopathology study (EDSP; exemplary publication on depression: Lieb et al., 2002).

Finally, at the end of the 1990s a cross-sectional study (The European Study of Epidemiology of Mental Disorders: the ESEMeD) has been carried out in six European countries (Belgium, France, Germany, Italy, the Netherlands and Spain) in order to evaluate the prevalence, the impact and the treatment patterns of mental disorders in Europe (Alonso et al., 2002). The results of this study assessing more than 20 000 adults over 18 allow interesting cross-national comparisons in terms of mental health (The ESEMeD-MHEDEA 2000 Investigators, 2004; The WHO World Mental Health Survey Consortium, 2004). For a review of available European studies since 1990 see Wittchen & Jacobi (in press).

ACKNOWLEDGEMENT

This chapter was supported by the European Program in Affective Neuroscience.

REFERENCES

Akiskal HS, Maser JD, Zeller PJ, Endicott J, Coryell W, Keller M, Warshaw M, Clayton P, Goodwin F (1995) Switching from 'unipolar' to bipolar II. An 11-year prospective study of clinical and temperamental predictors in 559 patients. *Arch Gen Psychiatry* **52**(2): 114–123.

Alonso J, Ferrer M, Romera B, Vilagut G, Angermeyer M, Bernert S, Brugha TS, Taub N, McColgen Z, De Girolamo G, Polidori G, Mazzi F, De Graaf R, Vollebergh WA, Buist-Bowman MA, Demyttenaere K, Gasquet I, Haro JM, Palacin C, Autonell J, Katz SJ, Kessler RC, Kovess V, Lepine JP, Arbabzadeh-Bouchez S, Ormel J, Bruffaerts R (2002) The European Study of the Epidemiology of Mental Disorders (ESEMeD/MHEDEA 2000) project: rationale and methods. *Int J Methods Psychiatr Res* **11**(2): 55–67.

American Psychiatric Association (1980) *Diagnostic and Statistical Manual of Mental Disorders* (3rd edition). Washington, DC: American Psychiatric Association.

American Psychiatric Association (1987) *Diagnostic and Statistical Manual of Mental Disorders* (3rd cdition, rcviscd). Washington, DC: Amcrican Psychiatric Association.

American Psychiatric Association (1994) *Diagnostic and Statistical Manual of Mental Disorders (4th edition). Washington, DC: American Psychiatric Association.*

Andrade L, Walters EE, Gentil V, Laurenti R, et al. (2002) Prevalence of ICD-10 mental disorders in a catchment area in the city of Sao Paulo, Brazil. *Soc Psychiatry Psychiat Epidemiol* **37**(7): 316–325.

Andrews G, Henderson S, Hall W (2001) Prevalence, comorbidity, disability and service utilisation. Overview of the Australian National Mental Health Survey. *Br J Psychiatry* **178**(2): 145–153.

Angst J (1996) Comorbidity of mood disorders: a longitudinal prospective study. *Br J Psychiatry* **168**(Suppl 30): 31–37.

Angst J, Dobler-Mikola A (1985) The Zurich study. A prospective epidemiological study of depressive, neurotic, and psychosomatic syndromes. IV. Recurrent and nonrecurrent brief depression. *Eur Arch Psychiatry Neurol Sci* **234**: 408–416.

Angst J, Dobler-Mikola A, Binder J (1984) The Zurich Study. A prospective epidemiological study of depressive, neurotic, and psychosomatic syndromes. I. Problem, methodology. *Eur Arch Psychiatry Neurol Sci* **234**: 13–20.

Angst J, Gamma A, Benazzi F, Ajdacic V, Eich D, Rossler W (2003a) Toward a re-definition of subthreshold bipolarity: Epidemiology and proposed criteria for bipolar-II, minor bipolar disorders and hypomania. *J Affect Disord* **73**: 133–146.

Angst J, Gamma A, Benazzi F, Ajdacic V, Eich D, Rossler W (2003b) Diagnostic issues in bipolar disorder. *Eur Neuropsychopharmacol* **13**(Suppl 2): 43–50.

Angst J, Merikangas K (1997) The depressive spectrum: diagnostic classification and course. *J Affect Disord* **45**: 31–39.

Ayuso-Mateos JL, et al. (2001) Depressive disorders in Europe: prevalence figures from the ODIN study. *Br J Psychiatry* **179**: 308–316.

Bebbington P (1994) Population surveys of psychiatric disorder and the need for treatment. *Soc Psychiatry Psychiatr Epidemiol* **25**: 33–40.

Bebbington PE (1996) The origins of sex differences in depressive disorder: Bridging the gap. *Int Rev Psychiatr* **8**: 295–332.

Bebbington PE (1998) Sex and depression. *Psychol Med* **28**: 1–8.

Bebbington P (2000) The need for psychiatric treatment in the general population. In Andrews G, Henderson S (eds) *Unmet Need in Psychiatry: Problems, Resources, Responses.* Cambridge, UK: Cambridge University Press, pp. 85–96.

Bebbington P, Hurry J, Tennant C, Sturt E, Wing JK (1981) Epidemiology of mental disorders in Camberwell. *Psychol Med* **11**: 561–579.

Ben-Arie O, Swartz L, Dickman BJ (1987) Depression in the elderly living in the community. Its presentation and features. *Br J Psychiatry* **150**: 169–174.

Berkman LF, Berkman CS, Kasl S, Freeman DH Jr, Leo L, Ostfeld AM, Cornoni-Huntley J, Brody JA (1986) Depressive symptoms in relation to physical health and functioning in the elderly. *Am J Epidemiol* **124**(3): 372–388.

Bijl RV, Ravelli A, van Zessen G (1998) Prevalence of psychiatric disorder in the general population: Results of The Netherlands Mental Health Survey and Incidence Study (NEMESIS). *Soc Psychiatry Psychiatr Epidemiol* **33**: 587–595.

Bijl RV, de Graaf R, Hiripi E, Kessler RC, Kohn R, Offord DR, Üstün TB, Vicente B, Vollebergh WAM, Walters EE, Wittchen H-U (2003) The prevalence of treated and untreated mental disorders in five countries. *Health Affairs* **22**(3): 122–133.

Bifulco A, Brown GW (1998) Cognitive coping response to crises and onset of depression. *Soc Psychiatry Psychiatr Epidemiol* **31**: 163–172.

Bland RC (1997) Epidemiology of affective disorders: a review. *Can J Psychiatry* **42**: 367–377.

Bland RC, Newman SC, Orn H (1988a) Period prevalence of psychiatric disorders in Edmonton. *Acta Psychiatr Scand* **338**(Suppl): 33–42.

Bland RC, Orn H, Newman SC (1988b) Lifetime prevalence of psychiatric disorders in Edmonton. *Acta Psychiatr Scand* **338**(Suppl): 24–32.

Blazer D, Williams CD (1980) Epidemiology of dysphoria and depression in an elderly population. *Am J Psychiatry* **137**(4): 439–444.

Blazer D, Burchett B, Service C, George LK (1991) The association of age and depression among the elderly: An epidemiologic exploration. *J Gerontol* **46**(6): M210–215.

Bridge JA, Brent DA, Johnson BA, Connolly J (1997) Familial aggregation of psychiatric disorders in a community sample of adolescents. *J Amer Acad Child Adolesc Psychiatry* **36**(5): 628–636.

Brown GW (1993) Life events and affective disorder: Replications and limitations. *J Psychosom Med* **55**: 248–259.

Brown GW, Andrews B (1986) Social support and depression. In Appley MH, Trumbull R (eds) *Dynamic of Stress.* New York: Plenum Press.

Brown GW, Harris TO (1993) Aetiology of anxiety and depressive disorders in an inner-city population. I. Early adversity. *Psychol Med* **23**: 143–154.

Brown GW, Harris TO, Hepworth C (1995) Loss, humiliation and entrapment among women developing depression: A patient and non-patient comparison. *Psychol Med* **25**: 7–21.

Brown GW, Harris TO (1993) Aetiology of anxiety and depressive disorders in an inner-city population. I. Early adversity. *Psychol Med* **23**: 143–154.

Brown GW, Moran PM (1997) Single mothers, poverty, and depression. *Psychol Med* **27**: 21–33.

Brugha TS, Bebbington PE, Jenkins R (1999a) A difference that matters: comparison of structured and semi-structured diagnostic interviews of adults in the general population. *Psychol Med* **29**: 1013–1020.

Brugha TS, Bebbington PE, Jenkins R, Meltzer H, Taub NA, Janas M, Vernon J (1999b) Cross validation of a general population survey diagnostic interview: A comparison of CIS-R with SCAN ICD-10 diagnostic categories. *Psychol Med* **29**: 1029–1042.

Canals J, Domenech-Llaberia E, Fernandez-Ballart J, et al. (2002) Predictors of depression at eighteen. A 7-year follow-up study in a Spanish nonclinical population. *European Child & Adolescent Psychiatry* **11** (5): 226–233.

Canino GJ, Bird HR, Shrout PE, et al. (1987) The prevalence of specific psychiatric disorders in Puerto Rico. *Arch Gen Psychiatry* **44**: 727–735.

Canino G, Shrout PE, Rubio-Stipec M, Bird HR, Bravo M, Ramirez R, Chavez L, Alegria M, Bauermeister JJ, Hohmann A, Ribera J, Garcia P, Martinez-Taboas A (2004) The DSM-IV rates of child and adolescent disorders in Puerto Rico: prevalence, correlates, service use, and the effects of impairment. *Arch Gen Psychiatry* **61** (1): 85–93.

Carpiniello B, Carta MG, Rudas N (1989) Depression among elderly people. A psychosocial study of urban and rural populations. *Acta Psychiatr Scand* **80** (5): 445–450.

Chen CN, Wong J, Lee N, Chan-Ho MW, Lau JT, Fung M (1993) The Shatin Community Mental Health Survey in Hong Kong. II. Major findings. *Arch Gen Psychiatry* **50**: 125–133.

Copeland JR, Dewey ME, Griffiths-Jones HM (1986) A computerized psychiatric diagnostic system and case nomenclature for elderly subjects: GMS and AGECAT. *Psychol Med* **16** (1): 89–99.

Copeland JR, Dewey ME, Wood N, Searle R, Davidson IA, McWilliam C (1987) Range of mental illness among the elderly in the community. Prevalence in Liverpool using the GMS-AGECAT package. *Br J Psychiatry* **150**: 815–823.

Coryell W, Winokur G (1992) Course and outcome. In Paykel ES (ed.) *Handbook of Affective Disorders* (2nd edition). New York: Guilford Press, pp. 89–108.

Costello EJ, Angold A, Burns BJ, Stangl DK, Tweed DL, Erkanli A, Worthman CM (1996) The Great Smoky Mountains Study of Youth. Goals, design, methods, and the prevalence of DSM-III-R disorders. *Arch Gen Psychiatry* **53** (12): 1129–1136.

Cramer D (1993) Living alone, marital-status, gender and health. *J Comm Appl Soc Psych* **3**: 1–15.

Cross-National Collaborative Group (1992) The changing rate of major depression. Cross-national comparison, **268** (21): 3098–3105.

Cutler SE, Nolen-Hoeksema S (1991) Accounting for sex differences in depression through female victimization: Childhood sexual abuse. *Sex Roles* **24**: 425–438.

de Girolamo G, Bassi M (2003) Community surveys of mental disorders: recent achievements and works in progress. *Curr Opin Psychiatry* **16**: 403–411.

del Barrio V (1993) The Children's Depression Inventory (CDI), 15 years later. *European Journal of Psychological Assessment* **9** (1): 51–53.

Dohrenwend BP, Dohrenwend BS (1982) Perspectives on the past and future of psychiatric epidemiology. *Am J Public Health* **72**: 1271–1279.

Endicott J, Spitzer RL (1978) A diagnostic interview: the schedule for affective disorders and schizophrenia. *Arch Gen Psychiatry* **35**: 837–844.

Ernst C, Angst J (1992) The Zurich Studie XII. Sex differences in depression. Evidence from longitudinal epidemiological data. *Eur Arch Psychiatry Clin Neurosci* **241**: 222–230.

Faravelli C, Abrardi L, Bartolozzi D, Cecchi C, Cosci F, D'Adamo D, Lo Iacono B, Ravaldi C, Scarpato MA, Truglia E, Rossi Prodi PM, Rosi S (2004a) The Sesto Fiorentino Study: Point and one year prevalences of psychiatric disorders in an Italian community sample using clinical interviewers. *Psychother Psychosom* **73**: 226–234.

Faravelli C, Abrardi L, Bartolozzi D, Cecchi C, Cosci F, D'Adamo D, Lo Iacono B, Ravaldi C, Scarpato MA, Truglia E, Rosi S (2004b) The Sesto Fiorentino Study: background, methods and preliminary results. Lifetime prevalence of psychiatric disorders in an Italian community sample using clinical interviewers. *Psychother Psychosom* **73**: 216–225.

Faravelli C, Bartolozzi D, Cimminiello L, Cecchi C, Cosci F, D'Adamo D, Di Matteo C, Di Primio C, Fabbri C, Lo Iacono B, Paionni A, Perone A, Rosi S, Scarpato MA, Serena A, Taberna A (2001) The Florence Psychiatric Interview. *Int J Methods Psychiatr Res* **10**: 157–171.

Feighner JP, Robins E, Guze SB, Woodruff RA Jr, Winokur G, Munoz R (1972) Diagnostic criteria for use in psychiatric research. *Arch Gen Psychiatry* **26**: 57–63.

First MB, Spitzer RL, Gibbon M, Williams JBW (1997) *Structured Clinical Interview for DSM-IV Axis I Disorders, Research Version, Non-patient Edition (SCID-I/NP)*. New York: Biometrics Research.

Fogarty F, Russell JM, Newman SC, Bland RC (1994) Epidemiology of psychiatric disorders in Edmonton. Mania. *Acta Psychiatr Scand* **376** (Suppl): 16–23.

Forsell Y, Jorm AF, von Strauss E, Winblad B (1995) Prevalence and correlates of depression in a population of nonagenarians. *Br J Psychiatry* **167** (1): 61–64.

Frances A (1998) Problems in defining clinical significance in epidemiological studies. *Arch Gen Psychiatry* **55**: 119.

Frerichs RR, Aneshensel CS, Clark VA (1981) Prevalence of depression in Los Angeles County. *Am J Epidemiol* **113** (6): 691–699.

Fuhrer R, Antonucci TC, Dartigues JF (1992) The cooccurrence of depressive symptoms and cognitive impairment in a French community – are there gender differences? *Eur Arch Psychiatry Clin Neurosci* **242**: 161–171.

Galbaud du Fort G, Newman SC, Bland RC (1993) Psychiatric comorbidity and treatment seeking. Sources of selection bias in the study of clinical populations. *Journal of Nervous and Mental Disease* **181**: 467–474.

Gater R, Tansella M, Korten A, Tiemens BG, Mavreas VG, Olatawura MO (1998) Sex differences in the prevalence and detection of depressive and anxiety disorders in general health care settings – Report from the World Health Organization collaborative study on Psychological Problems in General Health Care. *Arch Gen Psychiatry* **55**: 405–413.

Goldberg D, Huxley P (1980) *Mental Illness in the Community: The Pathway to Psychiatric Care*. London: Tavistock.

Goldberg EL, Van Natta P, Comstock GW (1985) Depressive symptoms, social networks and social support of elderly women. *Am J Epidemiol* **121** (3): 448–456.

Geller B, Fox LW, Clark KA (1994) Rate and predictors of prepubertal bipolarity during follow-up of 6- to 12-year-old depressed children. *J Am Acad Child Adolesc Psychiatry* **33** (4): 461–468.

Gurland BJ, Kuriansky JB, Sharpe L, et al. (1977) The Comprehensive Assessment and Referral Examination (CARE): rationale, development and reliability. *Int J Aging Hum Dev* **8**: 9–42.

Gurland B, Golden RR, Teresi JA, Challop J (1984) The SHORT-CARE: an efficient instrument for the assessment of depression, dementia and disability. *J Gerontol* **39** (2): 166–169.

Hagnell O, Lanke J, Rorsman B, Ojesjo L (1982) Are we entering an age of melancholy? Depressive illnesses in a prospective epidemiological study over 25 years: the Lundby Study, Sweden. *Psychol Med* **12**: 279–289.

Helzer JE, Pryzbeck TR (1988) The co-occurrence of alcoholism with other psychiatric disorders in the general population and its impact on treatment. *J Stud Alcohol* **49**: 219–224.

Henderson S (2000) Conclusion: the central issues. In Andrews G, Henderson S (eds) *Unmet Need in Psychiatry: Problems, Resources, Responses*. Cambridge, UK: Cambridge University Press, pp. 422–428.

Henderson S, Korten A, Medway J (2001) Non-disabled cases in a national survey. *Psychol Med* **31**: 769–777.

Hettema JM, Prescott CA, Kendler KS (2003) The effects of anxiety, substance use and conduct disorders on risk of major depressive disorder. *Psychol Med* **33**(8): 1423–1432.

Hobfoll SE, Dunahoo CL, Ben-Porath Y, Monnier J (1994) Gender and coping: the dual-axis model of coping. *Am J Community Psychol* **22**: 49–82.

Hodiamont P, Peer N, Syben N (1987) Epidemiological aspects of psychiatric disorder in a Dutch health area. *Psychol Med* **17**: 495–505.

Höfler M, Wittchen H-U (2000) Why do primary care doctors diagnose depression when diagnostic criteria are not met? *International Journal of Methods in Psychiatric Research* **9**(3): 110–120.

Horwath E, Weissman MM (1995) Epidemiology of depression and anxiety disorders. In Tsuang MT, Tohen M, Zahner GEP (eds) *Textbook in Psychiatric Epidemiology*. New York: John Wiley, pp. 317–344.

Horwath E, Johnson J, Weissman MM, Hornig CD (1992) The validity of major depression with atypical features based on a community study. *J Affect Disord* **26**: 117–126.

Hwu H-G, Yeh E-K, Chang L-Y (1989) Prevalence of psychiatric disorders in Taiwan defined by the Chinese Diagnostic Interview Schedule. *Acta Psychiatr Scand* **79**: 136–147.

Jacobi F, Höfler M, Meister W, Wittchen H (2002a) Prävalenz, Erkennens- und Verschreibungsverhalten bei depressiven Syndromen. Eine bundesdeutsche Hausarztstudie (Prevalence, Recognition and Prescription Behaviour in depressive syndromes. A German study). *Nervenarzt* **73**: 651–658.

Jacobi F, Wittchen H-U, Hölting C, Höfler M, Müller N, Pfister H, Lieb R (2004) Prevalence, comorbidity and correlates of mental disorders in the general population: Results from the German Health Interview and Examination Survey (GHS). *Psychol Med* **34**:597–611.

Jacobi F, Wittchen H-U, Müller N, Hölting C, Sommer S, Höfler M, Pfister H (2002b) Estimating the prevalence of mental and somatic disorders in the community: Aims and methods of the German National Health Interview and Examination Survey. *International Journal of Methods in Psychiatric Research* **11**(1): 1–18.

Jenkins R, Lewis G, Bebbington P, Brugha T, Farrell M, Gill B, Meltzer H (1997) The National Psychiatric Morbidity surveys of Great Britain – initial findings from the household survey. *Psychol Med* **27**(4): 775–789.

Joffe H, Cohen LS (1998) Estrogen, serotonin, and mood disturbance: Where is the therapeutic bridge. *Soc Biol Psychiatry* **44**: 798–811.

Kendler KS, Walters EE, Kessler RC (1997) The prediction of length of major depressive episodes: Results from an epidemiological sample of female twins. *Psychol Med* **27**(1): 107–117.

Kendler KS, Sheth K, Gardner CO, Prescott CA (2002) Childhood parental loss and risk for first-onset of major depression and alcohol dependence: The time-decay of risk and sex differences. *Psychol Med* **32**(7): 1187–1194.

Kendler KS, Hettema JM, Butera, F, et al. (2003) Life event dimensions of loss, humiliation, entrapment, and danger in the prediction of onsets of major depression and generalized anxiety. *Arch Gen Psychiatry* **60**(8): 789–796.

Kendler KS, Kuhn J, Prescott CA (2004) The interrelationship of neuroticism, sex, and stressful life events in the prediction of episodes of major depression. *Am J Psychiatry* **161**(4): 631–636.

Kennedy GJ, Kelman HR, Thomas C, Wisniewski W, Metz H, Bijur PE (1989) Hierarchy of characteristics associated with depressive symptoms in an urban elderly sample. *Am J Psychiatry* **146**(2): 220–225.

Kessler RC (1998) Sex differences in DSM-III-R psychiatric disorders in the United States: Results from the National Comorbidiy Survey. *J Am Med Wom Assoc* **53**: 148–158.

Kessler RC (2003) Epidemiology of women and depression. *J Affect Disord* **74**: 5–13.

Kessler RC, Berglund P, Demler O, Jin R, Koretz D, Merikangas KR, Rush AJ, Walters EE, Wang PS (2003) The epidemiology of major depressive disorder. Results from the National Comorbidity Survey Replication (NCS- R). *JAMA* **289**: 3095–3105.

Kessler RC, Brown RL, Broman CL (1981) Sex differences in psychiatric help-seeking: Evidence from four large-scale surveys. *J Health Soc Behav* **22**: 49–64.

Kessler RC, McGonagle KA, Swartz M, Blazer DG, Nelson CB (1993) Sex and depression in the National Comorbidity Survey I: Lifetime prevalence, chronicity and recurrence. *J Affect Disord* **29**: 85–96.

Kessler RC, McGonagle KA, Nelson CB, Hughes M, Swartz M, Blazer DG (1994a) Sex and depression in the National Comorbidity Survey 2. Cohort effects. *J Affect Disord* **30**: 15–26.

Kessler RC, McGonagle KA, Zhao S, Nelson CB, Hughes M, Ehleman S, Wittchen HU, Kendler KS (1994b) Lifetime and 12-month prevalence of DSM-III-R psychiatric disorders in the United States: Results from the National Comorbidity Survey. *Arch Gen Psychiatry* **51**: 8–19.

Kessler RC, Nelson CB, McGonagle KA, Liu J, Swartz M, Blazer DG (1996) Comorbidity of DSM-III-R major depressive disorder in the general population: Results from the US National Comorbidity Survey. *Br J Psychiatry* **168**(Suppl 30): 17–30.

Kessler RC, Wittchen HU, Abelson JM, McGonagle KA, Schwarz N, Kendler KS (1998) Methodological studies of the Composite International Diagnostic Interview (CIDI) in the US National Comorbidity Survey. *Int J Methods Psychiatr Res* **7**: 33–55.

Kessler RC, Wittchen H-U, Abelson J, Zhao S (2000) Methodological issues in assessing psychiatric disorders with self-reports. In Stone AA, Turkkan JS, Bachrach CA, Jobe JB, Kurtzman HS, Cain VS (eds) *The Science of Self-report. Implications for Research and Practice*. Mahwah, NJ: Lawrence Erlbaum Associates, pp. 229–255.

Kessler RC, Zhao S, Blazer DG, Swartz M (1997) Prevalence, correlates, and course of minor depression and major depression in the national comorbidity survey. *J Affect Disord* **45**: 19–30.

Kessler RC, Walters EE (1998) Epidemiology of DSM-III-R major depression and minor depression among adolescents and young adults in the National Comorbidity Survey. *Depress Anxiety* **7**(1): 3–14.

Klein DN, Lewinsohn PM, Rohde P, Seeley JR, Shankman SA (2003) Family study of co-morbidity between major depressive disorder and anxiety disorders. *Psychol Med* **33**(4): 703–714.

Klein DN, Lewinsohn PM, Seeley JR, Rohde P (2001) Family study of major depressive disorder in a community sample of adolescents. *Arch Gen Psychiatry* **58**: 13–20.

Klose M, Jacobi F (2004) Can gender differences in the prevalence of mental disorders be explained by sociodemographic factors? *Archives of Women's Mental Health* **7**(2): 133–148.

Kohn R, Dohrenwend BP, Mirotznik J (1998) Epidemiological findings on selected psychiatric disorders in the general population. In Dohrenwend BP (ed) *Adversity, Stress, and Psychopathology*. Cambridge, UK: Cambridge University Press, pp. 235–284.

Kornstein SG (1997) Gender differences in depression: implications for treatment. *J Clin Psychiatry* **58**: 12–18.

Knäuper B, Wittchen H-U (1994) Diagnosing major depression in the elderly: Evidence for response bias in standardized diagnostic interviews? *Journal of Psychiatric Research* **28**(2): 147–164.

Kraemer HC, Kazdin AE, Offord DR, Kessler RC, Jensen P, Kupfer DJ (1997) Coming to terms with the terms of risk. *Arch Gen Psychiatry* **54**: 337–343.

Kramer M (1969) Cross-national study of diagnosis of the mental disorders: Origin of the problem. *Am J Psychiatry* **125**(Suppl): 1–11.

Kringlen E, Torgersen S, Cramer V (2001) A Norwegian psychiatric epidemiological study. *Am J Psychiatry* **158**(7): 1091–1098.

Lee CK, Kwak YS, Yamamoto J, Rhee H, Kim YS, Han JH, et al. (1990a) Psychiatric epidemiology in Korea; Part I: Gender and age differences in Seoul. *J Nerv Ment Dis* **178**: 242–246.

Lee CK, Kwak YS, Yamamoto J, Rhee H, Kim YS, Han JH, et al. (1990b) Psychiatric epidemiology in Korea; Part II: Urban and rural differences. *J Nerv Ment Dis* **178**: 247–252.

Lehtinen V, Lindholm T, Veijola J, Vaisanen E, Puukka P (1991) Stability of prevalences of mental disorders in a normal population cohort followed for 16 years. *Soc Psychiatry Psychiatr Epidemiol* **26**: 40–46.

Leibenluft E (1999) *Gender Differences in Mood and Anxiety Disorders*. Washington, DC: American Psychiatric Press.

Lieb R, Isensee B, Höfler M, Pfister H, Wittchen H-U (2002) Parental major depression and the risk of depression and other mental disorders in offspring. A prospective-longitudinal community study. *Arch Gen Psychiatry* **59**(4): 365–374.

Lewinsohn PM, Rohde P, Seeley JR (1998) Major depressive disorder in older adolescents: prevalence, risk factors, and clinical implications. *Clin Psychol Rev* **18**(7): 765–794.

Lewis G, Pelosi AJ, Araya R, Dunn G (1992) Measuring psychiatric disorder in the community: A standardized assessment for use by lay interviewers. *Psychol Med* **22**: 465–486.

Loewenthal K, et al. (1995) Gender and depression in Anglo-Jewry. *Psychol Med* **25**: 1051–1063.

Maciejewski PK, Prigerson HG, Mazure CM (2001) Sex differences in event-related risk for major depression. *Psychol Med* **31**: 593–604.

Meltzer H, Baljit G, Petticrew M, Hinds K (1995) The prevalence of psychiatric morbidity among adults living in private households. OPCS Survey of psychiatric morbidity in Great Britain: Report 1. London: HMSO.

Merikangas KR, Angst J, Eaton W, Canino G, Rubio-Stipec M, Wacker H, Wittchen HU, Andrade L, Essau C, Whitaker A, Kraemer H, Robins LN, Kupfer DJ (1996) Comorbidity and boundaries of affective disorders with anxiety disorders and substance misuse: Results of an international task force. *Br J Psychiatry* **168**(Suppl 30): 58–67.

Murphy JM (1995) What happens to depressed men? *Harvard Rev Psychiatry* **3**: 47–49.

Murphy JM, Laird NM, Monson RR, Sobol AM, Leighton AH (2000) A 40-year perspective on the prevalence of depression: The Stirling County Study. *Arch Gen Psychiatry* **57**: 209–215.

Murray CJL, Lopez AD (eds) (1996) *The Global Burden of Disease: A Comprehensive Assessment of Mortality and Disability for Diseases, Injuries, and Risk Factors in 1990 and Projected to 2020*. Geneva: World Health Organization.

Murrell SA, Himmelfarb S, Wright K (1983) Prevalence of depression and its correlates in older adults. *Am J Epidemiol* **117**(2): 173–185.

Narrow WE, Rae DS, Robins LN, Regier DA (2002) Revised prevalence estimates of mental disorders in the United States. Using a clinical significance criterion to reconcile two surveys' estimates. *Arch Gen Psychiatry* **59**: 115–123.

Nazroo JY, Edwards AC, Brown GW (1997) Gender differences in the onset of depression following a shared life event: A study of couples. *Psychol Med* **27**: 9–19.

Nazroo JY, Edwards AC, Brown GW (1998) Gender differences in the prevalence of depression: Artefact, alternative disorders, biology or roles? *Soc Health Illn* **20**: 312–330.

Neugebauer R, Dohrenwend BP, Dohrenwend BS (1980) Formulation of hypotheses about the true prevalence of functional psychiatric disorders among adults in the United States. In Dohrenwend BP (ed) *Mental Illness in the United States*. New York: Praeger, pp. 45–94.

Nolen-Hoeksema S (1990) *Sex Differences in Depression*. Stanford, CA: University Press.

Nolen-Hoeksema S, Parker G, Larson J (1994) Ruminative coping with depressed mood following loss. *J Pers Soc Psychol* **67**: 92–104.

Oakley-Browne MA, Joyce PR, Wells JE, Bushnell JA, Hornblow AR (1989) Christchurch Psychiatric Epidemiology Study, Part I: Six month and other period prevalences of specific psychiatric disorders. *Aust NZ J Psychiatry* **23**: 327–340.

Offord DR, Boyle MH, Campbell D, Goering P, Lin E, Wong M, et al. (1996) One-year prevalence of psychiatric disorder in Ontarians 15–64 years of age. *Can J Psychiatry* **41**, 559–563.

Okwumabua JO, Baker FM, Wong SP, Pilgram BO (1997) Characteristics of depressive symptoms in elderly urban and rural African Americans. *J Gerontol A Biol Sci Med Sci* **52**(4): M241–246.

Pajer K (1995) New strategies in the treatment of depression in women. *J Clin Psychiatry* **56**: 30–37.

Parker G (1987) Are the lifetime prevalence rates in the ECA study accurate? *Psychol Med* **17**: 275–282.

Paykel ES (1991) Depression in women. *Br J Psychiatry* **151**: 22–29.

Paykel ES (2000) Not an age of depression after all? Incidence rates may be stable over time. *Psychol Med* **30**: 489–490.

Paykel ES (2001) Stress and affective disorders in humans. *Semin Clin Neuropsychiatry* **61**(1): 4–11.

Perugi G, Akiskal HS, Lattanzi L, et al. (1998) The high prevalence of 'soft' bipolar (II) features in atypical depression. *Comp Psychiatry* **39**: 1–9.

Pezawas L, Angst J, Gamma A, Ajdacic V, Eich D, Rossler W (2003) Recurrent brief depression – past and future. *Progr Neuropsychopharmacol Biol Psychiatry* **27**: 75–83.

Piccinelli M, Wilkinson G (2000) Gender differences in depression – Critical review. *Br J Psychiatry* **177**: 486–492.

Potter LB, Rogler LH, Moscicki EK (1995) Depression among Puerto Ricans in New York City: the Hispanic Health and Nutrition Examination Survey. *Soc Psychiatry Psychiatr Epidemiol* **30**(4): 185–193.

Rao U, Ryan ND, Birmaher B, Dahl RE, Williamson DE, Kaufman J, Rao R, Nelson B (1995) Unipolar depression in adolescents: Clinical outcome in adulthood. *J Am Acad Child Adolesc Psychiatry* **34**(5): 566–578.

Regier DA, Farmer ME, Rae DS, Locke BZ, Keith SJ, Judd LL, Goodwin FK (1990) Comorbidity of mental disorders with alcohol and other drug abuse. Results from the Epidemiologic Catchment Area (ECA) Study. *JAMA* **264**: 2511–2518.

Regier DA, Kaelber CT, Rae DS, Farmer ME, Knauper B, Kessler RC, Norquist GS (1998) Limitations of diagnostic criteria and assessment instruments for mental disorders. Implications for research and policy. *Arch Gen Psychiatry* **55**: 109–115.

Rihmer Z, Szadoczky E, Furedi J, Kiss K, Papp Z (2001) Anxiety disorders comorbidity in bipolar I, bipolar II and unipolar major depression: results from a population-based study in Hungary. *J Affect Disord* **67**: 175–179.

Roberts RE, Lewinsohn PM, Seeley JR (1995) Symptoms of DSM-III-R major depression in adolescence: evidence from an epidemiological survey. *J Am Acad Child Adolesc Psychiatry* **34**(12): 1608–1617.

Robins LN, Helzer JE, Croughan J, Ratcliff KS (1981) National Institute of Mental Health Diagnostic Interview Schedule. Its history, characteristics, and validity. *Arch Gen Psychiatry* **38**: 381–389.

Robins LN, Wing J, Wittchen H-U, Helzer JE, Babor TF, Burke J, Farmer A, Jablenski A, Pickens R, Regier DA, Sartorius N, Towle LH (1988) The Composite International Diagnostic Interview: an epidemiological instrument suitable for use in conjunction with different diagnostic systems and in different cultures. *Arch Gen Psychiatry* **45**: 1069–1077.

Rodgers B (1994) Pathways between parental divorce and adult depression. *J Child Psychol Psychiatry* **35**: 1289–1308.

Ryan ND, Puig-Antich J, Ambrosini P, Rabinovich H, Robinson D, Nelson B, Iyengar S, Twomey J (1987) The clinical picture of major depression in children and adolescents. *Arch Gen Psychiatry* **44**(10): 854–861.

Salokangas RKR, Vaahtera K, Pacriev S, Sohlman B, Lehtinen V (2002) Gender differences in depressive symptoms – An artefact caused by measurement instruments? *J Affect Disord* **68**: 215–220.

Sheehan DV, Lecrubier Y, Sheehan KH, Amorim P, Janavs J, Weiller E, Hergueta T, Baker R, Dunbar GC (1998) The Mini-International Neuropsychiatric Interview (MINI): The development and validation of a structured diagnostic psychiatric interview for DSM-IV and ICD-10. *J Clin Psychiatry* **59**(20): 22–33.

Silverstein B (1999) Gender differences in the prevalence of clinical depression: The role played by depression associated with somatic symptoms. *Am J Psychiatry* **156**: 480–482.

Simon GE, Goldberg DP, Von Korff M, Üstün TB (2002) Understanding cross-national differences in depression prevalence. *Psychol Med* **32**: 585–594.

Spitzer RL, Endicott J, Robins E (1978) Research diagnostic criteria: rationale and reliability. *Arch Gen Psychiatry* **35**: 773–782.

Steffens DC, Skoog I, Norton MC, Hart AD, Tschanz JT, Plassman BL, Wyse BW, Welsh-Bohmer KA, Breitner JC (2000) Prevalence of depression and its treatment in an elderly population: The Cache County study. *Arch Gen Psychiatry* **57**(6): 601–607.

Streiner DL (1998) Let me count the ways: Measuring incidence, prevalence, and impact in epidemiological studies. *Can J Psychiatry* **43**: 173–179.

Strober M, Lampert C, Schmidt S, Morrell W (1993) The course of major depressive disorder in adolescents: I. Recovery and risk of manic switching in a follow-up of psychotic and nonpsychotic subtypes. *J Am Acad Child Adolesc Psychiatry* **32**(1): 34–42.

Szadoczky E, Papp Z, Vitrai J, Rihmer Z, Furedi J (1998) The prevalence of major depressive and bipolar disorders in Hungary. Results from a national epidemiologic survey. *J Affect Disord* **50**: 153–162.

ten Have M, Vollebergh W, Bijl R, Nolen WA (2002) Bipolar disorder in the general population in The Netherlands: Prevalence, consequences and care utilisation: Results from The Netherlands Mental Health Survey and Incidence Study (NEMESIS). *J Affect Disord* **68**(2–3): 203–213.

The ESEMeD-MHEDEA 2000 Investigators (2004) Prevalence of mental disorders in Europe: Results from the European Study of Epidemiology of Mental Disorders (ESEMeD) Project. *Acta Psychiatr Scand* **109**(Suppl 420): 21–27.

The WHO World Mental Health Survey Consortium (2004) Prevalence, severity, and unmet need for treatment of mental disorders in the World Health Organization World Mental Health Surveys. *JAMA* **291**(21): 2581–2590.

Tohen M, Bromet E, Murphy JM, Tsuang MT (2000) Psychiatric epidemiology. *Harvard Rev Psychiatry* **8**(3): 111–125.

Tohen M, Goodwin FK (1995) Epidemiology of bipolar disorder. In Tsuang MT, Tohen M, Zahner GEP (eds) *Textbook in Psychiatric Epidemiology.* New York: John Wiley, pp. 301–315.

Turner CF, Ku L, Rogers SM, Lindberg LD, Pleck JH, Sonenstein FL (1998) Adolescent sexual behavior, drug use, and violence: Increased reporting with computer survey technology. *Science* **280**(5365): 867–873.

Uhlenhuth EH, Balter MB, Mellinger GD, Cisin IH, Clinthorne J (1983) Symptom checklist syndromes in the general population. Correlations with psychotherapeutic drug use. *Arch Gen Psychiatry* **40**(11): 1167–1173.

Üstün TB, Sartorius N (1995) Mental illness in General Health Care across the world. An international study. New York: John Wiley.

Vazquez-Barquero JL, Manrique JFD, Munoz J, Arango JM, Gaite L, Herrera S, Der GJ (1992) Sex-differences in mental illness – A community study of the influence of physical health and sociodemographic factors. *Soc Psychiatry Psychiatr Epidemiol* **27**: 62–68.

Warner V, Weissman MM, Mufson L, Wickramaratne PJ (1999) Grandparents, parents, and grandchildren at high risk for depression: a three-generation study. *J Amer Acad Child Adolesc Psychiatry* **38**(3): 289–296.

Weissman MM, Bland RC, Canino GJ, Faravelli C, Greenwald S, Hwu HG, Joyce PR, Karam EG, Lee CK, Lellouch J, Lepine JP, Newman SC, Rubio-Stipec M, Wells JE, Wickramaratne PJ, Wittchen H, Yeh EK (1996) Cross-national epidemiology of major depression and bipolar disorder. *JAMA* **276**: 293–299.

Weissman MM, Bland RC, Joyce PR, Newman SC, Wells JE, Wittchen HU (1993) Sex differences in rates of depression: Cross-national perspectives. *J Affect Disord* **29**: 77–84.

Weissman MM, Bruce LM, Leaf PJ, Florio LP, Holzer III C (1991) Affective disorders. In Robins LN, Regier DA (eds) *Psychiatric Disorders in America: The Epidemiologic Catchment Area Study.* New York: Free Press, pp. 53–80.

Weissman MM, Myers J (1978) Affective disorders in a U.S. urban community: The use of research diagnostic criteria in an epidemiological survey. *Arch Gen Psychiatry* **35**: 1304–1311.

Weissman MM, Myers JK, Tischler GL, Holzer CE 3rd, Leaf PJ, Orvaschel H, Brody JA (1985) Psychiatric disorders (DSM-III) and cognitive impairment among the elderly in a U.S. urban community. *Acta Psychiatr Scand* **71**(4): 366–379.

Wells KB, Stewart A, Hays RD (1989) The functioning and well-being of depressed patients: results from the Medical Outcomes Study. *JAMA* **262**: 916–919.

Wickramaratne PJ, Greenwald S, Weissman MM (2002) Psychiatric disorders in the relatives of probands with prepubertal-onset or adolescent-onset major depression. *J Amer Acad Child Adolesc Psychiatry* **39**(11): 1396–1405.

Wilhelm K, Parker G (1994) Sex differences in lifetime depression rates: fact or artefact? *Psychol Med* **24**: 97–111.

Whitaker A, Johnson J, Shaffer D, Rapoport JL, Kalikow K, Walsh BT, Davies M, Braiman S, Dolinsky A (1990) Uncommon troubles in young people: Prevalence estimates of selected psychiatric disorders in a nonreferred adolescent population. *Arch Gen Psychiatry* **47**(5): 487–496.

Wing JK, Cooper JE, Sartorius N (1974) *The Measurement and Classification of Psychiatric Symptoms: An Instruction Manual for the Present State Examination and CATEGO Programme.* London: Cambridge University Press.

Wing JK, Babor T, Brugha T, Burke J, Cooper JE, Giel R, Jablenski A, Regier D, Sartorius N (1990) SCAN. Schedules for Clinical Assessment in Neuropsychiatry. *Arch Gen Psychiatry* **47**: 589–593.

Wittchen H-U (1994) Reliability and validity studies of the WHO Composite International Diagnostic Interview (CIDI): a critical review. *J Psychiatric Res* **28**(1): 57–84.

Wittchen H-U (1996) Critical issues in the evaluation of comorbidity of psychiatric disorders. *Br J Psychiatry* **168**(Suppl 30): 9–16.

Wittchen HO, Essau CA, von Zerssen D, Krieg JC, Zaudig M (1992) Lifetime and six-month prevalence of mental disorders in the Munich Follow-up Study. *Eur Arch Psychiatry Clin Neurosci* **241**: 247–258.

Wittchen H-U, Jacobi F (in press) Size and burden of mental disorder in Europe: A critical review and appraisal of studies. *European Neuropsychopharmacology.*

Wittchen HU, Kessler RC, Pfister H, Lieb M (2000) Why do people with anxiety disorders become depressed? A prospective-longitudinal community study. *Acta Psychiatr Scand Suppl* **406**: 14–23.

Wittchen HU, Ustun TB, Kessler RC (1999a) Diagnosing mental disorders in the community: a difference that matters? *Psychol Med* **29**: 1021–1027.

Wittchen HU, Lieb R, Wunderlich U, Schuster P (1999b) Comorbidity in primary care: Presentation and consequences. *J Clin Psychiatry* **60**(Suppl 7): 29–36.

Wittchen H-U, Lachner G, Wunderlich U, Pfister H (1998) Test-retest reliability of the computerized DSM-IV version of the Munich-Composite International Diagnostic Interview (M-CIDI). *Social Psychiatry and Psychiatric Epidemiology* **33**(11): 568–578.

Wittchen H-U, Pittrow D (2002) Prevalence, recognition and management of depression in primary care in Germany: The Depression 2000 study. *Human Psychopharmacology – Clinical and Experimental* **17**(Suppl 1): 1–11.

World Health Organization (1978) *Mental Disorders: Glossary and Guide to their Classification in Accordance with the Ninth Revision of the International Classification of Diseases*. Geneva: World Health Organization.

World Health Organization (1993) *The ICD-10 Classification of Mental and Behavioural Disorders. Diagnostic Criteria for Research*. Geneva: World Health Organization.

Young MA, Scheftner WA, Fawcett J, Klerman GL (1990) Gender differences in the clinical features of unipolar major depressive disorder. *J Nerv Ment Dis* **178**: 200–203.

2

Genetics of Mood Disorders

Alessandro Serretti

Vita-Salute University, Milan, Italy

BACKGROUND

History

The idea that mood disorders are heritable disturbances may be dated back to Hippocrates theory of constitutional types. In fact, the hypothesis that psycho-pathological traits could be inherited (known as atavism) has been present since the origins of psychiatry, suggested by the observation that in some particular families there were more affected subjects than in the general population. The first authors to study this question in depth, were K. Lucas and B. A. Morel, in the first half of the nineteenth century, and R. Krafft-Ebing (Krafft-Ebing, 1939) at the end of the same century. More recently, scripts retrieved at the Bethlehem Hospital in London dated back to 1820, show that clinicians wondered if mental disorders were inheritable. However, a more precise hypothesis based on an interaction of causes, both predisposing and provoking, did not appear until the nineteenth century. Wilhelm Griesinger (1817–1868) distinguished in fact between traumatic external events and internal states (including hereditary predisposition), which could combine, in varying rates, to give rise to insanity. This causal model had a great success among his contemporary scientists and was adopted at that time by many authors, including Freud, the founding father of psychoanalysis, who divided neurotic states on this basis (Ackerknecht, 1959). With the beginning of the twentieth century and the rise of biological psychiatry the first twin studies were performed to investigate heritability of mental diseases and psychopathological traits. During the years between World Wars I and II there was a flourishing of experiments performed to demonstrate empirically the importance of inheritance in mental illness. Ernst Rudin and the Munich Research Institute improved the first statistical research techniques to quantify the familial concentration of some psychiatric diseases. But they tended to neglect completely the role of environmental influences, so their

Mood Disorders: Clinical Management and Research Issues. Edited by E. J. L. Griez, C. Faravelli, D. J. Nutt and J. Zohar.
©2005 John Wiley & Sons Ltd. ISBN 0 470 09426 5.

results were easily criticized by the so called 'environmentalists'. This widespread interest flowered particularly in Nazi Germany and research findings about heritability were at the basis of the eugenic movement. The term 'eugenic' was created by F. Galton in 1889. The followers of this doctrine had, as their main wish, to reduce illnesses and abnormality in humankind, through deliberate elimination and mating selection (Weber, 1997). They maintained that mental illness, feeble-mindedness, criminality, alcoholism and sexual promiscuity were all expressions of racial degeneracy, whose remedy lay in a policy of selective birth control, extending to the sterilization of those unfit to bear children. But first hopes received a setback when they understood that the necessary social laws would conflict with individual rights, and would therefore be difficult to apply. Ideas of this nature lead to the mass extermination of the mentally ill and handicapped under Hitler's regime (Meyer-Lindenberg, 1991). However recent knowledge has demonstrated that, from a purely genetic point of view, this strategy would be unfruitful and would, most probably, lead to deleterious consequences (CavalliSforza, 1997). In fact, selection of individuals based on phenotype appearance would never completely eliminate recessive factors that are carried by individuals without any negative phenotype trait. Moreover the reduction of genetic variability induced by selection has been shown to be disadvantageous for the species (CavalliSforza, 1997).

The following decades were strongly influenced by those events and psychiatric genetics, together with biological psychiatry as a whole, suffered from a long and widespread stigma during which phenomenology, psychoanalysis or, more recently, social approaches were favoured. Only in the late 1960s and the 1970s did the need to bridge the gap between psychiatry and the other rapidly advancing fields of medicine prompt many worldwide general and mental health authorities (World Health Organization, American Psychiatric Association) to turn psychiatric research to biological and genetic studies.

Key point: the origins of psychiatric genetics are very ancient but its greater development is very recent, dating back to the early 1960s, with family and twin studies, and having its full expansion since the 1980s, with the enormous progress of molecular biology.

Classification Issues

Mood disorders are characterized by a disturbance in mood as the predominant feature. This mood alteration may range from an extreme state of elation, called mania, to a severe state of dysphoria, named depression. In addition, these disorders are associated with some other signs and symptoms. The aim of nosologic researches has been to distinguish homogeneous subtypes of mood disorders corresponding to different clustering of these signs and symptoms, clearly delimited from other disorders. Modern psychiatric nosology follows Leonhard's (Leonhard, 1959) suggestion to subdivide mood disorders according to the type of mood disturbance experienced by the patient. A bipolar disorder (BP) is diagnosed when manic episodes or both manic and depressive episodes occur, and unipolar disorder when only depressive episodes occur. The most widely followed nosologic manual is currently the *Diagnostic and Statistical Manual of Mental Diseases* (DSM) which was compiled for the first time in 1951 by a special Committee (Committee on Nomenclature and Statistics) instituted by the American Psychiatric Association. It is periodically revised: the fifth revision is due to be published in the short term. According to DSM criteria, symptoms of a 'manic episode' are: expansive, elevated, or irritable mood, inflated self-esteem, decreased need for sleep, acceleration of speech and thoughts, distractibility, increased goal-directed activity and excessive involvement in reckless activities. Manic episodes are typically short, but they may have a more extended time course and, in rare cases, they may last for months. DSM (DSM-IV) distinguishes between BP type I (characterized by the occurrence of at least a full manic episode) and type II (characterized by a less severe manic episode, called 'hypomanic'). The symptomatology of a 'major depressive episode' consists of: depressed mood, diminished interest or pleasure in all activities, insomnia or hypersomnia, psychomotor agitation or retardation, fatigue and loss of energy, feelings of worthlessness or excessive guilt, inability to concentrate or act decisively, decreased appetite with weight loss and recurrent thoughts of death or suicide. Usually, major depressive episodes arise slowly, with an onset period varying from a week to some months. Each episode typically lasts for several months and ends gradually. The presence of both manic and depressed symptoms during the same episode characterized a 'mixed' episode. The different combinations of major depressive episodes, manic episodes, mixed episodes and hypomanic episodes define the diagnosis of mood disorders. Single episodes do not have their own diagnostic codes and cannot be diagnosed as separate entities, they serve as the building blocks for diagnoses. Finally, psychotic features such as delusions or hallucinations may occur during both manic or depressive episodes.

Do these definitions fit for genetic studies? In other words, are mood disorder subtypes genetically distinct? And are genes that cause a specific disorder completely different from those involved in other disorders, or do they overlap each other? Even though a clear diagnosis between typical schizophrenia and BP is possible, genetic distinction between other disorders is not so clear (Tsuang and Faraone, 1990; Winokur et al., 1993a).

Molecular genetic studies have tried to overcome this bias by using a stratified phenotype definition: from strict to broad. From family studies, in fact, there emerges a reasonable definition of a BP spectrum of mood disorders that would include, from narrow to broad, BP type I, BP type II, schizoaffective disorder, recurrent major depressive disorder (MD) and single episode major depression, this last being considered the disorder with the lowest genetic loading (Tsuang and Faraone, 1990). It is unclear, however, if this spectrum represents a pleiotropic expression of a single genetic susceptibility.

The overlap between different diagnostic phenotypes is even more extensive when less severe disorders are considered. The presence at the same time of several psychic disorders in a single subject is, for example, common. This phenomenon is called comorbidity. Do they really represent different nosologic entities or do they evidence deficits in the present diagnostic systems criteria? People suffering mood disorders often experience anxiety symptoms. Are the genes implicated in anxiety disorders the same as those involved in depression? Does the overlap between different diagnostic phenotypes reflect an overlap between the genes involved? Family and twin studies show a large overlap between them (Kendler et al., 1992b). A more careful twin study of comorbidity analysing different disorders found evidence of two clusters of genetic factors: one is related to MD and generalized anxiety disorder, the other is involved in panic disorder, bulimia and phobic disorder (Kendler et al., 1995). Even if comorbidity could represent a bias, molecular and genetic researches would provide some evidence for disentangling the overlap of these two pathologies.

As DSM is an atheoretical diagnostic manual, diagnoses made according to its criteria are based on phenotypic descriptions of symptoms and not on the probable cause of the symptoms. From the abovementioned description it is clear that the definition of an individual as an 'affected subject' is not based on biologically valid measurements, but mainly on clinical features. To face these difficulties, alternative phenotype definitions, based on symptomatology, neuropsychology, neuroimaging, time course or drug response have recently been developed (see later in this chapter).

Key point: because of the hazy phenotypes, psychiatric genetics research cannot use a 'gold standard' phenotype definition for its studies, and this is one of its most important limitations.

Epidemiology Issues

Mood disorders have a large impact on social health. They contribute to 11% of all the inabilities registered in the *International Classification of Disease* manual (ICD-9), and in the USA alone they cause a loss of 147 billion dollars per year taking into account both direct and indirect costs (Pincus and Pettit, 2001).

MD is twice as common in adolescent and adult females as in adolescent and adult males. Its point prevalence in adults in community samples varies from 5% to 9% for women and from 2% to 3% for men, while its lifetime prevalence ranges from 10% to 17% (Ustun, 2001; Weissman, 1987). These prevalence rates appear to be unrelated to ethnicity, education, income, or marital status, but culture may influence the experience and the communication of depressive symptoms. MD is associated with high mortality. Up to 17% of individuals with severe MD die by suicide. The mean age of onset is in the third decade of life, although onset in adolescence is increasingly common.

BP shows a mean age of onset in the second decade of life, and recent reports from population-based epidemiologic studies found age-corrected lifetime risks ranging from 0.3% to 1.5%, with equal risks for men and women (Weissman et al., 1996). The most widely accepted value of lifetime prevalence for general population is

1% (Weissman, 1987; Weissman and Myers, 1978). Lifetime rates for BP seem to be increasing in more recently born cohorts (Rice et al., 1987), but this is not a universal finding (Pauls et al., 1992). Moreover, a relatively sharp decrease in age at onset for individuals born after World War II was observed. One possible partial explanation for this observation among recent generations is anticipation. This term indicates the earlier occurrence and the greater severity of a genetic disorder in a younger generation. Anticipation is a phenomenon that is of substantial interest for genetic studies, though many doubts have been brought up about the methodological biases of anticipation studies (McInnis et al., 1993; Merette et al., 2000). Several molecular genetic studies on this issue will be reviewed later on in this chapter.

The reported prevalence for mood disorders may depend on diagnostic criteria. In fact, considering less severe forms such as 'minor depression' or 'brief recurrent depression', the lifetime rate may reach up to one-third of the population (Angst, 1995).

Key point: both classification and epidemiological issues show us that a valid definition for molecular genetic studies is not available. It is therefore clear that more stringent or alternative criteria are needed for genetic studies where the homogeneity of samples is crucial (Regier, 2000).

GENETIC STUDIES IN MOOD DISORDERS

The State of the Art

Psychiatric genetics uses different types of studies to determine the genetic influence in psychiatric disorders. They could be subdivided into clinical epidemiology (called formal genetics), which is based on family, twin, and adopted studies, and molecular genetics, which is aimed at finding the genetic variations predisposing to psychiatric diseases by using molecular biology modern techniques. A review of the most representative studies of each type of the genetics of mood disorders follows below.

Formal Genetics

Family Studies

Initial observations of familial aggregation for BP and 'unipolar depression' (UP) were followed by systematic twin, family, and adoption studies (conducted over the last 50 years) which undoubtedly indicated the importance of genetic predisposition (Goodwin and Jamison, 1990).

Convergent data from family studies showed that the risk for relatives of subjects affected by mood disorders is greater than that for relatives of normal controls (Tsuang and Faraone, 1990). McGuffin and Katz in 1986 analysed a dozen family studies of bipolar depression and calculated that the risk for relatives of probands was 8%, compared to a risk of 1% in general population (McGuffin and Katz, 1986). Major depression studies showed a family risk of 9%, compared to a general risk of 3% (Figure 2.1). These values are lower than those generally mentioned in most textbooks, mainly because these studies are focused on most severe depressions, often requiring hospitalization. Probably, the differences in familial risk ratios are due to different diagnostic methods.

The cross-risks for BP and UP are not symmetric; in fact, both bipolar and unipolar depressive disorders risks are higher in the relatives of bipolar probands, while the first-degree relatives of unipolar depressed probands have a higher rate only for unipolar depression (McGuffin and Katz, 1989; Moldin and Reich, 1993; Smeraldi et al., 1977; Tsuang and Faraone, 1990). Finally, the observation that major depression seems to be more common in pedigrees where parent's onset occurred when they were 20 years old or younger, prompted researchers to consider early age of onset a possible stratification factor (Weissman et al., 1988).

As a general rule, the risk for relatives of affected subjects decreases with genetic distance from the proband. In fact, for BP, while first-degree relatives show a risk of about 8, second-degree relatives have a risk of 2, and the risk rates decrease progressively to more distant relatives who show a risk near to that of the general population (Figure 2.2).

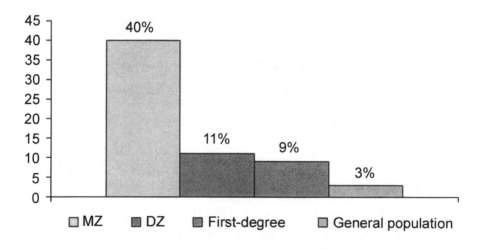

Figure 2.1 Family and twin studies results for major depressive disorder

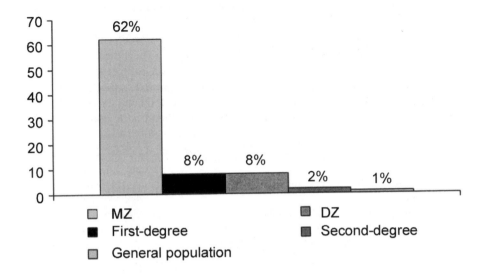

Figure 2.2   Family and twin studies results for bipolar disorder

Twin Studies

Twin studies make it possible to calculate heritability, that is to measure the influence of genetic factors on mood disorder liability. This aim is achieved by comparing the risk of being affected in monozygotic and dizygotic twins. In fact, while dizygotic twins share 50% of their genes, monozygotic twins share 100%. A comparison between the rate of affected co-twins in the two groups gives, with the help of mathematical models, a determination of heritability. Allen analysed some twin studies taken together and reported concordance rates of 40% and 11% for monozygotic (MZ) and dizygotic (DZ) twins respectively for major depression (Allen, 1976) (Figure 2.1). Following analysis substantially confirmed this finding with concordances of 40% (MZ) and 20% (DZ) (Bertelsen et al., 1977; McGuffin et al., 1996; Torgersen, 1986), even though concordance rates up to 67% were reported, but in a small sample of 12 monozygotic twins (Bertelsen, 1985). The heritability of major depression is therefore likely to be in the range of 31–42%. This value is probably the expression of the lower bound, and the level of heritability is likely to be substantially higher for reliably diagnosed major depression or for subtypes such as recurrent major depression (Sullivan et al., 2000).

   BP probandwise concordance rates range from 33% to 80% and 0% to 40% for MZ and DZ respectively, with heritability estimates ranging from 30% to 80% (Allen et al., 1974; Kringlen, 1967). The respective MZ and DZ probandwise concordance rates in the largest and most methodologically rigorous study were

62% and 8%, with an heritability estimate of 59% (Bertelsen et al., 1977) (Figure 2.2).

More recent twin studies conducted with modern diagnostic criteria, validated semi-structured interviews and blinded assessments, confirm these earlier reports, thought not without exception (Kendler et al., 1992a; McGuffin et al., 1996).

Interestingly, among MZ twin pairs concordant for mood disorder, 20% of the ill co-twins have major depression when one twin has a BP diagnosis (Allen et al., 1974; Bertelsen et al., 1977). This observation supports the hypothesis that BP and UP syndromes share some common genetic susceptibility factors. However, this is still a highly debated issue (Winokur et al., 1993a; Winokur et al., 1995).

Adoption Studies

Twin studies may be biased by environmental issues; in fact cultural influences could be responsible for the observed concordances, with monozygotic twins reared in a more homogeneous way, if compared to dizygotic twins. The ideal unbiased study would employ twins reared apart, but adoption studies may also overcome this bias. The basic strategy consists in studying the affection rate of biological parents of adopted affected subjects. A higher than expected rate in biological parents suggests heritable factors.

Results of adoption studies on mood disorders are heterogeneous. Wender (Wender et al., 1986) found that mood disorders are present in a rate of 8% in 387 biological relatives of probands, this risk value is weakly higher than the control one. Two other adoption studies, based on depression diagnosis, reported a small amount of evidence for genetic susceptibility (Cadoret et al., 1985; von Knorring et al., 1983). More interesting results were found by Mendlewicz in an adoption study on BP (Mendlewicz and Rainer, 1977). The rate of affected biological parents of probands was 7%, but it was null in biological parents of controls. In agreement with family studies biological parents of bipolar patients showed a larger number of subjects with major depression (21%) than biological parents of controls (2%); again this result suggests that major depression and BP share some common genetic susceptibility factors.

Mode of Inheritance

The knowledge of the mode of inheritance has substantial implications for aetiologic research and clinical practice. In fact, the finding of a single major locus (SML) involved (i.e. that a single locus is responsible for the transmission of the disorder), implies that a direct biochemical pathway from genotype to phenotype accounts for the pathophysiology of the disorders. On the other hand, if a multifactorial complex model (interaction of both genetic and environmental components) manages the mode of transmission, the search for a simple biochemical pathway is likely to be less fruitful. Unfortunately, converging evidence is consistent with a complex inheritance of mood disorders. In fact, some pedigree analyses yielded evidence for vertical familial transmission (Pauls et al., 1995a; Rice et al., 1987), but results in general were not consistent with inheritance under a single major gene (Tsuang and Faraone, 1990), even when families are subdivided according to clinical criteria.

Familial risks for BP are not consistent with either single locus models (Craddock et al., 1995), or two-locus/epistatic models (Neuman and Rice, 1992), although the epistatic models were the best-fitting ones. Multiplicative models involving three or more loci are more consistent (Craddock et al., 1995; Risch, 1990). A three-locus symmetric multiplicative model (in which each locus has an equal effect) offers a good fit, with a locus-specific recurrence risk ratio of about 2 (Craddock et al., 1995).

Segregation analyses on unipolar depression rejected SML inheritance (Crowe et al., 1981; Tsuang et al., 1985) but failed to discriminate between single major locus and multifactorial transmission (Price et al., 1987). In summary, the mode of inheritance for depression is complex, and transmission in most families does not follow simple Mendelian patterns. Multilocus genetic and not-shared environmental effects appear to play a significant role in influencing the risk of disease; heritability estimates (like prevalence and risk of recurrence) are highly susceptible to change in phenotypic definition. The potential involvement of epistatic multilocus transmission and locus heterogeneity have yet to be specified.

Finally, there is the possibility of an SML transmission of mood disorders that simulates a complex model. This could be considered in the case of:

(1) Reduced penetrance, that is when some individuals with the disease genotype do not express the illness phenotype, possibly because of polygenic effects, environmental events or variable age of onset
(2) Phenocopies, such as when individuals without a disease genotype show the syndrome for non-genetic causes
(3) Genetic heterogeneity for which mutation at different genetic loci can independently cause clinically indistinguishable disease forms.

Given the difficulty in homogeneity of mood disorder diagnoses, many authors have focused on markers that could identify more biologically homogeneous samples with a simpler transmission model.

One of these markers is represented by antidepressant and lithium treatment response. This choice spread from the observation that a first-degree relative of a responder to a specific antidepressant may be responsive to the same therapy (O'Reilly et al., 1994; Pare and Mack, 1971). In fact, families of probands responsive to tricyclics or SSRIs fitted in a better way with Mendelian models (Franchini et al., 1998; Orsini, 1987; Serretti et al., 1998a; Smeraldi et al., 1987). The prophylactic efficacy of lithium also allowed the identification of a more homogeneous group of subjects (Smeraldi et al., 1984) with a recessive SML mode of transmission (Alda et al., 1994). But no definite finding has been produced so far.

Key point: converging evidence is consistent with a complex inheritance of mood disorders. Also not-shared environmental effects appear to play a significant role in influencing the risk of disease; these facts, together with the difficulty in homogeneity of mood disorder diagnoses, have led many authors to direct their attention to markers that could identify more biologically homogeneous samples with a simpler transmission model, for example antidepressant and lithium treatment response. This choice spread from the observation that a first-degree relative of a responder to a specific antidepressant may be responsive to the same therapy.

Molecular Genetic Studies

Linkage Studies

Linkage studies are aimed at measuring the tendency of two genes to segregate together on the same chromosome through meiosis in families (LOD). The measurement unit is the LOD-score, which can vary from negative to positive values. A LOD-score of 3 or more is considered significant in fact it corresponds to a probability of 1000/1 in favour of linkage (Ott, 1991). The main limitations of linkage studies on mood disorders are connected to the complexity of this kind of disease: in fact genetic parameters, such as the mode of transmission and gene penetrance are unspecified, and, as was said above, phenotype definition is uncertain (Tsuang and Faraone, 1990). Several genetic loci have been studied; a review of the most important findings follows.

X-chromosome. Epidemiologic studies have consistently shown women to be at greater risk than men for developing mood disorders. Those findings, together with some studies on parent–child transmission of BP showing a father–child transmission less frequent than mother–child transmission, could be consistent with an X-linkage hypothesis of mood disorders. Table 2.1 shows a series of linkage studies based on the idea that at last one of the genes involved in the development of major depression and BP is located on chromosome X.

All the results of the reported studies are suggestive of X linkage, and, in particular, the Xq26–q28 region should be considered a strong candidate region for genetic studies about mood disorders. However, methodological criticisms have been raised about many of the earlier studies, and multiple failures to replicate have been reported. In particular, a LOD-score of 7.5 obtained in a methodologically rigorous study for linkage to colour-blindness and G6PD deficiency in five Israeli families (Baron et al., 1987) was not confirmed in those same pedigrees by methods employing relevant Xq28 DNA markers (Baron et al., 1993). There is no simple methodological explanation for why some studies are positive and other negative. Although there are more negative results, the positive ones cannot be discounted. Current literature suggests that consistent independent confirmation of reported linkages by molecular methods in novel kindred must remain the gold standard, regardless of the level of statistical significance achieved by a single report (Lander and Kruglyak, 1995).

Chromosome 6. On the short arm of chromosome 6 there is a tightly clustered group of genes known as the major histocompatibility complex (MHC). The MHC contains many genes involved in controlling the immune response to foreign antibodies and it is often called the HLA region. The region near to HLA has been hypothesized to be involved in the genesis of major depression and BP. We have summarized studies of HLA linkage to mood disorders in Table 2.2. Though more positive studies than expected have been performed, no unequivocal finding has been achieved.

Chromosome 11. The availability of new genetic markers has more recently allowed researchers to perform linkage studies on specific genes coding for enzymes involved in catecholamines metabolism or for amine receptors. A linkage study of Old Order Amish pedigrees described evidence (LOD-score > 4.0) for a BP locus on 11p15, where the tyrosine hydroxylase gene was located (Egeland et al., 1987), but the LOD-score (4.9) diminished to nonsignificance when pedigrees were extended and members reevaluated (Pauls et al., 1991). Similar weakly positive LOD scores were reported for this region by other investigators. Nevertheless, studies in numerous other pedigrees did not confirm the first results.

Linkage to the dopamine D2 receptor gene (11q22–q23) has been excluded in several analyses, while linkage to the dopamine D4 receptor gene (11p15.5) has not been excluded.

Chromosome 18. Suggestive evidence was found for BP linkage to chromosome 18p and more precisely to a pericentromeric susceptibility locus (Berrettini et al., 1997; Berrettini et al., 1994). Nonparametric analysis made on this study sample confirmed the observation of linkage (Gershon et al., 1996). In addition, a linkage study performed on nearly 30 pedigrees and using several of the same DNA markers and similar analyses confirmed previous findings (Stine et al., 1995). Moreover, Stine et al. (1995) noted that most of their positive 18p statistics derived from paternal pedigrees, that is from kindreds in which there was evidence for paternal transmission of the disease, like Berrettini et al. reported in the abovementioned study (Berrettini et al., 1994). However, the strong dependence of linkage by age correction employed in this sample (Cleves et al., 1997), makes these findings not easy to explain. On the other hand, in a study of rigorously defined high-density German families, no robust evidence for linkage for the pericentromeric region of chromosome 18 could be found (Maier et al., 1995). A suggestive evidence of an 18q locus was obtained in other analyses (Freimer et al., 1996), but the implicated region was over a 5 Mb region, and other markers in between provided evidence against linkage. Moreover, it was at least 15 Mb distant from the 18q region for which signif- icant evidence of linkage was previously reported (Stine et al., 1995). A further

TABLE 2.1   Studies of X-linkage in mood disorders

Study	Marker	Sample	Results
Mendlewicz et al., 1972	Colour blindness	9 pedigrees; all probands had BP but relatives had either unipolar or BP	Supported the presence of a dominant X-linked gene
Fieve et al., 1973	Blood group	6 pedigrees ascertained through bipolar proband	LOD-score: 1.12
Mendlewicz and Fleiss, 1974	Colour blindness	Additional family to that previously studied	LOD-score: 4.5 and 3.73
Mendlewicz and Fleiss, 1974	Blood group	25 families	LOD-score: 2.96
Mendlewicz et al., 1975	Blood group	12 families; all probands had BP but relatives had either unipolar or BP	LOD-score did not exceed 3
Johnson and Leeman, 1977	Colour blindness	2 pedigrees; all probands had BP but relatives had either unipolar or BP	No linkage
Baron, 1977	Colour blindness	One large pedigree ascertained through a schizoaffective proband, relatives had either unipolar or BP	LOD-score: 2.33
Leckman et al., 1979	Blood group	6 families ascertained through bipolar probands, relatives also had other mental disorders	Hypothesis of close linkage was not supported
Gershon, 1980	Colour blindness	International collaborative study in BP	LOD-score: 1.00
Mendlewicz et al., 1980	G6PD	Unipolar proband; relatives were considered ill if they had either unipolar or BP	LOD-score: 4.32
Del Zompo et al., 1984	G6PD	Major affective illness	LOD-score: 0.97
Del Zompo et al., 1984	Colour blindness	Major affective illness	LOD-score: 0.5
Kidd et al., 1984	Colour blindness	One bipolar family	LOD-score: 0.27
Kidd et al., 1984	Blood group	3 families	LOD-score: 0.36
Baron et al., 1987	G6PD, Colour	blindness	One large Israeli pedigree

Reference	Locus/marker	Sample	Result
Mendlewicz et al., 1987	F9	11 pedigrees with mood disorder	LOD-score: 3.1
Lucotte et al., 1992	F9	French pedigrees	LOD-score: 3.9
Berrettini et al., 1990	G6PD, Colour blindness	Bipolar pedigrees	No linkage
Gejman et al., 1990	F9	7 informative kindreds segregating for manic depressive illness	No linkage
Baron et al., 1993	G6PD	Multigeneration Israeli kindreds for manic depressive illness	No linkage
Craddock et al., 1994a	Fragile X syndrome Xq27.3	79 unrelated bipolar probands without fragile X syndrome and 77 unrelated controls	No linkage
De bruyn et al., 1994	F8, F9, DXS52	9 bipolar families	Data suggest linkage
Detera-Wadleigh et al., 1994	Pseudoautosomal region at Xpter	21 middle-sized pedigrees	Cumulative LOD-scores less than -2
Mendelbaum et al., 1995	Xq27	Previous X linkage data reanalysed	Confirm X-linked hypothesis
Pekkarinen et al., 1995	Xq26 region about 7 cM to the F9 locus	One large Finnish family	LOD-score: 3.5
Pekkarinen et al., 1995	Xq24–q27	Extended pedigree from Finland	Evidenced linkage
Stine et al., 1997	Xp22 and Xq26–q28	NIMH 97 pedigrees	Positive though small LOD-score
Smyth et al., 1997	Xq26.3–q28	23 large families	No linkage
Vallada et al., 1998	Xq25–q27	43 BP families	No linkage

TABLE 2.2   Studies of HLA-linkage

Study	Results
Smeraldi et al., 1978	Sib pair analysis suggests linkage
Smeraldi and Bellodi, 1981; Targum et al., 1979	Excludes close linkage
Weitkamp et al., 1980	Excludes close linkage
Weitkamp et al., 1981	Sib pair analysis suggests linkage
Johnson et al., 1981	Excludes close linkage
Suarez and Croughan, 1982	Sib pair analysis rejects linkage, but pooling with old data suggests linkage
Turner and King, 1981; Turner and King, 1983	Suggests linkage
Suarez and Reich, 1984	Sib pair analysis rejects linkage
Campbell et al., 1984	Excludes close linkage
Kidd et al., 1984	Excludes close linkage
Waters et al., 1988	Linkage was excluded
Stancer et al., 1988	Positive results
Payami et al., 1989	Sib pair analysis suggests linkage for UP
Price, 1989	No evidence for linkage

study supported the interest of the 18q23 region showing linkage with BP (Coon et al., 1996). Stine (Stine et al., 1995) also reported evidence for a susceptibility locus in 18q21, that is approximately 40 cM more telomeric than the region identified by Berrettini (Berrettini et al., 1994). In two large Belgian pedigrees, no linkage was found for a marker located in the pericentromeric region, but analysis in one family suggested that the 18q21.33–q23 region may contain a susceptibility locus for BP (De bruyn et al., 1996). Thus, an 80 Mb region encompassing most of both arms of chromosome 18 has been implicated. Several nonreplicating studies on chromosome 18 linkage have been reported, but some of these do not have adequate statistical power (Pauls et al., 1995b), even though other studies with adequate power have been described (Detera-Wadleigh et al., 1997; Knowles et al., 1998).

Cromosome 21. Straub et al. (1994) described evidence for linkage of BP to a region of chromosome 21q22.3, near the phosphofructokinase (PFLK) locus. A LOD-score of 3.41 (genome-wide *p* value 0.04) was found in 1 of 47 bipolar families for localization to 21q (Straub et al., 1994) and the analysis of the entire sample resulted in suggestive evidence of linkage (LOD-score=2.80). A confirmatory report has been described (Gurling et al., 1995), in which evidence for a two-locus BP disease model included an 11p and a 21q marker data. Further analyses confirmed this finding (Aita et al., 1999; Ewald et al., 1996; Smith and Rubin, 1997). Also a study made by Detera-Wadleigh et al. (Detera-Wadleigh et al., 1996, 1997) provide a confirmation of Straub's report (Straub et al., 1994), but, unfortunately, the evidence of linkage was to a region more than 15 Mb distant from that involved in Straub's study (Straub et al., 1994). Also, three non-replications have been published.

Other Chromosomes. Significant evidence of linkage to 4p was reported in a single pedigree (Blackwood et al., 1996), but a failure to replicate occurred in other pedigrees. Suggestive evidence has been reported for other linkages to 5p (Kelsoe et al., 1996), 6p (Ginns et al., 1996), 10q (Rice et al., 1997), 12q (Craddock et al., 1994b), 16p (Ewald et al., 1995), and 22q (Lachman et al., 1997). Other significant linkage studies were made by Straub (Straub et al., 1994) and Aita (Aita et al., 1999) on polymorphisms located on chromosome 21 and Blackwood (Blackwood et al., 1996) on chromosome 4p16.

Key point: no region has been convincingly identified as a locus of bipolar susceptibility, even if there are several confirmed reports of loci of smaller effect. The causes of this inability to obtain more compelling evidence may be multifaceted. Possibly, genes confer susceptibility to mood disorder, but they have such a small relative effect on risk that a very large sample is required for detection. Moreover, specific genes may confer susceptibility in a small number of families, so that failures to replicate reflect the confounding effects of genetic heterogeneity. Finally, the reported positive results may be due to chance.

Association Studies

The main goal of association studies is the detection of polymorphic genetic variants which occur more frequently in individuals with a disease compared to control subjects. The main advantages of this kind of study in mood disorders are the need to define a genetic model of the analysed disorder and the possibility of detecting genes with a minor effect on the affected phenotype (OR=2–5). The main disadvantages are the possible detection of spurious associations and the stratification biases due to the differences in allele frequency of the different ethnicities (Cardon and Bell, 2001). Similarly to linkage studies, association analyses have not yielded definite findings. Family-based association studies have been recently widely used to control for stratification biases (Falk and Rubinstein, 1987; Spielman et al., 1993). They are based on comparison of transmitted with non-transmitted alleles in families of affected subjects. However, this kind of study presents some recruitment difficulties, thus decreasing the power of the sample; in addition, the low age of probands may cause ascertainment biases (Khoury and Yang, 1998; Schulze et al., 2001).

HLA Complex and ABO System. Many studies have looked for a possible association between mood disorder and HLA antigens. The most conservative interpretation of these results is that mood disorder is not associated with HLA; however, if such an association exists, it is either very weak or limited to a subset of patients (Smeraldi and Bellodi, 1981; Suarez and Reich, 1984).

Like the HLA antigens, the ABO blood groups have been found to be associated with a variety of different diseases. The reported associations are in any case inconsistent with the negative ABO linkage studies. It is, however, notable that the gene for dopamine-beta-hydroxylase (DBH) is strongly suspected to be closely linked to the ABO locus on chromosome 9 (Goldin et al., 1982; Wilson et al., 1988). Since DBH is critical to the synthesis of catecholamines, it is a reasonable candidate to be involved in mood disorders.

Chromosome X: MAOA and MAOB genes and 5-HT$_{2C}$ Receptor Genes. The association between mood disorders and polymorphic markers on the X-chromosome have also been investigated. In fact Yoneda et al. (1992) reported an association with the marker DXYS20 in Japanese BP patients; this result has not, however, been replicated in European populations (Nothen et al., 1993; Parsian and Todd, 1994).

The MAOA and MAOB genes, which code for the enzymes that degrade biogenic amines, are both located on the X-chromosome in the Xp11.2–p11.4 region. Lim et al. (1994b, 1995) reported a weak but significant association between three different polymorphisms in the MAOA gene and mood disorders. An association has also been found between the MAOA gene and BP (Kawada et al., 1995), but the association concerned different alleles. A meta-analysis made by Rubinsztein in 1996 reported a significant difference between normal and bipolar allele frequencies (Rubinsztein et al., 1996). However, a series of negative reports followed.

The 5-HT$_{2C}$ receptor gene has been studied as a candidate gene for BP and MD. Two groups found a weak association with BP (Gutierrez et al., 1996; Oruc et al., 1997b) while Vincent and collaborators (Vincent et al., 1999) found no association. No association was found with major depression. Recently, a large data set from the European Collaborative Project on Affective Disorders has been analysed (Lerer et al., 2001). Significant associations of the 5-HT$_{2C}$ cys23ser polymorphism with both major depression ($p=0.006$) and BP ($p=0.02$) have been found.

Chromosome 5: Alpha1 GABA A Receptor, 5-HT$_{1A}$ Receptor and DT Genes. Preliminary evidence suggested linkage for the long arm of chromosome 5 with mood disorders. This region contains candidate genes for mood disorders, such as the alpha1 subunit of the GABA A receptor and the 5-HT$_{1A}$ receptor. In this case, as well, negative results were found (Curtis et al., 1993; Detera-Wadleigh et al., 1992). Also the dopamine transporter gene, located in a different region of chromosome 5, has been investigated, but no association with mood disorders has been found. In fact, evidence suggesting linkage disequilibrium between DT and BP has been reported by Waldman et al. (1997), even though other studies did not confirm this result.

Chromosome 11 and 17: Tyrosine Hydroxylase, D2 Receptor and D4 Receptor Genes, HTT, Tryptophan Hydroxylase. These two chromosomes received much interest because a series of candidate genes are included in them. Those are genes coding for proteins of serotonergic, dopaminergic, and adrenergic pathways that have been candidates because of their involvement in the pathophysiology of mood disorders (Willner, 1995). Chromosome 11 in particular has been largely investigated in psychiatric disorders because of the presence of tyrosine hydroxylase (TH), dopamine receptor D2 and dopamine receptor D4.

Several reports have described evidence for association of TH gene with BP (Leboyer et al., 1990; Meloni et al., 1995; Serretti et al., 1998c), although other groups have not confirmed this observation. Meta-analysis of the results of association studies (Furlong et al., 1999) do not support the TH gene having a major role in the aetiology of BP.

Most studies showed no association between the gene for the dopamine receptor D2 and mood disorders, while few studies investigating the dopamine receptor D4 gene have found positive results (Catalano et al., 1993; Kaiser et al., 2000; Lim et al., 1994a; Manki et al., 1996; Weiss et al., 1996) compared to many studies excluding associations.

One of the most widely studied candidate gene has been the serotonin transporter gene on chromosome 17q. Several positive results (Collier et al., 1996; Coyle et al., 2000) have been published, showing the association of BP with a polymorphism in the promoter region or an intronic polymorphism. Allelic association has also been suggested with MD; nevertheless, there have also been several negative reports for both BP and MD.

The tryptophan hydroxylase gene, located on chromosome 11, codes for the rate-limiting enzyme of serotonin metabolism and for this reason is a candidate gene for mood disorders. A significant association was found with BP by Bellivier and collaborators (Bellivier et al., 1998); but other studies did not confirm this positive result.

Other Candidate Genes. A large number of other candidate genes have been investigated, but to a lesser extent compared to the previous ones. Some of them are listed here. Catechol-*o*-methyl transferase (COMT) low activity polymorphic allele was associated with rapid-cycling BP (Lachman et al., 1996) and mood disorders in general (Ohara et al., 1998) but negative replications followed.

In 1995 Parsian and collaborators found an increased frequency of a specific transmitted allele of D3 receptor gene in bipolar families (Parsian et al., 1995), but several studies could not confirm it.

The 5-HT_{2A} receptor gene has been also studied as a candidate gene for mood disorders, but, again, ambiguous results have been reported.

Researchers had also investigated the possible association between genes coding for proteins involved in intraneuronal signal transduction and mood disorders. In fact, effects of mood stabilizers and antidepressants on G protein function have been observed (Manji et al., 1995). In addition, abnormalities in the expression of G protein have been demonstrated in patients affected by mood disorders. Zill et al. investigated whether the C825T Gbeta3 polymorphism was associated with mood disorders; they found a significantly higher frequency of mutant T allele in depressive patients than in healthy controls and schizophrenic patients (Zill et al., 2000) but another study could not confirm the finding in an oriental population (Lin et al., 2001).

Key point: a lot of association studies have been performed to investigate possible associations between mood disorders and genetic polymorphisms. The most attractive candidate gene studies would be those that test polymorphisms known to alter protein structure or to be expressed in genes which are simultaneously positional candidates and functional or structural candidates. Few candidate genes received independent confirmation and not one was unequivocally associated with mood disorders.

Anticipation

Molecular studies investigated also a different phenomenon called 'anticipation'. Anticipation implies that a disease occurs at a progressively earlier age of onset and with increased severity in successive generations. It has been found to correlate with a new class of mutations, expanded trinucleotide repeat sequences (CAG for example, in Huntington's disease). These repeat sequences are unstable and increase in size across generations. Evidence for anticipation has been reported in several family studies of BP (McInnis et al., 1993; Nylander et al., 1994) and of MD (Engstrom et al., 1995), but there are problems of ascertainment biases (Hodge and Wickramaratne, 1995). As an example, earlier age of onset and increase in severity may be related to increased sensitivity to diagnosis in offspring of affected parents. Researchers have investigated the presence of unstable expanding trinucleotide repeated sequences (Lindblad et al., 1995; O'Donovan et al., 1995; Oruc et al., 1997a), and a significant increase in CAG repeats between parents and offspring was observed (Mendlewicz et al., 1997; O'Donovan et al., 1996). However no definitive evidence for causative expansions has been found, so the hypothesis that unstable trinucleotide repeats represent a BP susceptibility factor deserves further studies (Saski et al., 1996).

Animal Studies

Given the difficulties encountered in human studies, many turned their efforts toward animal models. The term 'model' means that the animal behaviours are similar but not identical to some of the signs of the disorder. For example, in mice we can create a syndrome of 'learned helplessness' that could be considered as a model of depression. Biology and anatomical structures in different animals are homologous if they have similar evolutionary origins. In fact many human genes are homologous to genes found in the genomes of other animals: about 85% of genes found in mice are also found in humans. Moreover pharmacological studies routinely employ specific animal behaviours as models of human mental disorders.

Knockout strategies are the most widely used. The knockout mouse allows us to study the effects of mutations that prevent a gene from functioning. We can create a knockout mouse by removing both copies of a gene from its genome and therefore blocking the production of the correspondent specific protein. By studying these mice we learn about the effects of mutations that prevent normal gene functioning. As an example, a knockout mouse which was missing the dopamine transporter gene showed a prolonged clearance of dopamine of about 100 times. Interestingly, this knockout mouse exhibited hyperactivity, suggesting that the dopamine transporter plays an important role in influencing level of motor activity (Caron, 1996). Other findings include a quantitative trait locus QTL for a hyperactivity phenotype that has been localized in rat chromosome 8 and explains 29% of the variance (Moisan et al., 1996). More subtle traits such as memory have been studied as well. For example, mice that lack one of the isoforms of the protein kinase C show abnormal hippocampal 'long term potentiation'; similarly, a deletion of one of the subtypes of the metabotropic glutamate receptor results in impairment of LTP (Abeliovich et al., 1993; Aiba et al., 1994). Further, mice lacking monoamine oxidase A gene (Cases et al., 1995) show an abnormal mating behaviour, decreased thigmotaxis, increased resident intruder attacks and pup neurological abnormalities. On the other hand, mice without the D2 receptor gene have abnormal gait and hypoactivity on the rotarod. Finally, knockout mice for the tyrosine hydroxylase gene show a decrease of spontaneous activity and the cessation of eating and drinking (Zhou and Palmiter, 1995).

Key point: the study of knockout animals can help us to understand the connection between the genotype and the neurochemical modifications and the mechanisms of action involved in the pathogenesis of mood disorders, by giving us behavioural models reflecting human psychopathological phenotypes.

PERSPECTIVES IN TECHNIQUES AND GOALS FOR THE GENETICS OF MOOD DISORDERS

New Definitions of the Affected Phenotype

We have already mentioned that diagnoses in psychiatry are not based on biologically valid measurements, but mainly on clinical features. This lack of validity has probably been the reason for the lack of definite results in molecular genetic studies. Therefore, during recent years, researchers, prompted by inconclusive results, developed alternative phenotype definitions. This is a quite difficult issue because, before any phenotype can be used for the search for liability genes (e.g. symptomatology, neuropsychology), it must demonstrate a number of properties. First it should be a reliable measurement; then the pathway linking it to the underlying biological mechanism should be at least plausible; finally it should demonstrate a significant heritability in formal genetic studies. One approach used symptom clusters independently of diagnoses to be associated with specific gene variants. It has been reported that during illness episodes a number of symptoms may be similar across diagnoses (e.g. delusional symptoms). Those clusters of symptoms are receiving increasing interest as they may be reliably measured, have a plausible biological pathway, evidence a moderate but significant heritability (Cardno et al., 1997, 1998; Van Os et al., 1997), are stable over time and are correlated with regional anatomical brain abnormalities. As a result many recent studies reported genetic liabilities for symptom clusters or behavioural traits independently of psychiatric diagnosis. In particular DRD4 long variants have been associated with the novelty-seeking trait in normals, and the same DRD4 long variants have been associated with delusional and disorganized features in both mood disorders and schizophrenia (Benjamin et al., 1996; Ebstein et al., 1996; Serretti et al., 2000a, 2001a). Suicidality has also been studied, TPH*A variant was proposed as a liability factor for suicidal behaviour, but no unequivocal result has been reported.

Key point: psychiatric genetics could serve as an instrument to create new definitions and nosological criteria for the improvement of diagnostic and prognostic precision.

Pharmacogenetics

One of the most promising approaches is pharmacogenetics. This field has gained increasing attention in recent years and holds great promise for clinical medicine (Dettling et al., 2001; Pickar and Rubinow, 2001; Roses, 2000; Segman et al., 1999). Pharmacogenetic strategy studies how genetic variation could affect the response of patients to psychotropic drugs and their susceptibility to adverse drug reactions. The main goal would be the possibility for clinicians in the future to optimize the use of medications by choosing the drug most likely to work for a given patient according to its particular genetic profile. Pharmacogenetics could also be considered as a solution to bypass the problem of the biological heterogeneity of psychiatric diseases. In fact the heritability of response patterns to psychotropic drugs has been shown to be more homogeneous and not influenced by diagnostic biases (see the earlier section on 'Mode of inheritance').

Pharmacogenetic studies of mood disorder involving short-term antidepressant and long-term lithium response have only been performed in recent years (for a review see Serretti, 2002; Serretti et al., 2002). Drug response has the property of being reliably measurable (Hamilton, 1967), the involved pathway is, at least partly, known (Maes and Meltzer, 1995; Post and Weiss, 1995) and, finally, drug response has been shown to be heritable. In fact, affected relatives' response rate to a psychotropic drug should be taken into account in the choice of a patient therapy. Early reports have suggested that affected children of bipolar lithium responders showed a good response to lithium therapy (McKnew et al., 1981; Youngerman and Canino, 1978) and more recently Grof et al. have reported that lithium response in a sample composed by relatives of responder probands was 67% compared to 30% in a comparison group (Grof et al., 2000). Even studies of unipolar depression provide evidence of how antidepressant response runs in families (Franchini et al., 1998; O'Reilly et al., 1994; Pare and Mack, 1971). In Table 2.3 we report some recent psychopharmacogenetic association studies, with their findings. The most relevant finding is the repeatedly confirmed association between functional polymorphism (5-HTTLPR) in the upstream regulatory region of the serotonin transporter gene (SLC6A4) and the short-term response to various antidepressant treatments. Other genes have been proposed but they are to be confirmed.

Key point: pharmacogenetic studies could be useful to predict the patient response rate to the various psychopharmacological treatments, and thus facilitate therapeutic choices for the clinician. Moreover they shed light on mechanisms of antidepressant response and, eventually, on mechanisms of the diseases.

Illness Time Course

A prognostic factor for identifying specific patterns of recurrence in mood disorders would be useful to detect unfavourable outcomes during the early phases of the treatment (Merikangas et al., 1994) but currently, despite the efforts made in last recent decades, only few factors have been shown to be associated with specific illness time courses.

The time course of mood disorders can range from a single episode to a recurrent pattern with few or no intervals (Angst and Merikangas, 1997), and it is not stable over time; besides, cycle length appears to get progressively shorter, reaching after three to five episodes a frequency plateau of about one episode a year (Angst, 1981; Goodwin and Jamison, 1990; Keller et al., 1983; Kessing et al., 1998; Winokur et al., 1993b). Demographic and clinical features have been alternatively either associated with a worse prognosis or not (Cusin et al., 2000).

A possible association between the time course of mood disorders and genes involved in neurotransmission have been investigated, with the finding of a significant association between rapid cycling time course and the long 5-HTTLPR variant (Cusin et al., 2001; Smeraldi et al., 2002).

Neuropsychology Features

One approach that may improve power to find genes for complex disorders is to target biological traits found in ill subjects and in their unaffected relatives, so-called intermediate neuropsychological phenotypes (rather than clinical diagnosis) (Egan and Weinberger, 1997; Freedman et al., 1997; Kremen et al., 1994). Such traits may have a simpler genetic architecture and be more directly related to the biological effects of susceptibility genes (in comparison with the complex clinical syndrome). Up to now studies have principally concerned schizophrenic disorders, but they could be useful to hypothesize a similar approach to mood disorders. There is evidence that abnormal function of the prefrontal cortex may represent an intermediate phenotype related to genetic risk for schizophrenia (Cannon et al., 2000; Goldberg et al., 1990). Stable deficits in cognitive functions referable to the

TABLE 2.3   Psychopharmacogenetic studies

Author	Gene	Drug	Result
Smeraldi et al., 1998	Serotonin transporter (5-HTT)	Fluvoxamine	l allele subjects were more likely to respond (p=0.017)
Zanardi et al., 2001	5-HTT	Fluvoxamine	l allele subjects were more likely to respond (all sample p=0.029; without pindolol p=0.002)
Zanardi et al., 2000	5-HTT	Paroxetine	s allele associated with less favourable and slower response (p < 0.001)
Pollock et al., 2000	5-HTT	Paroxetine	s allele associated with slower response (p=0.028)
Kim et al., 2000	5-HTT	Fluoxetine and paroxetine	s/s genotype showed better response (p=0.007)
Yoshida et al., 2002a	5-HTT	Fluvoxamine	s allele associated with better response (p=0.010)
Arias et al., 2001	5-HTT	Citalopram	s/s genotype was significantly more frequent in no-remission group (p=0.006)
Rausch et al., 2002	5-HTT	Fluoxetine	l/l genotype subjects were more likely to respond (p=0.02)
Yu et al., 2002	SERTPR	Fluoxetine	l/l genotype shows a better response (p=0.013)
Ito et al., 2002	SERTPR	Fluvoxamine	No association
Serretti et al., 2001d	Tryptophan hydroxylase (TPH)	Fluvoxamine	A/A genotype was associated with slower response (no pindolol p=0.001)
Serretti et al., 2001c	TPH	Paroxetine	A/A and A/C genotypes were associated with slower response (no pindolol p=0.011)
Muller et al., 2000	Monoamine oxidase A (MAOA)	Moclobemide	No association
Yoshida et al., 2002b	MAOA, TPH	Fluvoxamine	No association in a Japanese sample
Zill et al., 2000	G-protein beta3	SSRI, TCA, ECT, combinations	TT homozygosity associated with response (p=0.01)
Serretti et al., 1999a	Dopamine receptor (DRD4)	S:eep deprivation	No association
Benedetti et al., 1999	5-HTT	S:eep deprivation	l/l patients showed better mood amelioration (p=0.05)
Schumann et al., 2001	Dopamine receptor (DRD3)	S:eep deprivation	No association
Mundo et al., 2001	5-HTT	SSRI, TCA	Patients with manic or hypomanic episodes induced by anti-depressant treatment had an excess of s alleles (p < 0001)

Reference	Gene/polymorphism	Drug	Result
Minov et al., 2001	Serotonin receptor ($5\text{-}HT_{2A}$)	SSRI, TCA, ECT, combinations	C containing variants associated with response ($p=0.023$)
Sato et al., 2002	$5\text{-}HT_{2A}$	Fluvoxamine	No association
Serretti et al., 1998b	DRD3	Lithium	No association
Serretti et al., 1999b	DRD2, DRD4, GABA A-alpha-1	Lithium	No association
Del Zompo et al., 1999	5-HTT	Lithium	l allele associated with nonresponders ($p=0.04$)
Serretti et al., 2001b	5-HTT	Lithium	s/s genotype associated with worse response ($p=0.005$)
Serretti et al., 1999c	TPH	Lithium	TPH*A/A variant showed a trend toward a worse response ($p=0.046$)
Serretti et al., 2000b	Serotonin receptor 2A, 2C, 1A	Lithium	No association
Steen et al., 1998	INPP1	Lithium	Difference between responders and nonresponders ($p=$n.s.)
Lovlie et al., 2001	PLC-gamma1	Lithium	No association
Zill et al., 2003	Beta 1 adrenergic receptor (ADRB1) G1165C polymorphism	TCA SSRI, NARI, NSRI	Tendency for association between CC homozygosity and better and faster antidepressant response
Yu et al., 2003b	NOS C276T polymorphism	Fluoxetine	No association
Yu et al., 2003a	Interleukin-1-beta (C-51IT) polymorphism	Fluoxetine	Homozygous for the −51IT lele had a trend of more favourable fluoxetine response

dorsolateral prefrontal cortex, such as working memory and so-called executive functions, and cortical physiological abnormalities during performance of such tasks, have been consistently reported in studies of patients with schizophrenia (Carter et al., 1998; Manoach et al., 1999; Weinberger et al., 1986). They may be reliably measured and recent evidence indicates that healthy siblings show cognitive and physiological abnormalities similar to affected subjects, suggesting that these traits may be heritable and could represent informative intermediate phenotypes for genetic studies of schizophrenia (Park et al., 1995). The relationship between a functional polymorphism in the COMT gene and prefrontal mediated cognition on the one hand and prefrontal cortical physiology on the other hand, was examined. Consistent with the enhancing effect of dopamine on prefrontal neuronal function demonstrated in experimental animals, the load of the low activity allele predicted enhanced cognitive performance (Egan et al., 2001).

Key point: association studies between genetic polymorphisms in candidate genes and neuropsychological task performances could evaluate the genetic contribution to the impairment of some functions, such as cognition, evidenced in mood disorders.

Chronobiology

Living organisms exist in an environment that varies regularly over a period of 24 hours. The endogenous source of the circadian control mechanism is what we refer to as its 'clock'. Given the importance of circadian rhythms in mood disorders (antidepressant efficacy of rhythm manipulation, abnormal rhythms observed in depression and mania) this field has recently interested researchers. About a decade ago, the first mammalian single-gene circadian mutant spontaneously appeared in a laboratory (tau mutant hamster). It exhibited a cluster of clock phenotypic abnormalities. Subsequently a mouse was found which showed an aberrant circadian period; this was the first carrier of a mutation in the clock gene. The clock gene was cloned and functionally confirmed to be responsible for the circadian phenotype by the transgenic insertion of copies of normal CLOCK into mutant mouse embryos, which was shown to rescue circadian rhythmic behaviour. Recent observations of clock genes and their role in the regulation of mammalian circadian rhythmicity raised interest in the possible role of genetic mechanisms in influencing the abnormalities of circadian rhythms that characterize major depressive episodes (Bunney and Bunney, 2000). Patients affected by a major depressive episode often report to the clinician an important variation in the intensity of perceived symptomatology during the day, with typical mood worsening in the morning. A single nucleotide polymorphism (T to C nucleotide substitution in position 3111) was identified, and a study on diurnal preferences of healthy human subjects showed that subjects carrying at least one copy of the C allele had a substantial 10- to 44-minute delay in preferred timing for activity or sleep (Katzenberg et al., 1998). Diurnal variations of mood are of great clinical relevance, because they have been shown to be a predictor of a good general clinical responsiveness both to antidepressant drugs (Fahndrich, 1987) and to antidepressant sleep deprivation therapy (Reinink et al., 1993). It has been recently reported that clock variants may influence recurrences of mood disorders (Benedetti et al., 2003), but further studies have yet to be performed.

Key point: the study of genes involved in circadian rhythm and their association with diurnal variations of mood, and dysfunctions in the sleep/wakefulness cycle, is a promising field for the better understanding of the neurobiology of mood disorders.

FINAL REMARKS

Clinical Implications of Psychiatric Genetics

Despite the large set of data produced, the practical implications of psychiatric genetic data for clinical work are not yet available. This reflects the natural progression of any scientific field: a long period of basic research and development usually precedes clinical applications by many years. In the future, as genes are discovered and their mechanisms of action are better understood, psychiatric genetics could have an important impact on clinical practice. In fact the delineation of subforms having different genetic and environmental contributions will allow clinicians to target treatments to specific causes. Present nosology could be largely reviewed and a new classification based on the genetic profile could be defined. Ultimately, the technology of gene therapy will allow physicians to prevent psychiatric disorders at the very earliest stages of life. Today, diagnostic tests are available for many genetic disorders. The development of such diagnostic instruments for psychiatric disorders and targeted therapies is a distant hope, but could be possible in the future.

New Approaches in Molecular Studies

Molecular genetic techniques are changing very rapidly. Until recently, a few hundred evenly spaced markers on the whole genome were used for a genome scan. But it has been shown that disequilibrium may be not detectable for distances larger than 60 kb, or even less in hot regions (Ardlie et al., 2002). This has led to the use of the single nucleotide polymorphism (SNP), the most abundant type of polymorphism in the genome. SNPs occur about once every 1000 base pairs; there are thus more than 3 million of them in the genome. A dense genome-wide map of SNPs has already been published (Marshall et al., 1999) and it is continuously being extended. Although these polymorphisms are mostly biallelic markers, thus providing relatively little information and, the majority of them, unlikely to influence either the structure or the function of coded proteins, they are useful because of their large number. The efficiency of this method is based on the ability to simultaneously perform large numbers of SNP genotypes using 'gene chips' (Shoemaker et al., 2001). These are small slides where thousands of genes may be analysed at one time. Despite their potential usefulness, the use is still limited by the high costs (about 1000 USD each) and the lack of adequate statistical analysis for the large amount of data they provide. In fact a simultaneous analysis of thousands of genes, many of which are nonfunctional or are not related to the trait under analysis, leads to an unacceptable risk of false positive findings.

A final step could be gene therapy: the gene product could be cloned and introduced, as has been done with blood clotting factor VIII (for haemophilia A) and growth hormone (for growth hormone deficiency). Alternatively, the gene itself could be directly a therapeutic target. Gene augmentation therapy could be the solution of problems concerning the loss of function of a specific gene; in this case, extra copies of the normal gene could be introduced. Target inhibition of gene expression could instead be employed if the inappropriate expression of a gene gives rise to a novel nonfunctional gene product. This may for example be accomplished using antisense therapeutics where gene-specific antisense sequences block transcription or translation of the susceptibility gene.

Key point: the most modern genetic techniques (for example gene chips) and the codification of the whole human genome, together with continuous progress in molecular genetic and biomedical knowledge, could make possible in the distant future a gene therapy also for psychiatric disorders. This technology would allow physicians to prevent psychiatric disorders at very earliest stages of life.

Conclusions

The inconsistent results of the different types of genetic studies support the hypothesis that mood disorders are both genetically and phenotypically heterogeneous. Genetic heterogeneity implies that more than one single genotype can cause mood disorders, while phenotypic heterogeneity suggests that a single pathogenic genotype can be expressed by several phenotypes. Future studies may have as their main target the provision of insight into these mechanisms.

A possible comprehensive explanation could be that gene abnormalities only confer susceptibilities to single phenotypic traits. For example, genetic liability may be also expressed as psychopathological traits shared by several psychiatric disorders. This is the case for DRD4*7, which, independently by categorical psychiatric diagnosis, has been reported to be associated with ADHD (Faraone et al., 1999), the novelty seeking personality trait (Ebstein and Belmaker, 1997), and delusions (Serretti et al., 2000a). This hypothesis is also valid for the genetics of treatment response. The polymorphism within the promoter of the serotonin transporter gene (5-HTTLPR*s) is hypothesized to confer susceptibility to anxiety features (Lesch et al., 1996) and a worse antidepressant response in subjects affected by mood disorder (Smeraldi et al., 1998).

In conclusion, genetic factors most probably influence mood disorders, the liability is most probably limited to traits such as psychopathology, time course or drug response. At the present time, knowledge does not allow us to formulate definitive hypotheses. The clinical utility of such researches in improving diagnosis and treatment could be more substantial once definite findings have been obtained.

ACKNOWLEDGEMENT

The author thanks Paola Artioli MD and Roberta Lilli for their help in writing the manuscript.

REFERENCES

Abeliovich A, Paylor R, Chen C, Kim JJ, Wehner JM, Tonegawa S (1993) PKC gamma mutant mice exhibit mild deficits in spatial and contextual learning. *Cell* **75**: 1263–1271.

Ackerknecht EH (1959) *A short history of psychiatry.* New York: Harper & Row.

Aiba A, Chen C, Herrup K, Rosenmund C, Stevens CF, Tonegawa S (1994) Reduced hippocampal long-term potentiation and context-specific deficit in associative learning in mGluR1 mutant mice. *Cell* **79**: 365–375.

Aita VM, Liu J, Knowles JA, Terwilliger JD, Baltazar R, Grunn A, Loth JE, Kanyas K, Lerer B, Endicott J, Wang Z, Penchaszadeh G, Gilliam TC, Baron M (1999) A comprehensive linkage analysis of chromosome 21q22 supports prior evidence for a putative bipolar affective disorder locus. *Am J Hum Genet* **64**: 210–217.

Alda M, Grof P, Grof E, Zvolsky P, Walsh M (1994) Mode of inheritance in families of patients with lithium-responsive affective disorders. *Acta Psychiatr Scand* **90**: 304–310.

Allen MG (1976) Twin studies of affective illness. *Arch Gen Psychiatry* **33**: 1476–1478.

Allen MG, Cohen S, Pollin W, Greenspan SI (1974) Affective illness in veteran twins: a diagnostic review. *Am J Psychiatry* **131**: 1234–1239.

Angst J (1981) Course of affective disorders. In Van Praag HM, Lader MH, Rafaelsen OJ, Sachar EJ (eds) *Handbook of Biological Psychiatry.* New York: Marcel Dekker, pp. 225–242.

Angst J (1995) The epidemiology of depressive disorders. *Eur Neuropsychopharmacol* **5** (Suppl): 95–98.

Angst J, Merikangas K (1997) The depressive spectrum: diagnostic classification and course. *J Affect Disord* **45**: 31–39; discussion 39–40.

Ardlie KG, Kruglyak L, Seielstad M (2002) Patterns of linkage disequilibrium in the human genome. *Nat Rev Genet* **2**: 299–309.

Arias B, Catalan R, Gasto C, Imaz ML, Gutierrez B, Pintor L, Fananas L (2001) Genetic variability in the promoter region of the serotonin transporter gene is associated with clinical remission of major depression after long term treatment with citalopram World Federation of Societies of Biological Psychiatry. Vol. 2 (1). *The World Journal of Biological Psychiatry,* Berlin, Germany, pp. 9S.

Baron M (1977) Linkage between an X-chromosome marker (deutan color blindness) and bipolar affective illness. Occurrence in the family of a lithium carbonate-responsive schizo-affective proband. *Arch Gen Psychiatry* **34**: 721–725.

Baron M, Freimer NF, Risch N, Lerer B, Alexander JR, Straub RE, Asokan S, Das K, Peterson A, Amos J, Endicott J, Ott J, Gilliam TC (1993) Diminished support for linkage between manic depressive illness and X-chromosome markers in three Israeli pedigrees. *Nature Genetics* **3**.

Baron M, Risch N, Hamburger R, Mandel B, Kushner S, Newman M, Drumer D, Belmaker RH (1987) Genetic linkage between X-chromosome markers and bipolar affective illness. *Nature* **326**: 289–292.

Bellivier F, Leboyer M, Courtet P, Buresi C, Beaufils B, Samolyk D, Allilaire JF, Feingold J, Mallet J, Malafosse A (1998) Association between the tryptophan hydroxylase gene and manic-depressive illness. *Arch Gen Psychiatry* **55**: 33–37.

Benedetti F, Serretti A, Colombo C, Barbini B, Lorenzi C, Campori E, Smeraldi E (2003) Influence of CLOCK gene polymorphism on circadian mood fluctuation and illness recurrence in bipolar depression. *Am J Med Genet* **123**B: 23–26.

Benedetti F, Serretti A, Colombo C, Campori E, Barbini B, Di Bella D, Smeraldi E (1999) Influence of a functional polymorphism within the promoter of the serotonin transporter gene on the effects of total sleep deprivation in bipolar depression. *Am J Psychiatry* **156**: 1450–1452.

Benjamin J, Li L, Patterson C, Greenberg B, Murphy D, Hamer D (1996) Population and familial association between the D4 dopamine receptor and measures of Novelty Seeking. *Nature Genetics* **12**: 81–84.

Berrettini WH, Ferraro TN, Goldin LR, Detera-Wadleigh SD, Choi H, Muniec D, Guroff JJ, Kazuba DM, Nurnberger JI Jr, Hsieh WT, Hoehe MR, Gershon ES (1997) A linkage study of bipolar illness. *Arch Gen Psychiatry* **54**: 27–35.

Berrettini WH, Ferraro TN, Goldin LR, Weeks DE, Detera-Wadleigh S, Nurnberger JI Jr, Gershon ES (1994) Chromosome 18 DNA markers and manic-depressive illness: evidence for a susceptibility gene. *Proc Natl Acad Sci USA* **91**: 5918–5921.

Berrettini WH, Goldin LR, Gelernter J, Gejman PV, Gershon ES, Detera-Wadleigh S (1990) X-chromosome markers and manic-depressive illness. Rejection of linkage to Xq28 in nine bipolar pedigrees. *Arch Gen Psychiatry* **47**: 366–373.

Bertelsen A (1985) Controversies and consistencies in psychiatric genetics. *Acta Psychiatr Scand Suppl* **319**: 61–75.

Bertelsen A, Harvald B, Hauge M (1977) A Danish twin study of manic-depressive disorders. *Br J Psychiatry* **130**: 330–351.

Blackwood DH, He L, Morris SW, McLean A, Whitton C, Thomson M, Walker MT, Woodburn K, Sharp CM, Wright AF, Shibasaki Y, St. Clair DM, Porteous DJ, Muir WJ (1996) A locus for bipolar affective disorder on chromosome 4p. *Nature Genetics* **12**: 427–430.

Bunney WE, Bunney BG (2000) Molecular clock genes in man and lower animals: possible implications for circadian abnormalities in depression. *Neuropsychopharmacology* **22**: 335–345.

Cadoret RJ, O'Gorman TW, Heywood E, Troughton E (1985) Genetic and environmental factors in major depression. *J Affect Disord* **9**: 155–164.

Campbell J, Crowe RR, Goeken N, Pfohl B, Pauls D, Palmer D (1984) Affective disorder not linked to HLA in a large bipolar kindred. *J Affect Disord* **7**: 45–51.

Cannon TD, Huttunen MO, Lonnqvist J, Tuulio-Henriksson A, Pirkola T, Glahn D, Finkelstein J, Hietanen M, Kaprio J, Koskenvuo M (2000) The inheritance of neuropsychological dysfunction in twins discordant for schizophrenia. *Am J Hum Genet* **67**: 369–382.

Cardno AG, Holmans PA, Harvey I, Williams MB, Owen MJ, McGuffin P (1997) Factor-derived subsyndromes of schizophrenia and familial morbid risks. *Schizophrenia Research* **23**: 231–238.

Cardno AG, Jones LA, Murphy KC, Sanders RD, Asherson P, Owen MJ, McGuffin P (1998) Sibling pairs with schizophrenia or schizoaffective disorder – associations of subtypes, symptoms and demographic variables. *Psychol Med* **28**: 815–823.

Cardon LR, Bell JI (2001) Association study designs for complex diseases. *Nat Rev Genet* **2**: 91–99.

Caron MG (1996) Images in neuroscience. Molecular biology, II. A dopamine transporter mouse knockout. *Am J Psychiatry* **153**: 1515.

Carter CS, Perlstein W, Ganguli R, Brar J, Mintun M, Cohen JD (1998) Functional hypofrontality and working memory dysfunction in schizophrenia. *Am J Psychiatry* **155**: 1285–1287.

Cases O, Seif I, Grimsby J, Gaspar P, Chen K, Pournin S, Muller U, Aguet M, Babinet C, Shih JC, De Maeyer E (1995) Aggressive behavior and altered amounts of brain serotonin and norepinephrine in mice lacking MAOA. *Science* **268**: 1763–1766.

Catalano M, Nobile M, Novelli E, Nothen M, Smeraldi E (1993) Distribution of novel mutation in the first exon of the human dopamine D4 receptor gene in psychotic patients. *Biological Psychiatry* **34**: 459–464.

CavalliSforza L (1997) *Genes, Peoples, and Languages.* Berkeley, CA: University of California Press.

Cleves MA, Dawson DV, Elston RC, Schnell AH (1997) A new test for linkage applied to bipolar disorder and marker D18S41. *Genetic Epidemiology* **14**: 581–586.

Collier D, Stöber G, Li T, Heils A, Catalano M, Di Bella D, Arranz M, Murray R, Vallada H, Bengel D, Müller-Reible C, Roberts G, Smeraldi E, Kirov G, Sham P, Lesh P (1996) A novel functional polymorphism within the promoter of the serotonin transporter gene: possible role in susceptibility to affective disorders. *Mol Psychiatry* **1**: 453–460.

Coon H, Hoff M, Holik J, Hadley D, Fang N, Reimherr F, Wender P, Byerley W (1996) Analysis of chromosome 18 DNA markers in multiplex pedigrees with manic depression. *Biol Psychiatry* **39**: 689–696.

Coyle N, Jones I, Robertson E, Lendon C, Craddock N (2000) Variation at the serotonin transporter gene influences susceptibility to bipolar affective puerperal psychosis. *Lancet* **356**: 1490–1491.

Craddock N, Daniels J, McGuffin P, Owen M (1994a) Variation at the fragile X locus does not influence susceptibility to bipolar disorder. *Am J Med Genet* **54**: 141–143.

Craddock N, Khodel V, Van Eerdewegh P, Reich T (1995) Mathematical limits of multilocus models: the genetic transmission of bipolar disorder. *Am J Hum Genet* **57**: 690–702.

Craddock N, Owen M, Burge S, Kurian B, Thomas P, McGuffin P (1994b) Familial cosegregation of major affective disorder and Darier's disease (keratosis follicularis). *Br J Psychiatry* **164**: 355–358.

Crowe RR, Namboodiri KK, Ashby HB, Elston RC (1981) Segregation analysis and linkage analysis of a large kindred of unipolar depression. *Neuropsychobiology* **7**: 20–25.

Curtis D, Brynjolfsson J, Petursson H, Holmes DS, Sherrington R, Brett P, Rifkin L, Murphy P, Moloney E, Holmes S, et al. (1993) Segregation and linkage analysis in five manic depression pedigrees excludes the 5HT1a receptor gene (HTR1A). *Ann Hum Genet* **57**: 27–39.

Cusin C, Serretti A, Lattuada E, Lilli R, Lorenzi C, Mandelli L, Pisati E, Smeraldi E (2001) Influence of 5-HTTLPR and TPH variants on illness time course in mood disorders. *J Psychiatric Res* **35**: 217–223.

Cusin C, Serretti A, Lattuada E, Mandelli L, Smeraldi E (2000) Impact of clinical variables on illness time course in mood disorders. *Psychiatry Res* **97**: 217–227.

De bruyn A, Raeymaekers P, Mendelbaum K, Sandkuijl LA, Raes G, Delvenne V, Hirsch D, Staner L, Mendlewicz J, Van Broeckhoven C (1994) Linkage analysis of bipolar illness with X-chromosome DNA markers: a susceptibility gene in Xq27-q28 cannot be excluded. *Am J Med Genet* **54**: 411–419.

De bruyn A, Souery D, Mendelbaum K, Mendlewicz J, Van Broeckhoven C (1996) Linkage analysis of families with bipolar illness and chromosome 18 markers. *Biol Psychiatry* **39**: 679–688.

Del Zompo M, Ardau R, Palmas MA, Bocchetta A, Reina A, Piccardi MP (1999) Lithium response: association study with two candidate genes. *Mol Psychiatry* **4**(Suppl 1): s66–s67.

Del Zompo M, Bocchetta A, Goldin LR, Corsini GU (1984) Linkage between X-chromosome markers and manic-depressive illness. Two Sardinian pedigrees. *Acta Psychiatr Scand* **70**: 282–287.

Detera-Wadleigh SD, Badner JA, Goldin LR, Berrettini WH, Sanders AR, Rollins DY, Turner G, Moses T, Haerian H, Muniec D, Nurnberger JI Jr, Gershon ES (1996) Affected-sib-pair analyses reveal support of prior evidence for a susceptibility locus for bipolar disorder, on 21q. *Am J Hum Genet* **58**: 1279–1285.

Detera-Wadleigh SD, Badner JA, Yoshikawa T, Sanders AR, Goldin LR, Turner G, Rollins DY, Moses T, Guroff JJ, Kazuba D, Maxwell ME, Edenberg HJ, Foroud T, Lahiri D, Nurnberger JI Jr, Stine OC, McMahon F, Meyers DA, MacKinnon D, Simpson S, McInnis M, DePaulo JR, Rice J, Goate A, Gershon ES, et al. (1997) Initial genome scan of the NIMH genetics initiative bipolar pedigrees: chromosomes 4, 7, 9, 18, 19, 20, and 21q. *Am J Med Genet* **74**: 254–262.

Detera-Wadleigh SD, Berrettini WH, Goldin LR, Martinez M, Hsieh WT, Hoehe MR, Encio IJ, Coffman D, Rollins DY, Muniec D, et al. (1992) A systematic search for a bipolar predisposing locus on chromosome 5. *Neuropsychopharmacology* **6**: 219–229.

Detera-Wadleigh SD, Hsieh WT, Berrettini WH, Goldin LR, Rollins DY, Muniec D, Grewal R, Guroff JJ, Turner G, Coffman D, et al. (1994) Genetic linkage mapping for a susceptibility locus to bipolar illness: chromosomes 2,3,4,7,9,10p,11p,22 and Xpter. *Am J Med Genet* **54**: 206–218.

Dettling M, Cascorbi I, Roots I, Mueller-Oerlinghausen B (2001) Genetic determinants of clozapine-induced agranulocytosis: recent results of HLA subtyping in a non-jewish caucasian sample. *Arch Gen Psychiatry* **58**: 93–94.

Ebstein RP, Belmaker RH (1997) Saga of an adventure gene: novelty seeking, substance abuse and the dopamine D4 receptor (D4DR) exon III repeat polymorphism. *Mol Psychiatry* **2**: 381–384.

Ebstein RP, Novick O, Umansky R, Priel B, Osher Y, Blaine D, Bennett ER, Nemanov L, Kats M, Belmaker RH (1996) Dopamine D4 receptor (D4DR) exon III polymorphism associated with the human personality trait of Novelty Seeking. *Nature Genetics* **12**: 78–80.

Egan MF, Goldberg TE, Kolachana BS, Callicott JH, Mazzanti CM, Straub RE, Goldman D, Weinberger DR (2001) Effect of COMT Val108/158 Met genotype on frontal lobe function and risk for schizophrenia. *Proc Natl Acad Sci USA* **98**: 6917–6922.

Egan MF, Weinberger DR (1997) Neurobiology of schizophrenia. *Curr Opin Neurobiol* **7**: 701–707.

Egeland JA, Gerhard DS, Pauls DL, Sussex JN, Kidd KK, Allen CR, Hostetter AM (1987) Bipolar affective disorders linked to markers on chromosome 11. *Nature* **325**: 783–787.

Engstrom C, Thornlund AS, Johansson EL, Langstrom M, Chotai J, Adolfsson R, Nylander PO (1995) Anticipation in unipolar affective disorder. *J Affect Disord* **35**: 31–40.

Ewald H, Eiberg H, Mors O, Flint T, Kruse TA (1996) Linkage study between manic-depressive illness and chromosome 21. *Am J Med Genet* **67**: 218–224.

Ewald H, Mors O, Flint T, Koed K, Eiberg H, Kruse TA (1995) A possible locus for manic depressive illness on chromosome 16p13. *Psychiatr Genet* **5**: 71–81.

Fahndrich E (1987) Biological predictors of success of antidepressant drug therapy. *Psychiatr Dev* **5**: 151–171.

Falk CT, Rubinstein P (1987) Haplotype relative risks: an easy reliable way to construct a proper control sample for risk calculations. *Ann Hum Genet* **51**: 227–233.

Faraone SV, Biederman J, Weiffenbach B, Keith T, Chu MP, Weaver A, Spencer TJ, Wilens TE, Frazier J, Cleves M, Sakai J (1999) Dopamine D-4 gene 7-repeat allele and attention deficit hyperactivity disorder. *Am J Psychiatry* **156**: 768–770.

Fieve RR, Mendlewicz J, Fleiss JL (1973) Manic-depressive illness: linkage with the Xg blood group. *Am J Psychiatry* **130**: 1355–1359.

Franchini L, Serretti A, Gasperini M, Smeraldi E (1998) Familial concordance of fluvoxamine response as a tool for differentiating mood disorder pedigrees. *J Psychiatr Res* **32**: 255–259.

Freedman R, Coon H, Myles-Worsley M, Orr-Urtreger A, Olincy A, Davis A, Polymeropoulos M, Holik J, Hopkins J, Hoff M, Rosenthal J, Waldo MC, Reimherr F, Wender P, Yaw J, Young DA, Breese CR, Adams C, Patterson D, Adler LE, Kruglyak L, Leonard S, Byerley W (1997) Linkage of a neurophysiological deficit in schizophrenia to a chromosome 15 locus. *Proc Natl Acad Sci USA* **94**: 587–592.

Freimer NB, Reus VI, Escamilla MA, McInnes A, Spesny M, Leon P, Service SK, Smith LB, Silva S, Rojas E, Gallegos A, Meza L, Fournier E, Baharloo S, Blankenship K, Tyler DJ, Batki S, Vinogradov S, Weissenbach J, Barondes SH, Sandkuijl LA (1996) Genetic mapping using haplotype, association and linkage methods suggests a locus for severe bipolar disorder (BPI) at 18q22-q23. *Nature Genetics* **12**: 436–441.

Furlong RA, Rubinsztein JS, Ho L, Walsh C, Coleman TA, Muir WJ, Paykel ES, Blackwood DHR, Rubinsztein DC (1999) Analysis and metaanalysis of two polymorphisms within the tyrosine hydroxylase gene in bipolar and unipolar affective disorders. *Am J Med Genet* **88**: 88–94.

Gejman PV, Detera-Wadleigh S, Martinez MM, Berrettini WH, Goldin LR, Gelernter J, Hsieh WT, Gershon ES (1990) Manic depressive illness not linked to factor IX region in an independent series of pedigrees. *Genomics* **8**: 648–655.

Gershon ES (1980) Genetic studies of manic-depressive illness. *Pharmakopsychiatr Neuropsychopharmakol* **13**: 55–61.

Gershon ES, Badner JA, Detera-Wadleigh SD, Ferraro TN, Berrettini WH (1996) Maternal inheritance and chromosome 18 allele sharing in unilineal bipolar illness pedigrees. *Am J Med Genet* **67**: 202–207.

Ginns EI, Ott J, Egeland JA, Allen CR, Fann CSJ, Pauls DL, Weissenbach J, Carulli JP, Falls KM, Keith TP, Paul SM (1996) A genome-wide search for chromosomal loci linked to bipolar affective disorder in the Old Order Amish. *Nature Genetics* **12**: 431–435.

Goldberg TE, Saint-Cyr JA, Weinberger DR (1990) Assessment of procedural learning and problem solving in schizophrenic patients by Tower of Hanoi type tasks. *J Neuropsychiatry Clin Neurosci* **2**: 165–173.

Goldin LR, Gershon ES, Lake CR, Murphy DL, McGinniss M, Sparkes RS (1982) Segregation and linkage studies of plasma dopamine-beta-hydroxylase (DBH), erythrocyte catechol-O-methyltransferase (COMT), and platelet monoamine oxidase (MAO): possible linkage between the ABO locus and a gene controlling DBH activity. *Am J Hum Genet* **34**: 250–262.

Goodwin F, Jamison K (1990) *Manic-depressive Illness*. New York: Oxford University Press.

Grof P, Duffy A, Cavazzoni P, Grof E, Garnham J, MacDougall M, O'Donovan C, Alda M (2000) Is response to prophylactic lithium a familial trait? *Int J Neuropsychopharmacol* **3**: 339.

Gurling H, Smyth C, Kalsi G, Moloney E, Rifkin L, O'Neill J, Murphy P, Curtis D, Petursson H, Brynjolfsson J (1995) Linkage findings in bipolar disorder. *Nature Genetics* **10**: 8–9.

Gutierrez B, Fananas L, Arranz MJ, Valles V, Guillamat R, van Os J, Collier D (1996) Allelic association analysis of the 5-HT2C receptor gene in bipolar affective disorder. *Neurosci Lett* **212**: 65–67.

Hamilton M (1967) Development of a rating scale for primary depressive illness. *Br J Soc Clin Psychol* **6**: 278–296.

Hodge S, Wickramaratne P (1995) Statistical pitfalls in detecting age-of-onset anticipation: the role of correlation in studying anticipation and detecting ascertainment bias. *Psychiatr Genet* **5**: 43–47.

Ito K, Yoshida K, Sato K, Takahashi H, Kamata M, Higuchi H, Shimizu T, Itoh K, Inoue K, Tezuka T, Suzuki T, Ohkubo T, Sugawara K, Otani K (2002) A variable number of tandem repeats in the serotonin transporter gene does not affect the antidepressant response to fluvoxamine. *Psychiatry Res* **111**: 235–239.

Johnson GF, Hunt GE, Robertson S, Doran TJ (1981) A linkage study of manic-depressive disorder with HLA antigens, blood groups, serum proteins and red cell enzymes. *J Affect Disord* **3**: 43–58.

Johnson GF, Leeman MM (1977) Analysis of familial factors in bipolar affective illness. *Arch Gen Psychiatry* **34**: 1074–1083.

Kaiser R, Konneker M, Henneken M, Dettling M, Muller-Oerlinghausen B, Roots I, Brock-moller J (2000) Dopamine D4 receptor 48-bp repeat polymorphism: no association with response to antipsychotic treatment, but association with catatonic schizophrenia. *Mol Psychiatry* **5**: 18–24.

Katzenberg D, Young T, Finn L, Lin L, King DP, Takahashi JS, Mignot E (1998) A CLOCK polymorphism associated with human diurnal preference. *Sleep* **21**: 569–576.

Kawada Y, Hattori M, Dai XY, Nanko S (1995) Possible association between monoamine oxidase A gene and bipolar affective disorder. *Am J Hum Genet* **56**: 335–336.

Keller MB, Lavori PW, Lewis CE, Klerman GL (1983) Predictors of relapse in major depressive disorder. *JAMA* **250**: 3299–3304.

Kelsoe JR, Sadovnick AD, Kristbjarnarson H, Bergesch P, Mroczkowski-Parker Z, Drennan M, Rapaport MH, Flodman P, Spence MA, Remick RA (1996) Possible locus for bipolar disorder near the dopamine transporter on chromosome 5. *Am J Med Genet* **67**: 533–540.

Kendler KS, Neale MC, Kessler RC, Heath AC, Eaves LJ (1992a) Familial influences on the clinical characteristics of major depression: a twin study. *Acta Psychiatr Scand* **86**: 371–378.

Kendler KS, Neale MC, Kessler RC, Heath AC, Eaves LJ (1992b) Major depression and generalized anxiety disorder. Same genes, (partly) different environments? *Arch Gen Psychiatry* **49**: 716–722.

Kendler KS, Walters EE, Neale MC, Kessler RC, Heath AC, Eaves LJ (1995) The structure of the genetic and environmental risk factors for six major psychiatric disorders in women. Phobia, generalized anxiety disorder, panic disorder, bulimia, major depression, and alcoholism. *Arch Gen Psychiatry* **52**: 374–383.

Kessing LV, Andersen PK, Mortensen PB (1998) Predictors of recurrence in affective disorder. A case register study. *J Affect Disord* **49**: 101–108.

Khoury MJ, Yang Q (1998) The future of genetic studies of complex human diseases: an epidemiologic perspective. *Epidemiology* **9**: 350–354.

Kidd KK, Egeland JA, Molthan L, Pauls DL, Kruger SD, Messner KH (1984) Amish study, IV: Genetic linkage study of pedigrees of bipolar probands. *Am J Psychiatry* **141**: 1042–1048.

Kim DK, Lim SW, Lee S, Sohn SE, Kim S, Hahn CG, Carroll BJ (2000) Serotonin transporter gene polymorphism and antidepressant response. *Neuroreport* **11**: 215–219.

Knowles JA, Rao PA, Cox-Matise T, Loth JE, de Jesus GM, Levine L, Das K, Penchaszadeh GK, Alexander JR, Lerer B, Endicott J, Ott J, Gilliam TC, Baron M (1998) No evidence for significant linkage between bipolar affective disorder and chromosome 18 pericentromeric markers in a large series of multiplex extended pedigrees. *Am J Hum Genet* **62**: 916–924.

Krafft-Ebing, Rv (1939) *Psychopathia Sexualis*. New York: Pioneer Publications.

Kremen WS, Seidman LJ, Pepple JR, Lyons MJ, Tsuang MT, Faraone SV (1994) Neuropsychological risk indicators for schizophrenia: a review of family studies. *Schizophr Bull* **20**: 103–119.

Kringlen E (1967) *Heredity and Environment in the Functional Psychoses*. Oslo: Universitetsforlaget.

Lachman HM, Kelsoe JR, Remick RA, Sadovnick AD, Rapaport MH, Lin M, Pazur BA, Roe AMA, Saito T, Papolos DF (1997) Linkage studies suggest a possible locus for bipolar disorder near the velo-cardio-facial syndrome region on chromosome 22. *Am J Med Genet* **74**: 121–128.

Lachman HM, Morrow B, Shprintzen R, Veit S, Parsia SS, Faedda G, Goldberg R, Kucherlapati R, Papolos DF (1996) Association of codon 108/158 catechol-O-methyltransferase gene polymorphism with the psychiatric manifestations of velo-cardio-facial syndrome. *Am J Med Genet* **67**: 468–472.

Lander E, Kruglyak L (1995) Genetic dissection of complex traits: guidelines for interpreting and reporting linkage results. *Nature Genetics* **11**: 241–247.

Leboyer M, Malafosse A, Boularand S, Campion D, Gheysen F, Samolyk D, Henriksson B, Denise E, Des Lauriers A, Lepine JP, Zarifian E, Clerget-Darpoux F, Mallet J (1990) Tyrosine hydroxylase polymorphism associated with manic-depressive illness. *Lancet* **335**: 1219.

Leckman JF, Gershon ES, McGinniss MH, Targum SD, Dibble ED (1979) New data do not suggest linkage between the Xg blood group and bipolar illness. *Arch Gen Psychiatry* **36**: 1435–1441.

Leonhard K (1959) *Aufteilung der Endopen psychosen*. Berlin: Akademic Verlag.

Lerer B, Macciardi F, Segman RH, Adolfsson R, Blackwood D, Blairy S, Del Favero J, Dikeos DG, Kaneva R, Lilli R, Massat I, Milanova V, Muir W, Noethen M, Oruc L, Petrova T, Papadimitriou GN, Rietschel M, Serretti A, Souery D, Van Gestel S, Van Broeckhoven C, Mendlewicz J (2001) Variability of 5-HT2C receptor cys23ser polymorphism among European populations and vulnerability to affective disorder. *Mol Psychiatry* **6**: 579–585.

Lesch K, Bengel D, Heils A, Sabol S, Greenberg B, Petri S, Benjamin J, Muller C, Hamer D, Murphy D (1996) Association of anxiety-related traits with a polymorphism in the serotonin transporter gene regulatory region. *Science* **274**: 1527–1530.

Lim L, Nothen M, Korner J, Rietschel M, Castle D, Hunt N, Propping P, Murray R, Gill M (1994a) No evidence of association between dopamine D4 receptor variants and bipolar affective disorder. *Am J Med Genet* **54**: 259–263.

Lim LC, Powell J, Sham P, Castle D, Hunt N, Murray R, Gill M (1995) Evidence for a genetic association between alleles of monoamine oxidase A gene and bipolar affective disorder. *Am J Med Genet* **60**: 325–331.

Lim LC, Powell JF, Murray R, Gill M (1994b) Monoamine oxidase A gene and bipolar affective disorder. *Am J Hum Genet* **54**: 1122–1124.

Lin CN, Tsai SJ, Hong CJ (2001) Association Analysis of a Functional G Protein beta3 Subunit Gene Polymorphism (C825T) in Mood Disorders. *Neuropsychobiology* **44**: 118–121.

Lindblad K, Nylander PO, De bruyn A, Sourey D, Zander C, Engstrom C, Holmgren G, Hudson T, Chotai J, Mendlewicz J, et al. (1995) Detection of expanded CAG repeats in bipolar affective disorder using the repeat expansion detection (RED) method. *Neurobiol Dis* **2**: 55–62.

Lovlie R, Berle JO, Stordal E, Steen VM (2001) The phospholipase C-gammal gene (PLCG1) and lithium-responsive bipolar disorder: re-examination of an intronic dinucleotide repeat polymorphism. *Psychiatr Genet* **11**: 41–43.

Lucotte G, Landoulsi A, Berriche S, David F, Babron MC (1992) Manic depressive illness is linked to factor IX in a French pedigree. *Ann Genet* **35**: 93–95.

Maes M, Meltzer HY (1995) The serotonin hypothesis of major depression. In Bloom FE, Kupfer DJ (eds) *Psychopharmacology: The Fourth Generation of Progress*. New York: Raven Press, pp. 933–944.

Maier W, Hallmayer J, Zill P, Bondy B, Lichtermann D, Ackenheil M, Minges J, Wildenauer D (1995) Linkage analysis between pericentrometric markers on chromosome 18 and bipolar disorder: a replication test. *Psychiatry Res* **59**: 7–15.

Manji HK, Potter WZ, Lenox RH (1995) Signal transduction pathways. *Arch Gen Psychiatry* **52**: 531–543.

Manki H, Kanba S, Muramatsu T, Higuchi S, Suzuki E, Matsushita S, Ono Y, Chiba H, Shintani F, Nakamura M, Yagi G, Asai M (1996) Dopamine D2, D3 and D4 receptor and transporter gene polymorphisms and mood disorders. *J Affect Disord* **40**: 7–13.

Manoach DS, Press DZ, Thangaraj V, Searl MM, Goff DC, Halpern E, Saper CB, Warach S (1999) Schizophrenic subjects activate dorsolateral prefrontal cortex during a working memory task, as measured by fMRI. *Biol Psychiatry* **45**: 1128–1137.

Marshall SE, Bird TG, Hart K, Welsh KI (1999) Unified approach to the analysis of genetic variation in serotonergic pathways. *Am J Med Genet* **88**: 621–627.

McGuffin P, Katz R (1986) Nature, nurture and affective disorder. In Royal College of Psychiatrists (ed) *The Biology of Affective Disorders*. London: Gaskell Press.

McGuffin P, Katz R (1989) The genetics of depression and manic-depressive disorder. *Br J Psychiatry* **155**: 294–304.

McGuffin P, Katz R, Watkins S, Rutherford J (1996) A hospital-based twin register of the heritability of DSM-IV unipolar depression. *Arch Gen Psychiatry* **53**: 129–136.

McInnis MG, McMahon FJ, Chase GA, Simpson SG, Ross CA, DePaulo JR Jr (1993) Anticipation in bipolar affective disorder. *Am J Hum Genet* **53**: 385–390.

McKnew DH, Cytryn L, Buchsbaum MS, Hamovit J, Lamour M, Rapoport JL, Gershon ES (1981) Lithium in children of lithium-responding parents. *Psychiatry Res* **4**: 171–180.

Meloni R, Leboyer M, Bellivier F, Barbe B, Samolyk D, Allilaire J, Mallet J (1995) Association of manic-depressive illness with tyrosine hydroxylase microsatellite marker. *Lancet* **345**: 932.

Mendelbaum K, Sevy S, Souery D, Papadimitriou GN, De Bruyn A, Raeymaekers P, Van Broeckhoven C, Mendlewicz J (1995) Manic-depressive illness and linkage reanalysis in the Xq27-Xq28 region of chromosome X. *Neuropsychobiology* **31**: 58–63.

Mendlewicz J, Fieve RR, Rainer J, Fleiss JL (1972) Manic-depressive illness: a comparative study of patients with and without family history. *Br J Psychiatry* **120**: 523–530.

Mendlewicz J, Fleiss JL (1974) Linkage studies with X-chromosome markers in bipolar (manic-depressive) and unipolar (depressive) illnesses. *Biol Psychiatry* **9**: 261–294.

Mendlewicz J, Fleiss JL, Fieve RR (1975) Linkage studies in affective disorders: the Xg blood group and manic-depressive illness. *Proc Annu Meet Am Psychopathol Assoc* 220–232.

Mendlewicz J, Lindbald K, Souery D, Mahieu B, Nylander PO, De Bruyn A, Zander C, Engstrom C, Adolfsson R, Van Broeckhoven C, Schalling M, Lipp O (1997) Expanded trinucleotide CAG repeats in families with bipolar affective disorder. *Biol Psychiatry* **42**: 1115–1122.

Mendlewicz J, Linkowski P, Wilmotte J (1980) Linkage between glucose-6-phosphate dehydrogenase deficiency and manic-depressive psychosis. *Br J Psychiatry* **137**: 337–342.

Mendlewicz J, Rainer JD (1977) Adoption study supporting genetic transmission in manic–depressive illness. *Nature* **268**: 327–329.

Mendlewicz J, Simon P, Sevy S, Charon F, Brocas H, Legros S, Vassart G (1987) Polymorphic DNA marker on X chromosome and manic depression. *Lancet* **1**: 1230–1232.

Merette C, Roy-Gagnon MH, Ghazzali N, Savard F, Boutin P, Roy MA, Maziade M (2000) Anticipation in schizophrenia and bipolar disorder controlling for an information bias. *Am J Med Genet* **96**: 61–68.

Merikangas KR, Wicki W, Angst J (1994) Heterogeneity of depression. Classification of depressive subtypes by longitudinal course. *Br J Psychiatry* **164**: 342–348.

Meyer-Lindenberg J (1991) The Holocaust and German psychiatry. *Br J Psychiatry* **159**: 7–12.

Minov C, Baghai TC, Schule C, Zwanzger P, Schwarz MJ, Zill P, Rupprecht R, Bondy B (2001) Serotonin-2A-receptor and -transporter polymorphisms: lack of association in patients with major depression. *Neurosci Lett* **303**: 119–122.

Moisan MP, Courvoisier H, Bihoreau MT, Gauguier D, Hendley ED, Lathrop M, James MR, Mormede P (1996) A major quantitative trait locus influences hyperactivity in the WKHA rat. *Nature Genetics* **14**: 471–473.

Moldin SO, Reich T (1993) The genetic analysis of depression: Future directions. *Clin Neurosci* **1**: 139–145.

Muller DJ, Schulze TG, Macciardi F, Ohlraun S, Gross MM, Bauer I, Scherk H, Kischkel E, Neidt H, Syagailo YV, Grassle M, Nothen MM, Maier W, Lesch KP, Rietschel M (2000) Moclobemide response in depressed patients: association study with a functional polymorphism in the monoamine oxidase-A promoter. Eighth World Congress on Psychiatric Genetics, Versailles, France, Vol. 96 (4): *Neuropsychiatric Genetics.* New York: Wiley-Liss, pp. 537.

Mundo E, Walker M, Cate T, Macciardi F, Kennedy JL (2001) The role of serotonin transporter protein gene in antidepressant-induced mania in bipolar disorder. *Arch Gen Psychiatry* **58**: 539–544.

Neuman RJ, Rice JP (1992) Two-locus models of disease. *Genet Epidemiol* **9**: 347–365.

Nothen MM, Cichon S, Erdmann J, Korner J, Rietschel M, Rappold GA, Fritze J, Propping P (1993) Pseudoautosomal marker DXYS20 and manic depression. *Am J Hum Genet* **52**: 841–842.

Nylander PO, Engstrom C, Chotai J, Wahlstrom J, Adolfsson R (1994) Anticipation in Swedish families with bipolar affective disorder. *J Med Genet* **31**: 686–689.

O'Donovan MC, Guy C, Craddock N, Bowen T, McKoen P, Machedo A, Maier W, Wildenauer W, Aschauer HN, Sorbi S, Feldman E, Mynett-Johnson L, Claffey E, Nacmias B, Valente J, Dourado A, Grassi E, Lenzinger E, Heiden AM, Moorhead S, Harrison D, Williams J, McGuffin P, Owen MJ (1996) Confirmation of association between expanded CAG/CTG repeats and both schizophrenia and bipolar disorder. *Psychol Med* **26**: 1145–1153.

O'Donovan MC, Guy C, Craddock N, Murphy KC, Cardno AG, Jones LA, Owen MJ, McGuffin P (1995) Expanded CAG repeats in schizophrenia and bipolar disorder. *Nature Genetics* **10**: 380–381.

Ohara K, Nagai M, Suzuki Y (1998) Low activity allele of catechol-o-methyltransferase gene and Japanese unipolar depression. *Neuroreport* **9**: 1305–1308.

O'Reilly RL, Bogue L, Singh SM (1994) Pharmacogenetic response to antidepressants in a multicase family with affective disorder. *Biol Psychiatry* **36**: 467–471.

Orsini A (1987) Antidepressant responses and segregation analyses in affective families. In Racagni G, Smeraldi E (eds) *Anxious Depression: Assessment and Treatment.* New York: Raven Press.

Oruc L, Lindblad K, Verheyen GR, Ahlberg S, Jakovljevic M, Ivezic S, Raeymaekers P, Van Broeckhoven C, Schalling M (1997a) CAG repeat expansions in bipolar and unipolar disorders. *Am J Hum Genet* **60**: 730–732.

Oruc L, Verheyen GR, Furac I, Jakovljevic M, Ivezic S, Raeymaekers P, Van Broeckhoven C (1997b) Association analysis of the 5-HT2C receptor and 5-HT transporter genes in bipolar disorder. *Am J Med Genet* **74**: 504–506.

Ott J (1991) *Analysis of Human Genetic Linkage.* Baltimore, MD: Johns Hopkins University Press.

Pare CM, Mack JW (1971) Differentiation of two genetically specific types of depression by the response to antidepressant drugs. *J Med Genet* **8**: 306–309.

Park S, Holzman PS, Goldman-Rakic PS (1995) Spatial working memory deficits in the relatives of schizophrenic patients. *Arch Gen Psychiatry* **52**: 821–828.

Parsian A, Chakraverty S, Todd RD (1995) Possible association between the dopamine D3 receptor gene and bipolar affective disorder. *Am J Med Genet* **60**: 234–237.

Parsian A, Todd RD (1994) Bipolar disorder and the pseudoautosomal region: an association study. *Am J Med Genet* **54**: 5–7.

Pauls DL, Bailey JN, Carter AS, Allen CR, Egeland JA (1995a) Complex segregation analyses of Old Order Amish families ascertained through bipolar I individuals. *Am J Med Genet* **60**: 290–297.

Pauls DL, Gerhard DS, Lacy LG, Hostetter AM, Allen CR, Bland SD, LaBuda MC, Egeland JA (1991) Linkage of bipolar affective disorders to markers on chromosome 11p is excluded in a second lateral extension of Amish pedigree 110. *Genomics* **11**: 730–736.

Pauls DL, Morton LA, Egeland JA (1992) Risks of affective illness among first-degree relatives of bipolar I Old-Order Amish probands. *Arch Gen Psychiatry* **49**: 703–708.

Pauls DL, Ott J, Paul SM, Allen CR, Fann CS, Carulli JP, Falls KM, Bouthillier CA, Gravius TC, Keith TP, et al. (1995b) Linkage analyses of chromosome 18 markers do not identify a major susceptibility locus for bipolar affective disorder in the Old Order Amish. *Am J Hum Genet* **57**: 636–643.

Payami H, Dubay C, Valenzuela RC (1989) HLA may be involved in resistance and susceptibility to affective disorders. *Genet Epidemiol* **6**: 293–298.

Pekkarinen P, Terwilliger J, Bredbacka PE, Lonnqvist J, Peltonen L (1995) Evidence of a predisposing locus to bipolar disorder on Xq24–q27.1 in an extended Finnish pedigree. *Genome Res* **5**: 105–115.

Pickar D, Rubinow K (2001) Pharmacogenomics of psychiatric disorders. *Trends Pharmacol Sci* **22**: 75–83.

Pincus HA, Pettit AR (2001) The societal costs of chronic major depression. *J Clin Psychiatry* **62** (Suppl 6): 5–9.

Pollock BG, Ferrell RE, Mulsant BH, Mazumdar S, Miller M, Sweet RA, Davis S, Kirshner MA, Houck PR, Stack JA, Reynolds CF, Kupfer DJ (2000) Allelic variation in the serotonin transporter promoter affects onset of paroxetine treatment response in late-life depression. *Neuropsychopharmacology* **23**: 587–590.

Post RM, Weiss SR (1995) The neurobiology of treatment-resistant mood disorders. In Bloom FE, Kupfer DJ (eds) *Psychopharmacology: The Fourth Generation of Progress.* New York: Raven Press, pp. 1155–1170.

Price RA (1989) Affective disorder not linked to HLA. *Genet Epidemiol* **6**: 299–304.

Price RA, Kidd KK, Weissman MM (1987) Early onset (under age 30 years) and panic disorder as markers for etiologic homogeneity in major depression. *Arch Gen Psychiatry* **44**: 434–440.

Rausch JL, Johnson ME, Fei Y-J, Li JQ, Shendarkar N, MacHobby H, Ganapathy V, Leibach FH (2002) Initial conditions of serotonin transporter kinetics and genotype: influence on ssri treatment trial outcome. *Biol Psychiatry* **51**: 723–732.

Regier DA (2000) Community diagnosis counts. *Arch Gen Psychiatry* **57**: 223–224.

Reinink E, Bouhuys AL, Gordijn MC, Van Den Hoofdakker RH (1993) Prediction of the antidepressant response to total sleep deprivation of depressed patients: longitudinal versus single day assessment of diurnal mood variation. *Biol Psychiatry* **34**: 471–481.

Rice J, Reich T, Andreasen N, Endicott J, Van Eerdewogh M, Fishman R, Hirschfield R, Klerman G (1987) The familial transmission of bipolar illness. *Arch Gen Psychiatry* **44**: 441–447.

Rice JP, Goate A, Williams JT, Bierut L, Dorr D, Wu W, Shears S, Gopalakrishnan G, Edenberg HJ, Foroud T, Nurnberger J Jr, Gershon ES, Detera-Wadleigh SD, Goldin LR, Guroff JJ, McMahon FJ, Simpson S, MacKinnon D, McInnis M, Stine OC, DePaulo JR, Blehar MC, Reich T (1997) Initial genome scan of the NIMH genetics initiative bipolar pedigrees: chromosomes 1, 6, 8, 10, and 12. *Am J Med Genet* **74**: 247–253.

Risch N (1990) Linkage strategies for genetically complex traits: I. Multilocus models. *Am J Med Genet* **46**: 222–228.

Roses AD (2000) Pharmacogenetics and the practice of medicine. *Nature* **405**: 857–865.

Rubinsztein DC, Leggo J, Goodburn S, Walsh C, Jain S, Paykel ES (1996) Genetic association between monoamine oxidase A microsatellite and RFLP alleles and bipolar affective disorder: analysis and meta-analysis. *Hum Mol Genet* **5**: 779–782.

Saski T, Billett E, Petronis A, Ying D, Parsons T, Macciardi FM, Meltzer HY, Lieberman J, Joffe RT, Ross CA, McInnis MG, Li SH, Kennedy JL (1996) Psychosis and genes with trinucleotide repeat polymorphism. *Hum Genet* **97**: 244–246.

Sato K, Yoshida K, Takahashi H, Ito K, Kamata M, Higuchi H, Shimizu T, Itoh K, Inoue K, Tezuka T, Suzuki T, Ohkubo T, Sugawara K, Otani K (2002) Association between −1438G/A promoter polymorphism in the 5-HT(2A) receptor gene and fluvoxamine response in Japanese patients with major depressive disorder. *Neuropsychobiology* **46**: 136–140.

Schulze TG, Muller DJ, Krauss H, Gross M, Bauer I, Fangerau-Lefevre H, Illes F, Ohlraun S, Fimmers R, Cichon S, Held T, Propping P, Nothen MM, Maier W, Rietschel M (2001) Caught in the trio trap? Potential selection bias inherent to association studies usings parent–offspring trios. *Am J Med Genet* **105**: 351–353.

Schumann G, Benedetti F, Voderholzer U, Kammerer N, Hemmeter U, Travers HW, Fiebich B, Holsboer-Trachsler E, Berger M, Seifritz E, Ebert D (2001) Antidepressive response to sleep deprivation in unipolar depression is not associated with dopamine D3 receptor genotype. *Neuropsychobiology* **43**: 127–130.

Segman R, Neeman T, Heresco-Levy U, Finkel B, Karagichev L, Schlafman M, Dorevitch A, Yakir A, Lerner A, Shelevoy A, Lerer B (1999) Genotypic association between the dopamine D3 receptor and tardive dyskinesia in chronic schizophrenia. *Mol Psychiatry* **4**: 247–253.

Serretti A (2002) Lithium long term treatment in mood disorders: clinical and genetic predictors. *Pharmacogenomics* **3**: 117–129.

Serretti A, Benedetti F, Colombo C, Lilli R, Lorenzi C, Smeraldi E (1999a) Dopamine receptor D4 is not associated with antidepressant activity of sleep deprivation. *Psychiatry Res* **89**: 107–114.

Serretti A, Franchini L, Gasperini M, Rampoldi R, Smeraldi E (1998a) Mode of inheritance in mood disorders families according to fluvoxamine response. *Acta Psychiatr Scand* **98**: 443–450.

Serretti A, Lattuada E, Lorenzi C, Lilli R, Smeraldi E (2000a) Dopamine receptor D2 ser/cys 311 variant is associated with delusion and disorganization symptomatology in major psychoses. *Mol Psychiatry* **5**: 270–274.

Serretti A, Lilli R, Lorenzi C, Franchini L, DiBella D, Catalano M, Smeraldi E (1999b) Dopamine receptor D2, D4, GABAA Alpha-1 subunit genes and response to lithium prophylaxis in mood disorders. *Psychiatry Research* **87**: 7–19.

Serretti A, Lilli R, Lorenzi C, Gasperini M, Smeraldi E (1998b) Dopamine receptor D3 gene and response to lithium prophylaxis in mood disorders. *Int J Neuropsychopharmacol* **1**: 125–129.

Serretti A, Lilli R, Lorenzi C, Gasperini M, Smeraldi E (1999c) Tryptophan hydroxylase gene and response to lithium prophylaxis in mood disorders. *J Psychiatr Res* **33**: 371–377.

Serretti A, Lilli R, Lorenzi C, Lattuada E, Smeraldi E (2001a) DRD4 exon 3 variants associated with delusional symptomatology in major psychoses: a study on 2,011 affected subjects. *Am J Med Genet* **105**: 283–290.

Serretti A, Lilli R, Mandelli L, Lorenzi C, Smeraldi E (2001b) Serotonin transporter gene associated with lithium prophylaxis in mood disorders. *Pharmacogenom J* **1**: 71–77.

Serretti A, Lilli R, Smeraldi E (2002) Pharmacogenetics in affective disorders. *Eur J Pharmacol* **438**: 117–128.

Serretti A, Lorenzi C, Lilli R, Smeraldi E (2000b) Serotonin receptor 2A, 2C, 1A genes and response to lithium prophylaxis in mood disorders. *J Psychiatr Res* **34**: 89–98.

Serretti A, Macciardi F, Verga M, Cusin C, Pedrini S, Smeraldi E (1998c) Tyrosine hydroxylase gene associated with depressive symptomatology in mood disorder. *Am J Med Genet* **81**: 127–130.

Serretti A, Zanardi R, Cusin C, Rossini D, Lorenzi C, Smeraldi E (2001c) Tryptophan hydroxylase gene associated with paroxetine antidepressant activity. *Eur Neuropsychopharmacol* **11**: 375–380.

Serretti A, Zanardi R, Rossini D, Cusin C, Lilli R, Smeraldi E (2001d) Influence of tryptophan hydroxylase and serotonin transporter genes on fluvoxamine antidepressant activity. *Mol Psychiatry* **6**: 586–592.

Shoemaker DD, Schadt EE, Armour CD, He YD, Garrett-Engele P, McDonagh PD, Loerch PM, Leonardson A, Lum PY, Cavet G, Wu LF, Altschuler SJ, Edwards S, King J, Tsang JS, Schimmack G, Schelter JM, Koch J, Ziman M, Marton MJ, Li B, Cundiff P, Ward T, Castle J, Krolewski M, Meyer MR, Mao M, Burchard J, Kidd MJ, Dai H, Phillips JW, Linsley PS, Stoughton R, Scherer S, Boguski MS (2001) Experimental annotation of the human genome using microarray technology. *Nature* **409**: 922–927.

Smeraldi E, Bellodi L (1981) Possible linkage between primary affective disorder susceptibility locus and HLA haplotypes. *Am J Psychiatry* **138**: 1232–1234.

Smeraldi E, Benedetti F, Zanardi R (2002) Serotonin transporter promoter genotype and illness recurrence in mood disorders. *Eur Neuropsychopharmacol* **12**: 73–75.

Smeraldi E, Macciardi F, Holmgren S, Perris H, von Knorring L, Perris C (1987) Age at onset of affective disorders in Italian and Swedish patients. *Acta Psychiatr Scand* **75**: 352–357.

Smeraldi E, Negri F, Melica AM (1977) A genetic study of affective disorders. *Acta Psychiatr Scand* **56**: 382–398.

Smeraldi E, Negri F, Melica AM, Scorza-Smeraldi R (1978) HLA system and affective disorders: a sibship genetic study. *Tissue Antigens* **12**: 270–274.

Smeraldi E, Petroccione A, Gasperini M, Macciardi F, Orsini A, Kidd KK (1984) Outcomes on lithium treatment as a tool for genetic studies in affective disorders. *J Affect Disord* **6**: 139–151.

Smeraldi E, Zanardi R, Benedetti F, Dibella D, Perez J, Catalano M (1998) Polymorphism within the promoter of the serotonin transporter gene and antidepressant efficacy of fluvoxamine. *Mol Psychiatry* **3**: 508–511.

Smith DJ, Rubin EM (1997) Functional screening and complex traits: human 21q22.2 sequences affecting learning in mice. *Hum Mol Genet* **6**: 1729–1733.

Smyth C, Kalsi G, Brynjolfsson J, O'Neill J, Curtis D, Rifkin L, Moloney E, Murphy P, Petursson H, Gurling H (1997) Test of Xq26.3–28 linkage in bipolar and unipolar affective disorder in families selected for absence of male to male transmission. *Br J Psychiatry* **171**: 578–581.

Spielman RS, McGinnis RE, Ewens WJ (1993) Transmission test for linkage disequilibrium: the insulin gene region and insulin-dependent diabetes mellitus (IDDM). *Am J Hum Genet* **52**: 506–516.

Stancer HC, Weitkamp LR, Persad E, Flood C, Jorna T, Guttormsen SA, Yagnow RL (1988) Confirmation of the relationship of HLA (chromosome 6) genes to depression and manic depression. II. The Ontario follow-up and analysis of 117 kindreds. *Ann Hum Genet* **52**: 279–298.

Steen VM, Lovlie R, Osher Y, Belmaker RH, Berle JO, Gulbrandsen AK (1998) The polymorphic inositol polyphosphate 1-phosphatase gene as a candidate for pharmacogenetic prediction of lithium-responsive manic-depressive illness. *Pharmacogenetics* **8**: 259–268.

Stine CO, Xu J, Koskela R, McMahon F, Gschwend M, Friddle C, Clark CD, McInnis MG, Simpson SG, Breschel TS, Vishio E, Riskin K, Feilotter H, Chen E, Shen S, Folstein S, Meyers DA, Botstein D, Marr TG, DePaulo JR (1995) Evidence for linkage of bipolar disorder to chromosome 18 with a parent-of-origin effect. *Am J Hum Genet* **57**: 1384–1394.

Stine OC, McMahon FJ, Chen L, Xu J, Meyers DA, MacKinnon DF, Simpson S, McInnis MG, Rice JP, Goate A, Reich T, Edenberg HJ, Foroud T, Nurnberger JI, Jr., Detera-Wadleigh SD, Goldin LR, Guroff J, Gershon ES, Blehar MC, DePaulo JR (1997) Initial genome screen for bipolar disorder in the NIMH genetics initiative pedigrees: chromosomes 2, 11, 13, 14, and X. *Am J Med Genet* **74**: 263–269.

Straub RE, Lehner T, Luo Y, Loth JE, Shao W, Sharpe L, Alexander JR, Das K, Simon R, Fieve RR, Lerer B, Endicott J, Ott J, Gilliam TC, Baron M (1994) A possible vulnerability locus for bipolar affective disorder on chromosome 21q22.3. *Nature Genetics* **8**: 291–296.

Suarez BK, Croughan J (1982) Is the major histocompatibility complex linked to genes that increase susceptibility to affective disorder? A critical appraisal. *Psychiatry Res* **7**: 19–27.

Suarez BK, Reich T (1984) HLA and major affective disorder. *Arch Gen Psychiatry* **41**: 22–27.

Sullivan PF, Neale MC, Kendler KS (2000) Genetic epidemiology of major depression: review and meta-analysis. *Am J Psychiatry* **157**: 1552–1562.

Targum SD, Gershon ES, Van Eerdewegh M, Rogentine N (1979) Human leukocyte antigen system not closely linked to or associated with bipolar manic-depressive illness. *Biol Psychiatry* **14**: 615–636.

Torgersen S (1986) Genetic factors in moderately severe and mild affective disorders. *Arch Gen Psychiatry* **43**: 222–226.

Tsuang M, Faraone S (1990) *The Genetics of Mood Disorders*. Baltimore, MD: Johns Hopkins University Press, pp. 1–31.

Tsuang MT, Bucher KD, Fleming JA, Faraone SV (1985) Transmission of affective disorders: an application of segregation analysis to blind family study data. *J Psychiatr Res* **19**: 23–29.

Turner WJ, King S (1981) Two genetically distinct forms of bipolar affective disorder? *Biol Psychiatry* **16**: 417–439.

Turner WJ, King S (1983) BPD2. An autosomal dominant form of bipolar affective disorder. *Biol Psychiatry* **18**: 63–88.

Ustun TB (2001) The worldwide burden of depression in the 21st century. In Weismann MM (ed) *Treatment of Depression: Bridging the 21st Century*. Washington, DC: American Psychiatric Press, pp. 35–45.

Vallada HP, Vasques L, Curtis D, Zatz M, Kirov G, Lauriano V, Gentil V, Murray RM, McGuffin P, Owen M, Gill M, Craddock N, Collier DA (1998) Linkage analysis between bipolar affective disorder and markers on chromosome X. *Psychiatr Genet* **8**: 183–186.

Van Os J, Marcelis M, Sham P, Jones P, Gilvarry K, Murray R (1997) Psychopathological syndromes and familial morbid risk of psychosis. *Br J Psychiatry* **170**: 241–246.

Vincent JB, Masellis M, Lawrence J, Choi V, Gurling HM, Parikh SV, Kennedy JL (1999) Genetic association analysis of serotonin system genes in bipolar affective disorder. *Am J Psychiatry* **156**: 136–138.

von Knorring AL, Cloninger CR, Bohman M, Sigvardsson S (1983) An adoption study of depressive disorders and substance abuse. *Arch Gen Psychiatry* **40**: 943–950.

Waldman ID, Robinson BF, Feigon SA (1997) Linkage disequilibrium between the dopamine transporter gene (DAT1) and bipolar disorder: extending the transmission disequilibrium test (TDT) to examine genetic heterogeneity. *Genet Epidemiol* **14**: 699–704.

Waters B, Sengar D, Marchenko I, Rock G, Lapierre Y, Forster-Gibson CJ, Simpson NE (1988) A linkage study of primary affective disorder. *Br J Psychiatry* **152**: 560–562.

Weber MM (1997) Ernest Rubin 1874–1952: a German psychiatrist and geneticist. *Am J Med Genet* **67**: 323–331.

Weinberger DR, Berman KF, Zec RF (1986) Physiologic dysfunction of dorsolateral prefrontal cortex in schizophrenia. I. Regional cerebral blood flow evidence. *Arch Gen Psychiatry* **43**: 114–124.

Weiss J, Magert HJ, Cieslak A, Forssmann WG (1996) Association between different psychotic disorders and the DRD4 polymorphism, but no differences in the main ligand binding region of the DRD4 receptor protein compared to controls. *Eur J Med Res* **1**: 439–445.

Weissman MM (1987) Advances in psychiatric epidemiology: rates and risks for major depression. *Am J Public Health* **77**: 445–451.

Weissman MM, Bland RC, Canino GJ, Faravelli C, Greenwald S, Hwu H-G, Joyce PR, Karam EG, Lee C-K, Lellouch J, Lepine J-P, Newman SC, Rubio-Stipec M, Wells JE, Wickramaratne PJ, Wittchen H-U, Yeh E-K (1996) Cross-national epidemiology of major depression and bipolar disorder. *J Am Med Assoc* **276**: 293–299.

Weissman MM, Myers JK (1978) Affective disorders in a US urban community: the use of research diagnostic criteria in an epidemiological survey. *Arch Gen Psychiatry* **35**: 1304–1311.

Weissman MM, Warner V, Wickramaratne P, Prusoff BA (1988) Early-onset major depression in parents and their children. *J Affect Disord* **15**: 269–277.

Weitkamp LR, Pardue LH, Huntzinger RS (1980) Genetic marker studies in a family with unipolar depression. *Arch Gen Psychiatry* **37**: 1187–1192.

Weitkamp LR, Stancer HC, Persad E, Flood C, Guttormsen S (1981) Depressive disorders and HLA: a gene on chromosome 6 that can affect behavior. *N Engl J Med* **305**: 1301–1306.

Wender P, Kety S, Rosenthal D, Schulsinger F, Ortmann J, Lunde I (1986) Psychiatric disorders in the biological and adoptive families of adopted individuals with affective disorders. *Arch Gen Psychiatry* **43**: 923–929.

Willner P (1995) Dopaminergic mechanisms in depression and mania. In Bloom FE, Kupfer DJ (eds) *Psychopharmacology: The Fourth Generation of Progress.* New York: Raven Press, pp. 921–931.

Wilson AF, Elston RC, Siervogel RM, Tran LD (1988) Linkage of a gene regulating dopamine-beta-hydroxylase activity and the ABO blood group locus. *Am J Hum Genet* **42**: 160–166.

Winokur G, Coryell W, Endicott J, Akiskal H (1993a) Further distinctions between manic-depressive illness (bipolar disorder) and primary depressive disorder (unipolar depression). *Am J Psychiatry* **150**: 1176–1181.

Winokur G, Coryell W, Keller M, Endicott J, Akiskal H (1993b) A prospective follow-up of patients with bipolar and primary unipolar affective disorder. *Arch Gen Psychiatry* **50**: 457–465.

Winokur G, Coryell W, Keller M, Endicott J, Leon A (1995) A family study of manic-depressive (bipolar I) disease. Is it a distinct illness separable from primary unipolar depression? *Arch Gen Psychiatry* **52**: 367–373.

Yoneda H, Sakai T, Ishida T, Inayama Y, Nonomura Y, Kono Y, Asaba H (1992) An association between manic-depressive illness and a pseudoautosomal DNA marker. *Am J Hum Genet* **51**: 1172–1173.

Yoshida K, Ito K, Sato K, Takahashi H, Kamata M, Higuchi H, Shimizu T, Itoh K, Inoue K, Tezuka T, Suzuki T, Ohkubo T, Sugawara K, Otani K (2002a) Influence of the serotonin transporter gene-linked polymorphic region on the antidepressant response to fluvoxamine in Japanese depressed patients. *Prog Neuropsychopharmacol Biol Psychiatry* **26**: 383–386.

Yoshida K, Naito S, Takahashi H, Sato K, Ito K, Kamata M, Higuchi H, Shimizu T, Itoh K, Inoue K, Tezuka T, Suzuki T, Ohkubo T, Sugawara K, Otani K (2002b) Monoamine oxidase: a gene polymorphism, tryptophan hydroxylase gene polymorphism and antidepressant response to fluvoxamine in Japanese patients with major depressive disorder. *Prog Neuropsychopharmacol Biol Psychiatry* **26**: 1279–1283.

Youngerman J, Canino IA (1978) Lithium carbonate use in children and adolescents. A survey of the literature. *Arch Gen Psychiatry* **35**: 216–224.

Yu YW, Chen TJ, Hong CJ, Chen HM, Tsai SJ (2003a) Association study of the interleukin-1beta (C-511T) genetic polymorphism with major depressive disorder, associated symptomatology, and antidepressant response. *Neuropsychopharmacology* **28**: 1182–1185.

Yu YW, Chen TJ, Wang YC, Liou YJ, Hong CJ, Tsai SJ (2003b) Association analysis for neuronal nitric oxide synthase gene polymorphism with major depression and fluoxetine response. *Neuropsychobiology* **47**: 137–140.

Yu YW, Tsai SJ, Chen TJ, Lin CH, Hong CJ (2002) Association study of the serotonin transporter promoter polymorphism and symptomatology and antidepressant response in major depressive disorders. *Mol Psychiatry* **7**: 1115–1119.

Zanardi R, Benedetti F, DiBella D, Catalano M, Smeraldi E (2000) Efficacy of paroxetine in depression is influenced by a functional polymorphism within the promoter of serotonin transporter gene. *J Clin Psychopharmacol* **20**: 105–107.

Zanardi R, Serretti A, Rossini D, Franchini L, Cusin C, Lattuada E, Dotoli D, Smeraldi E (2001) Factors affecting fluvoxamine antidepressant activity: influence of pindolol and 5-HTTLPR in delusional and nondelusional depression. *Biol Psychiatry* **50**: 323–330.

Zhou QY, Palmiter RD (1995) Dopamine-deficient mice are severely hypoactive, adipsic, and aphagic. *Cell* **83**: 1197–1209.

Zill P, Baghai TC, Engel R, Zwanzger P, Schule C, Minov C, Behrens S, Bottlender R, Jager M, Rupprecht R, Moller HJ, Ackenheil M, Bondy B (2003) Beta-1-adrenergic receptor gene in major depression: influence on antidepressant treatment response. *Am J Med Genet* **120B**: 85–89.

Zill P, Baghai TC, Zwanzger P, Schule C, Minov C, Riedel M, Neumeier K, Rupprecht R, Bondy B (2000) Evidence for an association between a G-protein beta3-gene variant with depression and response to antidepressant treatment. *Neuroreport* **11**: 1893–1897.

PART II
Syndromes and Nosology of Mood Disorders

3

Unipolar Depression

Carlo Faravelli, Claudia Ravaldi and Elisabetta Truglia

University of Florence, Florence, Italy

DEFINITION

All psychiatric classifications, both traditional and present, consider mood disorders in a unique, broad diagnostic category.

Mood is defined by DSM-IV as 'pervasive and sustained emotion that colours the perception of the world. In contrast with affect, which refers to more fluctuating changes in emotional "weather", mood refers to a more pervasive and sustained emotional *climate*' (DSM-IV).

The psychological, as well as philosophical, tradition describe mood as an affective/emotional state that colours, underlines, modulates, stands behind any psychic representation. A psychic representation is any content of the mind, whether conscious or not, such as ideas, memories, dreams, etc.

In other words mood has to be seen as coloured spectacles through which any individual sees the world, both external and internal. Such a similitude should remind those who are familiar with philosophy of Immanuel Kant's (1781) concept of space and time as 'categories'. In the same way, mood could be considered as an adjunctive categorical attitude that cannot be present and that is the necessary prerequisite to any form of cognition.

Mood is obviously modified by the events that occur in the real world. It is the common experience of each of us that negative events, losses and disappointments lower our mood, leading us into a state of depression, anger, pessimism . . . . Conversely, favourable occurrences, even the minor ones, tend to make us happier, positive, satisfied. On the other side, mood affects all of our cognitions, judgements, expectations. The same task that was seen as worthless, hard, useless when in low spirits, becomes positive, worthy, easy to achieve a few minutes later, after our mood has changed. Through these continuous variations, where mood is influenced by the ever-changing flow of life events, and in turn determines our attitude toward the life, remains the basic characteristic of normal mood, i.e. its mobility. Mood must

Mood Disorders: Clinical Management and Research Issues. Edited by E. J. L. Griez, C. Faravelli, D. J. Nutt and J. Zohar.
©2005 John Wiley & Sons Ltd. ISBN 0 470 09426 5.

MOOD 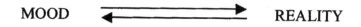 REALITY

Figure 3.1

be changeable, must vary, must have different colours. According to the classic psychopathology, mood disorders are characterized by the loss of the normal mobility and changeability of the mood: it remains blocked and fixed in a single, static condition.

Pathological mood is no longer influenced by changes in reality and remains steady and still, regardless of any occurrence. On the other hand, the state of mood continues to determine the cognition and the interpretation of reality. In the continuous inter-exchange mood <- -> reality the arrow 'mood towards reality' continues working, whereas the arrow < reality to mood > is interrupted (Figure 3.1).

Whether or not this condition represents an extreme of the continuum of mood (i.e. extreme depression or extreme euphoria) does not matter much to the psychopathologist. The simple fact that mood is no longer influenced by the events of everyday life, especially in relationships with others, is per se a dramatically painful experience for the sufferer. The incapability to 'feel with' is experienced as one of the most negative sensations that one can have. 'I cannot love my sons, and I can't stand it', 'I feel as though I were a fish in an aquarium, seeing the world through a glass, but without participating', 'I'm a rock in the river, the water flows and I remain stil', 'I'm flat, I cannot vibrate with the others' are some of the most typical sentences reported by sufferers from depressive illness.

The lack of response to the external stimuli is therefore the basis of the pathology of mood, rather than the intensity of the emotion

Basically, mood is usually considered to vary between euphoria and depression, with anger being present along the whole continuum of mood.

The word 'depression', however, is in itself a bad choice. First of all, 'de-pression' means loss of pressure, diminution, decrease. The use of the word 'depression' as a synonym of 'decrease' is clear, for instance, when we speak of 'an economic depression' or of 'a geographical depression'. Every clinician, however, is well aware that clinical pathological depression is far from being 'less': the level of the emotional arousal as well as the psychomotor agitation suggests instead the opposite.

Secondly, 'depression', even in its psychiatric use, is used with different meanings: it is in fact used to indicate a symptom (depressed mood), a set of symptoms (depressive syndrome) or a disease (depressive illness). These different uses may easily generate ambiguities. For lay people, for instance, the term 'depressed' as a synonym of 'sad', 'upset', 'low', allows pathological depression to be interpreted in comparison with their own subjective normal states of unhappiness, thus the vision of melancholia as a severe state is lost. For clinicians (and for patients), however, the 'erlebnis' of pathological depression is far from just 'feeling a little sad'. Hence the opinions that 'depression doesn't exist, it's just a matter of will', etc.

The term 'depression' can also indicate a group of symptoms and signs defining a syndrome, where having one symptom increases the probability of having other specific symptoms. This is the usual significance that psychiatrists give to the word 'depression'.

A third meaning that has been attached to the word 'depression' in psychiatry is that of an illness, assuming that all the aspects of the depressive syndrome should be attributed to a single, hidden pathological phenomenon, even if unknown at the moment. This interpretation was popular in Europe until a couple of decades ago.

At present, the commonly accepted meaning of the term 'depression' is that of a set of signs and symptoms, and the word used to mean it is 'disorder'.

PSYCHOPATHOLOGY

Four major clusters of symptoms and signs are recognized in the diagnosis of depression. These are: mood, cognition, psychomotricity and the neurovegetative area.

With regard to **mood**, the current diagnostic systems require the presence of the symptom 'depression'. Pathological depression differs from normal sadness because of the following characteristics:

- its 'erlebnis' is qualitatively different from that of sadness;
- there is no external trigger, or if there is, the depressive reaction is inadequate;
- it is not influenced by objective events or situations;
- it is quantitatively more severe;
- its duration is longer;
- it is often associated to other symptoms.

As said before, the main characteristic of pathological mood, depressive or manic, is its fixity: the patient's mood is unable to vary along the continuum ranging from sadness to euphoria. Normal external and internal events influence mood and mood influences the perception of reality. Reality, in pathological mood, loses its ability to influence mood, which indeed influences reality testing. Several characteristics of depression derive from this fixity of mood. Anhedonia (the inability to feel pleasure from formerly pleasant things) directly derives from the stasis of the mood. It might lead to 'the feeling of being absent' or affective depersonalization, experienced with great suffering, a sense of guilt and inadequacy. Patients do not take an interest or feel love for anyone, not even for those previously loved, such as family members. Sometimes regret becomes auto-sarcasm, described by German authors as 'galghenhumor' (gallows humour), comparing it to the witticisms of those condemned to death.

Patients perceive guilt and inadequacy in the present, irreparable faults in the past, and despair without any possibility in the future. Guilt and an alteration in temporality are depression's nuclear features.

According to the subjective phenomenological psychopathology (Jaspers, 1959), guilt is the nucleus of the internal experience of melancholic patients.

According to objective phenomenological psychopathology (Biswanger, 1960), the essence of the melancholic's internal world is an alteration of the time structure, with an abnormal prevalence of the past over the present and the future. This is the basis of other melancholic features, including a sense of guilt that is irreparable in the absence of a future when one might repair.

Sometimes the mood is prevalently dysphoric (depressed mood with irritability). Often anxiety accompanies depression, sometimes being dominant, especially in elderly patients.

Cognitive symptoms are considered (in classical phenomenological psychopathology) dependent on affective ones. This is evident in memory deficit: in depression, unlike that in dementia, the deficit is more subjective than objective and essentially depends on an attention deficit that is due to a typical lack of interest. The same goes for indecision: every decision seems difficult to make and the patient feels that making a choice is beyond his ability. A general lack of interest combined with a high sense of inadequacy manifests into a vicious cycle.

With regard to thought alterations, the typical depressive formal alteration is retardation in the flow of thinking, to the point of total inhibition. Sometimes thought tends to fix rigidly on the same themes, as in the case of ruminations or delusions. Typical depressive thought contents deal with sadness, hopelessness, lack of future, guilt, low self-esteem, ruin, disease and death. Depressed patients think about death in different ways, ranging from *taedium vitae* (boredom with life), to death desire without clear intention to kill themselves, to 'suicidal ideation', without a specific plan or with a structured programme of the modality and the instruments to realize the project. Actual self-harm (suicidal attempts and lethal suicides) are less frequent than suicidal ideation, because of the lack of will and energy typical of depressed patients. With regard to delusions, the classical psychopathology describes holothymic delusions (derivable from mood) as secondary delusions, but also acknowledges the possible presence of primitive delusions (not derivable from other psychopathological phenomena). DSM-IV (APA, 1994) distinguishes between mood-congruent and mood-incongruent delusions. Mood-congruent delusional themes are entirely consistent with the typical depressive feelings of personal inadequacy, guilt, disease, death, nihilism or deserved punishment. The extreme evolution of feelings of inadequacy and disease delusions is the 'nihilistic delusion', or Cotard's syndrome, in which negation is absolute and may concern the body, the spirit, the entire person, the whole universe, possibly reaching megalomania. Mood-incongruent delusions do not involve typical depressive themes, but refer to other themes, such as persecutory ideas, thought insertion, thought broadcasting and control experiences.

We can also find hallucinations, usually fragmentary and fluctuant, that might interest all the senses and are more similar to organic than to schizophrenic hallucinations. Even hallucinations can be mood-congruent or incongruent.

Regarding **psychomotricity**, the typical depressive feature is motor retardation: movements are reduced and slowed, speech is also reduced, slowed and polarized on the same restricted themes. The *facies* expresses lack of interest and sadness, mimics is rigid, patients complain of asthenia, loss of energy and fatigue to the point of psychomotor arrest, in which patients do not respond to any stimulation, do not eat, do not get up from bed even for their physiological needs. This condition is very severe and might worsen due to physical complications, especially linked to dehydration and denutrition.

Even if motor retardation is typical of depression, sometimes psychomotor agitation can also be present, especially in patients characterized by dysphoria or anxiety. The patients appear extremely restless and agitated.

Somatic symptoms and signs are usually linked to depressed mood and are sometimes the most prominent features ('depressive equivalents', 'masked depression') (Lopez-Ibor Alino, 1976; Lesse, 1977; Kielholz, 1979; Pichot, 1986; Cohen, 1987). These symptoms and signs refer to the areas of sleep, appetite, sexuality and biological rhythms. Depressed people can show both insomnia and hypersomnia, but the most characteristic pattern is terminal insomnia, with early morning waking (at least two hours before the usual time). Appetite can be decreased or increased with or without weight loss or gain; the most typical pattern is a decrease in appetite with weight loss. In the area of sexuality, desire is very usually severely impaired. Frequently men have erectile dysfunction and impotence, accompanied by loss of desire. Women experience loss of desire and menstrual cycle disturbances (retardation or arrest). Symptoms show a characteristic daily biological rhythm, with worsening in the morning, although an inverted rhythm with worsening in the evening is also possible. Sleep rhythm is altered in depressed people, with the already underlined early waking and typical electroencephalographic alterations (Hawkins and Mendels, 1966): reduced REM latency, augmented intensity REM sleep, REM prevalence in the early hours of the night and global reduction of sleep phases 3 and 4. Other circadian rhythms are altered, with a trend towards phase advancement, i.e. cortisol secretion (Carpenter and Bunney, 1971; Sachar et al., 1973) and bodily temperature patterns (Pflug et al., 1981; Faravelli et al., 1985). In addition to daily and circadian rhythms, rhythm alterations with longer periodicity can also be found, with recurrences in autumn or spring; when a clear seasonality is not recognizable, periodicity can usually still be found, being a characteristic and stable temporal pattern of recurrence.

According to DSM-IV, different kinds of depression can be distinguished: depressive episode with catatonic symptoms, with melancholic symptoms, with atypical symptoms, or with psychotic features (within the specifiers of severity).

Catatonic symptoms are peculiar alterations of voluntary movements that appear mood-incongruent: marked decrease in reactivity to the environment and/ or reduction in spontaneous movements and activity (catatonic stupor or catalepsy, including waxy flexibility); excited motor activity, apparently purposeless and not influenced by external stimuli (catatonic excitement); apparently motiveless resistance to all instructions or attempts to be moved (catatonic negativism) or mutism; voluntary assumption of inappropriate or bizarre postures, stereotypies, mannerisms; echolalia or echopraxia. Catatonic depression is a very severe picture, with possible physical complications due to malnutrition, dehydration or self-inflicted injuries.

Melancholic symptoms (biological symptoms in ICD-10) correspond to the endogenous symptoms of the psychopathological tradition. These seem to be the most specific symptoms of depression. The European psychopathological tradition indicates melancholy as the psychopathological nucleus of depression. It includes somatic symptoms and signs (worsening in the morning, early morning awakening, significant anorexia or weight loss), marked psychomotor retardation or agitation, guilty feelings and specific features of the mood (loss of interest or pleasure in all, or almost all, activities; lack of reactivity to usually pleasurable stimuli; peculiar characteristic of the depressed mood, qualitatively different from normal sadness).

With regard to melancholic vulnerability, Tellenbach defined the 'typus pre-melancolicus' and described the pathogenesis of its melancholic evolution. The main characteristics of the typus pre-melancolicus are the 'orderliness', which is a stressed version of order (rules in relationships with people and things), and the 'conscientiousness', which is the consideration of the consciousness as a means of avoiding any fault. The melancholic transformation of the typus is linked to certain situations, characterized by the constellations of 'includence' and 'remanence'. 'Includence' means to be contained or to close oneself within limits that the subject cannot overcome because of the regular actuation of its order ways. 'Remanence' means to remain back, which can slow the course of existence, until arrest. After Tellenbach (1960), other authors were interested in the characteristics of the typus. Kimura Bin (1992) defined the typus as a post-festum personality, i.e. oriented to the past. Kraus defined the typus as a hypernormic and etheronomic personality, which is a personality based much on external rules with a prevalence of the 'objective I' over the 'subjective I'.

Atypical symptoms are the opposite of melancholic ones: mood reactivity (i.e. mood brightens in response to actual or potential positive events) and inverse neurovegetative symptoms (significant weight gain or increase in appetite, hypersomnia). DSM-IV also reports leaden paralysis (i.e. heavy feelings in arms or legs) and a long-standing pattern of interpersonal sensitivity (not limited to episodes of mood disturbances).

Psychotic features considered by DSM-IV are delusions and hallucinations that might be mood-congruent or mood-incongruent, as already said.

Clinical and psychopathological traditions describe many other forms of depression: agitated depression, with predominant psychomotor agitation; anxious depression, with predominant psychic anxiety symptoms; hypochondriac depression, with predominant somatic complaints (defined also as 'masked depression', with symptoms of other psychopathological areas more evident than classical ones); amentia depression, with psychomotor arrest, confusion and medical complications; and Cotard's syndrome, with nihilistic delusions.

Depressive episodes usually start with unspecific prodromal symptoms and signs, such as anxiety, irritability, emotional lability, asthenia, impaired concentration, reduction in interests, anorexia or sleep disturbances. In this phase, a social or working impairment is not yet present. With the progression of the disease, other symptoms appear, becoming more severe, with a marked impairment in social and working activities. The state period of an untreated depressive episode lasts about 6–12 months, but longer periods have been frequently reported. Recovery from a depressive episode is usually gradual, and the persistence of residual symptoms is not infrequent. Often, residual symptoms are similar to prodromal ones (the rollback phenomenon; Detre and Jarecki, 1971; Fava, 1999) and in a minority of cases, depressive episodes have a chronic course (20%, according to Keller et al., 1984). Familial mood disorder, dysthymic temperament, early onset and high number of previous episodes are the better predictive factors of long-term poor outcome.

HISTORY

The existence of depression has been recognized since the origin of our culture. Hippocrates (fourth century BC) was the first to reject ethical-religious explanations of depression, considering the brain as the place of affectivity and other psychic manifestations. He thought that different combinations of the four humours that compose the human body (yellow bile, black bile, blood and phlegm) determine the different temperaments (choleric, melancholic, sanguine and phlegmatic), possibly leading to mental disease. According to his theory, melancholia was due to the prevalence of black bile. In the following century, Aristotle (third century BC) also defined melancholic temperament as a predisposing factor of depression.

Aretaeus from Cappadocia (first century BC) was the first to observe that depression and its opposite manifestation (mania) might be two aspects of the same disease.

In the Middle Ages, after the influence of Arabian culture (in particular, Avicenna), psychiatric diseases were seen as related to magical or religious causes. This view persisted for centuries until Vesalius (sixteenth century AD) once again defined depression as an organic illness.

In the seventeenth century, naturalistic observations found that the melancholic temperament predisposed one to depression, and that mood might change from depression to mania.

A major interest in illness classification was developed in the eighteenth century when many authors, emphasizing the characteristics of clinical course, such as recurrence with alternate cycles of mania, distinguished many clinical features on the basis of symptoms. Following this period, the relationship between depression and mania was studied. Failret, in 1854, described the 'folie circulaire', Baillarger in 1854, described the 'folie à double forme' and Kraepelin (1896) distinguished manic-depressive psychosis from 'dementia praecox', both within the category of the psychoses. Kraepelin's classification was based on a longitudinal criterion and, according to him, the cases with recurrent depression without mania had to be included in the same category as those presenting with both depression and mania. Not only were the depressive episodes perfectly alike, but course, onset, outcome, premorbid and personality characteristics were in fact the same.

After Kraepelin, for about half a century, there was little doubt that manic-depressive illness was a severe disease and that recurrent depression with no mania should be considered as an incomplete presentation of the same disorder that was bipolar in its typical course. To evaluate such a position the reader has to keep in mind the reality of psychiatry during the first half of the twentieth century. Psychiatric institutions were almost exclusively the mental hospitals and the kind of patients that could be observed were only of the most severe types. On the other hand, the possibility to treat depression effectively was almost none.

After World War II the situation of psychiatry changed dramatically. Efficacious treatments become available, namely ECT (discovered before the war but extensively used after 1950) and antidepressants. The number of admissions to psychiatric hospitals decreased; in the meantime the outpatient practice of psychiatrists increased tremendously. The field of observation of psychiatry underwent a major change: the relative number of severe, psychotic, melancholic depressed patients that had formed the typical samples diminished, whereas an ever-increasing number of non-psychotic, non-endogenous, non-bipolar affective cases made up the main bulk of the cases referred to the psychiatrists. Since 1960 psychiatric samples have come to be characterized by a majority of mild depressive states without severe/endogenous/psychotic features. This change in the composition of psychiatric samples led to the reconsideration of the formerly accepted nosographic concepts.

Basically, (a) the uniqueness of bipolar and unipolar cases was rejected and (b) the status of depression was disputed.

Leonhard (1957) divided the manic-depressive psychoses into monopolar (only depression or only mania) and bipolar forms (alternating bouts of depression and mania). Angst (1966) and Perris (1966a, 1966b) emphasized that the distinction between unipolar and bipolar disorders is supported by specific characteristics of clinical course and family history, confirming Leonhard's observation. At first, the unipolar/bipolar distinction was used to refer to only manic-depressive psychosis; afterwards 'unipolar' was used to define patients with depressive symptoms but without a history of manic episodes, becoming a heterogeneous category and confounding the boundaries between primary and secondary affective forms.

In addition to the unipolar/bipolar dichotomy, other problems arose in the classification of depression. As said above, before the 1960s, psychiatrists were considering depression as an illness because they were used to observing only the most severe cases. With the development of new theories (psychoanalytical and psychosocial) and with the introduction of new drugs, psychiatrists began observing even mild forms of the syndrome. Thus, between the mid-1960s and the mid-1970s a new debate on the nosography of depression was roused, based on the unitary and binary hypotheses. These hypotheses attempted to solve some dichotomies in the classification of depression:

- *Endogenous versus reactive*
  It is not easy to define the exact meaning of the term 'endogenous'. Tellenbach used this term to indicate expression of disease greatly based on physical factors. According to Weitbrecht, the use of the term 'endogenous' as an equivalent of 'somatogenous', meaning 'with a physical cause', is incorrect, and the opposing 'endogenous/exogenous' (the latter meaning 'with an environmental cause') is an over-simplification. Weitbrecht's interpretation of the causative aspects is negative, using 'endogenous' to mean not completely physical nor completely psychological, but cryptogenic, essential, unknown. The dichotomy endogenous/reactive refers to an aetiopathogenetic point of view. In endogenous depression, it is not possible to identify external physical or psychological factors implicated in the development of the disease; an internal unknown biological cause is implied. On the contrary, the onset of 'reactive depression' is linked to an event of great emotional impact. More logically, the opposite of endogenous would be the less used exogenous, including psychogenic forms, caused by psychological factors, and somatogenic forms, caused by physical factors.
- *Psychotic versus neurotic*
  Psychotic depression is characterized by gross impairment in reality testing, absence of insight, delusions, hallucinations and loosening of associative links. The expression 'neurotic depression' may mean both depression without severe (psychotic) symptoms and depression with some specific symptoms (mood reactivity, irritability, anxiety and long-term course). The dichotomy psychotic/neurotic was originally based on clinical features. Indeed, the term 'neurotic' was initially used with a descriptive meaning, but then it assumed an aetiopathogenetic meaning overlapping with the meaning of 'psychogenic'. American authors used 'psychotic depression' to refer to symptoms, and 'reactive' and 'endogenous depression' to emphasize the presence or absence of an external causing factor. According to European authors, 'psychotic' and 'endogenous' depression were instead the same, as well as 'neurotic' and 'reactive' depression.

If one acknowledges the existence of two types of depression, the problem of the relationship between the two forms is raised. The unitary hypothesis, presented by Kendell, contrasted the binary hypothesis, contended by Roth. According to Roth and the Newcastle school, there are points of rarity among affective disorders between depression and anxiety (Roth et al., 1972), and in depression between the endogenous form and the reactive one. The authors, therefore, proposed a model based on a categorical approach where depression is divided into two different and separate entities, 'endogenous' and 'reactive' (Kiloh and Garside, 1963; Carney et al., 1965; Garside et al., 1971, 1978; Roth et al., 1979). On the contrary, according to Kendell, depression cannot be divided into categories, being rather better described by a dimensional model; the simplest model has only one dimension, with endogenous depression at one side of the continuum and reactive depression at the other side (Kendell, 1969a, 1969b; Kendell and Gourlay, 1970; Kendell, 1970, 1972, 1976; Kendell et al., 1968). The debate on the unitary/binary classification of depression characterized the psychiatric literature of the times.

In 1972, the St. Louis group proposed the Feighner criteria (Feighner et al., 1972), in order to reduce the heterogeneity of depression and improve diagnostic reliability in research. They distinguished affective disorders into categories labelled 'primary' and 'secondary'. The secondary forms were defined as chronologically preceded by other mental diseases, or concomitant with physical diseases or pharmacological treatments. Although it was very restrictive, this description was homogeneous enough. It was the first 'atheoretic' description, based on an empirical-descriptive approach and using operational criteria. The authors opted for the criterion of severity, defined as a minimum number of symptoms and of chronology to define primary depression.

In 1975, a widening of the criteria was performed, leading in 1978 to the publication of the Research Diagnostic Criteria (RDC, Spitzer et al., 1978). The RDC changed the term 'primary depression' into 'major depression' (in opposition to 'minor depression') and abandoned the criterion of chronology.

This apparently small change actually implied an extremely important turning point: (a) the debate between qualitative and quantitative in the classification of depression was resolved, accepting the quantitative approach; (b) the criterion of severity was evaluated by counting the number of symptoms.

As the RDC were the basis for DSM-III, the choice of a quantitative model, based on the number of symptoms, became essential in defining both diagnosis and severity of depression.

THE CURRENT CLASSIFICATIONS

The *Diagnostic and Statistical Manual of Mental Disorders* (third edition) (DSM-III; APA, 1980) substantially referred to the RDC. The two following editions of the DSM (DSM III-R; APA, 1987; and DSM-IV; APA, 1994) made few modifications. The RDC were also the reference point for the *International Classification of Diseases* (10th edition) (ICD-10, World Health Organization, 1992). DSM-III brought some important changes to the classification of psychiatric disorders. It introduced diagnostic criteria and a multi-axial system of psychiatric pathology evaluation; it rejected the term 'neurosis', restricted the diagnosis of schizophrenia and enlarged the diagnosis of mood disorders. In the DSM-III-R and DSM-IV there were no substantial changes, apart from the increasing number of diagnostic categories and the definitive overcoming of the hierarchical principle (introduced by Jaspers and for a long time considered valid), by promoting multiple diagnoses (comorbidity).

DSM-IV classifies depressive disorders in the mood disorders, making a distinction between major depressive disorder, dysthymic disorder and depressive disorder not otherwise specified. Appendix B lists other depressive disorders that are not defined by diagnostic criteria but instead by research criteria: premenstrual dysphoric disorder, minor depressive disorder, recurrent brief depressive disorder and mixed anxiety–depressive disorder. The depressive episode can be characterized by some specifiers: mild, moderate, severe without psychotic symptoms, severe with psychotic symptoms, in partial remission, in full remission, chronic, with catatonic symptoms, with melancholic symptoms, with atypical symptoms, with post-partum onset.

Chapter V, section F of the ICD-10 is dedicated to the affective syndromes and classifies depressive syndromes as recurrent or persistent syndromes (dysthymia). According to ICD-10, a depressive episode might be mild (with or without biological symptoms), moderate (with or without biological symptoms) or severe (with or without psychotic symptoms). The ICD-10 specifies that 'biological' symp-

TABLE 3.1 Comparison between 'biological symptoms' of ICD-10 and DSM-IV criteria for 'melancholic features'

ICD-10 Biological symptoms

(1) loss of interest or pleasure in the activities that normally are a source of pleasure;
(2) lack of emotional reactivity to normally pleasant circumstances and events;
(3) waking early in the morning, two or more hours earlier than usual;
(4) worsening of symptoms in the morning;
(5) objective evidence of clear psychomotor retardation or agitation (observed or reported by other people);
(6) marked loss of appetite;
(7) loss of weight (often defined as a reduction of 5% or more of body weight in the last month);
(8) marked reduction in libido.

DSM-IV Criteria for melancholic features

(A) One of the following symptoms is present during the period of greatest severity of the current episode:
    (1) lack of interest in all or nearly all activities;
    (2) lack of reactivity to normally pleasant stimuli (subject does not feel better, not even temporarily, when something of good happens).
(B) Three (or more) of the following symptoms are present during the period of greatest severity of the current episode.
    (1) a particular quality of depressed mood (for example, patient perceives the depressed mood in a very different way compared to the sadness felt after the death of a loved one);
    (2) worsening of symptoms in the morning;
    (3) waking early in the morning (at least two hours earlier than usual);
    (4) marked motor retardation or agitation;
    (5) significant anorexia or weight loss;
    (6) excessive or inadequate feelings of guilt.

toms are also called 'melancholic', 'vital' or 'endogenomorphic'. Even if each symptom has an important clinical meaning, the clinical validity of the derived syndrome is not clear. The biological symptoms of ICD-10 are shown in Table 3.1.

In order to define a biological syndrome, at least four of these symptoms must be present. The biological symptoms of the ICD-10 are similar to those described in the DSM-IV, defining the depressive episode 'with melancholic symptoms' (Table 3.1)

In spite of the wide overlap of symptoms defining the biological syndrome in the ICD-10 and depression with melancholic characteristics in the DSM-IV, these two disorders are conceptually different: the DSM-IV classification is a categorical one, whereas the ICD-10 classification is a mixed one (both categorical and dimensional). In fact, according to the DSM-IV, the characterization 'with melancholic symptoms' is possible only within the diagnostic category 'major depressive episode', which means at least five symptoms. To the contrary, according to the ICD-10, it is possible to define as biological both the mild depressive episode, indicated by the presence of at least four symptoms out of ten, and the moderate depressive episode, indicated by the presence of at least five symptoms out of ten. In the severe depressive episode, characterized by the presence of at least seven out of ten symptoms, ICD-10 distinguishes between subtypes 'without psychotic symptoms' and 'with psychotic symptoms', assuming that the biological syndrome must always be present in a severe depressive episode.

Problems with the Current Classifications of Depression

(a) Number of Symptoms versus Type of Symptoms

As seen before, DSM-IV considers depression as a syndrome. Basically, major depressive episode is characterized by a minimum of five symptoms for two weeks, whereas dysthymic disorder has fewer than five symptoms, but with a longer duration.

In order to have a diagnosis of major depressive episode, the symptom depression or the symptom loss of interest or pleasure plus any four symptoms from the list are necessary and sufficient (once the exclusion and duration criteria are satisfied). As the symptoms listed in DSM-IV for major depressive episode are decidedly heterogeneous, subjects with very different patterns of symptoms may be included in the same category (Table 3.2).

The cases described by the two patterns of symptoms are obviously clinically different and do not seem to share any other characteristics apart from the inclusion criteria for the same category. With this classification system, we risk producing something similar to 'the category of objects with four legs, including tables, dogs and fourth degree equations' (Robert Musil, *The Man without Qualities*). This concept introduces the following: if a certain number of the listed symptoms is necessary and sufficient for diagnosing of major depression, all the symptoms hold the same weight in defining diagnosis and severity.

TABLE 3.2   Example of two subjects with very different patterns of symptoms included in the same category (depression) according to DSM-IV criteria

		Case 1
	Anhedonia	
	Psychomotor retardation	
	Inappropriate guilt	
Depressed mood	Weight loss	
Diminished interest or please	Early waking	
Weight loss/gain		
Insomnia/hypersomnia		
Psychomotor agitation/retardation		Case 2
Fatigue, loss of energy		
Worthlessness, inappropriate guilt	Depressed mood	
	Difficulty in falling asleep	
	Fatigue	
	Diminished concentration	
	Weight gain	

Faravelli et al. (1996) tried to verify this hypothesis. They evaluated: (i) whether a greater number of symptoms reflects increasing severity; (ii) whether all the symptoms have comparable weight in establishing the gradient of severity. If a greater number of symptoms reflected an increasing severity, the number of symptoms would be positively associated with other indicators of severity and the total number of symptoms would be correlated with other indicators of severity more than any single symptom. The external indicators of severity considered in this study were the Global Assessment of Functioning (GAF) scale (Endicott et al., 1976) and the Clinical Global Impression (CGI; APA, 1994). The GAF and CGI scores correlated with the number of symptoms, but the correlation rates were much higher with some specific symptoms. Moreover, in several stepwise regression analyses, severity was explained by a few specific symptoms, whereas the number of symptoms had marginal, nonsignificant weight. These symptoms were depressed mood, delusion, social withdrawal, psychic retardation and somatic retardation. In addition, melancholic depression differed from non-melancholic depression and psychotic depression differed from non-psychotic depression, even after correcting for the different number of symptoms. This study shows that certain depressive symptoms have greater weight in establishing the gradient of depression severity. Having these symptoms also increases the risk of having many other symptoms; this implies that certain symptoms alone are more specifically associated with the severity and pervasiveness of the disorder. The symptoms associated with a greater severity of the syndrome are generally considered a part of the melancholic (or somatic, or endogenous) pattern. Thus, according to the results of this study, ignoring the qualitative approach does not seem to be correct.

(b) Unipolar versus Bipolar

In the present classifications the first step is that of distinguishing the bipolar disorders from the unipolar ones. This decision is clearly impossible to achieve and causes bipolars to be classified as unipolars in most cases.

(a)   Depression precedes mania/hypomania in about 50% of the cases and the first episode of mania may occur even late in life. As a consequence, up to 30% of unipolars become bipolars during follow-up (Akiskal, 1995).

(b)   The diagnosis of mania/hypomania is ruled out if the patient manifests these symptoms during treatment with antidepressants. Since almost all the cases with depression are treated with antidepressants, one of the typical patterns of bipolarity, i.e. that where the episode starts with depression and naturally shifts into mania later (the so-called DM pattern) is by definition prevented from receiving the correct label.

(c)   There is consistent evidence that the phenomenon of mania may be graduated according to a gradient of severity, ranging from the most severe forms of delirious mania to the mildest forms, where bipolarity presents with hyperthymic temperament. All the studies on the bipolar spectrum seem to reach the conclusion that bipolarity may exist even in absence of manifest mania. This is in striking accordance with Kraepelin's original concept of manic-depressive illness.

Klerman (1981) identified the 'mania spectrum' in the early 1980s, including normal elation, neurotic elation, hypomania, mania and delirious mania. The presence, in the past, of a diagnosis from the mania spectrum (excluding normal elation) led to the concept of the 'bipolar disorder'. Among the subtypes of bipolarism, Klerman also included depressed subjects with a familial history of bipolar disorders. His work influenced the definition of the bipolar spectrum concept.

Later, Akiskal (1983) formulated the concept of the bipolar spectrum, placing different forms of recurrent depression, including type I bipolar, atypical bipolar, cyclothymic, dysthymic and other types with intermediate pictures. This concept of spectrum includes heterogeneous clinical pictures with a partially superimposed symptomatology, supposing that they are different expressions of a basic pathology, 'the bipolar disorder'.

(c) Sub-threshold Depression

Operational criteria require in order to qualify for a diagnosis: (a) certain symptoms, (b) in a given minimum number, (c) for a given period of time. Consequently, subjects with (a) a nontypical symptom pattern, (b) with an insufficient number of symptoms, (c) with a duration shorter than required cannot receive the diagnosis. This implies the existence of subthreshold disorders, where there are three different possibilities of being subthreshold (Table 3.3).

For major depression, let us imagine a patient presenting with depressed mood, delusion of guilt, psychomotor agitation, worse in the morning and lack of sexual desire. Since neither diurnal variation nor sexual desire are listed among the symptoms for major depressive episode diagnosis in DSM-IV, this patient does not meet criterion A and cannot be given a diagnosis of major depressive episode.

Another frequent possibility is that of a patient who satisfies the criteria, but the length of the episode is lesser than the required two weeks.

Subthreshold depression has been extensively studied. In particular, Angst proposed the diagnosis of recurrent brief depression (Angst et al., 1984, 1990). Recurrent brief depression shows the same number of the same symptoms as major depression, but with a duration of less than two weeks; the recurrence is defined by the occurrence 12 times over one year at least. Recurrent brief depression causes impairment and distress equivalent to major depression, is associated with considerable suicidality and treatment-seeking and is often comorbid with anxiety disorders. It may develop into major depression and vice versa in about the same percentage of cases (12% vs 15% in a seven-year follow-up made during the Zurich study). Patients with combined major and recurrent brief depression are more severely affected, have a higher suicide attempt rate and an increased frequency of treatment-seeking than patients with only one condition.

Appendix B of DSM-IV (dealing with research instead of diagnostic criteria) discusses the 'minor depressive disorder' and the 'recurrent brief depressive disorder': the first one differs from 'major depression' in the number of symptoms (less than five but at least two, at least one should be depressed mood or anhedonia) and the second one differs from 'major depression' in its duration (less than two weeks but at least two days), with the additional criterion of recurrence (at least once a month for 12 months, with no relationship in women to the menstrual cycle). Other subtypes of depressive disorders, not yet recognized by DSM-IV, are identified on the basis of the subthreshold concept: i.e. 'subsyndromal symptomatic depression', defined as a depressive state having two or more symptoms of major depressive episodes, excluding depressed mood and anhedonia; the symptoms must be present for more than two weeks and be associated with social impairment (Sadek and Bona, 2000). Some studies refer to 'depressive symptoms', that are not recognizable in any of these disorders, but are considered clinically meaningful.

TABLE 3.3   Possible definitions of subthreshold disorders

Subthreshold

1. Symptom(s) below the level of definite (very mild or fluctuating).
2. Fewer symptoms than required.
3. Duration shorter than required.

It has been found that the subthreshold forms of depression may be at least as disruptive, in terms of quality of life, suicide, mortality, as the full-blown forms.

DIFFERENT PERSPECTIVES IN THE CLASSIFICATION OF DEPRESSION

Spectrum

The concept of the 'spectrum' is similar to but conceptually different from that of the 'subthreshold'. In this case, the nearness to the central nucleus of the disorder is viewed as qualitative rather than quantitative (subthreshold is 'a bit less' than the typical disorder, while spectrum is 'similar' to the typical disorder).

The term 'spectrum' is at present used in psychopathology with various meanings, but it generally indicates a group of manifestations having something in common. We can essentially distinguish two principal meanings, spectrum as a combination of disorders and spectrum as a combination of symptoms and signs correlated to a disorder. In discussing depression the term 'spectrum' is also used to indicate a variety of meanings.

One way of using the expression 'depressive spectrum' was derived from the attempt of Winokur et al. (1975) to separate homogeneous forms from the heterogeneous picture of unipolar depression. This author distinguished, between familiar depression, sporadic depression and other heterogeneous forms, collected under the 'depressive spectrum' heading. These forms shared special personality traits. This concept of spectrum largely superimposed the concepts of neurotic and secondary depression.

Akiskal et al. (1980) similarly identified, among the 'characterial depressions', the 'character spectrum disorders', a heterogeneous group of personality disorders with secondary and inconstant dysphoria that is seen more frequently among women, is often complicated by alcohol and other substance use, and responds poorly to therapy.

Alarcon et al. (1987) attempted to better define the concept of 'affective spectrum'. The characteristics of spectrum are not only the heterogeneity and the presence of similar phenomena, but there are also some similarities at other levels, such as borderline or related to borderline personality, a tendency to be chronic, the possibility that depressive symptoms are influenced by environmental stimuli, familial predisposition, poor response to therapies. This concept of spectrum also provides a heterogeneous picture, in which there are some similar phenomena (linking partially superimposed clinical pictures) strongly linked to personality (often it is difficult to distinguish whether the phenomena observed are symptoms of illness or personality traits). The other characteristics mentioned above confirm the validity of the grouping, but they cannot be considered criteria for defining the spectrum.

These three concepts of the depressive spectrum were largely overlapping: they were based on the presence of similar phenomena and common characteristics of personality. Nevertheless, these personality characteristics have never been well defined and the clinical spectrum of depression has been delimited not because of unique personality characteristics, but as a concept that compiles the clinical entities that are not included in much better defined diagnostic categories of depression.

Hudson and Pope (1990) proposed another interpretation of the 'affective spectrum'. These authors grouped together many heterogeneous disorders, all responsive to SSRI therapy: major depression, bulimia nervosa, panic disorder, obsessive-compulsive disorder, attention deficit disorder with hyperactivity, cataplexy, migraine and irritable bowel syndrome. According to these authors, these different clinical forms share common pathogenetic pathways, which is the reason for their common response to the SSRI.

According to Angst et al. (1984, 1991, 1997a, 1997b), there is a *continuum* between normal and pathological depressed mood. He used the term 'depressive spectrum' to define a group of depressive disorders including major depression and dysthymia and syndromes that actually do not satisfy specific diagnostic criteria, but usually improve with antidepressant treatment and have a similar longitudinal course to depression. In fact, the different subtypes of depression above or under 'threshold' (major depressive disorder, dysthymia, brief recurrent depression, minor depression) have poor longitudinal stability. This suggests that depression is better defined by a continuous spectrum rather than as a group of discrete subtypes.

Some authors (Akiskal et al., 1989; Cassano et al., 1989) define the spectrum as including nuclear and subthreshold symptoms of the disorder, atypical symptoms, isolated symptoms and signs, temperamental and personality traits. Within the framework of this definition in regard to the mood spectrum, they classified a series of manifestations related to mood disorders as defined by the current diagnostic manuals: precursors, prodromes, typical forms, residual symptoms, subthreshold episodes, post-episodic modifications of character, post-episodic maladjustment, early onset persistent subthreshold symptoms, atypical forms and subthreshold unipolar or bipolar comorbidity.

Temperament/Premorbid Personality/Structure

The concepts of temperament/premorbid personality/structure are included in some concepts of spectrum and in the concept of subthreshold.

Temperament plays an important role in all of the European psychopathological tradition. Psychopathologists defined four major affective temperaments: cyclothymic, hyperthymic, depressive and irritable. The European psychopathological tradition looked with great emphasis at affective temperaments linked to mood, but there are also some models that do not specifically consider the relationship between temperament and mood (e.g. Cloninger's theory; Cloninger et al., 1993). The current classification systems do not take the concept of temperament into account. DSM-IV considers dysthymia and cyclothymia only when they reach the threshold to define a full axis I disorder, i.e. when they provoke a clinically meaningful subjective suffering or psychosocial impairment. There are different hypotheses regarding the relationship between affective temperaments and mood disorders: viewing temperament as an attenuated form of the illness, as a predisposing factor, as prodromes or sequelae, or as a factor with pathoplastic action.

Personality and character are two concepts similar to the notion of temperament. Personality is a pervasive pattern used by a subject in order to relate to, perceive and reflect on his environment and himself. Personality traits are prominent aspects of personality and do not imply a pathology. Personality disorders are pervasive and maladaptive patterns causing significant impairment in adaptive functioning or subjective distress. Personality includes temperament, which is the most biological aspect (innate, genetically determined) and character, which represents temperament coping with the environment. The premorbid personality, that represents personality characteristics before the onset of the disorder, tries to delineate temperamental traits of the subject. Studying the subthreshold of the various spectra tends to bring us back to the old concept of the premorbid personality.

By the term 'structure', we are referring to the structure of personality, which is similar to the basic nucleus of the individual, from which psychopathological traits may develop.

The description of temperamental/personality features has been one of the fundamental aspects in reporting the clinical picture of psychiatric disorders for over a century, and the base for developing some of the basic theories of mental illnesses (e.g. Kretschmer, 1936; Freud, 1917).

Paying greater attention to temperamental aspects and personality would probably improve the classification of mood and other psychiatric disorders.

'Functionalization' of Psychiatric Diagnoses

According to Van Praag (1997), psychiatric disorders are the resultants of the various combinations of psychological dysfunctions ('functionalization' of psychiatric diagnoses); each psychological dysfunction may be present in several disorders (see Chapter 17 by Van Praag).

Psychological dysfunctions are measurable, many of them quantitatively, by biological markers.

This trans-nosographical approach led to the only reliable finding of biological psychiatry, that is the reduction of the 5-hydroxyindolacetic acid in the liquor of patients with impulse discontrol (Van Praag 1982, 1986, 1995; Van Praag et al., 1986). According to Van Praag, serotoninergic functioning is disturbed in a subgroup of depression in which anxiety and/or aggressiveness are the primary psychopathological features (Van Praag, 1992a,b, 1996).

Following this approach, when a biological marker is identified, we could study all the subjects with this marker, independently of the diagnosis, to see whether they

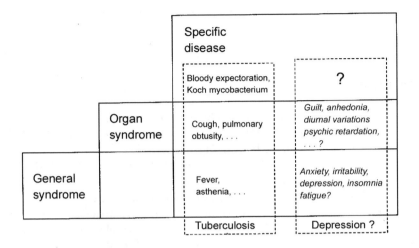

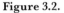

Figure 3.2.

have other common characteristics. For instance, the dexamethasone suppression test (DST) is positive in 40–60% of depressed patients (Carrol, 1982, 1984), 50% in patients with eating disorder, 30% in anxious patients and 10% in normal subjects (APA, 1987). Studying all the subjects who are non-suppressors to DST could hypothetically identify a homogeneous category (e.g. the category of stress-related disorders).

Different Organizational Models

In the current psychiatric classifications all the disorders are placed on the same level, say horizontally. However, in general medicine co-occurrent syndromes are usually placed according to a pyramidal shape (Fig 3.2): there is a general syndrome (e.g. fever, asthenia), an organ syndrome (e.g. cough and pulmonary obtusity stand for a respiratory syndrome) and specific symptoms (i.e. mean TBC). This concept is absent in psychiatry.

In our opinion, it could be worth exploring the possibility that even in psychiatry the simple transversal, 'either–or', 'separate box' model is improbable. For instance, in depression the symptoms could be distinguished into different levels:

- general symptoms: stress-related, unspecific, present in most psychiatric disorders, comparable to a general medical syndrome;

- some more specific (pathognomonic) symptoms and signs, comparable to a specific medical disease.

CONCLUSION

In this chapter, a series of criticisms of current classifications, and particularly of DSM-IV, have been raised. Actually, these criticisms involve the way DSM-IV is commonly used, rather than the body of the manual.

One of the most common mistakes is treating DSM-IV disorders as if they were illnesses (van Praag's 'premature nosologization').

The second mistake is confounding diagnostic criteria with the clinical description of a given disorder. The clinical picture is much more articulated and largely exceeds the simple list of criteria. DSM-IV is a multiaxial classification: using, in practice, only axis one consistently reduces the power of the instrument. Moreover, with regard to the use of axis one, codifying by the fifth digit and eventually characterizing by other specifiers of the clinical picture and of the clinical course is required and would ameliorate the quality of the diagnosis (e.g. reporting of 'major depressive disorder, severe with psychotic features' – 296.23 – implies much more information than the simple 'major depressive disorder, single episode' – 296.2. Another way to better describe a disorder is to take into account comorbid conditions. DSM-III was a hierarchical system, but DSM-III-R allowed comorbidity, and DSM-IV requires noting and reporting multiple diagnoses: a patient with major depressive episode comorbid with panic disorder is likely to be different from a case comorbid with, say, obsessive-compulsive disorder.

We believe that the proper and complete use of DSM-IV, would greatly improve our clinical and research practice.

REFERENCES

Akiskal HS (1995) Developmental pathways to bipolarity: are juvenile-onset depressions pre-bipolar? *J Am Acad Child Adolesc Psychiatry* **34**(6): 754–763.

Akiskal HS (1983) The bipolar spectrum: new concepts in classification and diagnosis. In Grispoon L (ed.) *Psychiatry Update*. Washington, DC: American Psychiatric Press.

Akiskal HS, Cassano GB, Musetti L, Perugi G, Tundo A, Mignani V (1989) Psychopathology, temperament, and past course in primary major depressions. 1. Review of evidence for a bipolar spectrum. *Psychopathology* **22**(5): 268–277.

Akiskal HS, Rosenthal TL, Haykal RF, Lemmi H, Rosenthal RH, Scott-Strauss A (1980) Characterological depressions. Clinical and sleep EEG findings separating 'subaffective dysthymias' from 'character spectrum disorders'. *Arch Gen Psychiatry* **37**: 777–783.

Alarcon RD, Walter-Ryan WG, Rippetoe PA (1987) Affective spectrum disorders. *Compr Psychiatry* **28**: 292–308.

Angst J, Dobler-Mikola A (1984) The Zurich study. II. The continuum from normal to pathological depressive mood swings. *Eur Arch Psychiatry Neurol Sci* **234**: 21–29.

Angst J, Merikangas K et al. (1990) Recurrent brief depression: a new subtype of affective disorder. *J Affect Dis* **19**: 97–98.

Angst J, Merikangas KR, Preising M (1997a) The depressive spectrum: diagnostic classification and course. *J Affect Disord* **45**: 31–39.

Angst J, Merikangas KR, Preisig M (1997b) Subthreshold syndromes of depression and anxiety in the community. *J Clin Psychiatry* **58**(Suppl 8): 6–10.

Angst J, Wicki W (1991) The Zurich Study. XI. Is dysthymia a separate form of depression? Results of the Zurich Cohort Study. *Eur Arch Psychiatry Clin Neurosci* **240**: 349–354.

Angst J (1966) Zur Etiologie und Nosologie Endogener Depressiver Psychosen. *Berlin: Springer.*

APA (1980) *Diagnostic and Statistical Manual of Mental Disorders* (DSM-III) 3rd edition. Washington, DC, APA.

APA (1987) *Diagnostic and Statistical Manual of Mental Disorders* (DSM-III-R) 3rd edition revised. Washington, DC, APA.

APA (1994) *Diagnostic and Statistical Manual of Mental Disorders* (DSM-IV) 4th edition. Washington, DC, American Psychiatric Association.

Biswanger L (1960) Melancholie und Manie: Phaenomenologische studien. Pfullingen: Guenter Nescher.

Carney MPW, Roth M, Garside RF (1965) The diagnosis of depressive syndromes and the prediction of ECT response. *Br J Psychiatry* **3**: 659–674

Carpenter WT, Bunney WE Jr (1971) Adrenal cortical activity in depressive illness. *Am J Psychiatry* **128**: 31–40.

Carrol BJ (1984) Dexamethasone suppression test: a review of contemporary confusion. *J Clin Psychiatry* **46**(2 sec 2): 13–24.

Carrol BJ (1982) The dexamethasone suppression test for melancholia. *Br J Psychopharmacology* **81**: 309.

Cassano GB, Akiskal HS, Musetti L, Perugi G, Soriani A, Mignani V (1989) Psychopathology, temperament, and past course in primary major depressions. 2. Toward a redefinition of bipolarity with a new semistructured interview for depression. *Psychopathology* **22**(5): 278–288.

Cloninger CR, Svrakic DGF, Przybeck TR (1993) A psychobiological model of temperament and character. *Arch Gen Psychiatry* **50**: 975–990.

Cohen IH (1987) Masked depression revisited. *Md Med J* **36**(7): 571.

Detre TP, Jarecki H (1971) *Modern Psychiatric Treatment. Philadelphia, PA: Lippincott.*

Endicott J, Spitzer RL, Fleiss J et al. (1976) The Global Assessment Scale: a procedure for measuring overall severity of psychiatric disturbance. *Arch Gen Psychiatry* **33**: 766–771.

Faravelli C, La Malfa G, Romano S. (1985) Circadian rhythm in primary affective disorder. *Compr Psychiatry* **26**: 364–389

Faravelli C, Servi P, Arends JA, Strik WK (1996) Number of symptoms, qualification, and quantification of depression. *Compr Psych* **37**(5): 307–315.

Fava G (1999) Subclinical symptoms in mood disorders: pathophysiological and therapeutic implications. *Psychol Med* **29**: 47–61.

Feighner JP, Robins E et al. (1972) Diagnostic criteria for use in psychiatric research. *Arch Gen Psych* **26**: 57–63.

Freud S (1917) *Trauer und Melancholie* (Trans *Lutto e Melanconia*). In Freud S *Opere 1915–17, vol 9. Turin: Boringhieri.*

Garside RF, Kay DV, Wilson IC, Deaton ID, Roth M (1971) Depressive syndromes and the classification of patients. *Psychol Med* **1**(4): 333–338.

Garside RF, Roth M (1978) Multivariate statistical methods and problems of classification in psychiatry. *Br J Psychiatry* **133**: 53–67.

Hawkins DR, Mendels J (1966) Sleep disturbance in depressive syndromes. *Am J Psychiatry* **123**(6): 682–690.

Hudson JI, Pope HG Jr (1990) Affective spectrum disorder: does antidepressant response identify a family of disorders with a common pathophysiology? *Am J Psychiatry* **147**: 552–564.

Jaspers K (1959) *Allgemeine Psychopathologie*. Berlin: Springer Verlag.

Kant I (1781) *Critica della ragion pura*.

Keller MB, Klerman GL, Lavori PV (1984) Long-term outcome of episodes of major depression. *JAMA* **252**: 761–768.

Kendell RE (1969a) The classification of depressive illness. The uses and limits of multivariate analysis. *Psychiatr Neurol Neurochir* **72**: 207–216.

Kendell RE (1969b) The continuum model of depressive illness. *Proc Roy Soc Med* **62**: 335–339.

Kendell RE (1970) The classification of depressive illness. *Br J Psychiatry* **117** (538): 347–348.

Kendell RE (1972) Endogenous and neurotic depression. *Br J Psychiatry* **121** (564): 575.

Kendell RE (1976) The classification of depression: a review of contemporary confusion. *Br J Psychiatry* **129**: 15–28.

Kendell RE, Everett B, Cooper JE, Sartorius N, David ME (1968) The reliability of the 'Present State Examination'. *Soc Psychiat* **3**: 123–129.

Kendell RE, Gourlay J (1970) The clinical distinction between psychotic and neurotic depression. *Br J Psychiatry* **117** (538): 257–260.

Kielholz P (1979) [The concept of masked depression (author's transl)]. *Encephale* **5** (5 Suppl): 459–462.

Kiloh LG, Garside RF (1963) The independence of neurotic depression and endogenous depression. *Br J Psychiatry* **109**: 451–463.

Kimura Bin (1992) *Écrits de Psychopathologie Phénomenologique*. Paris: Presses Universitaires de France.

Klerman GL (1981) The spectrum of mania. *Compr Psychiatry* **22**: 11–20.

Kraepelin E (1896) *Lehrbuch der Psychiatrie*. Leipzig: Barth.

Kretschmer E (1936) *Koerperbau und Charakter*. Berlin: Springer.

Leonhard K (1957) *Aufteilung der Endogenen Psychosen*. Berlin: Academic-Verlag.

Lesse S (1977) Masked depression and depressive equivalents [proceedings]. *Psychopharmacol Bull* **13** (1): 68–70.

Lopez-Ibor Alino JJ (1976) Depressive equivalents and masked depression. *Bibl Psychiatr* **152**: 35–75.

Perris C (1996a) A study of bipolar (manic-depressive) and unipolar recurrent depressive psychoses. Introduction. *Acta Psychiatr Scand* **194**: 9–14.

Perris C (1996b) A study of bipolar (manic-depressive) and unipolar recurrent depressive psychoses. XI Therapy and prognosis. *Acta Psych Scand* **42** (Suppl 194): 153–171.

Pflug B, Johnsson D, Tveito Ekse D (1981) Manic-depressive state and daily temperature. *Acta Psychiatr Scand* **63**: 277–289.

Pichot P (1986) Classification of depressive states. *Psychopathology* **19** (Suppl 2): 12–16.

Roth M, Garside RF, Gurney C, Kerr TA (1979) Psychotic and neurotic depression: a reply on method. *Br J Psychiatry* **135**: 94–96.

Roth M, Gurney C, Garside RF, Kerr TA (1972) Studies in classification of affective disorders. The relationship between anxiety state and depressive illnesses. I. *Br J Psychiatry* **121** (561): 147–171.

Sachar EJ, Hellman L, Roffwarg H, Halpern F, Fuskushima D, Gallagher T (1973) Disrupted 24-hour patterns of cortisol secretion in psychiatric depression. *Arch Gen Psychiatry* **28**: 19–24.

Sadek N, Bona J (2000) Subsyndromal symptomatic depression: a new concept. *Depress Anxiety* **12** (1): 30–39.

Spitzer RL, Endicott J, Robins E (1978) Research Diagnostic Criteria: rationale and reliability. *Arch Gen Psych* **35**: 773–779.

Tellenbach H (1960) *Melancholie*. Berlin: Springer.

Van Praag HM (1982) Depression, suicide and the metabolism of serotonin in the brain. *Affect Disord* **4**(4): 275–290.

Van Praag HM (1986) Affective disorders and aggression disorders: evidence for a common biological mechanism. *Suicide Life Threat Behav* **16**(2): 103-132.

Van Praag HM (1992a) About the centrality of mood lowering in mood disorders. *Eur Neuropsychopharmacol* **2**: 393–402.

Van Praag HM (1992b) *Make-believe in Psychiatry or the Perils of Progress.* New York: Brunner Mazel.

Van Praag HM (1995): Comorbidity (psycho-) analysed. *Br J Psychiatry* **168**: 129–134.

Van Praag HM (1996) Faulty cortisol/serotonin interplay: psychopathological and biological characterisation of a new hypothetical depression subtype (SeCa depression). *Psychiatry Res* **65**: 145–167.

Van Praag HM (1997) Over the mainstream: diagnostic requirements for biological psychiatric research. *Psychiatry Res* **72**: 201–212.

Van Praag HM, Plutchik R, Conte H (1986) The serotonin hypothesis of (auto)aggression. Critical appraisal of the evidence. *Ann N Y Acad Sci* **487**: 150–167.

Winokur G, Cadoret R, Baker M, Dorzab J (1975) Depression spectrum disease versus pure depressive disease: Some further data. *Br J Psychiatry* **127**: 75–77.

World Health Organization (1992) *The International Classification of Diseases* 10th revision (ICD-10). Geneva: OMS.

4

Bipolar Disorder

Leonardo Tondo
University of Cagliari, Cagliari, Italy

INTRODUCTION

Bipolar disorder (BPD), the current definition of the more classical manic-depressive illness, is an episodic disease marked by oscillations in mood of variable intensity from depression (melancholia) to hypomania or mania. Thinking, energy, and behaviour can also change in a way that affects the individual's occupational, social and interpersonal relationships (Goodwin and Jamison, 1990; Sadock and Sadock, 2000).

HISTORY

Mania and melancholia were sufficiently well defined by the Hippocratic school (ca. 400 BC), but Aretaeus of Cappadocia (AD 150) first described the occurrence of mania and melancholia in the same person (Adams, 1856). Further developments of the syndrome reappeared in Western medical literature in the second half of the nineteenth century with the descriptions of *folie circulaire* or *folie a double forme* by Baillarger and Falret. Kraepelin (1921) is credited for the most systematic, comprehensive and influential description of manic-depressive insanity (Baldessarini, 2000).

Kleist and Leonhard (Angst and Marneros, 2001) in the 1950s further classified the syndrome in bipolar (manic and depressive) and unipolar (depressive) forms of recurrent major mood disorders. Some twenty years later, Dunner and Fieve (1974) recognized the necessity of subdividing BPD into types I and II, in order to distinguish the syndromes according to the presence of mania vs. hypomania, respectively, in association with depressive episodes. In the same period, Akiskal et al. (1977) proposed the notion of bipolar spectrum disorder,

Mood Disorders: Clinical Management and Research Issues. Edited by E. J. L. Griez, C. Faravelli, D. J. Nutt and J. Zohar.
©2005 John Wiley & Sons Ltd. ISBN 0 470 09426 5.

ranging from minor cyclothymic syndromes to severe psychotic bipolar forms (Akiskal et al., 2000). Since Kraepelin, BPD has been known as a relatively benign illness but more recent reports show a rate of chronicity varying from 10% to 20% (Angst, 1995; Angst and Sellaro, 2000).

EPIDEMIOLOGY

The lifetime prevalence of BPD has been estimated at 1.6% (for mania), but may increase to 2–5% if bipolar II and cyclothymic cases are included (Angst, 1995), representing about 30% of all major mood disorders. The incidence per year of bipolar I disorder is at least 0.05%. Women tend to be affected more than men with a ratio of 1.4:1, which is inferior to that found in nonbipolar major depressive disorder. The median age-at-onset is about 20 years (Goodwin and Jamison, 1990; APA, 2000). It has been suggested that all major mood disorders are more common in recent years compared to the past (Klerman, 1976). It is still debated, however, whether this increase is due to a better recognition of the illness or whether it is associated with the impact of substance abuse and other environmental aspects. Predisposing factors to the development of BPD are cyclothymic and hyperthymic temperaments, as well as childhood attention deficit hyperactivity disorder.

GENETICS

The involvement of genetic factors in the transmission of BPD has been demonstrated in twin, adoption, and family studies (Tsuang and Faraone, 1990). The risk of depression, psychosis or suicide in first-degree relatives and fraternal twins of index cases of BPD is 5–10%, but it is about 40–70% in identical twins with a risk ratio for monozygotic:dizygotic of about 8:1 (Craddock and Jones, 1999). A study reported that 61% of first-degree family members of BPD patients had some type of mood disorder, and about 30% had a type of bipolar disorder (Tondo et al., 1998a). Reports from rare adoption studies show more affective illness and suicides among biological relatives than in the adopting family (Mitchell et al., 1993). Despite this epidemiological evidence, neither a specific mode of inheritance, nor a discrete genetic marker to BPD has yet been identified, more likely than not because the inheritance is associated with the interaction of more than one gene and of environmental factors. With the development of the human genome project it will be possible to identify the genes predisposing to BPD and the brain proteins coded for it. This will hopefully allow for the development of improved therapeutic and preventive strategies.

BIOLOGY

Other biological findings also are far from definitive (Nemeroff, 1999). The findings from structural and functional brain imaging techniques remain limited and inconclusive. Older biochemical findings in measurements of stress-sensitive neurotransmitters and neurohormones have proved nonspecific by diagnosis. The short REM sleep latency in mania and severe depression associated with a disregulation of the cholinergic system are mainly state-dependent and not necessarily clues to biological causes of the disorder (Nemeroff, 1999). A serotonergic deficiency associated with aggression and suicide has been reported but not found to be specific to BPD. Some cognitive and other neuropsychological deficits have also been identified in BPD, and some may be not associated with the acute episodes of illness (Mayberg et al., 1997). It has been hypothesized that a GABAergic deficiency may contribute to mood instability and that a manic state is sustained by increased noradrenergic and dopaminergic activity (Swann et al., 1994; McTavish et al., 2001). Brain imaging techniques have shown specific abnormalities in the white matter of the brain of BPD patients (Soares and Mann, 1997).

SYMPTOMS

Mania is characterized by an elevated or irritable mood, pressured speaking, increased physical activity, increased or uninhibited sexual drive, and decreased need for sleep. Cognitive disturbances include rapid, overproductive, semilogical thinking, the content of which may refer to increased self-esteem and grandiosity. Patients may continuously change topics and use loose connections; their attention may also be impaired by a high level of distractibility. Attempts to interrupt increased activities may provoke irritable or angry responses. Overactivity may include incessant, disorganized, or aimless motion. Social, interpersonal, and occupational functioning may be disturbed by excessive self-confidence, lack of inhibition, intrusiveness, impulsivity, recklessness, irritability, and sometimes aggressiveness. Risk-taking is common, and may include unrealistic plans or business initiatives, overspending, reckless driving, with or without abuse of alcohol or illicit drugs. Psychotic features may be present with grandiose delusions based on religion and power or persecutory ideation related to the belief of being an important person. Hallucinatory phenomena may more rarely occur with the same grandiose content. The mood-altered state is defined as being hypomanic if most of the described symptoms are present, with the exception of the psychotic features, and there is no substantial impairment in social, interepersonal, or occupational functioning. In both cases, but to a different extent, judgement may be impaired (APA, 2000).

The symptomatology of depression in a BPD does not differ from that in unipolar recurrent depression. It is mainly characterized by depressed mood, psychomotor retardation with a low level of energy, lassitude, decreased sexual drive, changes in appetite and weight loss, and sleep disturbances. Thinking processes are slow, attention is impaired by lack of interest, memory processes are impaired as well, reaction times are prolonged, problem-solving strategies are limited, and feelings of guilt, worthlessness, self-blame, despair, hopelessness may be present. Suicidal thoughts, gestures, or attempts may occur. Self-esteem is usually low with unrealistic, negative and pessimistic self-evaluation. Somatic complaints such as headaches, muscular aches, gastrointestinal, respiratory, cardiac, and other vegetative symptoms, may be present and more prominent than psychic symptoms. Psychotic features may be present with content of pessimism, nihilism, worthlessness, self-blame, and guilt. Persecutory ideation and delusions may stem from the idea of receiving a just punishment. Perception disturbances and hallucinations may more rarely occur. Depressive symptomatology may impair the persons' social, interpersonal, and occupational functioning, and their judgement capacity at various levels (APA, 2000).

A combination of depressive and manic symptoms occurring at the same time or in rapid alternation of hours or days is defined as a mixed episode. Agitated depression and dysphoric mania are the most common expressions of a mixed state (Cassidy et al., 1998; Koukopoulos and Koukopoulos, 1999). In the former case, a patient may communicate depressive feelings along with subjective or objective agitation, irritability, internal rage, and racing thoughts (Koukopoulos and Koukopoulos, 1999; Perugi et al., 2001). Koukopoulos and Koukopoulos (1999) propose three criteria for the diagnosis of agitated depression: motor agitation, psychic agitation with intense inner tension, and racing or crowded thoughts. A dysphoric manic patient may be dysphoric, agitated, aggressive, suicidal, with feelings of guilt, and irritable (McElroy et al., 1992; Cassidy et al., 1998; Cassidy and Carroll, 2001). This mood state has been considered either a form of mania, or a more severe form of mania, or a transitional state from mania to depression (McElroy et al., 1992). A correct diagnosis of mood mixed states is important because they tend to have more hospitalizations, a higher chance of suicidal behaviour, and a worse response to long-term treatments (Post et al., 1989).

BPDs are diagnosed when one or more depressive episodes are preceded or followed by one or more manic or hypomanic episodes over the years. Bipolar types I or II describe the occurrence of at least one episode of mania or hypomania, respectively. BP II disorder is found in 13–20% of all bipolar patients and is more frequent in women (Tondo et al., 1998a). The worldwide lifetime rate of BPD varies from 0.3% to 1.5% (Weissman et al., 1996). Both types are recognized in the World Health Organization's *International Classification of Diseases* (ICD-10; WHO 2000) and the American Psychiatric Association's *Diagnostic and Statistical Manual of Mental Disorders* (DSM-IV-TR; APA 2000). The latter also recognizes rapid-cycling BPD, with at least four episodes of mania or depression within 12 months of clinical assessment (Dunner and Fieve, 1974; APA, 2000).

COMORBIDITY

BPDs often show features of other psychiatric syndromes, especially anxiety disorders (Clayton, 1990; Angst, 1996; Pini et al., 1997; Angst, 1998; Cassano et al., 1999; McElroy et al., 2001; Yerevanian et al., 2001; Rihmer et al., 2001). A recent review shows an average of about 21% of co-occurrence of any anxiety disorder in patients with BPD (Tondo et al., 2003c). In addition, the co-occurrence of alcohol or drug abuse in BPD ranges between 40% and 60% (Regier et al., 1990; Strakowski et al., 1998; Sonne and Brady, 1999; McElroy et al., 2001). The comorbidity of BPD and other DSM-IV disorders from Axis I and II can severely complicate the clinical evaluation and treatment of the illness, and can increase suicide risk and worsen the overall prognosis (Young et al., 1993; Vieta et al., 2000; Freeman et al., 2002). Whether substance abuse is a contributing cause of BPD, or the disorder favours addictive behaviour remains unresolved. BPD is also frequently associated with attention deficit hyperactivity disorder (Milberger et al., 1995; Biederman et al., 1996; Pliszka, 1998; Sachs et al., 2001).

PSYCHOLOGY

From a psychological perspective, bipolar mood disorder is characterized by narcissistic features, lack of empathy, and unstable interpersonal relationships. The predominant defence mechanisms are denial in mania, and self-aggressiveness against internalized object loss in depression. Phenomenologically, mania has been interpreted as the result of an attempt to compensate for depressive feelings, while depression as an expression of guilt for the manic behaviour. Behaviouristic theories see depression as a consequence of learned helplessness after repeated unavoidable experiences, and cognitive approaches see it as an expression of negative self-evaluation and beliefs activated by stress. In both mood expressions, personality traits may include emotional dependence, lack of awareness of internal emotional responses in oneself or others, and of appreciation of differences between actual and idealized situations.

COURSE OF THE ILLNESS

The onset of BPD may not be easily recognized as such, and appropriate diagnosis and treatment may be delayed by several years. The illness may start in adolescence, more rarely before puberty with differential diagnostic challenges from attention/hyperactivity or conduct disorders (Papolos and Papolos, 2000). The initial typical episode is a mania or hypomania, particularly in men, whereas an initial depressive episode is more common in women. Women also tend to have more type II bipolar illness and prominent depressive episodes (Tondo et al., 1998a). In some cases of recurrent depression, mania or hypomania emerge later, sometimes during treatment with an antidepressant medicine.

The natural duration of untreated episodes of mania or bipolar depression is about 2–9 months, with approximately yearly recurrences (Angst and Sellaro, 2000; DSM-IV, 2000). With adequate medical treatments, the duration of acute episodes of mania is about 1–2 months, while depressive episodes may last 2–4 months. The frequency of untreated manic episodes may be more common than depressive episodes, but patients spend more time in depression than mania over years of bipolar illness (Angst, 1978; Tondo et al., 1998a).

Single episodes of mania and single cycles of depression accompanied by mania or hypomania occur in a few cases. Recurrent episodes, on the other hand, are more common and their frequency tends to increase over the years. It has been shown that about 90% of individuals with a single manic episode have future recurrences. Initial inter-episode time periods may average 2–3 years in young adults, but these intervals tend to shorten to 8–9 months after 6–8 recurrences; and the total time spent in illness is about 20–47% (Angst, 1978; Angst and Sellaro, 2000; Judd and Akiskal, 2002); and mainly in depression, 32% of the time (Judd and Akiskal, 2002). A minority of BPD patients estimated at about 15% eventually follow a more or less chronic course.

BPD with onset in childhood may involve mood instability and behavioural problems over months or years rather than a more defined recurrent course, which tends to become established during late adolescence or in young adults (Faedda et al., 1995; Shulman et al., 1995; Papolos and Papolos, 2000). Adolescent BPD affects about 1% of 14–18-year-olds, while about 6% of adolescents have experienced periods of irritability, mood disorder, and behavioural abnormalities without fulfilling the criteria for BPD or cyclothymia. All adolescents with these types of problems show higher rates of occupational, social, and interpersonal dysfunctioning as well as a higher chance of co-occurring anxiety, substance abuse, and other disruptive behaviours (Lewinsohn et al., 1995). The frequency of BPD with a later onset may be higher, and in many cases with an onset in the elderly the course may tend to chronicity more often and respond unfavourably to treatment (Shulman et al., 1995). The consequences of an early-onset BPD include poor academic functioning, interpersonal and family difficulties, increased risk of suicide attempts and use of alcohol, tobacco, and drugs, behavioural and legal problems (Birmaher and Heydl, 2001).

The sequence of manic and depressive episodes may follow a characteristic and repetitive pattern in some patients. The more frequent sequences are: manias or hypomanias preceding depressions (MDI) or vice versa (DMI), or with a continuously circular course (CC) with no free intervals (Angst, 1978; Kukopulos et al., 1980). Rapid-cycling course occurs in about 15% of reported treated cases, usually from specialized lithium clinics (Tondo and Baldessarini, 1998; Tondo et al., 2003a). The actual proportion of rapid cycling patients not attending such clinics has not been reported and is arguably lower. Rapid cycling is somewhat more common among women and persons with type II BPD (Tondo and Baldessarini, 1998). An uncertain proportion of cases of BPD follow a seasonal course, more commonly with depressions in autumn or winter and manias in spring or summer (Rosenthal and Wehr, 1987; Faedda et al., 1993a).

Since Kraepelin, BPD patients typically experience some degree of recovery between illness episodes; nevertheless, in a relevant proportion of them, the illness may lead to sustained functional problems in occupation, and social and interpersonal relationships, particularly in subjects with early onset, or psychotic symptoms (Tohen et al., 2000). The outcome may be less favourable if associated with either early or late onset age, presence of mixed or psychotic features, severe depression, and rapid cycling course (Goodwin and Jamison, 1990). The main reason for this poor outcome is attributable to a lower effect of medical treatments. Moreover, psychological and social consequences of the illness and its functional disturbances may profoundly affect the individual's self-esteem, and interpersonal relations which may worsen the illness itself.

MORTALITY

Premature mortality in BPD has to be associated mainly with suicide (Ahrens et al., 1995; Tondo et al., 2003b). Deaths attributed to suicide in mood disorders vary from the classical estimates of about 15% (Guze and Robins, 1970; Goodwin and Jamison, 1990; Angst and Preisig, 1995) to more recent and updated values of 6% (Inskip et al., 1998). Suicide attempts are frequent in bipolar disorder occurring in 20–40% of BPD patients (Tondo et al., 1998b; Weissman et al., 1996; Baldessarini et al., 2003) and their ratio with completed suicide is probably less than 5:1 compared to 20:1 in the general population (AAS, 2000). The implication is that BPD patients have a stronger intent to die and use methods of higher lethality than the general population. The depressive phase of a BPD carries the highest suicide risk, accounting for about three-quarters of all attempts and fatalities (Isometsá et al., 1994; Tondo et al., 1998b). Mixed states and agitated depressions may be at a higher risk for suicidal behaviour, but as they are less frequent than more typical episodes, they account for a lower proportion of suicidal behaviour (Koukopoulos and Koukopoulos, 1999). As in the general population, risk of completed suicide in BPD is greater in men than in women. Other risk factors include previous attempts, older age, family history of suicidal behaviour, and a comorbid abuse of alcohol or drugs.

Mortality rates in BPD are also elevated due to risk-taking behaviours, accidental deaths associated with alcohol and drug abuse, and the impact of stress-sensitive cardiovascular disorders with a mortality that is at least three times higher than in the general population (Ahrens et al., 1995; Baldessarini and Jamison, 1999).

CLINICAL MANAGEMENT

BPD requires careful clinical management. Manic patients need protection if they show impulsive, hostile or excessively uninhibited behaviour, or if they refuse treatment. They also need to be protected from others who may take advantage of their hypersexuality and prodigality. In extreme cases, patients may need to be committed to specialized hospital units. Hospitalization may be required for severely depressed patients because of a high risk of suicide or inability to care for themselves. Patients and their families also benefit from education about the illness, its treatment and expected course. Counselling is also useful to plan for the possible impact of the illness on career, financial and family planning.

DRUG TREATMENT

Treatment of acute bipolar episodes involves antidepressants for bipolar depression and mainly antipsychotics for mania (Baldessarini and Tarazi, 2000). Prolonged antidepressant treatments in bipolar depression may have a destabilizing effect in predisposed patients which manifests as an increased rate of mood-cycling or switching from depression to manic, mixed, or dysphoric states (Goodwin and Jamison, 1990). It has not been established whether tricyclic or monoamine oxidase inhibitors have a higher risk of inducing mood shifts than modern antidepressants. There is less evidence that antipsychotic or other sedatives used for the treatment of mania can induce depression in BPD. Electroconvulsive therapy may be a temporary alternative in severe cases and can be beneficial in manic, depressive and mixed episodes.

In addition to the treatment of acute episodes, BPD patients need to be treated for the prevention of the recurrences of mania and depression. Lithium salts are the best-established therapeutic strategy for this purpose (Cade, 1949; Baldessarini and Tarazi, 2000). The treatment tends to have a slow response at onset and may need to be adjuncted to an antipsychotic therapy in the treatment of acute mania. Lithium has complex and not completely explained effects on interneuronal signal transduction and on other molecular regulatory events in neurons (Nonaka et al., 1998; Manji et al., 2000). This agent is effective in prevention and delay of recurrences, and in lessening the intensity of manic and depressive states in about two-thirds of BPD patients over many years (Tondo et al., 1998a, 2001b). Owing to its limited safety margin, serum concentrations of lithium are monitored regularly, and are safe and effective in the range of 0.6–1.0 mEq/L. The frequency of adverse effects increase with higher lithium serum levels and may include tremor, polyuria, diarrhoea, nausea, weight gain, hypothyroidism and occasional severe impairment of renal function with uraemia. A serious problem of long-term lithium treatment is that abrupt or rapid discontinuation is often followed by a temporary greatly increased risk of recurrences of mania, depression, or suicidality, even after years of effective treatment (Faedda et al., 1993b; Baldessarini et al., 1999). Moreover, lithium treatment is the only long-term psychiatric treatment showing consistent evidence of reduction of suicidal behaviour of about 80% comparing periods of long-term treatment with lithium to periods without treatment (Tondo et al., 1998b, 2001a).

Alternative or adjunctive treatments to lithium include a growing number of anticonvulsants such as carbamazepine, valproic acid, lamotrigine, topiramate and gabapentin (De Leon, 2001; Macdonald and Young, 2002; Grunze and Walden, 2002). Valproic acid and its salts have been shown to have a particularly potent and rapid antimanic effect and are also employed empirically for maintenance treatment, although the long-term protective effects of this agent against recurrences of bipolar depression and mania are not fully proved (Bowden et al., 2000). Antipsychotic drugs in addition to their short-term antimanic effects, are also used to treat breakthrough episodes of mania, but their action in the prevention of recurrences of bipolar depression or mania for prolonged periods is not established. Clozapine has been tried for the treatment of resistant bipolar disorder (Suppes et al., 1999); olanzapine for the treatment of bipolar depression, especially with concomitant pscyhotic features (Rothschild et al., 1999), and for the acute treatment of mania (Tohen et al., 1999). Despite the testing and use of additional anticonvulsant, and of novel antipsychotics for the treatment of BPD, none has yet proved superior to lithium for long-term management of BPD.

PSYCHOSOCIAL INTERVENTIONS

Psychotherapeutic efforts are much less evaluated in bipolar than in depressive disorders, in part reflecting traditional views that bipolar patients are often less able to accept their condition as a disorder requiring treatment. The high rate of recurrences in many patients has, however, led to the use of psychotherapeutic interventions that seem to decrease the frequency of recurrences in adjunct to the pharmacological long-term treatments (Jamison, 1999). The most evaluated interventions include interpersonal psychotherapy (IPT), aimed at the improvement of coping strategies for social and interpersonal relationships; cognitive-behavioural therapy (CBT) which attempts to modify inappropriate, self-detrimental, or exaggerated concepts by encouraging development of more flexible schemas, and rehearsal of new cognitive and behavioural responses; interpersonal and social rhythm therapy (IPSRT), which helps to reorganize the everyday life, thus improving social relationships; family-focused therapy (FFT) aiming at reducing the level of distress within the patients' families. Psychoeducational and group-based or individual supportive treatments are also advisable (Huxley et al., 2000). In general, all psychosocial interventions should have a psychoeducational approach aimed at increasing knowledge and insight of the illness and recognizing the first symptoms before an acute episode occurs.

ACKNOWLEDGEMENTS

This study has been supported by the Stanley Medical Research Institute with an unlimited grant to Centro Lucio Bini, Cagliari; by NARSAD; and by private funders. Joseph P. Akeley provided editing assistance, and Giulio Ghiani provided valuable bibliographic assistance.

REFERENCES

Adams F (1856) *The Extant Works of Aretaeus, the Cappadocian.* The Sydenham Society, London.

Ahrens B, Müller-Oerlinghausen B, Schou M, Wolf T, Alda M, Grof E, Grof P, Lenz G, Simhandl C, Thau K, Vestergaard P, Wolf R, Möller HJ (1995) Excess cardiovascular and suicide mortality of affective disorders may be reduced by lithium prophylaxis. *J Affect Disord* **33**: 67–75.

Akiskal HS, Bourgeois ML, Angst J, Post R, Moller H, Hirschfeld R (2000) Re-evaluating the prevalence of and diagnostic composition within the broad clinical spectrum of BPDs. *J Affect Disord* **59** (Suppl 1): S5–S30.

Akiskal HS, Djenderedjian AM, Rosenthal RH, Khani MK (1977) Cyclothymic disorder: validating criteria for inclusion in the bipolar affective group. *Am J Psychiatry* **134**: 1227–1233.

AAS (2000) *Official 1998 Statistics.* American Association of Suicidology website, www.suicidology.org.

APA (2000) *Diagnostic and Statistical Manual of Mental Disorders*, 4th edition, text revision (DSM-IV-TR). Washington, DC: American Psychiatric Association.

Angst J (1978) The course of affective disorders: typology of bipolar manic-depressive illness. *Arch Psychiatrie Nervenkr* **226**: 65–73.

Angst J (1995) [Epidemiology of the bipolar spectrum.] *Encéphale* **21** (6): 37–42.

Angst J (1996) Comorbidity of mood disorders: a longitudinal prospective study. *Br J Psychiatry* **30** (Suppl): 31–37.

Angst J (1998) The emerging epidemiology of hypomania and bipolar II disorder. *J Affect Disord* **50**: 143–151.

Angst J, Marneros A. (2001) Bipolarity from ancient to modern times: conception, birth and rebirth. *J Affect Disord* **67**: 3–19.

Angst J, Preisig M (1995) Outcome of a clinical cohort of unipolar, bipolar and schizoaffective patients. Results of a prospective study from 1959 to 1985. *Schweiz Arch Neurol Psychiatr* **146**: 17–23.

Angst J, Sellaro R (2000) Historical perspectives and natural history of BPD. *Biol Psychiatry* **48**: 445–457.

Baldessarini RJ (2000) American biological psychiatry and psychopharmacology 1944–1994. In Menninger RW, Nemiah JC (eds) *American Psychiatry after World War II (1944–1994).* Washington, DC: American Psychiatric Press.

Baldessarini RJ, Jamison KR (1999) Effects of medical interventions on suicidal behavior: summary and conclusions. *J Clin Psychiatry* **60** (Suppl 2): 117–122.

Baldessarini RJ, Tarazi FI (2000) Drugs and the treatment of psychiatric disorders: antipsychotic and antimanic agents. In Hardman JG, Limbird LE, Molinoff PB, Ruddon RW, Gilman AG (eds) *Goodman & Gilman's The Pharmacological Basis of Therapeutics*, 10th edition. New York: McGraw-Hill.

Baldessarini RJ, Tondo L, Hennen J (2003) Lithium treatment and suicide risk in major affective disorders: update and new findings. *J Clin Psychiatry*, in press.

Baldessarini RJ, Tondo L, Viguera AC (1999) Effects of discontinuing lithium maintenance treatment. *Bipolar Disorder* **1**: 17–24.

Biederman J, Faraone S, Milberger S, Guite J, Mick E, Chen L, Mennin D, Marrs A, Ouellette C, Moore P, Spencer T, Norman D, Wilens T, Kraus I, Perrin J (1996) A prospective 4-

year follow-up study of attention-deficit hyperactivity and related disorders. *Arch Gen Psychiatry* **53**: 437–446.

Birmaher B, Heydl P (2001) Biological studies in depressed children and adolescents. *Int J Neuropsychopharmacol* **4**(2): 149–157.

Bowden CL, Calabrese JR, McElroy SL, Gyulai L, Wassef A, Petty F, Pope HG Jr, Chou JC, Keck PE Jr, Rhodes LJ, Swann AC, Hirschfeld RMA, Wozniak PJ (2000) Randomized, placebo-controlled trial of divalproex vs. placebo and lithium in maintenance therapy of bipolar disorders. *Arch Gen Psychiatry* **57**: 481–489.

Cade JFJ (1949) Lithium salts in the treatment of psychotic excitement. *Med J Austral* **2**: 349–352.

Cassano GB, Pini S, Saettoni M, Dell'Osso L (1999) Multiple anxiety disorder comorbidity in patients with mood spectrum disorders with psychotic features. *Am J Psychiatry* **156**: 474–476.

Cassidy F, Carroll BJ (2001) Frequencies of signs and symptoms in mixed and pure episodes of mania: implications for the study of manic episodes. *Prog Neuropsychopharmacol Biol Psychiatry* **25**(3): 659–665.

Cassidy F, Murry E, Forest K, Carroll BJ (1998) Signs and symptoms of mania in pure and mixed episodes. *J Affect Disord* **50**: 187–201.

Clayton PJ (1990) The comorbidity factor: establishing the primary diagnosis in patients with mixed symptoms of anxiety and depression. *J Clin Psychiatry* **51** (Suppl): 35–39.

Craddock N, Jones I (1999) Genetics of bipolar disorder. *J Med Genet* **36**: 585–594.

De Leon (2001) Antiepileptic drugs for the acute and maintenance treatment of bipolar disorder. *Harvard Rev Psychiatry* **9**(5): 209–222.

Dunner DL, Fieve RR (1974) Clinical factors in lithium carbonate prophylaxis failure. *Arch Gen Psychiatry* **30**: 229–233.

Faedda GL, Baldessarini RJ, Suppes T, Tondo L, Becker I, Lipschitz D (1995) Pediatric-onset BPD: a neglected clinical and public health problem. *Harvard Rev Psychiatry* **3**: 171–195.

Faedda GL, Tondo L, Teicher MH, Baldessarini RJ, Gelbard HA, Floris G (1993a) Seasonal mood disorders: patterns of seasonal recurrence in mania and depression. *Arch Gen Psychiatry* **50**: 17–23.

Faedda GL, Tondo L, Suppes T, Tohen M, Baldessarini RJ (1993b) Outcome after rapid vs gradual discontinuation of lithium treatment in bipolar disorders. *Arch Gen Psychiatry* **50**: 448–455.

Freeman MP, Freeman SA, McElroy SL (2002) The comorbidity of bipolar and anxiety disorders: prevalence, psychobiology, and treatment issues. *J Affect Disord* **68**: 1–23.

Goodwin FK, Jamison KR (1990) *Manic-Depressive Illness*. New York: Oxford University Press.

Grunze H, Walden J (2002) Relevance of new and newly rediscovered anticonvulsants for the atypical forms of bipolar disorder. *J Affect Disord* **72** (Suppl) :S15–21.

Guze SB, Robins E (1970) Suicide and primary affective disorders. *Br J Psychiatry* **117**: 437–438.

Huxley NA, Parikh SV, Baldessarini RJ (2000) Effectiveness of psychosocial treatments in BPD: state of the evidence. *Harvard Rev Psychiatry*, in press.

Inskip HM, Harris EC, Barraclough B (1998) Lifetime risk of suicide for affective disorder, alcoholism and schizophrenia. *Br J Psychiatry* **172**: 35–37.

Isometsä ET, Henriksson MM, Aro HM, Lonnqvist JK (1994) Suicide in bipolar disorder in Finland. *Am J Psychiatry* **151**: 1020–1024.

Jamison KR (1999) Suicide and manic-depressive illness: an overview and personal account. In Jacobs DG (ed.) *The Harvard Medical School Guide to Suicide Assessment and Intervention*. San Francisco, CA: Jossey-Bass.

Judd LL, Akiskal AS (2002) The long-term natural history of the weekly symptomatic status of bipolar I disorder. *Arch Gen Psychiatry* **59**: 530–537.

Klerman GL (1976) Age and clinical depression: today's youth in the twenty-first century. *J Gerontol* **31**: 318–323.

Koukopoulos A, Koukopoulos A (1999) Agitated depression as a mixed state and the problem of melancholia. *Psychiat Clin North Am* **22**: 547–564.

Kraepelin E (1921) *Manic-Depressive Insanity and Paranoia* (translation of the 1913 German edition by Barclay RM, edited by Robertson GM). E & S Livingstone, Edinburgh.

Kukopulos A, Reginaldi D, Laddomada P, Floris G, Serra G, Tondo L (1980) Course of the manic-depressive cycle and changes caused by treatments. *Pharmakopsychiatrie Neuropsychopharmakologie* **13**: 156–167.

Lewinsohn PM, Klein DN, Seeley JR (1995) Bipolar disorders in a community sample of older adolescents: prevalence, phenomenology, comorbidity, and course. *J Am Acad Child Adol Psychiatry* **34**(4): 454–463.

Macdonald KJ, Young LT (2002) Newer antiepileptic drugs in bipolar disorder: rationale for use and role in therapy. *CNS Drugs* **16**(8): 549–562.

Manji HK, Bowden CL, Belmaker RH (eds) (2000) *Bipolar Medications: Mechanisms of Action.* Washington, DC: American Psychiatric Press.

Mayberg HS, Mahurin RK, Brannan SK (1997) Neuropsychiatric aspects of mood and affective disorders. In Yudofsky SC, Hales RE (eds) *Textbook of Neuropsychiatry.* Washington, DC: American Psychiatric Press.

McElroy SL, Altshuler LL, Suppes T, Keck PE Jr, Frye MA, Denicoff KD, Nolen WA, Kupka RW, Leverich GS, Rochussen JR, Rush AJ, Post RM (2001) Axis I psychiatric comorbidity and its relationship to historical illness variables in 288 patients with BPD. *Am J Psychiatry* **158**: 420–426.

McElroy SL, Keck PE Jr, Pope HG Jr, Hudson JI, Faedda GL, Swann AC (1992) Clinical and research implications of the diagnosis of dysphoric or mixed mania and hypomania. *Am J Psychiatry* **149**: 1633–1644.

McTavish SF, McPherson MH, Harmer CJ, Clark L, Sharp T, Goodwin GM, Cowen PJ (2001) Antidopaminergic effects of dietary tyrosine depletion in healthy subjects and patients with manic illness. *Br J Psychiatry* **179**: 356–360.

Milberger S, Biederman J, Faraone SV, Murphy J, Tsuang MT (1995) Attention deficit hyperactivity disorder and comorbid disorders: issues of overlapping symptoms. *Am J Psychiatry* **152**: 1793–1799.

Mitchell P, Mackinnon A, Waters B (1993) The genetics of bipolar disorder. *Aust N Z J Psychiatry* **27**(4): 560–580.

Nemeroff CB (1999) *Mood disorders.* In Charney DS, Nestler EJ, Bunney BS (eds) *Neurobiology of Mental Illness.* New York: Oxford University Press.

Nonaka S, Hough CJ, Chuang DM (1998) Chronic lithium treatment robustly protects neurons in the central nervous system against excitotoxicity by inhibiting N-methyl-D-aspartate receptor-mediated calcium influx. *Proc Nat Acad Sc* **95**(5): 2642–2647.

Papolos D, Papolos J (2000) *The Bipolar Child.* New York: Broadway Books.

Perugi G, Akiskal HS, Micheli C, Toni C, Madaro D (2001) Clinical characterization of depressive mixed state in bipolar-I patients: Pisa–San Diego collaboration. *J Affect Disord* **67**: 105–114.

Pini S, Cassano GB, Simonini E, Savino M, Russo A, Montgomery SA (1997) Prevalence of anxiety disorders comorbidity in bipolar depression, unipolar depression and dysthymia. *J Affect Disord* **42**: 145–153.

Pliszka SR (1998) Comorbidity of attention-deficit/hyperactivity disorder with psychiatric disorder: an overview. *J Clin Psychiatry* **59**(Suppl 7): 50–58.

Post RM, Rubinow DR, Uhde TW, Roy-Byrne PP, Linnoila M, Rosoff A, Cowdry R (1989) Dysphoric mania. Clinical and biological correlates. *Arch Gen Psychiatry* **46**: 353–358.

Regier DA, Farmer ME, Rae DS, Locke BZ, Keith SJ, Judd LL, Goodwin FK (1990) Comorbidity of mental disorders with alcohol and other drug abuse. Results from the Epidemiologic Catchment Area (ECA) Study. *JAMA* **264**: 2511–2518.

Rihmer Z, Szadoczky E, Furedi J, Kiss K, Papp Z (2001) Anxiety disorders comorbidity in bipolar I, bipolar II and unipolar major depression: results from a population-based study in Hungary. *J Affect Disord* **67**: 175–179.

Rosenthal NE, Wehr TA (1987) Seasonal affective disorders. *Psychiatr Ann* **15**: 670–674.

Rothschild AJ, Bates KS, Boehringer KL, Syed A (1999) Olanzapine response in psychotic depression. *J Clin Psychiatry* **60**(2): 116–118.

Sachs GS, Baldassano CF, Truman CJ, Guille C (2000) Comorbidity of attention deficit disorder with early- and late-onset bipolar disorder. *Am J Psychiatry* **157**: 466–468.

Sadock BJ, Sadock VA (eds) (2000) *Kaplan & Sadock's Comprehensive Textbook of Psychiatry*, 7th edition. Philadelphia: Lippincott Williams & Wilkins.

Shulman K, Tohen M, Kutcher SP (eds) (1995) *Bipolar Disorder through the Life-Cycle*. New York: John Wiley.

Soares JC, Mann JJ (1997) The anatomy of mood disorders – review of structural neuroimaging studies. *Biol Psychiatry* **41**: 86–106.

Sonne SC, Brady KT (1999) Substance abuse and bipolar comorbidity. *Psychiatr Clin North Am* **22**: 609–627.

Strakowski SM, Sax KW, McElroy SL, Keck PE Jr, Hawkins JM, West SA (1998) Course of psychiatric and substance abuse syndromes co-occurring with BPD after a first psychiatric hospitalization. *J Clin Psychiatry* **59**: 465–471.

Suppes T, Webb A, Paul B, Carmody T, Kraemer H, Rush AJ (1999). Clinical outcome in a randomized 1-year trial of clozapine versus treatment as usual for patients with treatment-resistant illness and a history of mania. *Am J Psychiatry* **156**: 1164–1169.

Swann AC, Stokes PE, Secunda SK, Maas JW, Bowden CL, Berman N, Koslow SH (1994) Depressive mania versus agitated depression: biogenic amine and hypothalamic-pituitary-adrenocortical function. *Biol Psychiatry* **35**(10): 803–813.

Tohen M, Hennen J, Zarate CA Jr, Baldessarini RJ, Strakowski SM, Stoll AL, Faedda GL, Suppes T, Gebre-Medhin P, Cohen BM (2000) The McLean First Episode Project: two-year syndromal and functional recovery in 219 cases of major affective disorders with psychotic features. *Am J Psychiatry* **157**: 220–228.

Tohen M, Sanger TM, McElroy SL, Tollefson GD, Chengappa KN, Daniel DG, Petty F, Centorrino F, Wang R, Grundy SL, Greaney MG, Jacobs TG, David SR, Toma V (1999) Olanzapine versus placebo in the treatment of acute mania. Olanzapine HGEH Study Group. *Am J Psychiatry* **156**(5): 702–709.

Tondo L, Baldessarini RJ (1998) Rapid cycling in women and men with bipolar manic-depressive disorders. *Am J Psychiatry* **155**: 1434–1436.

Tondo L, Baldessarini RJ, Floris G (1998a) Lithium maintenance treatment: depression and mania in bipolar I and II disorders. *Am J Psychiatry* **155**: 638–645.

Tondo L, Baldessarini RJ, Floris G (2001b) Long-term clinical effectiveness of lithium maintenance treatment in types I and II bipolar manic-depressive disorders. *Br J Psychiatry* **178**(Suppl 40): S184–190.

Tondo L, Baldessarini RJ, Floris G, Silvetti F, Tohen M (1998b) Lithium treatment and risk of suicidal behavior in bipolar disorder patients. *J Clin Psychiatry* **59**: 405–414.

Tondo L, Hennen J, Baldessarini RJ (2001a) Reduced suicide risk with long-term lithium treatment in major affective illness: a meta-analysis. *Acta Psychiatr Scand* **104**: 163–172.

Tondo L, Hennen J, Baldessarini RJ (2003a) Rapid-cycling bipolar disorder: effects of long-term treatments. *Acta Psychiat Scand*, in press.

Tondo L, Isacsson G, Baldessarini RJ (2003b) Suicidal behavior in bipolar disorder: risk and prevention. *CNS Drugs*, in press.

Tondo L, Lai M, Salvatore P (2003c) I disturbi d'ansia e la comorbidità con i disturbi bipolari dell'umore. In Altamura CA (ed.) *I Disturbi d'Ansia e la Comorbidità con i Disturbi dell'Umore: Clinica e Trattamento.* Milan: McGraw Hill.

Tsuang MT, Faraone SV (1990) *The Genetics of Mood Disorders.* Baltimore, MD: Johns Hopkins University Press.

Vieta E, Colom F, Martinez-Aran A, Benabarre A, Reinares M, Gasto C (2000) Bipolar II disorder and comorbidity. *Compr Psychiatry* **41**: 339–343.

Weissman MM, Bland RC, Canino GJ, Faravelli C, Greenwald S, Hwu HG, Joyce PR, Karam EG, Lee CK, Lellouch J, Lepine JP, Newman SC, Rubio-Stipec M, Wells JE, Wickramaratne PJ, Wittchen H, Yeh EK (1996) Cross-national epidemiology of major depression and BPD. *JAMA* **276**: 293–299.

WHO (2000) *Manual of the International Statistical Classification of Diseases, Injuries, and Causes of Death*, 10th revision (ICD-10). Geneva: World Health Organization.

Yerevanian BI, Koek RJ, Ramdev S (2001) Anxiety disorders comorbidity in mood disorder subgroups: data from a mood disorders clinic. *J Affect Disord* **67**: 167–173.

Young LT, Cooke RG, Robb JC, Levitt AJ, Joffe RT (1993) Anxious and non-anxious BPD. *J Affect Disord* **29**: 49–52.

5

Subthreshold Mood Disorders

Stefano Pini, Nicolò Baldini-Rossi, Mario Miniati and Giovanni Battista Cassano

University of Pisa, Pisa, Italy

INTRODUCTION

Depressive and anxiety symptoms that fall below the threshold criteria for a mood or an anxiety disorder have been found to have considerable prevalence rates in the general population, as well as in the general health care sector and in psychiatric settings.

Early descriptions of depression by Kraepelin (1921) noted the presence of 'slight and slightest colouring of mood' which were thought mainly to represent rudimentary or prodromal symptoms of more severe affective disorders. Furthermore, depression not only could present in mild forms but also may reveal itself without any affective symptomatology, like somatization that may replace classic affective symptoms.

The initial problem with these forms of mood disorders is to come to terms with a definition of subthreshold depression that, indeed, has been described by using numerous labels such as 'minor', 'subsyndromal', 'incomplete', 'mild', 'attenuated', 'residual', 'masked', etc. In some cases, each of these labels provides only a partial definition and covers a limited number of the characteristics of subthreshold depression. Moreover, terms like 'depressive temperament' or 'depressive personality' were not rarely defined as primarily characterized by a particular constellation of personality traits indicating that the boundaries between 'depressive personality disorder' and 'chronic mild depressive features' are difficult to draw (Phillips et al., 1998). Other authors argued in favour of a distinction between a state and a trait depression, given that some symptoms (e.g. negative reactivity, remorsefulness, gloominess, pessimism, unassertiveness, etc.) differentiated depressed and non-depressed subjects, indicating that they are primarily belonging to depression, while low self-esteem, feeling burdened, and counterdependency manifested both state and trait components (Hartlage et al., 1998).

Mood Disorders: Clinical Management and Research Issues. Edited by E. J. L. Griez, C. Faravelli, D. J. Nutt and J. Zohar.
©2005 John Wiley & Sons Ltd. ISBN 0 470 09426 5.

While the earlier diagnostic and statistical manuals of mental disorders (DSM-I–III) limited the diagnosis of depression to a set of rigid criteria based on the number of symptoms present (at least five out of nine), the duration (at least two weeks), and the quality of these symptoms, more and more frequently patients present with symptoms of depression insufficient in number or duration to satisfy the DSM-III criteria, that result in significant impairment in social functioning. The interest in these so-called 'subthreshold' depressive states lead to the addition of three new categories of depression to the DSM as 'subthreshold forms of major depression'. Dysthymia was first added to DSM-III-R, and minor depression and recurrent brief depression were added to DSM-IV under the umbrella of depression NOS. Nevertheless, approximately two-thirds of patients with subthreshold depression continued to present with depressive symptoms, causing significant psychosocial impairment, but which still did not satisfy any DSM-IV diagnosis (Judd et al., 1994, 1997).

EPIDEMIOLOGICAL STUDIES

As stated by Angst and Merikangas (1997), the spectrum of depression 'is much wider than that reflected in the current diagnostic nomenclature'. Most recent epidemiological studies that confirmed the wide diffusion of depressive symptomatology in the general population derived essentially from the Epidemiologic Catchment Area (ECA) and the National Comorbidity Survey (NCS). The main objectives of these studies were essentially to evaluate the prevalence of subthreshold depression in the general population and to explore the relationship between this condition and individual's functional impairment and help-seeking behaviour patterns.

Judd et al. (1994), using the ECA database, described a potential clinical condition represented by 'any two or more simultaneous symptoms of depression, present for most or all of the time, of at least two weeks' duration, associated with evidence of social dysfunction, occurring in an individual that does not meet criteria for diagnoses of minor depression, major depression and/or dysthymia'. This condition has been defined as 'subsyndromal symptomatic depression' and had a prevalence of 11.8% during a one-year period. From a clinical viewpoint, these authors found that 'subsyndromal symptomatic depression' was associated with insomnia, fatigue and recurrent thoughts of death. However, they raised the question of whether subsyndromal depressive symptoms are associated with sufficient disruption in the domain of an individual's everyday functioning. In a more recent reappraisal of the ECA, Judd et al. (1996) restricted the analysis of ECA data to the Los Angeles site. These authors hypothesized that subjects with subsyndromal depressive symptoms reported more functional impairment than subjects with no depressive symptoms. They compared the social and functional impairment of subjects with and without subsyndromal depressive symptoms with that of subjects with major depression. Functional impairment was evaluated with questions regarding 10 domains of functional outcome and well-being, namely daily functions, high or low household strain, high or low social contacts, major financial loss, high or low financial strain, talked to someone about very personal problems, any day with restricted activity due to physical illness or any day in bed due to physical illness in previous two weeks, any chronic limitation in physical or job functioning due to physical illness, and general health status. Significantly more subjects with subsyndromal depressive symptoms than subjects with no depressive disorder or symptoms reported disability on seven out of 10 domains of function, namely high social irritability (62%), high household strain (45%), high financial strain (63%), restricted activity days due to physical illness (18%), bed days due to physical illness (11%), chronic limitation in physical or job functioning (18%) and self-rating of health scored as 'poor'.

Judd et al. (1997) classified all respondents from three out of five sites of the ECA overall sample into seven mutually exclusive categories based on the presence or absence of depressive symptoms or disorders. Overall, one-month prevalence of threshold or subthreshold depressive symptoms was found to be 22.6%, while that of a single depressive symptom was 8.7%, of subsyndromal depressive symptoms was 3.9% and of minor depressive disorder was 1.5%. From a clinical viewpoint, when compared to subjects without any depressive symptom, respondents with subsyndromal depressive symptoms were twice as likely to refer to mental health facilities and to have had disability benefits, and about four times more likely to have suicidal ideation or suicide attempts. A relevant proportion of these subjects with subsyndromal depressive symptoms experienced depressive symptoms as prodromal to the onset of a major or a minor depressive episode as well as residual to resolving episodes. These findings were consistent with the observation that subsyndromal depressive symptoms might be associated either with an history of past depressive episodes or with a relevant risk factor for future episodes.

Kessler et al. (1997) investigated subthreshold depression in the National Comorbidity Survey data. These authors adopted a modified definition of DSM-IV (APA, 1994) 'minor depression', that is only two to four criterion 'A' symptoms and no lifetime history of major depression or dysthymia. Furthermore, they considered two types of lifetime major depressive episode: the first was less severe (with five or six criterion 'A' symptoms) and the second more severe, characterized by seven to nine symptoms. The estimated lifetime prevalence of these forms of depression were 10% for minor depression, 8.3% for major depression with five to six symptoms and 7.5% for major depression with seven to nine symptoms. In this study, clinical correlates of minor and major depression were similar. Both minor and major depression appeared like recurrent disorders: the vast majority of subjects with lifetime minor depression and lifetime major depression reported having more than one episode (72.1% and 72.3% respectively), and only a minority of them, reported a persistent depression without remission from the time of first onset. As expected, a comparison of respondents whose worst lifetime episode had minor, major depression with five to six symptoms, and major depression with seven to nine symptoms, showed an increasing gradient in average number of lifetime episodes, average length of longest episodes, 30-day and 12-month prevalence. Nor were differences found across subsamples whose most recent episode ended more than 12 months ago, with approximately 16% of respondents reporting residual symptomatology.

Impairment associated with minor and major depression differed in the three subgroups. There was a clear gradient of increasing impairment expressed in terms of interference with everyday life and activities, the percentage who saw a doctor or some other professional, and the percentage who took medication for the depression. A substantial minority of those with minor depression (42%) and larger proportions of those with major depression with five to six symptoms (49.7%) and with seven to nine symptoms (68.2%) reported at least one of these indicators of impairment. Data on more recent impairment (during the past 30 days) showed that the average number of mental health work loss days is equal for those with recent minor and major depression with five to six symptoms, but much larger for those with recent major depressive episode with seven to nine symptoms. Kessler et al. (1997) concluded that whereas clinical correlates between minor and major depression were similar, differences in impairment were significant, implying that there is not a sharp divide between minor and major depression.

Sullivan et al. (1998) using the NCS data, identified six classes of subjects who endorsed different depressive conditions: namely, the *'severe typical and mild typical classes'* (subjects with a very high lifetime occurrence of major depression and preponderance of 'classical' depressive symptoms like weight and appetite loss, insomnia, psychomotor agitation, anergia and poor concentration), the *'severe and mild atypical classes'* (in which depressive episodes were characterized by appetite increase and weight gain), the *'intermediate class'* (intermediate lifetime occurrence of major depression with prominent symptoms of low mood, loss of interests, insomnia etc.), and finally the *'minimal symptoms class'* characterized by low rates of depressive symptoms endorsed and only 1% of subjects with a lifetime major depression. The overall prevalence of subthreshold forms of depression was 19% of the subjects in the NCS. These conditions, which were hypothesized to be quantitatively but not qualitatively different from major depression, were associated with social morbidity and an increased risk for first-onset major depression.

Angst and Merikangas (1997) investigated the presence and the prevalence of subthreshold depression in a community sample of 591 subjects, recruited over 15 years (Zurich cohort). Standard threshold criteria of dysthymia and major depression as defined by DSM-III-R (APA, 1987) were applied. Four subthreshold conditions were defined: depressive symptoms (one or two depressive symptoms for at least two weeks), minor depression (three or four depressive symptoms for at least two weeks), recurrent brief depression and recurrent brief depression without impairment. Lifetime recurrent brief depression and minor depression were found in 9.2% and in 6.2% of the overall sample respectively. Moreover, the majority of cases did not manifest a single subtype only: the presence of subthreshold forms of depression was a risk factor for the developing of a major disorder and a major

depressive episode might predispose to the development of a subthreshold symptomatology in almost 50% of cases as well.

Kendler and Gardner (1998) evaluated a group of female twins ascertained from
a large epidemiological sample denominated Population-based Virginia Twin
Registry and investigated the presence of 20 depressive symptoms during the year
before the evaluation. The aim of this study was to assess if major depression was 'a
discrete syndrome' qualitatively different from subthreshold depressive conditions
or if it was only a fictitious category superimposed on a continuum represented by
various depressive symptoms with different severity and duration. With the term
'minimal depressive syndrome' was defined a condition 'consisting of at least three
co-occurring depressive symptoms one of which had to be depressed mood or loss of
interest/pleasure during at least 5 days'. Subjects were interviewed on three consecutive occasions in order to assess whether the presence of depressive symptoms at
the baseline was predictive of the occurrence of a subsequent depressive episode.
The authors found that the risk of having a future major depressive episode was
related to the number of depressive symptoms observed at the first interview, but
they did not find a discontinuity between the risks related to subthreshold conditions
and those related to full-blown depressive conditions. The authors concluded that
subthreshold syndromes had predictive and familial validity as well as full-blown
forms of depression.

Studies in the General Health Care Sector

Probably, the largest effort to gain more insight into the phenomenology and course
of threshold and subthreshold depressive disorders in primary care using a refined
methodology was the multicentre WHO study denominated 'Psychological
Problems in General Health Care' (Sartorius et al., 1993; Ustun and Sartorius,
1995; Ormel and Tiemens, 1995). First longitudinal data from this study were
reported by Simon and VonKorff (1995) for the American site (Seattle, USA).
They found that the majority of patients with both major and minor depressive
disorders showed considerable improvement in depression and disability after 12
months. However, 30% of patients with major depression continued to fulfil criteria
for major depression after 12 months. Moreover, similar rates of recovery were
found among patients recognized by the physician as psychiatric cases (30.3%) as
compared to those unrecognized (30.4%), suggesting a lack of association between
identification by the physician and recovery (Simon and VonKorff, 1995).

Primary care subjects with subthreshold depressive symptoms may represent a
highly heterogeneous group. They may include not only individuals with partially
remitted or prodromal major depressive symptoms or subjects with transient
depressive symptomatology in response to stressful life-events, but also subjects
with depressive symptoms that are secondary to a general medical illness
(Sherbourne et al., 1994). In one study, Olfson et al. (1996) recruited a large
outpatient primary care sample (1001 subjects), in which subthreshold symptoma-

tology was defined for depression, panic disorder, OCD, drug, and alcohol abuse and dependence. A total of 30.1% of the subjects met the criteria for subthreshold symptoms, whereas 38.9% met the criteria for an axis I mental disorder. The criteria for depressive symptoms were met by 9.1% of the sample. Subjects with depressive symptoms were similar in mean age to patients with major depression but they were younger than patients with no symptoms. Social impairment, due to loss of work for mental health symptoms, marital distress and use of mental health services was significantly higher in subjects with subthreshold depression than in those without any depressive symptom (7.7 times increased risk for marital distress and 2.5 times increased risk for a recent loss of work or utilization of mental health services). Furthermore, one-third of subjects with subthreshold depression met the full criteria for another mental disorder, in particular drug abuse or dependence. Among subthreshold symptomatology, only depressive symptoms and panic symptoms seemed strongly associated with a significant impairment. However, Olfson (1996) noted that it was difficult to detect the clinical significance of subthreshold depressive symptomatology in primary care patients, because of the widespread prevalence of comorbidity with other psychiatric and non-psychiatric disorders or symptoms.

Rapaport and Judd (1998) recruited 15 subjects with subthreshold depression and minor depression, from a general practice sample and from the community. They quantified functional impairment and depressive symptomatology in these subjects before and after eight weeks of pharmacological treatment. All subjects were medically stable, they were not on psychotropic medication, and they met criteria for either minor depression or subthreshold depression but no other psychiatric disorder. Minor depression was defined as 'feeling sad or blue or anhedonic' plus at least one other symptom of depression as presented in the DSM-IV (APA, 1994) list of symptoms. Subthreshold depression was defined as having two or more symptoms of depression excluding the A criteria as defined by DSM-IV (feeling sad, blue or anhedonic) and a Global Assessment Score (GAS) < 75. Subjects with a current or past history of major depression in the last year were excluded from the sample. When confronted with a general population sample without depressive symptomatology, subjects with minor and subthreshold depression showed lower scores for physical role functioning, emotional role, energy/fatigue, emotional well-being and social functioning. After the treatment with fluvoxamine, depressive symptomatology decreased in minor depressives as well as in subjects with subthreshold depressive symptoms and approximately 30% of the patients had complete resolution of all depressive symptoms. However, these results derived from an open label pilot study on a small sample.

Studies in Clinical Settings

As stated previously, most recent epidemiological surveys in the general population and in primary care have shown that a substantial proportion of disabling depressive syndromes do not meet the criteria for major forms of depression. These findings have driven the clinicians to propose less restrictive boundaries and definitions for depressive conditions. In some recent studies conducted in clinical settings, subthreshold depressive symptomatology was mainly described from two different perspectives that reported different aspects of the same phenomenon. One approach consisted in considering subthreshold depressive conditions as expressions of 'prodromal' or 'partial or incomplete remission' or 'residual symptomatology' of a depressive episode. The other approach was that of conceptualizing subthreshold depressive conditions as alternative forms of different symptomatic phases of the same disease on a 'symptomatic continuum' (Judd, 1997).

The high prevalence of residual depressive symptomatology after the treatment of a major depressive episode in clinical samples, their role as a predictor of subsequent depressive recurrences, the impact on therapy choices, and the degree of enduring psychosocial impairment subsequent to the partial remission of a depressive episode have been well investigated.

Paykel (1998) reports the course and the levels of symptomatological remission of 64 major depressives with an examination of residual symptoms. This study revealed that 32% of patients who remitted below major depression showed 8 or more on the Hamilton Depression Scale. The pattern was of 'mild atypical depressive symptoms' without major biological symptoms. According to Paykel (1998) residual symptoms were more common in subjects with more severe initial depression and with passive dependent personality traits; in these subjects, residual symptoms were strong predictors of subsequent relapse.

Agosti and Stewart (1998) investigated the clinical profile of depressed psychiatric patients who responded to acute treatment and had a sustained six-month period of recovery (n=48), and they compared their social functioning with that of a psychiatrically normal community sample (n=974). Symptom scores of the recovered group were significantly higher than the community control group but not clinically significant: 94% of the recovered patients had a mean SCL-90-R total score of less than 1 ('a little bit'). Nevertheless, the recovered group was more impaired in social and leisure functioning than the non-psychiatric sample.

Fava et al. (1998), in a follow-up assessment investigated if cognitive-behavioural treatment of residual symptoms of depression might have a significant effect on relapse rate. Forty consecutive depressed outpatients who met the Research Diagnostic Criteria for a major depressive disorder were treated for at least three months with full doses of antidepressants. Subjects who completed the treatment period were randomly assigned to a specific cognitive-behavioural treatment of residual symptoms or to a clinical routine management. Cognitive-behavioural treatment seemed to show a substantial effect on relapse rate only in the first four years of follow-up. In particular, at the two-year follow-up, CBT resulted in a relapse rate of 25%, significantly lower than did clinical management (80%). CBT efficacy faded at a six-year follow-up. These results are concordant with those of a previous study (Blackburn and Moore, 1997) in which 75 patients with recurrent depression, were subdivided into three groups: short-term and maintenance (two years) treatment with antidepressant drugs, CBT in the short-term as well as in the maintenance phase and antidepressant use in the short-term phase plus CBT for maintenance. Cognitive therapy displayed a similar prophylactic effect to maintenance medication (Blackburn and Moore, 1997).

Judd et al. (1998a) in a naturalistic study, investigated the weekly symptomatic course of 431 patients with unipolar major depressive disorder and they considered the influence of mood disorder history on the course of illness, during a 12-year follow-up. Judd et al. (1998a) subdivided the overall sample into three mutually exclusive groups: patients in their first lifetime major depressive episode (MDE) in the absence of ongoing dysthymia (28% of the sample), patients with one or more prior MDEs in the absence of ongoing dysthymia (47%) and patients with double depression (24%). Follow-up weeks were assigned to one of four mutually exclusive depressive symptoms severity levels that represented states of illness activity: 1 – depressive symptoms at the threshold for MDD, 2 – depressive symptoms at the threshold for minor depressive or dysthymic disorder (MinD), 3 – 'subthreshold' or 'subsyndromal' depressive symptoms (below the thresholds for MinD and MDD), and 4 – no depressive symptoms. Subjects of the study with MDD spent 41.5% and 15.3% of follow-up weeks asymptomatic and with depressive symptoms at the MDD level respectively. For approximately one-quarter of the follow-up weeks (26.7%) patients showed minor depression level symptoms, whereas subthreshold depression was present during 16.5%. Patients in the double depression group spent significantly more time with minor depressive symptoms (34.6%) than patients in the other subgroups. Moreover, weekly analyses of unipolar MDD revealed prolonged chronic symptoms in the course of illness, with only 41.5% of asymptomatic weeks for an average of 8.7 years. Patients with double depression had the most symptomatic course.

BIPOLAR–UNIPOLAR DICHOTOMY

Since the bipolar–unipolar dichotomy of the DSM era replaced the unitary vision proposed by Kraepelin in the early twentieth century, the bipolar–unipolar distinction has represented a major advance in the classification and description of mood disorders, providing a basis for the evaluation of genetic, clinical and therapeutic differences, rather than representing a 'purely descriptive sub-grouping' (Goodwin and Jamison, 1990). However, the ambiguities regarding the boundaries between unipolar and bipolar disorders, and the definition of relationships between polarity and cyclicity still stands, raising practical problems for research and treatment choices. The original contribution by Dunner et al. (1976) in the early '70s in differentiating bipolar I and II conditions was paramount for including in the bipolar spectrum those patients presenting with clinical depression whose hypomanic phases, not requiring hospitalization or treatment, or not impairing individual's functioning, are only detectable by clinical history (Coryell et al., 1987).

Subsequently, the contribution of Akiskal and Cassano in the 1980s indicated that about 50% of mood disorders seen in clinical settings might pertain to the bipolar spectrum. This widening of bipolarity to the detriment of unipolar forms was corroborated by Angst (1995) who demonstrated through epidemiological data that more than 5% of the general population might be affected by bipolar spectrum conditions.

Akiskal and Pinto (1999) and Akiskal et al. (2000) reappraised the bipolar spectrum in a conceptual and clinical context using case material. The authors argue that many major depressions in the DSM-IV schema are, in reality, part of the bipolar spectrum. This approach led to the formulation of a list of prototypes (BP-I, BP-I$\frac{1}{2}$, BP-II, BP-II$\frac{1}{2}$, BP-III, BP-III$\frac{1}{2}$, BP-IV) along the continuum of mood dysregulations. The major implication of this theory is that the extension of the concept of the bipolar spectrum would defend a depressed patient unprotected by mood stabilizers from possible negative effects of antidepressants. Second, recognition of some attenuated forms of bipolarity pursuing a subacute or chronic course may obviate a more prognostically unfavourable diagnosis such as borderline or antisocial personality disorder or schizophrenia.

Furthermore, this model has shed light on the true prevalence of bipolar spectrum conditions, and challenged the conservative figure of 1% usually reported in the traditional literature for bipolar disorder (Weissman et al., 1998).

However, there are a series of limitations in this model. First, prototypes are mostly based on individual case reports rather than systematic evaluations of representative samples of subjects. One risk in following this approach is that it may produce, at least theoretically, a myriad of subcategories based on individual anecdoctal cases, one phenomenologically different from another, which do not necessarily reflect independent clinical entities. Furthermore, there may be patients who present some features of one prototype and some others belonging to another prototype. These cases would be forced to enter into one prototype rather than into the other, to the detriment of a more precise phenomenic characterization.

A second limitation of this model concerns treatment implications. A strict hierarchical approach to prototypes in terms of the severity of the bipolar component of the illness has not been posited, and the use of a mood stabilizer for each prototype does not follow precise guidelines. For example, gabapentin at doses of 1200 mg/day has been reported as successful monotherapy for 'depression with protracted hypomania' (bipolar I$\frac{1}{2}$). However, there are a number of recent studies that do not give strong support to the use of this drug for bipolar spectrum conditions, especially the more severe forms, unless it is employed as an adjunct to other mood-stabilizing medications of proven efficacy (Knoll et al., 1998; Ghaemi and Goodwin, 2001). On the contrary, a more classical combination of lithium (600 mg/day) and divalproex (600 mg/day) has been proposed to treat 'depression with hypomania' (bipolar II); such a treatment does not differ substantially from that proposed for the treatment of typical bipolar I conditions. Moreover, the adoption of rigid therapeutic schema based on anticonvulsants often interferes with the establishment of an optimal treatment paradigm for bipolar depression. Substantial proportions of depressed patients with a history of episodes of attenuated hypomania (bipolar II spectrum) may show a satisfactory and stable long-term outcome with antidepressants not necessarily associated with mood stabilizers (MacQueen and Young, 2001). Conversely, mood stabilizers, either alone or combined with antidepressants, may leave these patients in a mild depression with hypersedation, a condition that is subjectively unpleasant for the individual. Finally, no clear treatment indications are provided for 'hyperthymic depression' (bipolar IV), though reported to be at high risk of manic switches (Henry et al., 2001).

More recently, prompted by various considerations, Joffe et al. (1999) proposed a different conceptualization of bipolar spectrum. The central thesis is that the current notion of bipolar spectrum, as a discrete entity distinct from unipolar depression, is artificial, not theoretically and clinically useful and not supported by the literature.

When mania and depression coexist in the form of bipolar disorder, further episodes of depression, which tend to worsen the illness, may lead to a chronic course and poor prognosis. This model may have theoretical and clinical implications. From a theoretical point of view, mania and depression are proposed as two entities to be studied separately in their clinical and psychopathological characteristics. A unitarian 'spectrum' view of bipolar illness is not contemplated by the authors. This may lead to a better characterization of the two conditions.

Actually, these recent extreme conceptualizations suggested to us the need for assessing manic and depressive features within a more unitary framework encompassing the broad range of mood spectrum manifestations. We aimed at studying the mood spectrum, avoiding rigid theoretical positions that might lead, on the one hand, to excessive diagnostic fragmentation of the bipolar and unipolar spectrum and, on the other, to drastic separation between bipolar and unipolar forms.

THE MOOD-SPECTRUM APPROACH

Baldessarini (2000) has speculated on the extreme and inappropriate widening of the schizophrenia rubric in the middle of the twentieth century. Based on loose clinical criteria and on a psychodynamic stereotyped conceptualization, the expansion of the diagnosis of schizophrenia was detrimental to the diagnosis of various forms of psychoses pertaining to the realm of mood disorders and, in some cases, of personality disorders. As a consequence, chlorpromazine in variable doses was given to a large number of subjects in which clinicians recognized vague expressions of bizarre thinking and behaviour. Analogously – clinicians and researchers today should avoid that – the expansion of criteria for bipolar spectrum conditions would be reflected in a similar uncontrolled and widespread use of lithium and anticonvulsants in the absence of clear scientific evidence of their efficacy in bipolar conditions other than bipolar I disorder. At present, for instance, controlled studies and clinical experience do not support, with some exceptions, a favourable cost–benefit ratio for the systematic use of mood stabilizers in individuals with subsyndromal bipolar features, cyclothymia, and bipolar II disorder (MacQueen and Young, 2001).

Nevertheless, the definition of the cut-off point between unipolar and bipolar forms – if it exists at all – still stems from a purely descriptive approach to the varying degrees of loading for depressive and manic dimensions. Clinicians often face a complex array of co-occurring isolated or clustered mood symptoms that may be associated with one or more axis I or axis II conditions, giving rise to complex clinical situations. Moreover, the DSM-IV approach tends to trivialize or neglect such symptoms as 'background noise' interfering with the primary task of matching symptoms to diagnostic criteria. Conversely, there is evidence that failure to recognize such symptoms may have prognostic implications.

Also, DSM-IV imposes a rigid and inflexible approach to the nosology of depression. DSM-certified main depressive categories, namely major depression and dysthymia, do not suffice and therefore many new entities have been added. Examples are categories such as minor depression, subsyndromal depression, recurrent brief depression, subaffective personality disorder and mixed anxiety–depression disorder. Such categories are often introduced without rigorous validating studies; yet they are being considered as if they were valid entities. The study of under-validated concepts runs a considerable risk of yielding invalid results that are hard to reproduce (Van Praag, 1998).

We argue that systematic study, not only of the core symptoms of depression and mania but also of the associated aura of subthreshold and atypical manifestations, the importance of which is usually underestimated, may be relevant to diagnosis and treatment, and may have important theoretical significance. The term 'spectrum' has been previously used to describe relationships among clusters and symptoms or to place a group of defined syndromes in relation to one another (Kety, 1987; Akiskal et al., 1980; Akislal, 1983a; Hollander, 1993). We use the term spectrum to refer to a broad area of psychopathological phenomena relating to a single mental disorder including: (a) core atypical symptoms of the primary axis I disorder, (b) signs, isolated symptoms, symptom clusters and behavioural patterns related to the core symptoms that may be _prodromal_, may represent _precursors_ of not yet fully expressed conditions, or may be _sequelae_ of a previously experienced disorder, and (c) temperamental or personality traits (Cassano et al., 1997).

Within the context of mood disorders, our mood-spectrum approach was primarily conceived to shed light on and reorganize the relatively undefined area of symptoms which stretches from mania (bipolar) toward the depression (unipolar) realm. We hypothesize that this area of mood disorders should be better defined by fostering a unitary dimensional model as opposed to a fragmentation into multiple subcategories, such as, for example, depression with psychotic features, post-partum depression, protracted attenuated depressive mixed states, depression with hyperthymic or cyclothymic temperament, depression with very brief hypomanic episodes, isolated manic symptoms, early onset and highly recurrent depression, seasonal depression, atypical depression, depression with family loading for bipolar disorders (Akiskal et al., 2000).

We argue that the detection of these less classical mixtures of manic-depressive and unipolar depressive symptoms needs subtle diagnostic tools and can be improved by the introduction of refined assessment procedures also aimed at identifying vulnerability to recurrences or to the emergence of more severe forms of psychopathology.

In this perspective, rather than coming to a net (clear-cut) diagnostic categorization of bipolar and unipolar conditions, we first try to conceive a spectrum model of mood disorders that might encompass not only subthreshold and threshold manic and depressive phenomenologies in their various presentations, but also those symptoms that may have occurred through an individual's childhood, adolescence, and adult life that may have represented precursor, prodromal, and residual forms of a full-fledged manic or a depressive episode (Fagiolini et al., 1999).

We will discuss the major implications of detecting such mood-spectrum manifestations within the framework of the process of construction and validation of a structured clinical interview, the Structured Clinical Interview for Mood Spectrum (SCI-MOODS™).

SCI-MOODS™ not only includes typical and diagnostic symptoms of manic, mixed and depressive episodes but also symptoms and signs that represent precursors, prodromals, residuals and other subdiagnostic conditions which may have occurred across an individual's lifespan. The choice of each of these elements has been made on the basis of the existing literature integrated with clinical experience.

The Structured Clinical Interview for Mood Spectrum: SCI-MOODS™

The last three decades, representing the 'DSM era' of psychiatry, have been strongly characterized by a 'splitting' attitude of researchers toward diagnosis and classification of mood and anxiety disorders. Though such an approach has produced important progress, at present a reappraisal of the 'lumping' approach seems to be a more suitable process for exploring and defining the phenomenology of the broad area of mood disorders. In this perspective, we conceived the spectrum model, based on an integration of both dimensional and categorical approaches. We tried to give empirical support to our concept of the spectrum by designing a structured clinical interview for mood disorders. The principal aim of SCI-MOODS™ and MOODS-SR, its self-rated version, is to capture the patient's lifetime continuity of mood dysregulations through a systematic, longitudinal assessment of mood psychopathology. In the research field, as in clinical practice, the SCI-MOODS™ systematic approach offers a conceptual frame of reference for the clinician to explore extensively different depression and mania dimensions. Moreover, this approach should enable us to better recognize and express quantitatively threshold and subthreshold psychopathology. Therefore, the wide area of subthreshold and of atypicality within the context of mood disorders should be better and more homogeneously defined for research and treatment aims.

The Structured Clinical Interview for Mood Spectrum (SCI-MOODS™) has been designed to assess a wide variety of lifetime mood signs and symptoms, in order to explore their predictive value and clinical relevance. Unlike the Structured Clinical interview for DSM-IV (SCID-IV™), which is used to test specific criteria of axis I and II disorders, SCI-MOODS™ provide an assessment of a wide range of mood dysregulation, as well as of the more classical symptom criteria (Fagiolini et al., 1999). The interview was not originally designed to enable clinicians to make operationalized diagnoses according to the DSM criteria. A structured categorical interview like the SCID, would be preferable for this purpose.

SCI-MOODS™ is currently composed of 161 items, grouped into four domains (or clusters). (1) The first domain (Rhythmicity and Vegetative Functions) considers disturbances and rhythmic changes in feelings and behaviour associated with physical experiences such as eating, sexual activity, and sleep, including rhythmic variations in affective and sub-affective symptoms. (2) The second domain is devoted to energy levels (Energy) and changes in everyday activities, with particular attention to work, hobbies and social life. (3) The third domain explores mood phenomenology from sub-clinical unipolar and bipolar depressive symptoms to severe mixed and manic symptoms (Mood). (4) The fourth domain explores the cognitive changes that often occur with energy and mood dysregulations (Cognition). The four domains of SCI-MOODS™ include a large number of symptoms, signs and behaviours that may have occurred during the individual's lifespan. Some of these manifestations may configure typical forms of mood disorders, as described in the DSM or ICD. More interestingly they may occur in isolation and represent precursors or prodromals of a major episode of illness, as well as residuals or post-episodic maladjustment phenomena (see Table. 5.1).

Mood-spectrum Components

In the following paragraphs, we will review the different areas from which the items of SCI-MOODS™ were derived (see Table 5.2). Each area is analysed by exploring systematically the relative literature and on the basis of our clinical experience in the field. In order to better clarify the psychopathological and clinical bases of our mood-spectrum model, the definition and short description of each area has been reported in separate paragraphs.

Precursors

'Precursors' are commonly defined as 'signs and symptoms from a diagnostic cluster that precede a disorder, but do not predict its onset' (Eaton et al., 1995) (see Table 5.3).

TABLE 5.1   The mood disorders spectrum

Typical forms (described in DSM or ICD)

Atypical forms

- Early onset
- Late onset
- Chronic forms
- Masked or covered by full-blown or spectrum comorbidity
- In 'spcial populations'

Subthreshold manifestations

- Precursors
- Prodromals
- Residuals
- Early onset (<20 years) subthreshold persistent forms
- Mono/oligo-symptomatic forms

Complicated forms

- Alcohol or substance use/abuse
- AIDS, HBV, HCV
- Illegal or 'antisocial' behaviours

Forms with comorbidity

- Full-blown comorbidity
- Subthreshold comorbidity

Some dysregulations of energy/activity levels that characterize an individual's lifestyle may have the role of precursors of a mood disorder. SCI-MOODS™ should allow us to recognize and depict these features: nine items explore depressive manifestations, which can precede by many years the onset of a mood disorder, such as, for example, brief or protracted periods of subjective feeling of slowness, slight tiredness or weakness, or a certain difficulty in starting the day. These symptoms are relatively aspecific, if they are not considered within the context of a broader array. Precursors are especially difficult for patients to recall when they are the expression of a subthreshold hypomanic state and are related to a subjective feeling of well-being (e.g., becoming overconfident, assertive, or more talkative and creative than usual). Subthreshold mood fluctuations may precede the onset of a full-blown mood episode by many years, and are labelled as 'personality or affective temperamental traits' (the so-called 'hyperthymic–cyclothymic' background).

The SCI-MOODS™ first domain (Rhythmicity and Vegetative Functions), explores levels of productivity, physical energy, and cognitive performance. The items of this section depict disturbances or rhythmic changes in feelings and behaviours, often associated with the dysregulation of physical experiences, for instance eating and sexual behaviours, sleep patterns.

TABLE 5.2   The mood disorders spectrum components (unipolar and bipolar)

1. Precursors
2. Prodromals
3. Typical forms
4. Residuals
5. Subthreshold episodic (incomplete expressions, subsyndromal, isolated, recurrent or continuous manifestations)
6. Post-episodic characterological changes
7. Post-episodic maladjustment
8. Early-onset subthreshold persistent ('lifelong') forms (the so-called 'affective temperament')
9. Atypical forms
    - Atypical mania
    - Masked depression
    - Neurotic depression
    - Age-related atypical forms
    - Primary vs. secondary
10. Unipolar and bipolar sub-threshold comorbidity
    - Axis I and Axis II psychiatric comorbidity
    - Neurological comorbidity
    - Other comorbidities

Prodromal Symptoms

The prodromal phase of a mood episode has been defined as 'the time interval between the onset of prodromal symptoms and the onset of the characteristic manifestations of a full-fledged mood episode' (Fava, 1999).

The proper appreciation of the significance of prodromals grew up two decades ago, with the emergence of studies conducted on subjects in the community, and the organization of mood clinics dedicated to the long-term treatment of mood disorders (Barrett et al., 1978). Most findings are consistent in showing a high prevalence of prodromal symptoms in patients with both unipolar and bipolar disorder: manic prodromals have been identified in nearly 75% of subjects with mood disorders; depressive prodromals have been described in 85% (Smith and Tarrier, 1992; Keitner et al., 1996) (see Table 5.4). Prodromals seem to be

TABLE 5.3   The mood disorders spectrum precursors[a]

- Hyper/hypo-somnia
- Migraine
- Sleep dysregulations
- Biological rhythm dysregulations
- Pseudo-ADHD
- Premenstrual syndrome
- Early onset persistent subthreshold mood dysregulation

[a]Not necessarily followed by a full-blown mood episode.

characterized by a remarkable consistency within each subject in successive episodes of the same polarity; the concordance in different subjects is lower. For this reason, the patient and his/her relatives are often able to recognize a new mood episode of illness approaching days or even weeks beforehand, from the presence of isolated symptoms already experienced in previous episodes of the same polarity. These symptoms certainly constitute in most cases a sort of 'warning sign' of a new episode with a full-blown symptomatology, but they can also remain stable for a long period, in the absence of 'major' episodes. In this case, the given definition of prodromal, that implies the heralding of a full-blown episode, clearly limits the real impact of the so-called prodromals in the individual clinical history, which can result in his/her being affected in a severe way, even if these symptoms are not directly related to a mood episode. For this reason, the assessment of isolated symptoms recurring in a cyclical pattern and belonging to both the manic and the depressive side, is one of the targets of SCI-MOODS[TM]. In the interview, mood symptoms are listed without any relationship to the presence of a 'full-blown' episode. According to the authors' mood-spectrum model, prodromals, residuals and sub-clinical protracted fluctuations of mood, energy, cognitive performance and neurobehavioural patterns may represent three essential components of a persistent subthreshold phenomenology, which may also exist in the absence of a full-blown mood episode (Fava, 1999; Cassano et al., 1999; Chien and Dunner, 1996). The lifetime assessment proposed by SCI-MOODS[TM], as well as the last month's MOOD-SR may help the clinician to detect symptoms observed during prodromal or residual phases. Moreover, following a lifetime perspective, those residual symptoms that may become prodromals of a mood relapse may be captured (Fava, 1999). Subthreshold mood phenomenology in the similar forms of precursors and prodromals can be equally detected in the various affected and non-affected members of the same family. In these subjects, these partial expressions of mood disorders may represent different levels of vulnerability to the same psycho-pathology.

Residual Symptoms and Post-episodic Maladjustment

Residuals have been defined as 'the persistence of symptoms and signs of a definite disorder, despite apparent remission or recovery of the full-blown episode' (Fava, 1999). During primarily hospital-based psychiatry, the major focus of treatment was getting the patient out of his severe episode, back into the community; so, psychiatrists devoted little effort to detecting and treating residuals, either because it was felt that they were 'an acceptable part of the illness' or because adequate treatment tools did not exist in those days (Judd et al., 1998b). Mood episodes are frequently followed by a persistent constellation of symptoms: 30% of bipolar I patients and 37% of patients with bipolar II disorder, or unipolar depression have only a partial resolution of major episodes (Cassano and Savino, 1993). Residuals appear to be related to an increased duration of index episode, and to higher risks

TABLE 5.4   Prodromals

Manic side
• Increased psychomotor activity
• Decreased need for sleep
• Elevated mood
(Carlson and Goodwin, 1973; Keitner et al., 1996)

Depressive side
• Loss of energy
• Impaired concentration
• Anergia
• Decreased self-confidence
• Morbid thoughts
(Molnar et al., 1988; Sclare and Creed, 1990; Smith and Tarrier, 1992)

Manic and depressive side
• Unusual thought content
• Conceptual disorganization, from one to four months before
(Altman et al., 1992)

of chronic course and recurrences (76%) (Cassano and Savino, 1997), and to be inversely related to therapeutic success (Fava, 1999; Angst, 1986; Frank and Thase, 1999). Residual manic symptoms are related with lower levels of insight, and with a higher potential for dangerous behaviours, if compared to the depressive ones (Pini et al., 2001). As noted before, residuals may also represent a risk factor for the onset of a new episode, acting as prodromals. The systematic assessment of residuals permits us to identify a wide range of mood phenomenology, which may also arise during the lifetime of subjects who never have had (nor will develop) a full-blown mood disorder. In fact, an intriguing point is to understand the significance of such a kind of residual mood phenomenology, when it is not preceded or followed by a full-blown mood episode. Some patients, for example, seem to present with a long-lasting residual mood symptomatology, after having experienced what we could call 'a subthreshold mood episode'. In these cases, residual symptomatology may consist in isolated symptoms that may reduce subjective and objective levels of work and social adjustment, and may be interpreted as an individual's temperamental background. In some other cases, these isolated symptoms may continue completely unrecognized, if they are not specifically investigated.

The recognition and systematic assessment of these symptoms, which in most cases are likely to be different from the 'classical' DSM-IV symptoms constituting criteria for diagnosis (e.g., low self-esteem, lack of interest in work and hobbies, low energy levels) (Paykel and Weissman, 1973; Paykel, 1998), submissive dependency and abnormal levels of family attachment, long-lasting inhibited interpersonal relationships and communications (Bauwens et al., 1991; Goering et al., 1992; Coryell et al., 1993), rigidity in routines, resignation from leisure activity, inhibited interpersonal communication and irritable disposition (Akiskal, 1981, 1983), autonomic system irregularities, such as decreased libido, mono-symptomatic pain, easy fatigability, or fear of coping/facing daily activities) should be part of the routine clinical assessment, independently of the occurrence of a full-blown episode (see Table 5.5). The last one to six months MOODS-SR evaluation forms give clinicians a tool for multiple systematic assessment of residual mood-spectrum phenomenology, which is often related to post-episodic levels of functional impairment, adjustment and quality of life.

Subthreshold Episodic Mood Changes

Studies on the clinical and heuristic value of so-called 'partial', 'incomplete', 'subliminal' or 'subthreshold' forms of mood disorders have been extensively reported in the literature. We have decided to include under the term 'subthreshold' those conditions which do not fulfil the diagnostic criteria of the international classifications for mood disorders. Subthreshold depressive features are mostly associated with subjective distress, and are more easily recognized by patients and clinicians; indeed, a subthreshold manic mood is often pleasant, and associated with periods of improved productivity and better functioning: its perception is ego-syntonic even when cognitive and behavioural patterns have changed significantly from the individual baseline (Cassano et al., 1999). Higher levels of productivity, sociability and energy, are not remembered by the patient as 'harmful', and, for this reason, are never mentioned to the clinician.

SCI-MOODS™ explores in a systematic manner the presence of subthreshold expressions of mood-spectrum disorders, along the entire lifetime. The instrument assesses mood, energy, psychomotor and neurovegetative dysregulations, on both the depressive and the manic side. The organization of SCI-MOODS™ into the four abovementioned domains, reflects this *a priori* approach. Patients are questioned as to whether they feel extremely clever, happy, productive, confident, exuberant, irritable or arrogant, only at certain times of the day, or night, or in

TABLE 5.5   Mood residuals in patients with a manic or mood episode in remission

Manic residuals	
• Behavioural	persistent hyperactivity, energy levels
• Cognitive	feeling guilty, fear of relapse/recurrences
• Mood	sadness, feeling worried
• Neurovegetative	sleep dysregulations
• Social	poor capability in establishing good interpersonal relationships
Depressive residuals	
• Behavioural	slowness in everyday activities (especially in work)
• Cognitive	fear of relapse/recurrences, low self-esteem
• Mood	irritability, anxiety
• Neurovegetative	low energy levels
• Social	reduced social interaction capability

Modified from Keitner et al. (1996).

certain seasons. Variations in interests, efficiency, sleep patterns or physical energy are explored over the course of the year or even over the course of the day, from childhood to adulthood, in relation to the change of seasons, to jet-lag, or over the course of the menstrual cycle (see Table 5.6). Such mood, energy, psychomotor and neurovegetative episodic subthreshold dysregulations, even if ego-syntonic and adaptive, may represent a background vulnerability for a full-fledged mood episode of both manic and depressive polarity. The spectrum approach to sub-clinical mood changes overcomes the rigid unipolar–bipolar distinction: at this level of severity, the dimensional model responds better to clinical and heuristic needs.

Subthreshold Mood Dysregulations: from Persistent Lifelong Characterological Changes to Acquired Lifestyles

We argue that mood spectrum symptoms and behaviours may occur as early-onset, prodromal, and residual symptoms, and as persistent subthreshold conditions related to the full-blown manifestations of a mood disorder. From such a perspective, the individual's lifestyle may result as partially determined by the presence of long-lasting, unrecognized areas of mood psychopathology, responsible for dys/functional marital, work, and other psychosocial relationships (Frank et al., 1998). Paradigmatic is the case of a gloomy person with a joyless disposition, guilt-prone, with low levels of sexual drive, lethargy, and instability of self-esteem, the consequence of an enduring subthreshold depressive form, which never reached the threshold of a full-blown episode. Conversely, when subthreshold bipolar manifestations are present, they can be experienced as ego-syntonic, and not even noticed. Many of these subjects, define themselves as 'unreliable', absolutely 'unpredictable' regarding the quality of their social, sexual and work performances, but they do not want to be called 'moody'. Their lifestyle is mainly characterized by 'day in–day out', often related to sleep patterns. However, the ego-syntonic perception of these manifestations does not reduce the risk of the appearance of a fully syndromal disorder.

SCI-MOODS^{TM} assesses in a systematic manner the so-called individual acquired lifestyle or temperamental traits in a different perspective. This assessment in most cases may reveal subthreshold mood dysregulations that usually range from a subsyndromal depressive state to an attenuated manic condition. In most of these subjects, the 'constant in life' is represented by one (or more) of the following conditions: (1) a sub-continuous up and down, from lethargy, anergia, hypersomnia, to intense activity, energy and hyposomnia; from the 'fast way of thinking' and 'over-confidence' to 'slowness' and 'indecisiveness' (Akiskal's 'cyclothymic temperament'); (2) a stable subthreshold depressive condition (Akiskal's 'depressive temperament'); (3) a stable hypomanic mood (Akiskal's 'hyperthymic temperament').

The complexity of the picture offered by the single patient can be adequately described by SCI-MOODS^{TM}, which detects and records a wide number of traits

TABLE 5.6   SCI-MOODS™ items exploring subthreshold episodic mood changes

- Feel a strong desire to reconnect with people you had not seen or spoken with for a long time
- Overly talkative, speak rapidly or loudly, or be difficult to interrupt
- Constantly active and have the pleasant sensation of never getting tired
- Overactive and have such high energy that it sometimes exhausted or irritated others
- Enjoy making many jokes (even if inappropriate or out of place)
- Wear clothing or a hairstyle that is dramatic, extravagant, very high fashion or very unusual
- Tend to behave in an oppositional way or play the devil's advocate
- Rarely have periods free of abrupt shifts from one brief subthreshold bipolar phase to another
- Feel as if others were causing all of your problems
- Behave overconfidently and in an uninhibited manner
- Have diurnal and/or seasonal rhythmic variations of any or all of the above

and symptoms and provides the clinician with a refined descriptive 'profile' of the single individual leading to a profound sense of 'being understood' on the part of the patient.

The 'Atypical Side' of Mood Spectrum

The various categories of mood disorders are defined by the presence of easily recognizable mood symptoms. However, their stereotypic rigidity has resulted in the failure to identify the full range of symptoms and syndromes with which patients may present. So the term 'atypical' has been utilized to describe those conditions which were difficult to accommodate in the DSM or ICD diagnostic criteria, and 'liable to be consigned to some wastepaper basket category' or even ignored (Roth, 1992). Therefore, recognizing and assessing atypical mood signs/symptoms and atypical mood syndromes may represent a valuable adjunct to categorical methods of diagnosis and classification. On the atypical side of the mood spectrum are included: (1) mood symptoms, signs, or behaviours not listed in the DSM-IV criteria for hypo/manic, mixed or depressive episodes, but commonly seen in clinical populations (Cassano and Savino, 1997); (2) subthreshold mood dysregulations: forms with a limited number of symptoms (oligo- or mono-symptomatic forms) or with brief duration (e.g., three to five days); (3) subthreshold mood disorders mixed, covered or masked by threshold or subthreshold comorbidity for other psychiatric disorders; (4) mood symptoms in comorbidity with drugs or substance or alcohol abuse, mainly characterized by impulsive risk-taking traits, and cyclicity of manifestations. They may lead to dangerous behaviours (Geller and Luby, 1997; Brady et al., 1998; Pliszka et al., 2000; Perretta et al., 1996; Cassano et al., 2000) when poor development of judgement abilities, the feeling of being untouchable by any peril, and low levels of harm avoidance tend to prevail (Pliszka et al., 2000); (5) mood symptoms and signs combined with or masked by physical (e.g., neurological) disorders or physiological conditions (e.g. pregnancy); (6) age-related forms: presentations of mood spectrum in infancy, childhood or the elderly. In fact, during childhood and adolescence, mood disorders may be characterized by temporary forms of psychomotor agitation in the absence of evident mood symptoms, abrupt antisocial behaviours (young people suddenly transformed into 'wild people') (Carlson, 1990), episodic outburst of rage in situations of overstimulation ('episodic irritability'), fluctuations of energy levels with pseudo-conduct features, or phases of psychomotor hyperactivity alternating with phases in which neurovegetative altera- tions tend to be prominent (Egeland, 2000).

Among the elderly, atypical features are mainly related to medical diseases preceding and triggering (or following and complicating) the course of both condi- tions (Catinci et al., 1997; Mayou et al., 2000).

All these atypical presentations of mood spectrum may characterize 'special populations' of patients, with less predictable clinical course and response to treat- ment, or peculiar (often dangerous) behaviours and lifestyles (Cassano et al., 2000). In these subjects, mood symptoms may remain undetected, masked or misdiag- nosed by more 'visible' manifestations. So, an accurate detection of mood, psychomotor, vegetative and cognitive dysregulations may be useful to centre clin- ician attention, and to recognize the presence of a mood-spectrum disorder. Nevertheless, the use of SCI-MOODS™ in atypical populations needs to be tested. We envision a number of potential uses of the interview in this specific area, from the improvement of treatment selection, to the development of better strategies for outcomes measurement, to monitoring the course of different patterns of mood symptoms.

CONCLUDING REMARKS

The insufficiency of threshold psychiatry is clearly demonstrated by the frequency and clinical relevance of the so-called 'subthreshold depressive syndromes'. Although data from epidemiological literature are in general consistent in showing the relatively more favourable outcome of minor mental disorders as compared to threshold ones, a considerable proportion of cases with subthreshold forms of depression may have a negative outcome or a tendency to transit into a threshold mental disorder (Simon and VonKorff, 1995; Tiemens et al., 1996). However, there seems to be a clear tendency on the part of physicians to detect patients with more severe psychiatric illness, while minor psychiatric conditions tend to remain unrec- ognized and unmanaged (Ormel et al., 1991; Coyne et al., 1995; Pini et al., 1997).

In psychiatric settings, depressive symptoms, though of low severity, are easily recognized as such. However, these subthreshold syndromes are, at best, defined in a negative light, i.e. as cases not meeting the threshold for any DSM-IV (APA, 1994) or ICD-10 (WHO, 1992) diagnosis; they should, instead, be defined 'positively' on the basis of the subtle symptomatology, clinical course and functional impairment that they may produce.

Subthreshold and enduring symptomatology, with an onset in childhood or adolescence, turned out to be linked with subsequent, later-onset major episodes so that the hypothesis which has been proposed represents the subtle symptomatology as the basic nuclear core that, by interacting with the environment, generates the full-blown disorder (Akiskal, 1983b). According to this view, the disease is initially expressed at a 'temperamental' level or, more precisely, as a subthreshold symptom pattern. Whether an early detection of such subtle background phenomenology is of value for predicting subsequent more serious, life-disrupting symptomatology remains unclear.

The findings described in this chapter should also be interpreted in the light of recent debate and a reappraisal of the importance of mental illness in non-psychiatric settings. It has been argued that minor mental disorders seen in primary care have a high likelihood of spontaneous recovery (Goldberg, 1992; Katon et al., 1994; Katon, 1995; Simon and VonKorff, 1995). Some recent studies suggest that outcomes of mental disorders in primary care are not simply related to their initial severity and that recognition is not always associated with a better outcome. Future efforts by researchers in the field should not be only addressed to improve physicians' ability to detect and treat formal mental disorders. A better understanding of what comprises the definition of subthreshold forms of depression and what psychopathological conditions are considered to deserve attention and treatment should be taken into account.

Subthreshold psychopathology and comorbidity undermine current nosologies, from two opposite viewpoints: comorbidity seems not to leave space for 'pure' or sharp and delimited diagnostic categories. The description of subthreshold forms is continuously lowering the cut-off point of each 'discrete' disorder. We believe that a spectrum approach, thus in no way rejecting the DSM categories, may contribute to better face these two problems. From typical to atypical presentations, from full-blown to subthreshold forms, from 'pure disorders' to full-blown or subthreshold comorbidity, a spectrum approach could provide an operational conceptual model useful to improve the description of each categorical entity.

In the area of mood disorders, the spectrum approach may contribute to the solution of another problem: how to override the unipolar–bipolar distinction (Cassano et al., 2002). In fact, cut-off between bipolar and unipolar disorders is still undefined, with relevant impact on research as on treatment. Several cut-off points have been posed, but, in the absence of a list of reliable external validators, their validity is related only to operational criteria, and to the capacity to represent clinical reality. So, current categorical approaches are still partially reliable and clinically weak. The combination between the categorical and the dimensional approach seems to be the most suitable solution to overcome such a practical problem. The assessment of mood dysregulations in a lifelong perspective, by focusing on distinct evolving steps of mood phenomenology, reduces the 'entropy level' produced by the effort of splitting mood symptoms into 'unipolar' versus 'bipolar'. If implemented and integrated with the categorical approach, the dimensional model permits us to direct the effort to a different aim, and to promote a unitary view of mood disorders.

As an atheoretical and strictly operational model, our mood spectrum permits us to discriminate between a depressive episode 'tout-court' and a depressive episode on a subthreshold bipolar background, or vice versa, to improve the recognition of signs and symptoms of both manic and depressive dimensions. These two main mood dimensions are commonly considered in clinical practice, when co-occurring with other mental disorders, namely schizophrenia, anxiety disorders, drug abuse or personality disorders. During the course of an anxiety disorder, mood symptoms can manifest themselves as threshold or subthreshold, manic or depressive dysregulations, triggered by the drugs (e.g., antidepressants for the manic dimension or antipsychotics for the depressive dimension) administered for the treatment of the 'primary' disorder.

As a paradox, the co-occurrence of subthreshold manic features into the area of the traditionally defined 'unipolar' disorders, such as MDE and dysthymia, provided only a growing constellation of categories, splitting what could be better defined with a unitarian dimensional approach.

Fluctuations of energy levels, neurovegetative changes, psychological drives, dysregulations in psychomotor activity, rhythmic and seasonal patterns of symptoms can be utilized to unify, instead of separate, the unipolar and the bipolar side. Greater clinical weight needs to be attributed to subthreshold and atypical manic features during the lifetime course of unipolar depression, with a reevaluation of subthreshold bipolar manic components both in treatment and in research perspectives. This process will not lead to a continuous erosion of the unipolar categorical subtypes, because of the progressive widening of bipolar symptoms, but not of the depressive dimension 'per se', which, conversely, will result in being better defined.

The mood-spectrum model described in this chapter is based on a dimensional approach to mood disorders and permits a unitarian assessment of the global mood phenomenology, though maintaining most of the traditional categorical nomenclature. The SCI-MOODS™, that we are proposing, has turned out to be suitable for such purposes. In fact, this instrument could provide clinical and experimental foundations with a conceptual operational frame of reference to a model – the mood spectrum – whose borders should be continuously subject to dynamic revision.

REFERENCES

Agosti V, Stewart JW (1998) Social functioning and residual symptomatology among outpatients who responded to treatment and recovered from major depression. *J Affect Disord* **48**: 207–210.

Akiskal HS (1981) Subaffective disorders: dysthymic, cyclothymic and bipolar II disorders in the 'borderline' realm. *Psychiatr Clin North Am* **4**: 25–46.

Akiskal HS (1983a) The bipolar spectrum: new concepts in classification and diagnosis. In Grinspoon L (ed.) *Psychiatry Update: The American Psychiatric Association Annual Review*, Vol. 2. Washington, DC: American Psychiatric Press, pp. 271–292.

Akiskal HS (1983b) Dysthymic disorder: psychopathology of proposed chronic depressive subtypes. *Am J Psychiatry* **140**: 11–20.

Akiskal HS, Bourgeois ML, Angst J, Post R, Moller H, Hirschfeld R (2000) Re-evaluating the prevalence of and diagnostic composition within the broad clinical spectrum of bipolar disorders. *J Affect Disord* **59**(Suppl 1): S5–S30.

Akiskal HS, Pinto O (1999) The evolving bipolar spectrum. Prototypes I, II, III, and IV. *Psychiatr Clin North Am* **22**(3): 517–534.

Akiskal HS, Rosenthal TL, Haykal RF, Lemmi H, Rosenthal RH, Scott-Strauss A (1980) Characterological depressions. Clinical and sleep EEG findings separating 'subaffective dysthymias' from 'character spectrum disorders'. *Arch Gen Psychiatry* **37**(7): 777–783.

Altman ES, Rea MM, Mintz J, Miklowitz DJ, Goldstein MJ, Hwang S (1992) Prodromal symptoms and signs of bipolar relapse: a report based on prospectively collected data. *Psychiatry Res* **41**(1): 1–8.

Angst J (1986) The course of affective disorders. *Psychopathology* **2**(Suppl 19): 47–52.

Angst J (1995) Epidémiologie du spectre bipolaire. *Encéphale* **6**: 37–42.

Angst J, Merikangas K (1997) The depressive spectrum: diagnostic classification and course. *J Affect Disord* **45**: 39–40.

APA (1987) *Diagnostic Statistical Manual of Mental Disorders*, 3rd edition, revised. Washington, DC: American Psychiatric Association.

APA (1994) *Diagnostic and Statistical Manual of Mental Disorders*, 4th Edition. Washington, DC: American Psychiatric Association.

Baldessarini RJ (2000) A plea for integrity of the bipolar disorder concept. *Bipolar Disord* **2**(1): 3–7.

Barrett J, Hurst MW, DiScala C, Rose RM (1978) Prevalence of depression over a 12-month period in a nonpatient population. *Arch Gen Psychiatry* **35**(6): 741–744.

Bauwens F, Tracy A, Pardoen D, Vander Elst M, Mendlewicz J (1991) Social adjustment of remitted bipolar and unipolar out-patients. A comparison with age- and sex-matched controls. *Br J Psychiatry* **159**: 239–244.

Blackburn IM, Moore RG (1997) Controlled acute and follow-up trial of cognitive therapy in outpatients with recurrent depression. *Br J Psychiatry* **171**: 328–334.

Brady KT, Myrick H, McElroy S (1998) The relationship between substance use disorders, impulse control disorders, and pathological aggression. *Am J Addict* **7**(3): 221–230.

Carinci F, Nicolucci A, Ciampi A, Labbrozzi D, Bettinardi O, Zotti AM, Tognoni G (1997) Role of interactions between psychological and clinical factors in determining 6-month mortality among patients with acute myocardial infarction. Application of recursive partitioning techniques to the GISSI-2 database. Gruppo Italiano per lo Studio della Sopravvivenza nell'Infarto Miocardico. *Eur Heart J* **18**(5): 835–845.

Carlson GA (1990) Child and adolescent mania – diagnostic considerations. *J Child Psychol Psychiatry* **31**(3): 331–341.

Carlson GA, Goodwin FK (1973) The stages of mania. A longitudinal analysis of the manic episode. *Arch Gen Psychiatry* **28**(2): 221–228.

Cassano GB, Dell'Osso L, Frank E, Miniati M, Fagiolini A, Shear K, Pini S, Maser J (1999) The bipolar spectrum: a clinical reality in search of diagnostic criteria and an assessment methodology. *J Affect Disord* **54**(3): 319–328.

Cassano GB, McElroy SL, Brady K, Nolen WA, Placidi GF (2000) Current issues in the identification and management of bipolar spectrum disorders in 'special populations'. *J Affect Disord* **59**(Suppl 1): S69–S79.

Cassano GB, Michelini S, Shear MK, Coli E, Maser JD, Frank E (1997a) The panic agoraphobic spectrum: a descriptive approach to the assessment and treatment of subtle symptoms. *Am J Psychiatry* **154**(Suppl 6): 27–38.

Cassano GB, Savino M (1993) Chronic major depressive episode and dysthymia: comparison of demographic and clinical characteristics. *Eur Psychiatry* **8**: 277–279.

Cassano GB, Savino M (1997b) Chronic and residual major depressions. In Akiskal HS, Cassano GB (eds) *Dysthymia and the Spectrum of Chronic Depressions.* New York: Guilford Press, pp. 54–65.

Cassano GB, Frank E, Miniari M, Rucci P, Fagiolini A, Pini S, Shear MK, Maser JD (2002) Conceptual underpinnings and empirical support for mood spectrum. *Psychiatric Clinic of North America* **25**(4): 699–712.

Cassano GB, Rucci P, Frank E, Fagiolini A, Dell'Osso L, Shear MK, Kupfer DJ (2004) The mood spectrum in unipolar and bipolar disorder: arguments for a unitary approach. *American Journal of Psychiatry* **161**(7): 1264–1269.

Chien AJ, Dunner DL (1996) The Tridimensional Personality Questionnaire in depression: state versus trait issues. *J Psychiatr Res* **30**(1): 21–27.

Coryell W, Andreasen NC, Endicott J, Keller M (1987) The significance of past mania or hypomania in the course and outcome of major depression. *Am J Psychiatry* **144**: 309–315.

Coryell W, Scheftner W, Keller M, Endicott J, Maser J, Klerman GL (1993) The enduring psychosocial consequences of mania and depression. *Am J Psychiatry* **150**(5): 720–727.

Coyne JC, Schwenk TL, Fechner-Bates S (1995) Nondetection of depression by primary care physicians reconsidered. *Gen Hosp Psychiatry* **17**: 3–12.

Dunner DL, Fleiss JL, Fieve RR (1976) The course of development of mania in patients with recurrent depression. *Am J Psychiatry* **133**: 905–908.

Eaton WW, Badawi M, Melton B (1995) Prodromes and precursors: epidemiologic data for primary prevention of disorders with slow onset. *Am J Psychiatry* **152**(7): 967–672.

Egeland JA, Hostetter AM, Pauls DL, Sussex JN (2000) Prodromal symptoms before onset of manic-depressive disorder suggested by first hospital admission histories. *J Am Acad Child Adolesc Psychiatry* **39**(10): 1245–1252.

Fagiolini A, Dell'Osso L, Pini S, Armani A, Bouanani S, Rucci P, Cassano GB, Endicott J, Maser JD, Shear MK, Grochocinski V, Frank E (1999) Validity and reliability of a new instrument for assessing mood symptomatology: the Structured Clinical Interview for Mood Spectrum (SCI-MOODS). *J Meth Psychiatr Res* **8**: 71–82.

Fava GA (1999) Subclinical symptoms in mood disorders: pathophysiological and thera-peutic implications. *Psychol Med* **29**(1): 47–61.

Fava GA, Rafanelli C, Grandi S, Canestrari R, Morphy MA (1998a) Six-year outcome for cognitive behavioral treatment of residual symptoms in major depression. *Am J Psychiatry* **155**: 1443–1445.

Fava GA, Rafanelli C, Grandi S, Conti S, Belluardo P (1998b) Prevention of recurrent depression with cognitive behavioral therapy. Preliminary findings. *Arch Gen Psychiatry* **55**: 816–820.

Frank E, Cassano GB, Shear K, Rotondo A, Dell'Osso L, Mauri M, Maser JD, Grochocinski V (1998) The spectrum model: a more coherent approach to the complexity of psychiatric symptomatology. *CNS Spectrums* **4**: 23–34.

Frank E, Thase ME (1999) Natural history and preventative treatment of recurrent mood disorders. *Annu Rev Med* **50**: 453–468.

Geller B, Luby J (1997) Child and adolescent bipolar disorder: a review of the past 10 years. *J Am Acad Child Adolesc Psychiatry* **36**(9): 1168–1176.

Ghaemi SN, Goodwin FK (2001) Gabapentin treatment of the non-refractory bipolar spec-trum: an open case series. *J Affect Disord* **65**(2): 167–171.

Goering PN, Lancee WJ, Freeman SJ (1992) Marital support and recovery from depression. *Br J Psychiatry* **160**: 76–82.

Goldberg D (1992) The treatment of mental disorders in general medical settings. *Gen Hosp Psychiatry* **14**: 83–85.

Goodwin FK, Jamison KR (1990) *Manic-depressive Illness.* New York: Oxford University Press.

Hartlage S, Arduino K, Alloy LB (1998) Depressive personality characteristics: state dependent concomitants of depressive disorder and traits independent of current opinion. *J Abnorm Psychol* **197**: 349–354.

Henry C, Sorbara F, Lacoste J, Gindre C, Leboyer M (2001) Antidepressant-induced mania in bipolar patients: identification of risk factors. *J Clin Psychiatry* **62**(4): 249–255.

Hollander E (1993) Obsessive-compulsive spectrum disorders: an overview. *Psychiatr Ann* **23**: 355–358.

Joffe RT, Young LT, MacQueen GM (1999) A two-illness model of bipolar disorder. *Bipolar Disord* **1**(1): 25–30.

Judd LL (1997) Pleomorphic expressions of unipolar depressive disease: summary of the 1996 CINP President's workshop. *J Affect Disord* **45**: 109–116.

Judd LL, Akiskal HS, Maser J, Zeller PJ, Endicott J, Coryell W, Paulus M, Kunovac JL, Leon AC, Mueller TI, Rice JA, Keller MB (1998a) A prospective 12-year study of subsyndromal and syndromal depressive symptoms in unipolar major depressive disorders. *Arch Gen Psychiatry* **55**: 694–700.

Judd LL, Akiskal HS, Maser JD, Zeller PJ, Endicott J, Coryell W, Paulus MP, Kunovac JL, Leon AC, Mueller TI, Rice JA, Keller MB (1998b) Major depressive disorder: a prospective study of residual subthreshold depressive symptoms as predictor of rapid relapse. *J Affect Disord* **50**(2–3): 97–108

Judd LL, Akiskal HS, Paulus MP (1997) The role and clinical significance of subsyndromal depressive symptoms (SSD) in unipolar major depressive disorder. *J Affect Disord* **45**: 5–18.

Judd LL, Paulus MP, Wells KB, Rapaport MH (1996) Socioeconomic burden of subsyndromal depressive symptoms and major depression in a sample of the general population. *Am J Psychiatry* **153**: 1411–1417.

Judd LL, Rapaport MH, Paulus MP, Brown JL (1994) Subsyndromal symptomatic depression: a new mood disorder? *J Clin Psychiatry* **55**(Suppl 4): 18–28.

Katon W (1995) Will improving detection of depression in primary care lead to improved depressive outcomes? *Gen Hosp Psychiatry* **17**: 1–2.

Katon W, Lin E, Von Korff M, Bush T, Walker E, Simon G, Robinson P (1994) The predictors of persistence of depression in primary care. *J Affect Disord* **31**: 81–90.

Keitner GI, Solomon DA, Ryan CE, Miller IW, Mallinger A, Kupfer DJ, Frank E (1996) Prodromal and residual symptoms in bipolar I disorder. *Compr Psychiatry* **37**(5): 362–367.

Kendler SK, Gardner CO (1998) Boundaries of major depression: an evaluation of DSM-IV criteria. *Am J Psychiatry* **155**: 172–177.

Kessler RC, Zhao S, Blazer DG, Swartz M (1997) Prevalence, correlates and course of minor depression and major depression in the National Comorbidity Survey. *J Affect Disord* **45**: 30–32.

Kety SS (1987) The significance of genetic factors in the etiology of schizophrenia: results from the national study of adoptees in Denmark. *J Psychiatr Res* **21**: 423–429.

Knoll J, Stegman K, Suppes T (1998) Clinical experience using gabapentin adjunctively in patients with a history of mania or hypomania. *J Affect Disord* **49**(3): 229–233.

Kraepelin, E (1921) *Manic-depressive Illness and Paranoia*. Edinburgh: E & S Livingstone.

MacQueen GM, Young LT (2001) Bipolar II disorder: symptoms, course, and response to treatment. *Psychiatr Serv* **52**(3): 358–361.

Mayou RA, Gill D, Thompson DR, Day A, Hicks N, Volmink J, Neil A (2000) Depression and anxiety as predictors of outcome after myocardial infarction. *Psychosom Med* **62**(2): 212–219.

Molnar G, Feeney MG, Fava GA (1988) Duration and symptoms of bipolar prodromes. *Am J Psychiatry* **145**(12): 1576–1578.

Olfson M, Broadhead WE, Weissman MM, Leon AC, Farber L, Hoven C, Kathol R (1996) Subthreshold psychiatric symptoms in a primary care group practice. *Arch Gen Psychiatry* **53**: 880–886.

Ormel J, Tiemens B (1995) Recognition and treatment of mental illness in primary care. Towards a better understanding of a multifaceted problem. *Gen Hosp Psychiatry* **17**: 160–164.

Ormel J, Koeter MWJ, van den Brink W, van de Willige G (1991) Recognition, management, and course of anxiety and depression in general practice. *Arch Gen Psychiatry* **48**: 700–706.

Paykel ES (1998) Remission and residual symptomatology in major depression. *Psychopathology* **31**: 5–14.

Paykel ES, Weissman MM (1973) Social adjustment and depression. A longitudinal study. *Arch Gen Psychiatry* **28**(5): 659–663.

Perretta P, Nisita C, Zaccagnini E, Lorenzetti C, Nuccorini A, Cassano GB, Akiskal HS (1996) Psychopathology in 90 consecutive human immunodeficiency virus-seropositive and acquired immune deficiency syndrome patients with mostly intravenous drug use history. *Compr Psychiatry* **37**(4): 267–272.

Perretta P, Nisita C, Zaccagnini E, Lorenzetti C, Nuccorini A, Cassano GB, Akiskal HS (1996) Psychopathology in 90 consecutive human immunodeficiency virus-seropositive and acquired immune deficiency syndrome patients with mostly intravenous drug use history. *Compr Psychiatry.* **37**(4):267–272.

Phillips KA, Gunderson JG, Triebwasser J, Kimble CR, Faedda G, Lyoo IK, Renn J (1998) Reliability and validity of depressive personality disorder. *Am J Psychiatry* **155**: 1044–1048.

Pini S, Berardi D, Rucci P, Piccinelli M, Neri C, Tansella M, Ferrari G (1997) Identification of psychiatric distress by primary care physician. *Gen Hosp Psychiatry* **19**: 411–418.

Pini S, Cassano GB, Dell'Osso L, Amador XF (2001) Insight into illness in schizophrenia, schizoaffective disorder, and mood disorders with psychotic features. *Am J Psychiatry* **158**(1): 122–125.

Pliszka SR, Sherman JO, Barrow MV, Irick S (2000) Affective disorder in juvenile offenders: a preliminary study. *Am J Psychiatry* **157**(1): 130–132.

Rapaport MH, Judd LL (1998) Minor depressive disorder and subsyndromal depressive symptoms: functional impairment and response to treatment. *J Affect Disord* **48**: 227–232.

Roth M (1992) The classification of affective disorders. *Pharmacopsychiatry* **25**(1): 18–21.

Sartorius N, Ustun TB, Costa e Silva JA, Goldberg D, Lecrubier Y, Ormel J, VonKorff M, Wittchen HU (1993) An international study of psychological problems in primary care. *Arch Gen Psychiatry* **50**: 819–824.

Sclare P, Creed F (1990) Life events and the onset of mania. *Br J Psychiatry* **156**: 508–514.

Sherbourne CD, Wells KB, Hays RD, Rogers W, Burnam MA, Judd LL (1994) Subthreshold depression and depressive disorder: clinical characteristics of general medical and mental health specialty outpatients. *Am J Psychiatry* **151**: 1777–1784.

Simon GE, VonKorff M (1995) Recognition, management, and outcome of depression in primary care. *Arch Fam Med* **4**: 99–105.

Smith JA, Tarrier N (1992) Prodromal symptoms in manic depressive psychosis. *Soc Psychiatry Psychiatr Epidemiol* **27**(5): 245–248.

Sullivan PF, Kessler RC, Kendler KS (1998) Latent class analysis of lifetime depressive symptoms in the National Comorbidity Survey. *Am J Psychiatry* **155**: 1398–1406.

Tiemens BG, Ormel J, Simon GE (1996) Occurrence, recognition and outcome of psychological disorders in primary care. *Am J Psychiatry* **153**: 636–644.

Ustun TB, Sartorius N (eds) (1995) *Mental Illness in General Health Care: An International Study.* New York: John Wiley.

Van Praag HM (1998) The diagnosis of depression in disorder. *Aust NZ J Psychiatry* **32**(6): 767–772.

Weissman MM, Leaf PJ, Tischler GL, Blazer DG, Karno M, Bruce ML, Florio LP (1988) Affective disorders in five United States communities. *Psychol Med* **18**(1): 141–153.

WHO (1992) *International Statistical Classification of Diseases and Related Health Problems*, 10th revision (ICD-10). Geneva. World Health Organization.

6

Suicidal Behaviour

Diego De Leo and Kym Spathonis

Australian Institute for Suicide Research and Prevention, Griffith University, Queensland, Australia

Between 1950 and 1995 suicide rates have increased by 60% worldwide, and in 1998 represented 1.8% of the total global burden of disease (WHO, 1999). Suicidal behaviour constitutes a significant public health problem, and in many countries, suicide rates, particularly those among younger age groups, equal or exceed the number of deaths caused by road accidents (WHO, 1999). Suicide currently stands as one of the three leading causes of death among individuals aged 15–34 years in all countries that report mortality data on suicide to the World Health Organization (WHO, 1999).

Premature death through suicide results not only in the direct loss of life, but also places a burden upon national economic productivity and resources in both primary and secondary health care settings (Schmidtke, 1997). Those bereaved by suicide (e.g., family, friends and work colleagues) may also endure emotional, social and economic turmoil, and in some cases the impact of suicide on survivors may manifest itself in suicidal behaviour.

Attempted suicide is 10–20 times more frequent than completed suicide, and in many cases results in the need for medical attention (Moscicki, 1985). However, suicidal behaviours, which extend from feelings that 'life is not worth living' to suicide attempts and completed suicide, are provoked by a multiplicity of factors that, to date, have hindered efforts to predict and obstruct their occurrence.

ON DEFINITIONS OF SUICIDAL BEHAVIOUR

Originally, the term *suicide* was devised by Sir Thomas Browne and first published in *Religio Medici* in 1643. Albeit little used at first, the term was founded on Latin *sui* (of oneself) *caedes* (killing), and had become an established

Mood Disorders: Clinical Management and Research Issues. Edited by E. J. L. Griez, C. Faravelli, D. J. Nutt and J. Zohar.
©2005 John Wiley & Sons Ltd. ISBN 0 470 09426 5.

noun and verb by the mid-eighteenth century. Over time, there has been much disagreement about the appropriate conditions which satisfy the classification of suicide. Since *Religio Medici*, the gamut of clauses that exist to define suicide synonymously acknowledge that death is both self-inflicted and intentional. For example, Emile Durkheim (1897) suggested that suicide constitutes 'all those death cases directly or indirectly resulting from a positive or negative act of the victim, who is aware of the consequences of its behaviour'. In 1973, Edwin Shneidman defined suicide as 'the act of intentionally self-inflicting one's own life cessation' (Shneidman, 1985) – a definition that has been quoted extensively over time. More recently, the World Health Organization adopted 'fatal suicidal behaviour' as the result of an act deliberately initiated and performed by a person in the full knowledge or expectation of its fatal outcome. Yet, not all individuals who die by suicide may have intended to die and not all individuals who survive a suicide attempt may have intended to live.

'Passive suicidal behaviours' such as the refusal to eat or drink, or comply with medication regime, which may result in death, may not necessarily be synonymous with the intent to die. The complexities associated with determining deaths as suicides are also heightened in the absence of clear verbal indications before death, or suicide notes found after death.

Attempted suicide (non-fatal suicidal behaviour) has been defined as a potentially self-injurious action with a non-fatal outcome for which there is evidence, either explicit or implicit, that the individual intended to kill him/herself. The action may or may not result in injuries (O'Carroll et al., 1996). The outcome of non-fatal suicidal behaviour varies depending on intention, preparation, knowledge of the lethality of the chosen method and coincidental factors (e.g. rescue or intervention) (Kerkhof, 2000). Other terms such as *parasuicide, self-injury* or *deliberate self-harm* are not implicitly associated with the intent to die, nor are they conceived as suicidal acts or gestures in the patient's perception of the event, the proposed function of the behaviour, and the associated features (Firestone and Seiden, 1990).

Suicidal ideation may be associated with suicidal thoughts and feelings ranging from a dissatisfaction with life, thoughts of death and killing oneself, feeling that life is not worth living, being tired of life, and wishing to die. Suicidal ideation is thought to constitute part of a continuum ranging from death wishes, suicidal ideation and planning, to suicide attempts and completed suicide.

THE RELIABILITY OF SUICIDE STATISTICS

On a worldwide scale, there is an absence of standardized criteria for the classification of deaths by suicide. In the absence of routine, scientific procedures which can provide 'objective' evidence to classify a death as a suicide (e.g. autopsies), officials are not likely to record a 'borderline' suspicious death as a suicide. Stigma on the family, legal sanctions against suicide, political pressures, or practical considerations of insurance compensation may predispose coroners and medical examiners to avoid the classification of suicide (Pescosolido and Mendelsohn, 1986). Hence, suicide is often under-reported (Tsuang and Simpson, 1985) and many actual suicides are recorded by coroners as accidental death (Brooke and Atkinson, 1974) or open verdicts, that is, verdicts indicating possible but not proven suicide (Shaw and Sims, 1984).

Suicide statistics are reported by many nations to the World Health Organization (WHO); however, several countries, particularly from Africa, the Middle East, and Central and South America, do not have available epidemiological data. For countries that do report mortality statistics to the WHO, the validity of official suicide data is wide-ranging.

Variability in defining and reporting cases has called into question the reliability of official rates in some countries (Sainsbury and Jenkins, 1982; Farmer, 1988). In particular, countries like Austria and the Netherlands generate suicide data of high quality, whereas other countries, most notably Finland, Greece, Israel, Ireland, and the United Kingdom, provide data of a nature that is subject to misclassification within certain sub-populations, especially the 15–24 and 75 years and older age groups (Rockett and Thomas, 1999).

Social implications of suicide may reduce the likelihood of the reporting of suicidal behaviour in some regions, particularly where religious and cultural sanctions condemn suicidal behaviour and stigmatize relatives of individuals who die by suicide or make a suicide attempt. In other cases, suicide may be deliberately masked as an accident, particularly in the case of one-occupant motor vehicle crashes and drug overdoses. In such circumstances the death may often be misclassified as 'accidental'.

Studies conducted on populations undifferentiated by age, however, suggest that official suicide data are spatially and temporally reliable enough for comparative scientific research (Sainsbury and Jenkins, 1982). Nonetheless, taking these aforementioned factors into consideration, the interpretation of available suicide statistics, in any context, must be construed with extreme caution and a discernment of the reliability and sensitivity of suicide certification.

EPIDEMIOLOGY OF SUICIDAL BEHAVIOURS

Suicide

International rates of suicide differ significantly; however, epidemiological studies have observed elevated rates of suicide in some Asian and Western Pacific regions, and highest rates in Eastern European nations. Table 6.1 presents the rates of suicide by year and gender for countries reporting suicide statistics to the World Health Organization, for the most recent year available (WHO, 2003).

Suicide rates in Eastern Europe have increased in recent years and are in general substantially higher than countries in Western Europe (Sartorius, 1995). However, the rank ordering of suicide rates in European countries has remained remarkably

TABLE 6.1   Suicide rates (per 100 000), by country, year and gender for the most recent year available (WHO, 2003)

Country	Year	Total	Males	Females
African countries				
Mauritius	1999	15.3	21.1	9.5
São Tomé and Principe	1987	0.9	0.0	1.8
Seychelles	1987	13.2	9.1	0.0
Zimbabwe	1990	7.9	10.6	5.2
American countries				
Argentina	1996	6.4	9.9	3.0
Bahamas	1995	1.1	2.2	0.0
Barbados	1995	6.5	9.6	3.7
Belize	1995	6.5	12.1	0.9
Brazil	1995	4.1	6.6	1.8
Canada	1997	12.3	19.6	5.1
Chile	1994	5.7	10.2	1.4
Colombia	1994	3.5	5.5	1.5
Costa Rica	1995	5.9	9.7	2.1
Cuba	1996	18.3	24.5	12.0
Ecuador	1995	4.8	6.4	3.2
El Salvador	1993	7.9	10.4	5.5
Guatemala	1984	0.5	0.9	0.1
Guyana	1994	10.5	14.6	6.5
Jamaica	1985	0.3	0.5	0.2
Mexico	1995	3.1	5.4	1.0
Nicaragua	1994	3.4	4.7	2.2
Panama	1987	3.8	5.6	1.9
Paraguay	1994	2.3	3.4	1.2
Peru	1989	0.5	0.6	0.4
Puerto Rico	1992	8.7	16.0	1.9
Saint Lucia	1988	7.5	9.3	5.8
Surinam	1992	11.9	16.6	7.2
Trinidad and Tobago	1994	11.6	17.4	5.0
United States of America	1998	11.3	18.6	4.4
Uruguay	1990	10.3	16.6	4.2
Venezuela	1994	5.1	8.3	1.9
Southeast Asian countries				
India	1998	10.7	12.2	9.1
Republic of Korea	2000	13.6	18.8	8.3
Sri Lanka	1991	31.0	44.6	16.8
Thailand	1994	4.0	5.6	2.4
European countries				
Albania	1998	4.9	6.3	3.6
Armenia	2000	1.6	2.5	0.7
Austria	2000	19.6	29.3	10.4
Azerbaijan	2000	0.8	1.2	0.4
Belarus	1999	34.0	61.1	10.0
Belgium	1995	21.3	31.3	11.7
Bulgaria	1999	15.9	24.1	8.1
Croatia	2000	21.1	32.9	10.3
Czech Republic	2000	16.1	26.0	6.7
Denmark	1998	14.4	20.9	8.1
Estonia	1999	32.5	56.0	12.1
Finland	1999	23.4	37.9	9.6

TABLE 6.1   (*Continued*)

Country	Year	Total	Males	Females
European Countries (continued)				
France	1998	17.9	27.1	9.2
Georgia	2000	2.9	4.8	1.2
Germany	1999	13.6	20.2	7.3
Greece	1998	3.8	6.1	1.7
Hungary	2000	32.6	51.5	15.4
Iceland	1997	12.2	19.1	5.2
Ireland	1998	13.4	23.1	3.9
Israel	1997	6.5	10.5	2.6
Italy	1998	7.8	12.3	3.6
Kazakhstan	1999	26.8	46.4	8.6
Kyrgyzstan	1999	11.6	19.3	4.0
Latvia	2000	32.4	56.6	11.9
Lithuania	2000	44.1	75.6	16.1
Luxembourg	2000	14.4	22.2	6.7
Macedonia FYR	2000	7.4	10.3	4.5
Malta	1999	7.1	11.7	2.6
Netherlands	1999	9.6	13.0	6.3
Norway	1998	12.4	18.2	6.7
Poland	1999	15.0	26.1	4.5
Portugal	2000	5.1	8.5	2.0
Republic of Moldova	2000	14.9	26.7	4.1
Romania	2000	12.6	21.2	4.5
Russian Federation	1998	35.5	62.6	11.6
Slovakia	2000	13.5	22.6	4.9
Slovenia	1999	29.9	47.3	13.4
Spain	1998	8.3	13.0	3.8
Sweden	1998	13.9	20.1	7.8
Switzerland	1996	20.2	29.2	11.6
Tajikistan	1995	3.5	5.1	1.8
Turkmenistan	1998	8.6	13.8	3.5
Ukraine	2000	29.6	52.1	10.0
United Kingdom	1999	7.5	11.8	3.3
Uzbekistan	1998	6.8	10.5	3.1
Yugoslavia	1990	15.3	21.6	9.2
Eastern Mediterranean Countries				
Bahrain	1988	3.1	4.9	0.5
Egypt	1987	0.0	0.1	0.0
Iran	1991	0.2	0.3	0.1
Kuwait	2000	1.6	1.6	1.6
Syrian Arab Republic	1985	0.1	0.2	0.0
Western Pacific Countries				
Australia	1999	13.1	21.2	5.1
China (selected rural and urban areas)	1998	14.1	13.4	14.8
China (Hong Kong SAR)	1999	13.2	16.7	9.8
China (mainland, selected rural areas)	1998	23.3	21.9	24.8
China (mainland, selected urban areas)	1998	6.8	6.8	6.8
Japan	1999	25.1	36.5	14.1
New Zealand	1998	15.1	23.7	6.9
Philippines	1993	2.1	2.5	1.7
Singapore	2000	9.5	12.5	6.4

stable over time (Makinen and Wasserman, 1997). The highest rates of suicide in Eastern Europe have been observed in Lithuania (44.1 per 100 000), Russian Federation (35.5 per 100 000), Belarus (34.0 per 100 000), Hungary (32.6 per 100 000), Estonia (32.5 per 100 000), Slovenia (29.9 per 100 000) and Ukraine (29.6 per 100 000).

In Southeast Asia, Sri Lanka also report high levels of completed suicide (31.0 per 100 000), as do Western Pacific countries China (mainland) (23.3 per 100 000) and Japan (25.1 per 100 000). Overall, the lowest rates of suicide observable are located among the general population in Eastern Mediterranean, American and African regions. For the most recent year available, Egypt (0.0 per 100 000), Syrian Arab Republic (0.1 per 100 000) and Iran (0.2 per 100 000) reported the lowest rates of suicide, followed by São Tomé and Principe (combined) (0.9 per 100 000). American nations reporting low rates of suicide include Jamaica (0.3 per 100 000), Guatemala (0.5 per 100 000) and Peru (0.5 per 100 000) (WHO, 2003).

Male rates of suicide are highest in European countries Lithuania (75.6 per 100 000), Russian Federation (62.6 per 100 000), Belarus (61.1 per 100 000), Latvia (56.6 per 100 000), and Hungary (51.5 per 100 000). Lowest rates are reported in Africa: São Tomé and Principe (0.0 per 100 000); the Eastern Mediterranean: Egypt (0.0 per 100 000), Syrian Arab Republic (0.1 per 100 000) and Iran (0.2 per 100 000); and America: Jamaica (0.5 per 100 000), Peru (0.6 per 100 000) and Guatemala (0.9 per 100 000).

China reports the highest rates of suicide among females across all age bands (24.8 per 100 000) followed by Sri Lanka (16.8 per 100 000), Lithuania (16.1 per 100 000) and Hungary (15.4 per 100 000). Currently China is the only world nation where female rates exceed the rates of suicide for males, particularly in rural regions. Over the period 1987–1996, rural Beijing reported higher rates of suicide among women aged 15–24, 25–34, and 35–44 years compared to men (Yip, 2001), and female rates in urban areas exceeded those of males in the 45–54 and 55–64 year age brackets (Yip, 2001). Recent evidence also shows a disproportionate number of women aged 75 years and older in rural China at a heightened risk of completing suicide compared to women in English-speaking countries (Qin and Mortensen, 2001; Pritchard and Baldwin, 2002). Lowest rates of suicide among women are reported in Eastern Mediterranean countries Egypt (0.0 per 100 000), Syrian Arab Republic (0.0 per 100 000) and Iran (0.1 per 100 000); in Seychelles, Africa (0.0 per 100 000); and in American nations Guatemala (0.1 per 100 000) and Peru (0.4 per 100 000).

The most striking epidemiological feature of suicidal behaviour in many nations is the increasing rate of suicide with age; however, this pattern is not found in every nation (see Figure 6.1). Until recently, suicide was a phenomenon with rates ubiquitously peaking in the elderly, and mainly among men. However, current rates of suicide among young people are the highest in a third of all countries, both developed and developing (WHO, 1999). In recent time, an increase in suicide among individuals aged 15–24 years and a subsequent decline in the rates of suicide among the elderly has been observed, particularly in Anglo-Saxon nations such as

Australia, New Zealand, Canada and the USA (Gulbinat, 1995). Contrary to this, suicide rates over the last 30 years have observed a relevant increase in suicide in old age in a number of Asian and Latin nations, with an almost parallel decrease in suicide rates in Anglo-Saxon countries.

Despite the high rates of suicide reported in older age, the absolute numbers of suicides reported are highest among those aged 25–44 years, a trend which is currently observable worldwide (De Leo et al., 2002a). This observation has changed remarkably over the last half-century, when also the absolute number of cases of suicide roughly increased with age (De Leo et al., 2002a).

In general, the male female ratio of suicide increases with age, from approximately 3:1 in young people up to 12:1 among those over the age of 85 (De Leo, 1997). However, the gender ratio differs somewhat between countries. In Anglo-Saxon nations (e.g. New Zealand, Canada, Australia, and also Scotland and Ireland), the male–female ratio is typically 4–5 times higher in men in both young and old age groups. On the contrary, Latin nations have experienced a lower male–female ratio of suicide in younger age (approximately 3:1), which increases to a higher ratio in older age (e.g. 6:1 in Portugal, 4:1 in Italy and Spain and 5:1 in Belgium and France) (De Leo, 1997). This phenomenon, however, does not extend to every Latin or Anglo-Saxon nation.

Attempted Suicide

Attempted suicide may occur 10–20 times more frequently than completed suicide (Moscicki, 1985), with rates more elevated among females compared to males. In the general population, several studies have investigated the lifetime prevalence of

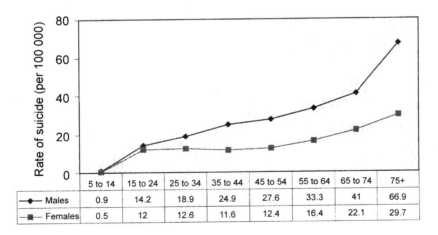

	5 to 14	15 to 24	25 to 34	35 to 44	45 to 54	55 to 64	65 to 74	75+
Males	0.9	14.2	18.9	24.9	27.6	33.3	41	66.9
Females	0.5	12	12.6	11.6	12.4	16.4	22.1	29.7

Figure 6.1 Global suicide rates (per 100 000) by gender and age, selected countries, 1995 (WHO, 1999)

attempted suicide. Paykel and colleagues (1974) observed a 1.1% lifetime prevalence of suicide attempts in the general population of New Haven, USA. The NIMH Epidemiologic Catchment Area Study (Moscicki et al., 1988), Maryland, USA, found a 2.9% lifetime prevalence of attempted suicide among the general population of adults aged 18 years and older. Other studies indicate a lifetime prevalence of 4.6% among individuals aged 15–54 years in Boston, USA (Kessler et al., 1999), and 5.1% among individuals aged 18 years and older in Latvia (Rancans et al., 2003).

Significantly higher rates of attempted suicide have been reported in hospital settings, with some regions reporting rates of 124.7 per 100 000 (USA) (Birkhead et al., 1993), 149 per 100 000 (Latvia) (Rancans et al., 2001), and 335 per 100 000 (Réunion Island, France) (Duval et al., 1997). The WHO-EURO Multicentre Study on Suicidal Behaviour (Schmidtke et al., 1996) investigated the epidemiology of suicide attempts in 16 centres in 13 European countries during the period 1989–92. The average age-standardized rates of attempted suicide among males were highest in Helsinki, Finland (314 per 100 000), and the lowest rates in Guipuzcoa, Spain (45 per 100 000), representing a seven-fold difference. The highest average female age-standardized rates were found in Cergy-Pontoise, France (462 per 100 000), and the lowest also in Guipuzcoa, Spain (69 per 100 000).

Attempted and completed suicide incidence rates exhibit opposing tendencies with respect to age: whilst the incidence of suicide rises as age increases, attempted suicide tends to decrease reaching lowest levels among the elderly (De Leo et al., 2001). Suicide attempts are four times more frequent among women aged 15–34 years compared to women 65 years and older, and the young/elderly ratio in males is approximately 3 to 1 (Schmidtke et al., 1996).

Suicide attempt methods employed by women of all ages most frequently involve drug overdose, particularly benzodiazepines and hypnotics in older age (De Leo et al., 2001), and analgesics among youth (Michel et al., 2000). In general, men employ 'harder' suicide attempt methods such as hanging, jumping from a height and firearms (De Leo et al., 2001). Few studies have investigated the cross-cultural variation of methods employed in suicide attempts.

Internationally, suicide attempt rates may be grossly underestimated. A measure of the true prevalence or incidence of suicide attempts may be difficult to gauge due to the fact that many calculations are derived from populations of suicide attempters who are admitted to hospital or present to a health care facility. Moreover, the lethality of a suicide attempt may not necessitate immediate medical attention, nor may the individual wish to seek mental health services in the time subsequent to a suicide attempt. As well as this, reporting of suicide attempts may also be affected by the age of the attempter, access to health care, and a cultural condemnation of suicidal behaviour; factors, which may both mask suicidal behaviour and lessen the likelihood of health care service utilization.

Suicidal Ideation

Epidemiological studies indicate that lifetime experience of life weariness and death wishes may be prevalent among 12.5% of the general population (Renberg, 2001), and between 4.8% (Paykel et al., 1974) and 15.9% (Schwab et al., 1972) may experience suicidal ideation in a lifetime. Higher rates of suicidal ideation have been observed among younger and older age groups in the community compared to the general population. For example, Wunderlich and colleagues (2001) found that of a total sample of 4263 subjects aged 15–24 years, 22.6% had thoughts about suicide, and 15% had the wish to die for a period of two weeks or more, with significantly higher rates observed among females in both realms. Overall, studies have found that the lifetime prevalence of suicidal ideation among adolescents ranges from 15% to 53% (Diekstra and Gulbinat, 1993). Death thoughts and suicidal ideation among the elderly aged 65 years and older in the general community population reportedly range from 2.3% to 15.9% (Jorm et al., 1995; Skoog et al., 1996).

RISK FACTORS FOR SUICIDE

Demographic and Sociocultural Factors

Gender

Between genders, the risk of suicide is greater among males. With the sole exception of China, male suicide rates in all nations outnumber rates for females. In Western nations such as Greece, Mexico and the United States, male suicides outnumber female suicides three- to five-fold (WHO, 2001). In Asia, the gender gap is narrower, where the difference tends to be less than twofold (WHO, 2001).

The gender difference in suicide risk may be attributed to a range of factors, which, on the one hand, render males at a higher risk, and on the other, operate to protect women. Compared to females, a higher rate of alcoholism (Rich et al., 1988) and comorbid depression, alcohol and/or substance abuse disorder (Rihmer et al., 1995) has been observed among males. In accord, men are also more likely to use alcohol during suicide completion, and alcohol intoxication has been associated with the increased likelihood of the use of a gun in suicides completed by males, but not for females (Brent et al., 1999). A greater likelihood of men employing irreversible methods of suicide (e.g. firearm) compared to common methods used by women (e.g. drug overdose) may also significantly increase suicide risk (Stengel, 1964).

In a study conducted by Murphy (1998), women were more likely to experience episodes of major depression, but were 25% less likely than men to complete suicide. This may be explained by a greater tendency for women to verbally express psychological pain, seek help for psychiatric symptoms and receive treatment as a result (Murphy, 1998). A lesser tendency for men to verbalize feelings of depression, hopelessness and suicidality, particularly in older age, may be related to social norms which foster the internal harbouring of psychological pain, and perceive help-seeking as an act of weakness (Murphy, 1998) and a declaration of incompetence (Tannen, 1990).

Ethnicity

Suicide rates vary between countries and across various racial and ethnic groups. In many countries, the prevalence of suicide among Caucasians is approximately twice that observed in other races (Moscicki, 1985). For example, a higher prevalence of completed suicide has been documented among Caucasians in South Africa and Zimbabwe (Lester, 1998) and among African Americans recently in the United States (NCIPC, 2003). This pattern, however, is not observed in nations such as the former Soviet republics of Armenia, Azerbaijan and Georgia (Wasserman et al., 1998).

Within countries, suicide rates may also differ between ethnic groups. In the United States the rate of suicide among Indians and Alaska Natives exceeds the rate observed among the general population (Indian Health Service, 1999). In Singapore, different ethnicities, although living in the same place, have nonetheless very different rates, with the Chinese and Indian having much higher rates than Malayan (Yip and Tan, 1998). In Kuala Lumpur, Malaysia, suicide rates are remarkably higher in Chinese people than in Indian and Malay, mirroring the report from Singapore (Yip and Tan, 1998).

Socioeconomic Status

A review of studies in the last 30 years on socioeconomic status and suicide concluded that the lower the socioeconomic status, the higher the suicide risk (Boxer et al., 1995). Several other studies have also shown that regions characterized by high levels of socioeconomic deprivation have increased rates of suicide (Gunnell et al., 1995; Congdon, 1996). Of relevance, Whitley and colleagues (1999) found that higher rates of suicide in parliamentary constituencies of Great Britain were associated with higher levels of social fragmentation, and that over a succession of years (1981–1991), areas experiencing the greatest absolute increase in social fragmentation also had the greatest increase in suicide. Sustained unemployment may damage social relations and reinforce the effect of social isolation (Burnley, 1995). In rural regions, economic distress and family discord may contribute to higher levels of suicide (Burnley, 1995). Moreover job loss may also weaken social integration and deprive an individual of his/her status and social role that may, in turn, elevate the risk of suicide (Durkheim, 1897).

TABLE 6.2   Risk factors for suicide

Category of risk	Risk factor
Demographic and sociocultural factors	Male Caucasian Unemployment Low socioeconomic status Social isolation Lack/loss of social support Immigration Type of religion, atheism Economic recession Political coercion and violence
Psychopathological and personological factors	Major depressive disorder Bipolar disorder Schizophrenia Alcohol abuse disorder Substance abuse disorder Personality disorder Post-traumatic stress disorder Comorbid psychiatric conditions Previous suicide attempts Suicidal ideation Hospital inpatient or recently discharged Hopelessness, helplessness Impulsivity, aggression Cognitive rigidity Shame
Biological and medical factors	Genetic predisposition to suicide Family history of suicide Abnormal serotonergic functioning Severe, painful and disabling physical illness; fear of illness Comorbid physical illness/psychiatric disorder
Life events	Separation/divorce, widowed Family discord Interpersonal relationship problems Violent, physical and mental trauma Physical and sexual abuse in childhood Early parental loss Problems with sexual orientation
Environmental factors	Access to, and availability of, lethal means of suicide Rural residential location Media portrayal of suicidal behaviour

Political Factors

Evidence suggests that women's access to social, economic and political power may contribute to suicide. This was demonstrated through findings from Portugal where the rise of the female independence movement correlated with a significantly increased risk in female suicide rates, particularly among professional women living in urban areas. This change in the rate may have been mediated through an increase in alcohol use among professional women subsequent to achieving greater independence (De Castro et al., 1988).

Stronger social integration during political activity and presidential elections may also correlate with decreased suicide rates (Boor, 1981); however, this finding is not supported by all studies (Wasserman, 1983). During time of war, suicide among the population is generally reduced (Lester, 1993) but political coercion or violence can increase suicide. For example, the Singhalese majority of Sri Lanka's population have generally experienced a low rate of suicide until the start of the civil war two decades ago, when its rate increased greatly (Marecek, 1998). Altruistic suicides during war also increases suicide rates. For example, in ancient times in China, those soldiers thought to be particularly brave stepped forward in front of battle lines to complete suicide as a demonstration of the fierceness of their loyalty and determination against invading armies from Central Asia (Lin, 1990).

Economic recession may significantly elevate suicide rates in many regions. For example, high suicide rates during economic recession in Japan were documented during the post World War II period 1975–90 (Goto et al., 1994). During the economic upswing in Finland between 1985 and 1990, Hintikka and colleagues (1999) observed a significant increase in suicide among both males and females, followed by a subsequent decline in rates during economic recession from 1990 to 1995. With economic recession, unemployment might result in loss of identity and self-respect with suicide a possible outcome (Platt, 1984).

Unemployment

Aggregate-level longitudinal studies have found that unemployment is positively correlated with suicide rates in many Western countries (Brenner and Mooney, 1982). A number of case–control analyses have also found significantly greater 'unemployment, job instability or occupational problems' among people who had committed or attempted suicide than among those who had not (Durkheim, 1897; Platt, 1984). In a longitudinal survey conducted in Britain, Lewis and Sloggett (1998) found that, compared to employed counterparts, those who were unemployed were over 2.5 times more likely to kill themselves than their employed counterparts (OR = 2.58, 95% CI = 1.97–3.38). In younger generations suicide risk is also elevated through unemployment, and studies conducted in Denmark (Agerbo et al., 2002), Puerto Rico (McQuillan and Rodriguez, 2000), the United Kingdom (Hawton et al., 1999) and Australia (Morrell et al., 1998) support this premise. However, future research is needed to determine whether unemployment per se provokes suicide in unemployed individuals or whether additional factors, for example psychiatric illness, contribute a more profound impact.

Social Integration, Support and Isolation

According to Durkheim (1897), suicide varies inversely with the degree of social integration of the social groups of which the individual forms a part. Hence, when social integration fails, the suicide rate usually rises (Maris, 1997b). Completed suicide occurs more often in those who are more socially isolated and lack supportive family and friendships (Appleby et al., 1999a). In a study conducted by Maris (1981), individuals who completed suicide tended to be the most inter-personally isolated, and experienced the highest degree of non-participation in organizations and social groups. Individuals who live alone may also be at an increased risk for suicide (Maris et al., 1997b). Earlier studies have found a higher correlation between suicide and living alone in the old than in the young population (Sainsbury, 1955) and in the general community (Waern et al., 2002). Moreover, suicide rates may be associated with the percentage of persons who live alone, live alone in just one room, or live in hotel rooms (Sainsbury, 1955).

The absence (Nisbet, 1996) or loss of social support may increase the risk of suicide (Maris et al., 1997a). In a comparative study conducted among individuals who died from natural causes and by suicide, Maris (1981) observed that on average, those who died natural deaths had about twice as many close friends as suicide completers despite the fact that the former sample of deaths were on average 20 years older. Studies of youth at risk for adverse outcomes, including suicide, have demonstrated that social support potently buffers the effects of negative life events (Carbonell et al., 1998; Vance et al., 1998). The benefits of social support have also been documented in an enhanced ability to cope with stresses, including bereave-ment, rape, job loss, physical illness, and overall enhanced psychological and physical health (IOM, 2001; Sarason et al., 1990). Social support may also attenuate severity of depression and can speed remission of depression in at-risk groups such as immigrants and the physically ill (Barefoot et al., 2000; Shen and Takeuchi, 2001).

Immigration

In some countries, higher rates of suicide have been reported for immigrants and, in general, such rates tend to reflect that of the country of origin, with convergence toward that of the host country over time (Singh and Siahpush, 2001). This phenom-enon has been observed among immigrants from Finland to Sweden (Ferrada-Noli et al., 1995), and among immigrants to the United States (Sorenson and Shen, 1996), Britain and Australia (Lester, 1972).

In a study of suicide rates among ethnic-immigrant groups to Canada (English/ Welsh, American Scottish, Irish, German, Italian, Portuguese and foreign-born), Trovato (1986) observed a higher suicide rate among ethnic-immigrant groups who experienced a greater degree of social assimilation and a lower level of commu-nity cohesiveness (Trovato, 1986). Other factors that may be associated with suicidality among immigrant groups include disagreement with the decision to migrate and poor expectations for the future (Hovey, 2000a,b), social isolation, low social class (Ferrada-Noli et al., 1995) and language barriers (Hovey, 2000a,b). Additional acculturative stressors may impact upon psychological health such as disrupted social and family support networks, pre-migration variables such as adaptive functioning (self-esteem, coping ability, psychiatric status), spiritual beliefs, and tolerance and acceptance of the host country towards immigrants (Berry and Kim, 1988; Williams and Berry, 1991).

Religion

In some cultures where major religious beliefs assert theological sanctions against suicide, correspondingly low rates of suicide have been reported. For example, a number of studies suggest lower suicide rates in countries with less social or religious tolerance of suicide (Pescosolido and Georgianna, 1989). Church membership (Breault, 1986) may protect against suicide, and regular church attendance may reduce the risk of suicide (Stack, 1992) by up to four times (Comstock and Partridge, 1972). As well as this, religion may decrease suicide risk in proportion to the extent to which it facilitates friendship networks among coreligionists (Pescosolido and Georgianna, 1989).

Among individuals aged 50 years and older, participation in religious activities may reduce the odds of suicide (Nisbet et al., 2000). Of relevance, older persons who practise their faith have frequently lower rates of depression, alcoholism, and hopelessness (Koenig, 1994), all prominent risk factors for suicidal behaviour (Rifai et al., 1994). However, older-age women tend to be more religious than men, attend church more, and have lower suicide rates (Weaver and Koenig, 1996). Hence, the propensity for religious affiliations to benefit suicide rates in old age may be differentiated by gender.

Fewer studies have investigated the impact of religion on suicide among younger age samples. Some studies have found that church attendance among youths of various ethnic/racial backgrounds reduces suicide risk, including suicide attempts (Conrad, 1991; Kirmayer et al., 1996, 1998). In a large meta-analysis of studies undertaken on religion and suicidality among youth in the United States, Donahue (1995) found that religiousness decreases risk of suicide ideation and attempts in youth.

Psychopathological Factors

Psychiatric Conditions

Retrospective research shows that close to 90% of individuals who complete suicide have diagnosable psychiatric disorders at the time of death (Appleby et al., 1999a; Cavanagh et al., 1999a; Henriksson et al., 1993). However, only a small proportion of individuals with major psychopathology take their own life (Hendin, 1991; Moscicki, 1995), and psychiatric disorders alone are not sufficient predictors of suicide.

Depressive disorders are found in 30–90% of completed suicides (with bipolar disorders representing 5% of depressive disorders) (Lönnqvist, 2000). The lifetime risk of suicide in individuals with major and bipolar depression is approximately 12–15% (Guze and Robins, 1970; Harris and Barraclough, 1997). An elevated prevalence of suicide among affective disorder patients with a history of hospitalization, particularly when suicidal, has also been documented (Bostwick and Pankratz, 2000). As well as this, suicide may occur at different points in the natural course of affective illness (Pokorny, 1983; Goldacre et al., 1993) and the risk of suicide decreases as the time from the most recent hospitalization, or treatment, increases (Davies et al., 1998; Simon and VonKorff, 1998). Suicide risk is highest during the years immediately following the onset of affective disorders (Amaddeo et al., 1995).

In patients with schizophrenia, suicide is the major cause of premature death (Allebeck, 1989; Tsuang et al., 1990). It has been estimated that 10–15% of individuals with schizophrenia die by suicide (Caldwell and Gottesman, 1992; Westermeyer et al., 1991). The relative risk for suicide appears to be highest at the time when schizophrenia is first diagnosed (Rossau and Mortensen, 1997). The risk of dying by suicide in patients with psychosis is also increased by the presence of depression (Axelsson and Lagerkvist-Briggs, 1992; Westermeyer et al., 1991), and alcohol abuse disorder (Meltzer, 1998).

The risk of suicide among patients with anxiety disorders, regardless of diagnostic type, is higher than in the general population by a factor of ten or more (Khan et al., 2002). Among individuals with a diagnosis of panic disorder (Schmidt et al., 2000) or post-traumatic stress disorder (Kessler, 2000), the risk for suicide is greater when compared to other diagnosable anxiety disorders. As well as this, the presence of anxiety may further increase suicide risk among patients with other psychiatric illness such as bipolar mood disorder or cyclothymia (Young et al., 1993).

Approximately 2–4% of individuals with an alcohol use disorder will complete suicide and approximately 25% of individuals who complete suicide are alcohol-dependent (Murphy et al., 1992). Comorbid psychiatric conditions, particularly depressive (Murphy et al., 1992) and anxiety disorders (Arikan et al., 1999) significantly increase the risk of suicide among alcoholic individuals (Murphy et al., 1992). Abuse of illicit substances may significantly increase the risk of suicide; even more when comorbid Axis I and II disorders are present (Flavin et al., 1990). For example, heroin users are 14 times more likely than peers to die by suicide and deaths among heroin users attributed to suicide range from 3% to 35% (Darke and Ross, 2002). The relationship of substance abuse disorders and comorbid psychiatric diagnoses to suicidal behaviour is complex, since it is often unclear in what order the conditions arose, what causal links exist, and whether other characteristics may mediate the relationship (IOM, 2002).

Psychological autopsy studies have reported that approximately one-third of suicide victims meet the criteria for a diagnosis of personality disorder (Henriksson et al., 1993). In particular, borderline personality disorders (BPD), and to a lesser extent antisocial personality disorders (ASPD), present a significant risk of suicide. A diagnosis of personality disorder is found in 9–28% of completed suicides and follows depression, schizophrenia, and alcoholism in order of importance as a major risk factor (Hirschfeld and Davidson, 1988). Longitudinal investigations report suicide rates in BPD ranging from 3% to 9%, comparable to affective and schizophrenic disorders (Mehlum et al., 1994). A diagnosis of antisocial personality disorders has been reported in 5% of completed suicides (Frances et al., 1988).

Hospitalization and Recent Discharge

Suicide risk is especially high during hospitalization (Mortensen et al., 2000), with the majority of inpatients who suicide suffering from schizophrenia or affective disorders (Proulx et al., 1997; Wolfersdorf, 1996; Roy and Draper, 1995). The risk of suicide in hospital also increases with higher cumulative length of stay, previous suicide attempts (Spießl et al., 2002), previous hospital admissions, suicidal ideation at the time of admission and during the admission, suicide attempts during the admission, and a greater number of ward transfers (Shah and Ganesvaran, 1997).

After discharge from psychiatric hospital the risk of suicide is very high within the first weeks (Axelsson and Lagerkvist-Briggs, 1992; Lawrence et al., 1999) and remains elevated for up to six months (Appleby et al., 1999b). The risk of suicide after discharge from hospital may be associated with drug and alcohol abuse, loss of contact with the primary mental health professional, living alone, hopelessness, relationship difficulties, lack/loss of a job, history of attempted suicide, and a diagnosis of depression (King et al., 2001; McKenzie and Wurr, 2001).

Previous Suicidal Behaviour

A previous history of non-fatal suicidal behaviour ranks with discharge from inpatient psychiatric care as the major risk factor for suicide (Gunnell and Frankel, 1994). The highest risk of completed suicide occurs during the six months following a suicide attempt (Suokas et al., 2001); however, risk also remains high in the years following. Approximately one-quarter of suicides are preceded by non-fatal suicidal behaviour in the previous year (Owens and House, 1994) and approximately 1% of individuals who attempt suicide end their own life during the 12 months subsequent to the index event (Hawton and Fagg, 1988; Kreitman, 1977). In the years following an initial suicide attempt, studies indicate a suicide risk that ranges from 3.2% (Suokas and Lönnqvist, 1991) to 11.6% (Nielsen et al., 1990) within 5 years, 4.8% (Beck and Steer, 1989) to 12.1% (Nielsen et al., 1995) within 10 years, 6.7% within 18 years (De Moore and Robertson, 1996), and 10–15% within a lifetime (Fremouw et al., 1990).

Long-term risk factors for suicide mortality after attempted suicide include multiple episodes of deliberate self-harm, male sex, somatic disease, self-reported 'wish to die' motive for the index suicide attempt (Suokas et al., 2001), alcoholism, high suicidal intent and taking more precautions against discovery at the time of their index attempt (Beck and Steer, 1989). As well as this, social class, unemployment, previous inpatient psychiatric treatment, substance misuse, and personality disorder may predict suicide among individuals aged between 15–24 years who have a previous history of non-fatal suicidal behaviour (Hawton et al., 1993).

Psychological Constructs

Several psychological vulnerabilities are found to distinguish suicide completers from controls; however, other variables frequently moderate the relationship. Despite this difficulty, the importance of psychological vulnerabilities lies in the likelihood that they engender or exacerbate other psychiatric and social risk factors to establish an individual's unique risk profile (Conner et al., 2001). Hopelessness is a significant risk factor for suicide and may arise separately from mood disorders, occur across psychiatric diagnoses (Bonner and Rich, 1991; Joiner et al., 2001a), be experienced continuously and chronically over the course of mental illness, and remain even after remission of major depression (Brent et al., 1998; Minkoff et al., 1973; Rifai et al., 1994). Hopelessness may predict as many as 91–94% of suicides in both inpatient and outpatient samples (Beck et al., 1974). A high level of hopelessness during one psychiatric episode may also predict high hopelessness in later episodes (Beck et al., 1985). Feelings of hopelessness may derive from a low level of self-esteem combined with interpersonal losses and a lack of confidence in one's ability to regulate mood or solve personal problems (Catanzaro, 2000; Dieserud et al., 2001).

Other psychological vulnerabilities associated with completed suicide may include impulsivity and aggression, depression, cognitive rigidity (dichotomous thinking), anxiety, and self-consciousness/social disengagement (Conner et al., 2001). 'Psychache' or a state of psychic pain (Shneidman, 1993), which has been likened to feelings of anxiety, depression and agitation (IOM, 2002), may also present a particular risk for suicide.

Biological and Medical Factors

Genetic Influences

Only a limited number of studies have investigated the genetic influence in the realm of suicide, and many studies have lacked adequate control for psychiatric disorders. However, since the psychiatric disorders associated with increased risk for suicidal behaviour are heritable, the genetic influences on these psychiatric diagnoses and suicidal behaviour may also be transmitted within families (Fu et al., 2002). This has been confirmed by studies that have found that a family history of suicide increases suicide risk irrespective of psychiatric illness and for people with and without a psychiatric history (Qin et al., 2002; Fu et al., 2002). Hence, a positive family history of suicide is considered to be an important risk factor for completed suicide (Roy et al., 1999), and attempted suicide (Brent et al., 1994, 1996; Mann et al., 1999). Some research findings also suggest a positive association between violent suicide methods such as hanging and a familial predisposition (Linkowski et al., 1985; Roy, 1993).

Twin and adoption studies of the genetic contribution to completed suicide have been conducted. Roy and colleagues (1991) combined their own results with published data from other studies to find a significantly higher concordance: 11.5%, in monozygotic twins (who have 100% of their genes in common) versus 2% in dizygotic or non-identical twins (who share 50% of their genes). In another review of genetic studies of suicide, Roy and colleagues (1997) examined data from 399 twin pairs (129 monozygotic, 270 dizygotic) from different countries. A higher concordance for suicide was reported in monozygotic (13.2%) than in dizygotic twins (0.7%). A more recent study (Fu et al., 2002) also found that once controlling for the effects of psychiatric disorders, the genetic effects specific to suicidal behaviour are not mediated by common psychiatric risk factors such as major depression, childhood conduct disorder, ASPD, panic disorder, PTSD, and alcohol and drug dependence.

Schulsinger et al. (1979) found that 4.5% of the biological relatives of adopted away suicides also died by suicide compared with just 0.7% of the biological relatives of controlled adoptees. Half of all suicides were not associated with major depression. In another study of suicide among adopted patients, it was found that biological relatives of adoptees with affective disorder who had made an impulsive suicide attempt had significantly higher rates of suicide than those of matched control adoptees without affective disorders (Wender et al., 1986).

Neurobiological Processes

Evidence suggests that serotonin mediates inhibition of impulsive action to the extent that deficient functioning may predispose individuals to suicidal and other potentially harmful impulsive acts. Low serotonin metabolite (5-hydroxy-indoleacetic acid 5-HIAA) levels in cerebrospinal fluid (CSF) have been significantly associated with suicide (Du et al., 2000; Bondy et al., 2000), violent suicide attempts (Banki and Arato, 1983; Lester, 1995), and aggression and/or impulsivity (Virkkunen et al., 1994; Zalsman et al., 2001). A blunted prolactin response to fenfluramine may be a second index of serotonergic dysfunction that is related to both a history of suicidal behaviour in proportion to its seriousness and to impulsive aggression (Coccaro et al., 1989; Mann et al., 1992; Mann and Malone, 1997).

Physical Illness

The prevalence of medical illness among suicides ranges from 30% to 40% (Mackenzie and Popkin, 1987; Whitlock, 1986), and escalates to as high as 88% in elderly suicide victims (Henriksson et al., 1995). A number of studies have documented a significantly higher rate of suicide among individuals suffering from somatic illnesses including cancer, human immunodeficiency virus (HIV) infection and AIDS, stroke, juvenile diabetes mellitus, delirium, epilepsy, Parkinson's disease, traumatic brain injury, spinal cord injury, multiple sclerosis, Huntington's disease, and amyotrophic lateral sclerosis (Harris and Barraclough, 1994; Stenager and Stenager, 2000). Somatic conditions that are chronic, disabling, and painful, and have negative prognoses, are also correlated with suicide (Lönnqvist, 2001). A hypochondrial syndrome or intense fear related to severe illnesses such as blindness (De Leo et al., 1999), cancer or HIV/AIDS may also contribute to increased psychiatric disorders and completed suicide (Lönnqvist, 2001).

Much speculation surrounds the impact of physical illness upon completed suicide, and whether or not physical illness contributes to suicide independently or is mediated by other (risk) factors. In particular, individuals with somatic conditions encounter comorbid psychiatric illnesses, usually depression or anxiety, or both. Various studies have found that the risk of suicide is high with physical illness, especially when symptoms of depression are also present (Fawcett, 1972; Farberow et al., 1963; Whitlock, 1978; Stensman and Sundqvist-Stensman, 1989). As well as this, the rates of major depression rise when serious medical illness is present (Cassem, 1995) which may in turn, lead to an increased risk of suicide. Moreover, the additional failure of physicians to detect depression in the medically ill, or perceiving depressive symptoms as 'appropriate' to the patient's condition can also heighten the risk of suicide (Cassem, 1995).

Precipitating Life Events

Singlehood, Widowhood and Divorce

In general, married persons experience lower suicide rates compared to single and never-married persons, with the highest rates observed among divorced, separated and widowed persons (Smith et al., 1988). Individuals who are divorced and separated may be twice as likely to commit suicide compared to married persons, with a pronounced risk observed among men (Kposowa, 2000). An elevated risk of suicide among men aged 25–39 years who have never been married or divorced has also been observed (Burnley, 1995). Widowhood in the first half of life may present a particularly high risk for suicide (Kreitman, 1988; Buda and Tsuang, 1990), and an 8–50% (Kreitman, 1988; Buda and Tsuang, 1990) increase in mortality among young widows and widowers compared to the general population has also been observed (Stroebe and Stroebe, 1993).

Marriage may serve as a protective factor against suicide, particularly for men, by providing social and emotional stability (Durkheim, 1897; Kposowa et al., 1995), enhancing social and community integration, and reducing social isolation (Durkheim, 1897; Kposowa et al., 1995; Breault, 1986). On the other hand, divorce may render the loss of social support and family integration as an inherently stressful life crisis that may lead to severe psychological distress, which could culminate in suicide (Verbrugge, 1979).

Loss of a Significant Other

After the death of a parent or spouse, suicide risk rises more among men than women and remains elevated for 4–5 years (Wasserman, 2001). Bereavement is very frequently represented as a stressful life event for elderly persons, and particularly for men, especially when the death of a spouse is sudden (McIntosh et al., 1994). After suicide of a close family member, the risk of suicide is elevated for other family members during the grief process (Wasserman, 2001).

It has been suggested that what differentiates a suicidal reaction to a loss from a non-suicidal one is the frequency and timing of these experiences (Slater and Depue, 1981). That is, some individuals may be unable to resolve grief prior to the experience of another loss. Unresolved grief has been identified in 13–44% of cases of attempted suicide, chiefly owing to death of the spouse (Schmid et al., 1994).

Interpersonal Relationships

Often, suicide is immediately preceded by various types of relationships problems involving close family members, friends and colleagues (Freud, 1957). Suicide among children and adolescents may also be related to family discord, through findings where adolescents living in single-parent families or who were exposed to parent–child discord were more likely to complete suicide than matched controls (Brent et al., 1994; Trovato, 1992). Family discord has also been found to increase the risk of suicide in patients with mental disorders approximately ninefold (Cavanagh et al., 1999b). School and workplace bullying, victimization and harassment may also heighten suicidality, particularly when threats or acts of violence are implicated (Wasserman, 2001).

Violent, Physical and Mental Trauma

A significant risk of suicide is represented by traumatic events such as sexual molestation and assault, rape, and physical and mental abuse. Moreover, incest, torture, and any occurrence that brings to the fore memories thereof, may be associated with suicide (Ferrada-Noli et al., 1998). A significant body of evidence suggests that of the many types of childhood trauma, child sexual abuse is a strong risk factor for attempted suicide (Santa Mina and Gallop, 1998; Fergusson et al., 2000; Molnar et al., 2001; Paolucci et al., 2001) and completed suicide (Brent et al., 1999). Child sexual abuse accounts for 9–20% of suicide attempts in adults (Brown et al., 1999; Fergusson et al., 1996; Molnar et al., 2001), and is a risk factor for attempted suicide independent of psychopathology (Molnar et al., 2001). Sexual abuse also carries an extremely high risk (OR = 30.3) for repeated suicide attempts in adolescents (Brown et al., 1999). Early childhood adversity may also increase the likelihood of developing mental illnesses associated with suicide risk, such as substance use, posttraumatic stress disorder and depression (Fergusson et al., 2000; Molnar et al., 2001).

Sexual Orientation

While there is no clear evidence that homosexuality may increase at any age the risk of completing suicide, many studies have demonstrated a higher risk of attempted suicide among bisexual and homosexual youth, particularly males (DuRant et al., 1998; Garofalo et al., 1999). A somewhat less pronounced yet significantly elevated risk of attempted suicide has also been observed among young adult and middle-aged homosexuals compared to controls (Cochran and Mays, 2000; Herrell et al., 1999). Among homosexual and bisexual males aged between 18 and 40 years, the risk of a suicide attempt may be up to 5–14 times higher than for heterosexual males of the same age (Bagley and Tremblay, 1997; Cochran and Mays, 2000).

Environmental Factors

Geographical Location

Suicide rates in a number of rural regions, such as Australia (Baume and Clinton, 1997; Yip et al., 2000), Beijing, China (Yip et al., 2000), Finland (Pesonen et al., 2001), Scotland (Crombie, 1991), the USA (American Association of Suicidology, 1999) and the United Kingdom (Gregoire, 2002) have been found to be significantly higher than in urban areas. The increased risk of suicide in rural regions may be attributable to a range of factors. Compared with high-density populations, rural areas often receive a lack of public health services, have higher rates of unemployment, lower levels of education and limited social support networks (Pesonen, 2001). Among young rural people, suicide risk may be increased via media representations of suicides (Hassan, 1995), greater availability of lethal suicide methods such as firearms or herbicides/pesticides (Brent et al., 1991; Cantor and Slater, 1995), and problems in accessing and using mental health services (Baume, 1994). As well as this, limited skills of rural primary health care professionals in detecting and managing depression may increase the risk of suicide in these areas (Rutz et al., 1992).

Suicide Method

Methods chosen for suicide vary considerably in terms of 'lethality', that is, the probability of death (McIntosh, 1992). Firearms, hanging and carbon monoxide poisoning are considered to be the most lethal methods of suicide as they are more likely to be immediately fatal, are associated with a high level of impulsivity, are absolutely or relatively equal in their degree of accessibility, and are difficult to reverse. Drug overdose, poisoning with other gases, and drowning are less immediately fatal, leave time for someone to intervene, and vary in degree of accessibility (Marzuk et al., 1992). In part, the greater propensity for males to employ more violent and lethal means of suicide compared to females may account for a higher suicide rate. In older age, the lethality of the suicide method chosen may also reflect a greater determination and intent to die (De Leo and Ormskerk, 1991).

Fluctuations in suicides within and between countries at any single point in time may reflect changes or differences in the cultural acceptability of suicide methods (Cantor and Baume, 1998). For example, the declining use of particular methods of suicide in Australia (e.g. drug overdose) and a rise in others (e.g. hanging) may reflect sociocultural acceptability, since hanging has always remained a highly accessible method of suicide (Cantor and Baume, 1998; De Leo et al., 2002b).

Method availability may be considerably associated with method-specific rates of suicide. In a study conducted in the United States, firearm ownership was significantly correlated with suicide rates among individuals aged 15–24 years and 65–84 years (Birckmayer and Hemenway, 2001). In a comparison of five counties in the United States, Marzuk and colleagues (1992) found that counties had similar suicide rates for those methods that were equally accessible to the populations, but significantly different rates for methods that were differentially accessible. In England and Wales, deaths from paracetamol overdose has also largely paralleled sales figures (Gunnell et al., 1997), indicating that the extent of self-poisoning with paracetamol largely reflects its availability. However, evidence suggests that suicidal persons may use alternative methods that are more widely available if one or more means are restricted or unavailable in that community (Marzuk et al., 1992). For example, Rich and colleagues (1990) found that in Toronto, stricter gun control laws led to a decrease in suicide using guns, but led to a matching increase in suicide using other methods (e.g. jumping).

Media Coverage of Suicide

Media portrayal of lethal means of suicide may contribute significantly to increase both the rate of suicide and the incidence of suicides that adopt the same method. For example, during 1984 and 1985, the number of deaths that resulted from drinking the poison paraquat in Japan increased dramatically from 594 to 1021. Among the 1021 deaths in 1985, 96.5% were suicides (National Police Agency, 1986). The sharp increase in suicide by paraquat was attributed to the extensive media presentation of a criminal act in which 17 innocent victims consumed soft drinks, from vending machines, contaminated by paraquat.

Media-based coverage of suicides may also trigger copycat suicides in the mass public. For example, during the 12 months following the publication of *Final Exit*, a guide to suicide by asphyxiation for terminally ill persons, the number of suicides by asphyxiation in NewYork rose by 313% from 8 to 33. In 27% of suicide cases, a copy of the guide was found at the place of abode (Stack, 2000). Media reports of suicides in newspapers may also impact upon the rate of suicide. The propensity for newspaper stories to be saved, reread, displayed, and studied may result in a greater risk of copycat suicides compared to stories that are televised (Stack, 2002). It has also been found that studies based on real suicide stories are approximately four times more likely to report copycat effects than studies based on fictional suicides (Stack, 2002). Other evidence from a recent meta-analysis has found that the suicide of celebrity entertainers may have the greatest impact upon copycat suicides in the mass public, presenting a 14.3 times higher risk of copycat effect (Stack, 2002).

SUICIDE PREVENTION

As suicide is considered to be a multi-determined behaviour, it would be unrealistic to expect that any single preventive effort may reduce the risk of suicide and overall suicide mortality rates. In general, the array of preventive efforts that have been initiated in a number of multidisciplinary settings operate to target risk factors for suicide. However, to date there has been no significant decline in the overall rates of suicide as a direct outcome of preventive initiatives (De Leo, 2002). Nonetheless, initiatives to prevent suicide fall into three major realms, namely *prevention*, *intervention*, and *aftercare*, which are summarized in Table 6.3.

Prevention

Public Policy

The potential for applying comprehensive general population strategies to suicide prevention has been apparent for more than 100 years, since Durkheim observed that the frequency of suicide varied inversely with social integration (Durkheim, 1897). Socioeconomic determinants of psychiatric illness and suicide, such as unemployment and low levels of formal education, poverty and poor social welfare and housing systems, decreased social support, legal sanctions, drug and alcohol use, and community attitudes including stigma need also to be addressed by large-scale governmental initiatives. In 1989, the World Health Organization recommended that member states should develop national preventive programmes, where possible linked to other public health policies, and establish national coordinating committees. Its approach was based on the identification of groups at risk and restricting access to means of suicide (WHO, 1990). According to the United Nations (1996), only a minority of world nations have implemented nationally based suicide prevention initiatives with easily identifiable intervention targets. The formulation of official guidelines for national suicide prevention strategies by the United Nations in 1996 resulted in the development of suicide prevention programmes in several European and American countries. In 1992, Finland was the first country to establish a nationally implemented, research-based comprehensive suicide prevention programme. Since then, national suicide prevention programmes have been implemented in many countries including Australia, New Zealand, Norway, Sweden, Denmark and England.

Mental Health Promotion and Public Education

The promotion of optimal mental health through the learning and development of personal resources necessary to cope with the stressors presented in everyday life may be an effective way in which to facilitate a sense of mental well-being. Specifically, mental health promotion efforts endeavour to develop coping, problem-solving, decision-making and communication skills, which may enable individuals to overcome situational life difficulties, and control and even improve health status. Mental health promotion may form part of a comprehensive suicide prevention strategy and may be incorporated through government (e.g. school health curriculum) and/or non-government (e.g. religious organizations) education systems, as well as through the mass media.

Education of the public is an important suicide prevention strategy that is incorporated into all existing national suicide prevention strategies. In general, public education strategies operate to curtail the impact of social stigma relating not only to suicidal behaviour, but also to psychiatric illnesses. Community stigma surrounding suicide and psychiatric illness may reduce the likelihood that individuals will seek help when they are suicidal, and discourage the accurate reporting of actual suicides. Moreover, social stigma may limit the attention focused on suicide prevention at local, regional and national government levels. Some evidence suggests, however, that the social stigma of suicide may in fact reduce the ease with which people will actually contemplate suicide when under duress (Shaffer et al., 1998). The accessibility and availability of pertinent information regarding suicide is relevant for large-scale community awareness campaigns, school-based programmes, clinical treatment settings, research endeavours, programme administration and service delivery, as well as for members of the general community.

Media Guidelines for the Coverage and Reporting of Suicides

Media sources such as television, radio and newspapers play a critical role in influencing community attitudes and perceptions of social norms. In recent times, specific guidelines for media sources have been released in order to sanction the portrayal of mental health issues, including psychiatric illnesses and suicide, in conjunction with efforts to educate and raise awareness of such issues among media personnel. Many countries including Australia, Austria, Canada, Germany, Japan, New Zealand, Switzerland, and the United States, and organizations including the World Health Organization (United Nations, 1996; WHO,

TABLE 6.3   Overview of suicide prevention realms and initiatives

Realm	Description	Initiatives
Prevention	Preventive efforts taken to minimize the possible future development of suicidal tendencies and behaviour among members of the general population who are not currently experiencing suicidality	• Public policy initiatives • Media guidelines for the coverage and reporting of suicides • Mental health promotion and education • School-based education campaigns
Intervention	Preventive efforts targeted to assist individuals who manifest suicidal tendencies or conditions that carry an associated high suicide risk	• Detection and treatment of psychiatric disorders • Psychotherapeutic and psychosocial interventions • Improved assessment of non-fatal suicidal behaviour • Crisis intervention and telephone hotlines • Suicide prevention centres • Suicide prevention training for professional and lay-workers • Restriction of access to, and availability of lethal means • School-based programmes
Aftercare	Prevention efforts taken to minimize the risk of further suicidal behaviour among suicide attempters, and/or to reduce the impact of suicide and suicidal behaviour among survivors	• Monitoring of hospitalized suicide attempters • Aftercare programmes for hospital-treated suicide attempters • Bereavement services for survivors of suicide • Media guidelines for the coverage and reporting of suicides

2000) have formulated guidelines for media coverage of suicides. Various stipulations of media guidelines indicate that accounts of suicide should neither romanticize nor normalize suicide, particularly in the case of celebrity death by suicide; should include factual information on suicide contagion and mental illness; should avoid terminology such as 'successful suicide' which may downplay the dire loss of life; and should address suicide as an issue in its own right, reporting on stigma, treatment, and trends in suicide rates, rather than only in response to a tragedy.

Intervention

Pharmacotherapy

The early detection of psychiatric illnesses that contribute to a heightened suicide risk (i.e. major depression, schizophrenia, alcohol and substance abuse and personality disorders) is considered to be a vital measure in preventing suicide. However, the validity of assessment tools utilized in clinical settings to determine acute suicide risk or to predict when a person will attempt or complete suicide are inadequate. Nonetheless, pharmacological agents are predominantly utilized in the treatment of suicidal patients and include those which are diagnosis-specific and aim to regulate the biochemistry associated with predisposing, potentially suicidogenic pathologies. Newer generation pharmacological agents may also indirectly affect suicidality through the tendency to produce fewer side effects and more specific therapeutic profiles, resulting in increased compliance with treatment regimes and enhanced symptomatological outcomes. The use of lithium to treat bipolar disorder patients may reduce rates of suicide and attempted suicide. However, such findings are only observed among fully compliant patients treated for a minimum of two years (Baldessarini and Tondo, 1999). The efficacy of clozapine in reducing the risk of suicidality among patients with schizophrenia and schizoaffective disorder has been put forth by recent internationally based findings (Meltzer et al., 2002). However, through a lack of randomized controlled studies, the efficacy of anti-anxiety agents or electroconvulsive therapy in preventing sucidality has not yet been determined.

Despite the fact that the vast majority of individuals who commit suicide suffer from an underlying psychopathology, new developments in psychiatry, medicine and pharmacology have not yet resulted in a significant decline in suicide rates (De Leo, 2002). Several variables, however, have hindered the confirmation of the effectiveness of pharmacological treatments in reducing suicidality. Pharmacological treatments may require a minimum of six weeks to exert maximal efficacy (Fenton, 2000), and individuals during that time may be discharged into the community while symptoms are still quite intense. As well as this, unpleasant side effects may occur during the initial treatment period. As a result, individuals who become non-compliant with treatment regimes shortly after discharge may not be medicated for a long enough period of time to experience symptom relief. Another issue to consider relates to the reduction of psychiatric hospital beds which has led to shorter and more frequent hospital admissions, and thus to an increased risk of suicide, corresponding to the duplication of high-risk illness phases (Rossau and Mortensen, 1997).

Psychosocial Interventions

Risk factors for suicide indicate that necessary attention must be paid to factors outside the realm of psychiatric illnesses. Hence, desirable approaches to suicide prevention tend to acknowledge and utilize psychosocial interventions in order to reduce the risk of suicide through the enhancement of social, cognitive, and behavioural skills and functioning. Often, short-term psychosocial interventions in combination with psychiatric medication are incorporated in the treatment of suicidal patients. However, evaluations of long-term therapeutic interventions are rare, and not all investigations utilize randomized procedures. Linehan and colleagues (1991) conducted one of the only randomized trials investigating the long-term impact of therapeutic interventions on suicidality. In the study it was found that dialectic behavioural therapy (DBT) consisting of weekly individual therapy, group skills training, and as-needed phone calls led to a greater reduction in the rate of suicide attempts and the number of hospitalized days for suicidal behaviours. In addition, a greater treatment adherence over a 12-month follow-up, as compared to a group who received a referral to other outpatient treatment, was observed.

Although numerous studies document the efficacy of therapeutic interventions, especially cognitive-behavioural therapy (CBT), in treating high-risk psychiatric disorders such as depression and post-traumatic stress disorder, far fewer studies document the direct effects of therapy on suicidal behaviour and intent (IOM, 2002). Nonetheless, four controlled studies of suicidal adolescents and young adults suggest that CBT with problem-solving components and general problem-solving therapy reduces suicidal ideation and symptomatology such as depressive symptoms, hopelessness, and loneliness for at least two years (Harrington et al., 1998; Joiner et al., 2001b; Lerner and Clum, 1990; Rudd et al., 1996). However, such interventions may not have a long-term impact upon the rate of future suicide attempts or completed suicide.

Crisis Intervention Services and Suicide Prevention Centres

During the early 1960s, the establishment of the Samaritans in London and the first Suicide Prevention Centre in Los Angeles stimulated the growth of a number of crisis services and suicide prevention centres. Currently, over 350 Befrienders International Centres, associated with the Samaritans, exist in over 40 countries (Scott, 2000). Crisis services for suicidal individuals comprise a broad scope of 24-hour suicide and crisis telephone services that are directly linked to mental health care facilities, medical and psychiatric back-up (inpatient and outpatient), crisis counselling, mobile outreach, and short-term stay facilities. Evidence suggests some efficacy of such services in reducing suicide rates (Bagley, 1986). However, due to the fact that consumers of such services actively seek out assistance, question has been raised as to whether or not centres attract individuals with an elevated risk for suicidal behaviour, and whether they prevent these individuals' suicide or suicide attempt (Lester, 1974; Bridge et al., 1977).

Suicide Prevention Training for Professional and Lay-workers

Rutz and colleagues (1992) conducted a study in Gotland, Sweden, between 1984 and 1986, to determine whether education of primary care physicians can improve treatment of depression and reduce suicide rates. After completing the training programme, primary care physicians were more likely to prescribe antidepressants and less likely to prescribe anxiolytics. Accordingly, the rate of hospital admission for depression and the suicide rate decreased during the study. However, the decrease in suicides was reflected mostly by a decrease in suicides among women with depression (Rihmer et al., 1995). The suicide rate rose two years after the completion of the study, but due to the small number of suicides observed, it was difficult to distinguish whether or not the rise and fall was spontaneous or occurred as a response to the intervention per se (Szanto et al., 2002).

Accurate clinical assessment of attempted suicide is also important in the emergency care setting, particularly in light of the increasing proportion of patients who are directly discharged home from such departments. Although the management of individuals admitted to hospital places a considerable strain on services, particularly those afforded by psychiatrists, other disciplines in emergency departments, including nurses, medical teams (junior doctors and nurses), and social workers, should be confidently equipped to manage suicidal patients.

Environmental Measures

Stengel (1964) was the first to acclaim that efforts to control the environment may impact upon decreasing the incidence of suicide. According to a previous report produced by the World Health Organization (1998) regarding the prevention of suicide, the majority of the basic principles recommended incorporated measures to control the environment. These included the control of gun possession, the detoxification of domestic gas, the detoxification of car exhaust emissions, the control of toxic substance availability (e.g. appropriate dosage units and packages for medications) and toning down media reports of suicide. Moreover, other measures prescribed to prevent suicide included the fencing of high buildings and bridges. To date, controlling the environment has been shown to be an effective strategy in preventing suicide.

School-based Interventions

The need for suicide prevention initiatives to be developed in school settings has sprung from an increasing trend in youth suicide (particularly during the 1990s), which has placed a consequent strain upon the resources of the mental health care system. School settings provide a unique environment for the implementation of suicide prevention strategies featured by the potential to access a large proportion of the youth population. However, the ability of school-based initiatives to reach the most socially disadvantaged youth, who are perhaps the most at risk of suicide, is limited due to the fact that such individuals are not likely to be in regular attendance of formal education. Nevertheless, school-based suicide prevention policies must be developed in collaboration with schools and staff, students and parents, the local community and the professional community (e.g. psychiatrists, psychologists, researchers). Training and education of such stakeholders and predefined links to community mental health care services are essential to efficient suicide risk identification and the concurrent referral of students who may be at risk. A comprehensive postvention suicide plan coordinated by a mental health expert is also essential.

Aftercare

Monitoring and Aftercare of Hospitalized Suicide Attempters

The efficacy of psychosocial interventions (e.g., psychotherapy, case management, community-based interventions), particularly during the first three to six months after discharge from hospital may critically determine the outcomes of symptomatology, compliance with medication and suicidality. Follow-up of suicidal patients admitted to the emergency room three months after discharge from hospital has been shown to reduce suicide attempt and treatment adherence rates (Termansen and Bywater, 1975). Motto and Bostrum (2001) found that among suicidal patients who refused ongoing treatment after discharge from hospital, those who were sent regular follow-up letters from hospital staff, compared to patients who were not, were less likely to suicide during the first two years after discharge. Other findings supported the benefit of a suicide intervention counsellor working with patients from within 48 hours of admission until six weeks post-discharge (Aoun, 1999). In this study, patients who received treatment from the suicide intervention counsellor had significantly lower rates of hospital readmission for suicide attempts over a 22-month follow-up period, compared to readmission rates among patients who received treatment as usual and patients admitted prior to the start of the intervention.

Postvention for Survivors of Suicide

The increased risk of suicide among survivors during the aftermath of suicide draws particular attention to the need for therapeutic interventions that ultimately aspire to develop the means to assist suicide survivors to return to a level of functioning comparable to that before the attempt. Elements of a postvention intervention may incorporate education about grief, demystifying suicide, and eliminating excessive guilt, shame and blaming, as well as assessing and responding to potential suicide risk in the survivors. Postvention strategies should operate to identify those affected, and assist survivors by offering a continuum of immediate and follow-up services specifically designed to assist them in adjusting to the loss (Paul, 1995). Monitoring of grieving processes in the months following a suicide, particularly in relation to the onset of depressive symptoms among survivors, is particularly pertinent. Generally, it is considered that if depressive symptomatology persists for longer than six months after bereavement, then that depression should be treated in its own right rather than simply being considered part of a grief and mourning process that will resolve spontaneously (I.A.S.P. Executive Committee, 1999). In the long-term follow-up of survivors of suicide, particular attention should also be attended to death anniversaries, which may provoke suicidal impulses in survivors.

RECOMMENDATIONS IN RESPONSE TO SUICIDE PREVENTION ISSUES

National and international data that exist on suicide and non-fatal suicidal behaviour may be grossly underestimated.

- Enhanced monitoring and recording of suicide mortality statistics should be encouraged through the development of death classification criteria and definitions of suicide and suicidal behaviour that are comparable within and across nations. Improved training of coroners and medical examiners is also required.
- Registries of non-fatal suicidal behaviour for clinical surveillance and research purposes need also to be developed. National registries documenting non-fatal suicidal behaviour may enable the regional, national and international comparison of data.
- Increased detection, referral and monitoring of suicidal persons in a diversity of settings (e.g. medical and health, school, police, community and welfare) may improve data related to suicide and attempted suicide.
- Efforts to link suicide data across a variety of realms including hospitals, psychiatric and medical institutions, coroners and police may improve data accessibility.

Further research efforts are required to clarify risk and protective factors for suicide.

- Clinical trials are required to determine the specific effects on suicide of reducing hopelessness.
- Biological predictors of suicidal behaviour should be sought through prospective studies examining changes in brain functioning over time.
- Genetic studies are required to examine the relationship between genetic predisposition and family history of suicide. Studies searching for genes associated with suicidal behaviour, aggression and impulsivity should also be undertaken.

Many countries lack comprehensive nationally based suicide prevention strategies.

- Suicide prevention programmes should be adopted at a national level and supported by public policies that address the social determinants of suicidal behaviour.
- Overthrowing legal sanctions against suicide and suicidal behaviour in some cultures may reduce social stigma associated with psychiatric illness and suicide and consequently benefit suicide rates.
- Prevention and intervention initiatives should be based on research, carefully designed with appropriate controls, and rigorously evaluated with long-term follow-up.
- National suicide prevention programmes should provide direction for the development and implementation of regional and local level services and programmes.

- Suicide prevention and intervention initiatives must be assessed in order to determine whether or not particular programmes may be applicable to other population groups.

The primary health care and mental health care professions are in a particularly relevant position to prevent suicide.

- Funding should be directed toward the clinical development and evaluation of screening tools that assess risk factors for suicide.
- Evidence-based guidelines for suicide risk identification, assessment and referral should be implemented in the primary health care setting.
- Improved training of health care professionals in suicide risk assessment may impact significantly upon suicide rates.
- Physicians should refer patients with multiple risk factors for suicide to consultation with a mental health professional.
- Mental health services should be easily accessible, affordable, and culturally appropriate for all members of the community, particularly in under-serviced, at-risk populations.

The efficiency of pharmacological treatment interventions in preventing suicidality is largely unknown.

- Randomized controlled trials stand as the best form of methodological investigation that may determine the impact of pharmacological interventions upon suicide.
- Future clinical trials are needed to investigate the long-term effects of a range of pharmacological agents that are used in the treatment of suicidal individuals. Particular focus should be placed upon the effect of psychiatric medications on suicide and non-fatal suicidal behaviour, as well as on factors related to symptomatology, side effects, relapse rates and compliance with medications prescribed.

The efficiency of psychosocial treatment interventions in preventing suicidality is largely unknown.

- Psychosocial interventions are essential in the treatment and rehabilitation of suicidal individuals. Such interventions may reduce the impact of psychological and social risk factors for suicide and inadvertently reduce suicidality, particularly when treatment is combined with psychiatric medication.
- Randomized controlled trials are necessary to determine the direct impact of psychosocial interventions on suicide rates.
- Clinical trials of future suicidal behaviour among hospital-treated suicide attempters in relation to treatment effectiveness are required.

Measures to alter the environment may contribute significantly to reduce suicide rates.

- Access to lethal means of suicide should be addressed through legislative efforts and national suicide prevention guidelines. Such efforts should attend to the availability of firearms, domestic gases, gun possession, the detoxification of domestic gas, the detoxification of car exhaust emissions, the control of toxic substance availability and the media portrayal of suicide events.

Community-based efforts comprise a significant component in the suicide prevention agenda.

- Community-based suicide prevention initiatives should be developed and implemented in association with nationally defined suicide prevention targets and outcomes.
- Appropriate government funding is essential for the development, implementation and evaluation of community-based programmes and services.
- Community-based suicide prevention efforts should engender educational campaigns, support groups for survivors of suicide, and suicide prevention centres, as well as crisis intervention services.
- The training of lay-workers such as police officers, ambulance and emergency personnel, teachers, youth workers, clergy, and other community members is also an important suicide prevention initiative.

REFERENCES

Agerbo E, Nordentoft M, Mortensen PB (2002) Familial, psychiatric, and socioeconomic risk factors for suicide in young people: nested case-control study. *British Medical Journal* **325**: 74.

Allebeck P (1989) Schizophrenia: a life-shortening disease. *Schizophrenia Bulletin* **15**: 81–89.

Amaddeo F, Bisoffi G, Bonizzato P, Micciolo R, Tansella M (1995) Mortality among patients with psychiatric illness. *British Journal of Psychiatry* **166**: 783–788.

American Association of Suicidology (1999) *Rates of Suicide throughout the County: Fact Sheet*, Washington, DC: American Association of Suicidology.

Aoun S (1999) Deliberate self-harm in rural Western Australia: results of an intervention study. *Australian and New Zealand Journal of Mental Health Nursing* **8**: 65–73.

Appleby L, Cooper J, Amos T, Faragher B (1999a) Psychological autopsy study of suicides by people aged under 35. *British Journal of Psychiatry* **175**: 168–174.

Appleby L, Shaw J, Amos T, McDonnell R, Harris C, McCann K, Kiernan K, Davies S, Bickley H, Parsons R (1999b) Suicide within 12 months of contact with mental health services: national clinical survey. *British Medical Journal* **318**: 1235–1239.

Arikan Z, Cepik-Kuruoğlu A, Eltutan H, Işik E (1999) Alkol bağimliliği ve depresyon. *Düşünen Adam* **12**: 22–26.

Axelsson R, Lagerkvist-Briggs M (1992) Factors predicting suicide in psychotic patients. *European Archives of Psychiatry and Clinical Neuroscience* **241**: 259–266.

Bagley C (1986) The evaluation of a suicide prevention scheme by an ecological method. *Social Science and Medicine* **2**: 1–14.

Bagley C, Tremblay P (1997) Suicide behaviors in homosexual and bisexual males. *Crisis* **18**: 24–34.

Baldessarini RJ, Tondo L (1999) Antisuicidal effect of lithium treatment in major mood disorders, in Jacobs DG (ed) *The Harvard Medical School Guide to Suicide Assessment and Intervention*. San Francisco: Jossey-Bass, pp. 355–371.

Banki C, Arato M (1983) Amine metabolites and neuroendocrine responses related to depression and suicide. *Journal of Affective Disorders* **5**: 223–232.

Barefoot JC, Brummett BH, Helms MJ, Mark DB, Siegler IC, Williams RB (2000) Depressive symptoms and survival of patients with coronary artery disease. *Psychosomatic Medicine* **62**: 790–795.

Baume PJM (1994) *Strategy for the Prevention of Suicide*. Canberra: Australian Government Publishing Service.

Baume PJM, Clinton ME (1997) Social and cultural patterns of suicide in young people in rural Australia. *Australian Journal of Rural Health* **5**: 115–120.

Beck AT, Steer RA (1989) Clinical predictors of eventual suicide: a 5- to 10-year prospective study of suicide attempters. *Journal of Affective Disorders* **17**: 203–209.

Beck AT, Steer RA, Kovacs M, Garrison B (1985) Hopelessness and eventual suicide: a 10-year prospective study of patients hospitalised with suicidal ideation. *American Journal of Psychiatry* **142**: 559–563.

Beck AT, Weissman A, Lester D, Trexler L (1974) The measurement of pessimism: the hopelessness scale. *Journal of Consulting and Clinical Psychology* **42**: 861–865.

Berry JW, Kim U (1988) Acculturation and mental health. In Dasen P, Berry JW, Sartorius N (eds) *Health and Cross-Cultural Psychology: Towards Application*. London: Sage, pp. 207–236.

Birckmayer J, Hemenway D (2001) Suicide and firearm prevalence: are youth disproportionately affected? *Suicide and Life Threatening Behavior* **31**: 303–310.

Birkhead GS, Galvin VG, Meehan PJ, O'Carroll PV, Mercy JA (1993) The emergency department in surveillance of attempted suicide: findings and methodological considerations. *Public Health Report* **108**: 323–331.

Bondy B, Erfurth A, de Jonge S, Kruger M, Meyer H (2000) Possible association of the short allele of the serotonin transporter promoter gene polymorphism (5-HTTLPR) with violent suicide. *Molecular Psychiatry* **5**: 193–195.

Bonner RL, Rich AR (1991) Predicting vulnerability to hopelessness. A longitudinal analysis. *Journal of Nervous and Mental Disease* **179**: 23–32.

Boor M (1981) Effects of United States presidential elections on suicides and other causes of death. *American Sociological Review* **46**: 616–618.

Bostwick JM, Pankratz VS (2000) Affective disorders and suicide risk: a reexamination. *American Journal of Psychiatry* **157**: 1925–1932.

Boxer PA, Burnett C, Swanson N (1995) Suicide and occupation: a review of the literature. *Journal of Occupational and Environmental Medicine* **37**: 442–452.

Breault KD (1986) Suicide in America: a test of Durkheim theory of religious and family integration. *American Journal of Sociology* **92**: 628–656.

Brenner MH, Mooney A (1982) Economic change and sex-specific cardiovascular mortality in Britain, 1955–1976. *Social Science and Medicine* **16**: 431–436.

Brent DA, Baugher M, Bridge J, Chen T, Chiappetta L (1999) Age- and sex-related risk factors for adolescent suicide. *Journal of the American Academy of Child and Adolescent Psychiatry* **38**: 1497–1505.

Brent DA, Bridge J, Johnson BA, Connolly J (1996) Suicidal behavior runs in families: a controlled family study of adolescent suicide victims. *Archives of General Psychiatry* **53**: 1145–1152.

Brent DA, Kolko DJ, Birmaher B, Baugher M, Bridge J, Roth C, Holder D (1998) Predictors of treatment efficacy in a clinical trial of three psychosocial treatments for adolescent depression. *Journal of the American Academy of Child and Adolescent Psychiatry* **37**: 906–914.

Brent DA, Perper JA, Allman CJ, Moritz GM, Wartella ME, Zelenak JP (1991) The presence and accessibility of firearms in the homes of adolescent suicides: a case control study. *Journal of the American Medical Association* **266**: 2989–2995.

Brent DA, Perper JA, Moritz G, Liotus L, Schweers J, Balach L, Roth C (1994) Familial risk factors for adolescent suicide: a case-control study. *Acta Psychiatrica Scandinavica* **89**: 52–58.

Bridge TP, Potkin SG, Zung WW, Soldo BJ (1977) Suicide prevention centers: ecological study of effectiveness. *Journal of Nervous and Mental Disease* **164**: 18–24.

Brooke E, Atkinson M (1974) Ascertainment of death from suicide. In Breeks EM (ed) *Suicide and Attempted Suicide*. Geneva: World Health Organization.

Brown J, Cohen P, Johnson JG, Smailes EM (1999) Childhood abuse and neglect: specificity of effects on adolescent and young adult depression and suicidality. *Journal of the American Academy of Child and Adolescent Psychiatry* **38**: 1490–1496.

Buda M, Tsuang MT (1990) The epidemiology of suicide: implications for clinical practice. In Blumenthal SI, Kupfer DJ (eds) *Suicide over the Life Cycle: Risk Factors, Assessments, and Treatment of Suicide Patients*. Washington, DC: American Psychiatric Press, pp. 17–38.

Burnley IH (1995) Socioeconomic and special differentials in mortality and means of committing suicide in New South Wales, Australia, 1985–91. *Social Science and Medicine* **41**: 687–698.

Caldwell CB, Gottesman II (1992) Schizophrenia – a high risk factor for suicide: clues to risk education. *Suicide and Life Threatening Behavior* **22**: 479–493.

Cantor C, Baume P (1998) Changing methods of suicide by young Australians 1974–1994. *Archives of Suicide Research* **4**: 41–50.

Cantor C, Slater P (1995) The impact of firearm control legislation on suicide in Queensland: preliminary findings. *Medical Journal of Australia* **162**: 583–585.

Carbonell DM, Reinherz HZ, Giaconia RM (1998) Risk and resilience in late adolescence. *Child and Adolescent Social Work Journal* **15**: 251–272.

Cassem E (1995) Depressive disorders in the medically ill: an overview. *Psychosomatics* **36**: S2–S10.

Catanzaro SJ (2000) Mood regulation and suicidal behavior. In Joiner TE, Rudd DM (eds) *Suicide Science: Expanding the Boundaries*. Norwell, MA: Kluwer, pp. 81–103.

Cavanagh JTO, Owens CG, Johnstone EC (1999a) Suicide and undetermined death in southeast Scotland. A case-control study using the psychological autopsy method. *Psychological Medicine* **29**: 1141–1149.

Cavanagh JTO, Owens CG, Johnstone EC (1999b) Life events in suicide and undetermined death in south-east Scotland: a case-control study using the method of psychological autopsy. *Social Psychiatry and Psychiatric Epidemiology* **34**: 645–650.

Coccaro EF, Siever LJ, Lkar HM, Maurer G, Cochrane K, Cooper TB, Mohs RC, Davis KL (1989) Serotonergic studies in patients with affective and personality disorders. *Archives of General Psychiatry* **46**: 587–599.

Cochran SD, Mays VM (2000) Lifetime prevalence of suicide symptoms and affective disorders among men reporting same-sex sexual partners: results from NHANES III. *American Journal of Public Health* **90**: 573–578.

Comstock GW, Partridge KB (1972) Church attendance and health. *Journal of Chronic Diseases* **25**: 665–672.

Congdon P (1996) Suicide and parasuicide in London: a small area-study. *Urban Studies* **33**: 137–158.

Conner KR, Duberstein PR, Conwell Y, Seidlitz L, Caine ED (2001) Psychological vulnerability to completed suicide: a review of empirical studies. *Suicide Life Threatening Behavior* **31**: 367–385.

Conrad N (1991) Where do they turn? Social support systems of suicidal high school adolescents. *Journal of Psychosocial Nursing and Mental Health Services* **29**: 14–20.

Crombie IK (1991) Suicide among men in the highlands of Scotland. *British Medical Journal* **302**: 761–762.

Darke S, Ross J (2002) Suicide among heroin users: rates, risk factors and methods. *Addiction* **97**: 1383–1394.

Davies S, Naik PC, Lee AS (1998) Lifetime risk of suicide in affective disorders (letter). *British Journal of Psychiatry* **173**: 185.

De Castro EF, Pimenta F, Martins I (1988) Female independence in Portugal: effect on suicide rates. *Acta Psychiatrica Scandinavica* **78**: 147–155.

De Leo, D (1997) I comportamenti suicidari negli anziani: fattori demografici, psicosociali, malattie croniche. [Suicidal behaviour in the elderly: demographic, psychosocial, and chronic illness-related factors]. *Italian Journal of Suicidology* **9**: 277–290.

De Leo D (2002) Why are we getting any closer to preventing suicide? (editorial). *British Journal of Psychiatry* **181**: 372–374.

De Leo D, Diekstra RF (1990) *Depression and Suicide in Late Life.* Toronto/Bern: Hogrefe and Huber.

De Leo D, Ormskerk S (1991) Suicide in the elderly: general characteristics. *Crisis* **12**: 3–17.

De Leo D, Bertolote JM, Lester D (2002a) *Self-directed Violence,* World Report on Violence and Health. Geneva: World Health Organization.

De Leo D, Evans R, Neulinger K (2002b) Hanging, firearm, and non-domestic gas suicides among males: a comparative study. *Australian and New Zealand Journal of Psychiatry* **36**: 183–189.

De Leo D, Hickey P, Meneghel G, Cantor CH (1999) Blindness, fear of sight loss, and suicide. *Psychosomatics* **40**: 339–344.

De Leo D, Padoani W, Scocco P, Lie D, Bille-Brahe U, Arensman E, Hjelmeland H, Crepet P, Haring C, Hawton K, Lönnqvist J, Michel K, Pommereau X, Querejeta I, Phillipe J, Salander-Renberg E, Schmidtke A, Fricke S, Weinacker B, Tamesvary B, Wasserman D, Faria S (2001) Attempted and completed suicide in older subjects: results from the WHO/EURO multicentre study of suicidal behaviour. *International Journal of Geriatric Psychiatry* **16**: 300–310.

De Moore GM, Robertson AR (1996) Suicide in the 18 years after deliberate self-harm: a prospective study. *British Journal of Psychiatry* **169**: 489–494.

Diekstra RFW, Gulbinat W (1993) The epidemiology of suicidal behaviour: a review of three continents. *WHO Statistical Quarterly* **46**: 52–68.

Dieserud G, Roysamb E, Ekeberg O, Kraft P (2001) Toward an integrative model of suicide attempt: a cognitive psychological approach. *Suicide and Life Threatening Behavior* **31**: 153–168.

Donahue MJ (1995) Religion and the well-being of adolescents. *Journal of Social Issues* **51**: 145–160.

Du L, Bakish D, Lapierre YD, Ravindran AV, Hrdina PD (2000) Association of poly-morphism of serotonin 2A receptor gene with suicidal ideation in major depressive disorder. *American Journal of Medical Genetics* **96**: 56–60.

DuRant RH, Krowchuk DP, Sinal SH (1998) Victimization, use of violence, and drug use at school among male adolescents who engage in same-sex sexual bahavior. *Journal of Paediatrics* **133**: 113–118.

Durkheim E (1897/1951) *Suicide: A Sociological Study.* Glencoe, IL: Free Press.

Duval G, Baillet A, Catteau C (1997) Epidemiology of suicide attempts in Reunion Island [in French]. *Rev Epidémiol Santé Publique.* **45**: 23–28.

Farberow NL, Schneidman ES, Leonard NN (1963) Suicide among general medical and surgical hospital patients with malignant neoplasm. *VA Bulletin* **9**: 1–11.

Farmer RT (1988) Assessing the epidemiology of suicide and parasuicide. *British Journal of Psychiatry* **153**: 16–20.

Fawcett J (1972) Suicidal depression and physical illness. *Journal of the American Medical Association* **219**: 1303–1305.

Fenton WS (2000) Depression, suicide and suicide prevention in schizophrenia. *Suicide and Life Threatening Behaviour* **30**: 34–39.

Fergusson DM, Horwood LJ, Lynskey MT (1996) Childhood sexual abuse and psychiatric disorder in young adulthood: II. Psychiatric outcomes of childhood sexual abuse. *Journal of the American Academy of Child and Adolescent Psychiatry* **35**: 1365–1374.

Fergusson DM, Woodward LJ, Horwood LJ (2000) Risk factors and life processes associated with the onset of suicidal behaviour during adolescence and early adulthood. *Psychological Medicine* **30**: 23–39.

Ferrada-Noli M, Asberg M, Ormstad K (1998) Suicidal behaviour after severe trauma Part 2. The association between methods of torture and of suicidal ideation in posttraumatic stress disorder. *Journal of Trauma and Stress* **11**: 113–124.

Ferrada-Noli M, Asberg M, Ormstad K, Nordstrom P (1995) Definite and undetermined forensic diagnoses of suicide among immigrants in Sweden. *Acta Psychiatrica Scandinavica* **91**: 130–135.

Firestone RW, Seiden RH (1990) Suicide and the continuum of self-destructive behavior. *Journal of American College Health* **38**: 207–213.

Flavin DK, Franklin, JE, Frances RJ (1990) Substance abuse and suicidal behavior. In Blumenthal SJ, Kupfer DJ (eds) *Suicide over the Life Cycle: Risk Factors, Assessment, and Treatment of Suicidal Patients*. Washington, DC: American Psychiatric Press, pp. 177–204.

Frances A, Fyer M, Clarkin J (1988) Personality and suicide. *Annals of the New York Academy of Sciences* **487**: 281–293.

Fremouw WJ, Fremouw MP, Ellis TE (1990) *Suicide Risk: Assessment and response Guidelines*, New York: Pergamon Press, p 25.

Freud S (1957) Mourning and melancholia. In Strachey J (ed) *The Standard Edition of the Complete Psychological Works of Sigmund Freud*, Vol. XIV. London: Hogarth Press, pp. 243–258.

Fu Q, Heath AC, Bucholz KK, Nelson EC, Glowinski AL, Goldberg J, Lyons, MJ, Tsuang MT, Jacob T, True MR, Eisen SA (2002) A twin study of genetic and environmental influences on suicidality in men. *Psychological Medicine* **32**: 11–24.

Garofalo R, Wolf RC, Wissow LS, Woods ER, Goodman E (1999) Sexual orientation and risk of suicide attempts among a representative sample of youth. *Archives of Paediatrics and Adolescent Medicine* **153**: 487–493.

Goldacre M, Seagroat V, Hawton K (1993) Suicide after discharge from psychiatric inpatient care. *Lancet* **342**: 283–286.

Goto H, Nakamura H, Miyoshi T (1994) Empirical studies on regional differences in suicide mortality and its correlation with socio-economic factors. *Tokushima Journal of Experimental Medicine* **41**: 115–132.

Gregoire A (2002) The mental health of farmers. *Occupational Medicine* **52**: 471–476.

Gulbinat W (1996) The epidemiology of suicide in old age. *Archives of Suicide Research* **2**: 31–42.

Gulbinat W (1995) The epidemiology of suicide in old age. In Diekstra RF, Gulbinat W, Kienhorst I, De Leo D (eds) *Preventive Strategies on Suicide*. Leiden: WHO–EJ Brill.

Gunnell D, Frankel S (1994) Prevention of suicide: aspirations and evidence. *British Medical Journal* **308**: 1227–1233.

Gunnell D, Hawton K, Murray V, Garnier R, Bismuth C, Fagg J, Simkin S (1997) Paracetamol and aspirin. *Current Problems in Pharmacovigilance* **23**: 9.

Gunnell D, Peters T, Kammerling R, Brooks J (1995) Relation between parasuicide, suicide, psychiatric admissions, and socio-economic deprivation. *British Medical Journal* **311**: 226–230.

Guze SB, Robins E (1970) Suicide and primary affective disorders. *British Journal of Psychiatry* **117**: 437–438.

Harrington R, Kerfoot M, Dyer E, McNiven F, Gill J, Harrington V, Woodham A, Byford S (1998) Randomized trial of a home-based family intervention for children who have deliberately poisoned themselves. *Journal of the American Academy of Child and Adolescent Psychiatry* **37**: 512–518.

Harris EC, Barraclough BM (1994) Suicide as an outcome for medical disorders. *Medicine* **73**: 281–296.

Harris EC, Barraclough BM (1997) Suicide as an outcome for mental disorders. A meta-analysis. *British Journal of Psychiatry* **170**: 205–228.

Hassan R (1995) *Suicide Explained: The Australian Experience.* Melbourne: Melbourne University Press.

Hawton K, Fagg J (1988) Suicide, and other causes of death following attempted suicide. *British Journal of Psychiatry* **152**: 359–366.

Hawton K, Fagg J, Platt S, Hawkins M (1993) Factors associated with suicide after parasuicide in young people. *British Medical Journal* **306**: 1641–1644.

Hawton K, Houston K, Shepperd R (1999) Suicide in young people. Study of 174 cases, aged under 25 years, based on coroners' and medical records. *British Journal of Psychiatry* **175**: 271–276.

Hendin H (1991) Psychodynamics of suicide, with particular reference to the young. *American Journal of Psychiatry* **148**: 1150–1158.

Henriksson MM, Aro HM, Marttunen MJ, Heikkinen ME, Isometsä ET, Kuoppasalmi KI, Lönnqvist JK (1993) Mental disorders and comorbidity in suicide. *American Journal of Psychiatry* **150**: 935–940.

Henriksson MM, Marttunen MJ, Isometsä ET, Heikkinen ME, Aro HM, Kuoppasalmi KI, Lönnqvist JK (1995) Mental disorders in elderly suicide. *International Psychogeriatrics* **7**: 275–286.

Herrell R, Goldberg J, True WR, Ramakrishan V, Lyons M, Eisen S, Tsuang MT (1999) Sexual orientation and suicidality: a co-twin control study in adult men. *Archives of General Psychiatry* **56**: 867–874.

Hintikka J, Saarinen PI, Viinamaki H (1999) Suicide mortality in Finland during an economic cycle, 1985–1995. *Scandinavian Journal of Public Health* **27**: 85–88.

Hirschfeld RMA, Davidson L (1988) Risk factors for suicide. In Frances AJ, Hales RE (eds) *American Psychiatric Press Review of Psychiatry*, Vol. 7, Washington, DC: American Psychiatric Press.

Hovey JD (2000a) Acculturative stress, depression, and suicidal ideation among Central American immigrants. *Suicide and Life Threatening Behavior* **30**: 125–139.

Hovey JD (2000b) Acculturative stress, depression, and suicidal ideation in Mexican immigrants. *Cultural Diversity and Ethnic Minority Psychology* **6**: 134–151.

I.A.S.P. Executive Committee (1999) I.A.S.P. guidelines for suicide prevention. *Crisis* **20**: 155–163.

Indian Health Service (1999) *Trends in Indian Health, 1998–1999.* Rockville, MD: US Department of Health and Human Services.

IOM (Institute of Medicine) (2001) *Health and Behavior: The Interplay of Biological, Behavioral, and Societal Influences.* Washington, DC: National Academy Press.

IOM (Institute of Medicine) (2002) *Reducing Suicide: National Imperative.* Washington, DC: National Academy Press.

Joiner TE Jr, Steer RA, Abramson LY, Alloy LB, Metalsky GI, Schmidt NB (2001a) Hopelessness depression as a distinct dimension of depressive symptoms among clinical and non-clinical samples. *Behaviour Research and Therapy* **39**: 523–536.

Joiner TE Jr, Voelz ZR, Rudd MD (2001b) For suicidal young adults with comorbid depressive and anxiety disorders, problem-solving treatment may be better than treatment as usual. *Professional Psychology Research and Practice* **32**: 278–282.

Jorm AF, Henderson AS, Scott R, Korten AE, Christensen H, Mackinnon AJ (1995) Factors associated with the wish to die in elderly people. *Age and Ageing* **25**: 389–392.

Kerkhof AJ (2000) Attempted suicide: patterns and trends. In Hawton K, van Heeringen K (eds) *The International Handbook of Suicide and Attempted Suicide*. Chichester, UK: John Wiley.

Kessler RC (2000) Posttraumatic stress disorder: the burden to the individual and to society. *Journal of Clinical Psychiatry* **61** (Suppl 5): 4–12; discussion 13–14.

Kessler RC, Borges G, Walters EE (1999) Prevalence of and risk factors for lifetime suicide attempts in the National Comorbidity Survey. *Archives of General Psychiatry* **56**: 617–626.

Khan A, Leventhal RM, Khan S, Brown WA (2002) Suicide risk in patients with anxiety disorders: a meta-analysis of the FDA database. *Journal of Affective Disorders* **68**: 183–190.

King EA, Baldwin DS, Sinclair JM, Baker NG, Campbell MJ, Thompson C (2001) The Wessex Recent In-patient Suicide Study, 1. Case–control study of 234 recently discharged psychiatric patient suicides. *British Journal of Psychiatry* **178**: 531–536.

Kirmayer LJ, Boothroyd LJ, Hodgins S (1998) Attempted suicide among Inuit youth: psychosocial correlates and implications for prevention. *Canadian Journal of Psychiatry* **43**: 816–822.

Kirmayer LJ, Malus M, Boothroyd LJ (1996) Suicide attempts among Inuit youth: a community survey of prevalence and risk factors. *Acta Psychiatrica Scandinavica* **94**: 8–17.

Koenig HG (1994) *Aging and God*. New York: Haworth Press.

Kotler M, Iancu I, Efroni R, Amir M (2001) Anger, impulsivity, social support, and suicide risk in patients with posttraumatic stress disorder. *Journal of Nervous and Mental Disease* **189**: 162–167.

Kposowa AJ (2000) Marital status and suicide in the National Longitudinal Mortality Study. *Journal of Epidemiological and Community Health* **54**: 254–261.

Kposowa AJ, Breault KD, Singh GK (1995) White male suicide in the United States: a multivariate individual-level analysis. *Social Forces* **74**: 315–323.

Kreitman N (1977) *Parasuicide*. Chichester: John Wiley.

Kreitman N (1988) Suicide, age, and marital status. *Psychological Medicine* **18**: 121–128.

Lawrence DM, Holman CD, Jablensky AV, Fuller SA (1999) Suicide rates in psychiatric in-patients. An application of record linkage to mental health research. *Australian and New Zealand Journal of Public Health* **23**: 468–470.

Lerner MS, Clum GA (1990) Treatment of suicide ideators: a problem-solving approach. *Behavior Therapy* **21**: 403–411.

Lester D (1972) Migration and suicide. *Medical Journal of Australia* **1**: 941–942.

Lester D (1974) Effect of suicide prevention centres on suicide rates in the United States. *Health Services Reports* **89**: 37–39.

Lester D (1993) The effect of war on suicide rates. A study of France from 1826 to 1913. *European Archives of Psychiatry and Clinical Neuroscience* **242**: 248–249.

Lester D (1995) The concentration of neurotransmitter metabolites in the cerebrospinal fluid of suicidal individuals: a meta-analysis. *Pharmacopsychiatry* **28**: 77–79.

Lester D (1998) *Suicide in African Americans*. Commack, NY: Nova Science.

Lewis G, Sloggett A (1998) Suicide, deprivation, and unemployment: record linkage study. *British Medical Journal* **317**: 1283–1286.

Lin YH (1990) *The Weight of Mount T'Ai: Patterns of Suicide in Traditional Chinese History and Culture*. Doctoral Dissertation, University of Wisconsin Madison.

Linehan MM, Armstrong HE, Suarez A, Allmon D, Heard HL (1991) Cognitive-behavioral treatment of chronically parasuicidal borderline patients. *Archives of General Psychiatry* **48**: 1060–1064.

Linkowski, P, de Maertelaer V, Mendlewicz J (1985) Suicidal behavior in major depressive illness. *Acta Psychiatrica Scandinavica* **72**: 233–238.

Lönnqvist J (2000) Psychiatric aspects of suicidal behaviour: depression. Hawton K, van Heeringen K (eds). *The International Handbook of Suicide and Attempted Suicide*. Chichester, UK: John Wiley, pp. 107–120.

Lönnqvist J (2001) Physical illness and suicide. In Wasserman D (ed.) *Suicide: An Unnecessary Death*. London: Martin Dunitz, pp. 93–98.

Mackenzie PB, Popkin MK (1987) Suicide in the medical patient. *International Journal of Psychiatry and Medicine* **17**: 3–22.

Makinen IH, Wassermann D (1997) Suicide prevention and cultural resistance: stability in European countries' suicide ranking, 1970–1988. *Italian Journal of Suicidology* **7**: 73–86.

Mann JJ, Malone KM (1997) Cerebrospinal fluid amines and higher lethality suicide attempts in depressed inpatients. *Biological Psychiatry* **41**: 162–171.

Mann JJ, McBride PA, Brown RP, Linnoila M, Leon AC, DeMeo M, Mieczkowski T, Myers JE, Stanley M (1992) Relationship between central and peripheral serotonin indexes in depressed and suicidal psychiatric inpatients. *Archives of General Psychiatry* **49**: 442–446.

Mann JJ, Oquendo M, Underwood MD, Arango,V (1999) The neurobiology of suicide risk: a review for the clinician. *Journal of Clinical Psychiatry* **60**(Suppl 2): 7–11.

Marecek J (1998) Culture, gender, and suicidal behavior in Sri Lanka. *Suicide and Life Threatening Behavior* **28**: 69–81.

Maris RW (1981) *Pathways to Suicide: A Survey of Self-Destructive Behaviors*. Baltimore, MD: Johns Hopkins University Press.

Maris RW (1997a) Social and familial risk factors in suicidal behavior. *The Psychiatric Clinics of North America* **20**: 519–550.

Maris RW (1997b) Social suicide. *Suicide and Life Threatening Behavior* **27**: 41–49.

Marzuk PM, Leon AC, Tardiff K, Morgan EB, Stajic M, Mann JJ (1992) The effect of access to lethal methods of injury on suicide rates. *Archives of General Psychiatry* **49**: 451–458.

McIntosh JL (1992) Methods of suicide. In Maris RW, Berman AL, Maltsberger JT, Yufit RI (eds) *Assessment and Prediction of Suicide*. New York: Guilford Press, pp. 381–397.

McIntosh JL, Santos JF, Hubbard RW (1994) *Elderly Suicide Research, Theory and Treatment*. Washington, DC: American Psychological Association.

McKenzie W, Wurr C (2001) Early suicide following discharge from a psychiatric hospital. *Suicide and Life Threatening Behavior* **31**: 358–363.

McQuillan CT, Rodriguez J (2000) Suicide, adolescents and Puerto Rico. *Boletin de la Association Medica de Puerto Rico* **92**: 22–29.

Mehlum L, Friis S, Vaglum P, Karterud S (1994) The longitudinal pattern of suicidal behaviour in borderline personality disorder: a prospective follow-up study. *Acta Psychiatrica Scandinavica* **90**: 124–130.

Meltzer HY (1998) Suicide in schizophrenia: risk factors and clozapine treatment. *Journal of Clinical Psychiatry* **59**(Suppl 3): 15–20.

Meltzer HY, Alphs L, Anand R, et al. (2002) *The InterSePT trial: reduced suicidality with clozapine treatment*. Presented at the 155th annual meeting of the American Psychiatric Association, May 22, Philadelphia, PA.

Michel K, Ballinari P, Bille-Brahe U, Bjerke T, Crepet P, De Leo D, Haring C, Hawton K, Kerkhof A, Lönnqvist J, Querejeta I, Salander-Renberg E, Schmidtke A, Temesvary B, Wasserman D (2000) Methods used for parasuicide: results of the WHO/EURO Multicentre Study on Parasuicide. *Social Psychiatry and Psychiatric Epidemiology* **35**: 156–163.

Minkoff K, Bergman E, Beck AT, Beck R (1973) Hopelessness, depression, and attempted suicide. *American Journal of Psychiatry* **130**: 455–459.

Molnar BE, Berkman LF, Buka SL (2001) Psychopathology, childhood sexual abuse and other childhood adversities: relative links to subsequent suicidal behaviour in the US. *Psychological Medicine* **31**: 965–977.

Morrell SL, Taylor RJ, Kerr CB (1998) Jobless. Unemployment and young people's health. *Medical Journal of Australia* **168**: 236–240.

Mortensen PB, Agerbo E, Erikson T, Qin P, Westergaard-Nielsen N (2000) Psychiatric illness and risk factors for suicide in Denmark. _Lancet_ **355**: 9–12.

Moscicki EK (1985) Epidemiology of suicidal behavior. In Silverman MM, Maris RW (eds) _Suicide Prevention: Toward the Year 2000_. New York: Guilford Press, pp. 22–35.

Moscicki EK (1995) Epidemiology of suicidal behavior. _Suicide and Life Threatening Behavior_ **25**: 22–35.

Moscicki EK, O'Carroll P, Rae DS, Locke BZ, Roy A, Regier DA (1988) Suicide attempts in the Epidemiologic Catchment Area Study. _Yale Journal of Biological Medicine_ **61**: 259–268.

Motto JA, Bostrom AG (2001) A randomised controlled trial of postcrisis suicide prevention. _Psychiatric Services_ **52**: 828–833.

Murphy GE (1998) Why women are less likely than men to commit suicide. _Comprehensive Psychiatry_ **39**: 165–175.

Murphy GE, Wetzel RD, Robins E, McEvoy L (1992) Multiple risk factors predict suicide in alcoholism. _Archives of General Psychiatry_ **49**: 459–463.

National Police Agency (1986) _National Police Agency's 1985 Annual Report_. Tokyo: Printing Section of Ministry of Finance.

NCIPC (National Centre for Injury Prevention and Control). _Web-based Injury Statistics Query and Reporting System_. [Online.] Available: http://www.cdc.gov/ncipc/wisqars/ [accessed March 6, 2003].

Nielsen B, Petersen P, Rask PH, Krarup G (1995) Suicide and other causes of death in patients admitted for attempted suicide. 10-year follow-up [in Danish]. _Ugeskr Laeger_ **157**: 2149–2153.

Nielsen B, Wang AG, Bille-Brahe U (1990) Attempted suicide in Denmark. IV. A five-year follow-up. _Acta Psychiatrica Scandinavica_ **81**: 250–254.

Nisbet PA (1996) Protective factors for suicidal black females. _Suicide and Life Threatening Behavior_ **26**: 325–341.

Nisbet PA, Duberstein PR, Conwell Y, Seidlitz L (2000) The effect of participation in religious activities on suicide versus natural death in adults 50 and older. _Journal of Nervous and Mental Disease_ **188**: 543–546.

O'Carroll PW, Berman AL, Maris RW, Moscicki EK, Tanney BL, Silverman MM (1996) Beyond the Tower of Babel: a nomenclature for suicidology. _Suicide and Life Threatening Behavior_ **26**: 237–252.

Owens D, House A (1994) General hospital services for deliberate self-harm. _Journal of the Royal College of Physicians of London_ **28**: 370–371.

Paolucci EO, Genuis ML, Vialato C (2001) A meta-analysis of the published research on the effects of child sexual abuse. _Journal of Psychology_ **135**: 17–36.

Paul P (1995) The development process of a community postvention protocol. In Mishara B (ed) _The Impact of Suicide_. New York: Springer, pp. 64–72.

Paykel ES, Myers LK, Lindenthal JJ, Tanner J (1974) Suicidal feelings in the general population: a prevalence study. _British Journal of Psychiatry_ **124**: 460–469.

Pescosolido BA, Georgianna S (1989) Durkheim, suicide, and religion: toward a network theory of suicide. _American Sociological Review_ **5**: 33–48.

Pescosolido BA, Mendelsohn R (1986) Social causation or social construction of suicide? An investigation into the social organization of official rates. _American Sociological Review_ **51**: 80–100.

Pesonen TM, Hintikka J, Karkola KO, Saarinen PI, Antikainen M, Lehtonen J (2001) Male suicide mortality in eastern Finland: urban/rural changes during a 10-year period between 1988 and 1997. _Scandinavian Journal of Public Health_ **29**: 189–193.

Platt S (1984) Unemployment and suicidal behavior: a review of the literature. _Social Science and Medicine_ **19**: 93.

Pokorny AD (1983) Prediction of suicide in psychiatric patients. _Archives of General Psychiatry_ **40**: 249–257.

Pritchard C, Baldwin DS (2002) Elderly suicide rates in Asian and English-speaking countries. *Acta Psychiatrica Scandinavica* **105**: 271–275.

Proulx F, Lesage AD, Grunberg F (1997) One hundred in-patient suicides. *British Journal of Psychiatry* **171**: 247–250.

Qin P, Agerbo E, Mortensen PB (2002) Suicide risk in relation to family history of completed suicide and psychiatric disorders: a nested case-control study based on longitudinal registers. *Lancet* **360**: 1126–1130.

Qin P, Mortensen PB (2001) Specific characteristics of suicide in China. *Acta Psychiatrica Scandinavica* **103**: 117–121.

Rancans E, Alka I, Renberg ES, Jacobsson L (2001) Suicide attempts and serious suicide threats in the city of Riga and resulting contacts with medical services. *Nordic Journal of Psychiatry* **55**: 279–286.

Rancans E, Lapins J, Salander Renberg E, Jacobsson L (2003) Self-reported suicidal and help seeking behaviours in the general population in Latvia. *Social Psychiatry and Psychiatric Epidemiology* **38**: 18–26.

Renberg ES (2001) Self-reported life-weariness, death-wishes, suicidal ideation, suicidal plans and suicide attempts in general population surveys in the north of Sweden 1986 and 1996. *Social Psychiatry and Psychiatric Epidemiology* **36**: 429–436.

Rich CL, Ricketts JE, Fowler RC, Young D (1988) Some differences between men and women who commit suicide. *American Journal of Psychiatry* **145**: 718–722.

Rich C, Young J, Fowler R, Wagner J, Black N (1990) Guns and suicide. *American Journal of Psychiatry* **147**: 342–346.

Rifai AH, George CJ, Stack JA, Mann JJ, Reynolds CF (1994) Hopelessness in suicide attempters after acute treatment of major depression in later life. *American Journal of Psychiatry* **151**: 1687–1690.

Rihmer Z, Rutz W, Pihlgren H (1995) Depression and suicide on Gotland: an intensive study of all suicides before and after a depression-training program for general practitioners. *Journal of Affective Disorders* **35**: 147–152.

Rockett IR, Thomas BM (1999) Reliability and sensitivity of suicide certification in higher-income countries. *Suicide Life Threatening Behavior* **29**: 141–149.

Rossau CD, Mortensen PB (1997) Risk factors for suicide in patients with schizophrenia: nested case-control study. *British Journal of Psychiatry* **171**: 355–359.

Roy A (1993) Features associated with suicide attempts in depression: a partial replication. *Journal of Affective Disorders* **27**: 35–38.

Roy A, Draper R (1995) Suicide among psychiatric hospital in-patients. *Psychological Medicine* **25**: 199–202.

Roy A, Nielsen D, Rylander G, Sarchiapone M, Segal N (1999) Genetics of suicide in depression. *Journal of Clinical Psychiatry* **60** (Suppl 2): 12–17.

Roy A, Rylander G, Sarchiapone M (1997) Genetics of suicides. Family studies and molecular genetics. *Annals of the New York Academy of Sciences* **836**: 135–157.

Roy A, Segal NL, Centerwall BS, Robinette CD (1991) Suicide in twins. *Archives of General Psychiatry* **48**: 28–32.

Rudd MD, Rajab MH, Orman DT, Joiner T, Stulman DA, Dixon W (1996) Effectiveness of an outpatient problem-solving intervention targeting suicidal young adults: preliminary results. *Journal of Consulting and Clinical Psychology* **64**: 179–190.

Rutz W, von Knorring L, Walinder J (1992) Long term effects of an educational program for general practitioners given by the Swedish Committee for Prevention and Treatment of Depression. *Acta Psychiatrica Scandinavica* **85**: 457–465.

Sainsbury P (1955) *Suicide in London.* London: Chapman and Hall.

Sainsbury P, Jenkins JS (1982) The accuracy of officially reported suicide statistics for purposes of epidemiological research. *Journal of Epidemiology and Community Health* **36**: 43–48.

Santa Mina EE, Gallop RM (1998) Childhood sexual and physical abuse and adult self-harm and suicidal behaviour: a literature review. *Canadian Journal of Psychiatry* **43**: 793–800.

Sarason IG, Sarason BR, Pierce GR (1990) Social support, personality, and performance. *Journal of Applied Sport Psychology* **2**: 117–127.

Sartorius N (1995) Recent changes in suicide rates in selected eastern European and other European countries. *International Psychogeriatrics* **7**: 301–308.

Schmid H, Manjee K, Shah T (1994) On the distinction of suicide ideation versus attempt in elderly psychiatric inpatients. *Gerontology* **34**: 332–339.

Schmidt NB, Woolaway-Bickel K, Bates M (2000) Suicide and panic disorder: integration of the literature and new findings. In Joiner TE, Rudd MD (eds) *Suicide Science: Expanding the Boundaries*. Norwell, MA: Kluwer, pp. 117–136.

Schmidtke A (1997) Perspectives: suicide in Europe. *Suicide and Life Threatening Behavior* **27**: 127–135.

Schmidtke A, Bille-Brahe U, De Leo D, Kerkhof A, Bjerke T, Crepet P, Haring C, Hawton K, Lonqvist J, Michel K, Pommereau X, Querejeta I, Phillipe I, Salander-Renberg E, Temesvary B, Wasserman D, Fricke S, Weinacker B, Sampaio-Faria JG (1996) Attempted suicide in Europe: rates, trends and sociodemographic characteristics of suicide attempters during the period 1989–1992. Results of the WHO/EURO Multicentre Study on Parasuicide. *Acta Psychiatrica Scandinavica* **93**: 327–338.

Schulsinger R, Kety S, Rosenthal D, Wender P (1979) A family study of suicide. In Schou M, Stromgren E (eds) *Origins, Prevention and Treatment of Affective Disorders*. New York: Academic Press, pp. 277–287.

Schwab JJ, Warheit GJ, Holzer CE (1972) Suicidal ideation and behavior in a general population. *Diseases of the Nervous System* **33**: 745–748.

Scott V (2000) Crisis services: Befrienders International: volunteer action in preventing suicide. In Lester D (ed) *Suicide Prevention: Resources for the Millennium*. Ann Arbor, MI: Sheridan Books, pp. 265–273.

Shaffer D (1998) Epidemiological aspects of some problems in child and adolescent psychiatry. *Epidemiology Psychiatric Sociology* **7**: 151–155.

Shah AK, Ganesvaran T (1997) Inpatient suicides in an Australian mental hospital. *Australian and New Zealand Journal of Psychiatry* **31**: 291–298.

Shaw S, Sims A (1984) A survey of unexpected deaths among psychiatric patients. *British Journal of Psychiatry* **145**: 473–476.

Shen BJ, Takeuchi DT (2001) A structural model of acculturation and mental health status among Chinese Americans. *American Journal of Community Psychology* **29**: 387–418.

Shneidman ES (1985) *Definitions of Suicide*. New York: John Wiley.

Shneidman ES (1993) Suicide as psychache. *Journal of Nervous and Mental Disease* **181**: 147–149.

Simon GE, Von Korff M (1998) Suicide mortality among patients treated for depression in an insured population. *American Journal of Epidemiology* **147**: 155–160.

Singh GK, Siahpush M (2001) All-cause and cause-specific mortality of immigrants and native born in the United States. *American Journal of Public Health* **91**: 392–399.

Skoog I, Aevarsson O, Beskow J, Larsson L, Palsson S, Waern M, Landahl S, Ostling S (1996) Suicidal feelings in a population sample of nondemented 85-year-olds. *American Journal of Psychiatry* **153**: 1015–1020.

Slater J, Depue R (1981) The contribution of environmental events and social support to serious suicide attempts in primary depressive disorder. *Journal of Abnormal Psychology* **40**: 275–285.

Smith JC, Mercy JA, Conn JM (1988) Marital status and the risk of suicide. *American Journal of Public Health* **78**: 78–80.

Sorenson SB, Shen H (1996) Youth suicide trends in California: an examination of immigrant and ethnic group risk. *Suicide and Life Threatening Behavior* **26**: 143–154.

Spießl H, Hübner-Liebermann B, Cording C (2002) Suicidal behaviour of psychiatric in-patients. *Acta Psychiatrica Scandinavica* **106**: 134–138.

Stack S (1992) Marriage, Family, Religion And Suicide. In Maris RW (ed) *Assessment and Prediction of Suicide*. New York: Guilford Press, pp. 540–553.

Stack S (2000) Media impacts on suicide: a quantitative review of 293 findings. *Social Science Quarterly* **81**: 957–971.

Stack S (2002) Media coverage as a risk factor in suicide. *Injury Prevention* **8**: 430–432.

Stenager EN, Stenager E (2000) Physical illness and suicidal behaviour. In Hawton K, van Heeringen K (eds) *Suicide and Attempted Suicide*. Chichester, UK: John Wiley, pp. 405–420.

Stengel E (1964) *Suicide and Attempted Suicide*. Baltimore, MD: Penguin.

Stensman R, Sundqvist-Stensman UB (1989) Physical disease and disability among 416 suicide cases in Sweden. *Canadian Journal of Social Medicine* **16**: 149–153.

Stroebe MS, Stroebe W (1993) The mortality of bereavement: a review. In Stroebe MS, Stroebe W, Hansson RO (eds) *Handbook of Bereavement: Theory, Research, and Intervention*. Cambridge, UK: Cambridge University Press, pp. 175–195.

Suokas J, Lönnqvist J (1991) Outcome of attempted suicide and psychiatric consultation: risk factors and suicide mortality during a five-year follow-up. *Acta Psychiatrica Scandinavica* **84**: 545–549.

Suokas J, Suominen K, Isometsä E, Ostamo A, Lönnqvist J (2001) Long-term risk factors for suicide mortality after attempted suicide – findings of a 14-year follow-up study. *Acta Psychiatrica Scandinavica* **104**: 117–121.

Szanto K, Gildengers A, Mulsant BH, Brown G, Alexopoulos GS, Reynolds CF. 3rd (2002) Identification of suicidal ideation and prevention of suicidal behaviour in the elderly. *Drugs and Aging* **19**: 11–24.

Tannen D (1990) *You Just Don't Understand. Women and Men in Conversation*. New York: Ballantine.

Termansen PE, Bywater C (1975) S.A.F.E.R.: a follow-up service for attempted suicide in Vancouver. *Canadian Psychiatric Association Journal* **20**: 29–34.

Trovato F (1986) A time series analysis of international immigration and suicide mortality in Canada. *International Journal of Social Psychiatry* **32**: 38–46.

Trovato F (1992) A Durkheimian analysis of youth suicide: Canada, 1971 and 1981. *Suicide and Life Threatening Behavior* **22**: 413–427.

Tsuang MT, Lyons MJ, Faraone SV (1990) Heterogeneity of schizophrenia. Conceptual models and analytic strategies. *British Journal of Psychiatry* **156**: 17–26.

Tsuang MT, Simpson JC (1985) Mortality studies in psychiatry: should they stop or proceed? *Archives of General Psychiatry* **42**: 98–103.

United Nations (1996) *Prevention of Suicide: Guidelines for the Formulation and Implementation of National Strategies*, New York: United Nations.

Vance JE, Fernandez G, Biber M (1998) Educational progress in a population of youth with aggression and emotional disturbance: the role of risk and protective factors. *Journal of Emotional and Behavioral Disorders* **6**: 214–221.

Verbrugge LM (1979) Marital status and health. *Journal of Marriage and the Family* **41**: 267–285.

Virkkunen M, Rawlings R, Tokola R, Poland RE, Guidotti A, Nemeroff CB, Bissette G, Kalogeras K, Karonen SL, Linnoila M (1994) CSF biochemistries, glucose metabolism, and diurnal activity rhythms in alcoholic, violent offenders, fire setters, and healthy volunteers. *Archives of General Psychiatry* **51**: 20–27.

Waern M, Runeson BS, Allebeck P, Beskow J, Rubenowitz E, Skoog I, Wilhelmsson K (2002) Mental disorder in elderly suicides: a case-control study. *American Journal of Psychiatry* **159**: 450–455.

Wasserman D (1983) Political business cycles, presidential elections, and mortality patterns. *American Sociological Review* **48**: 711–720.

Wasserman D (2001) Negative life events (losses, changes, traumas and narcissistic injury) and suicide. InWasserman D (ed) *Suicide: An Unnecessary Death*. London: Martin Dunitz, pp. 111–118.

Wasserman D, Varnik A, Dankowicz M (1998) Regional differences in the distribution of suicide in the former Soviet Union during perestroika, 1984–1990. *Acta Psychiatrica Scandinavica* **394**: 5–12.

Weaver AJ, Koenig HG (1996) Elderly suicide, mental health professionals, and the clergy: a need for clinical collaboration, training, and research. *Death Studies* **20**: 495–508.

Wender P, Kety S, Rosenthal D, Schulsinger F, Ortmann J, Lunde I (1986) Psychiatric disorders in the biological and adoptive families of adopted individuals with affective disorder. *Archives of General Psychiatry* **43**: 923–929.

Westermeyer JF, Harrow M, Marengo JT (1991) Risk for suicide in schizophrenia and other psychotic and nonpsychotic disorders. *Journal of Nervous and Mental Disease* **179**: 259–266.

Whitley E, Gunnell D, Dorling D, Davey Smith G (1999) Ecological study of social fragmentation, poverty, and suicide. *British Medical Journal* **319**: 1034–1037.

Whitlock FA (1978) Suicide, cancer, and depression. *British Journal of Psychiatry* **132**: 269–274.

Whitlock FA (1986) Suicide and physical illness. In Roy A (ed) *Suicide*. Baltimore, MD: Williams & Wilkins.

WHO (World Health Organization) (1990) *Consultation on Strategies for Reducing Suicidal Behaviour in the European Region. Summary Report*. Geneva: World Health Organization.

WHO (World Health Organization) (1998) *Primary prevention of mental, neurological and pyschosocial disorders: Suicide*. Geneva: World Health Organization, pp. 75–90.

WHO (World Health Organization) (1999) *Health for All Data Base*. Geneva: World Health Organization.

WHO (World Health Organization) (2000) *Preventing Suicide: A Resource for Media Professionals*. Geneva: World Health Organization.

WHO (World Health Organization) (2001) *Mental Health and Brain Disorders. Suicide Rates (per 100 000)*. Geneva: World Health Organization. [Online.] Available:http://www.who.int/mental_health/Topic_Suicide/Suicide?rates.html. Accessed March 6, 2003.

WHO (World Health Organization) (2003) *Country Report*. Available at: http://www5.who.int/mental_health/main.cfm?p = 0000000515. Accessed February 13, 2003.

Williams CL, Berry JW (1991) Primary prevention of acculturative stress mong refugees: application of psychological theory and practice. *American Psychologist* **46**: 632–641.

Wolfersdorf M (1996) In-patient suicide in psychiatric hospitals. Selected results of an in-patient suicide study (KSV I/II), 1970–1992 of the working group 'suicidality and psychiatric hospital' [in German]. *Psychiatrische Praxis* **23**: 84–89.

Wunderlich U, Bronisch T, Wittchen HU, Carter R (2001) Gender differences in adolescents and young adults with suicidal behaviour. *Acta Psychiatrica Scandinavica* **104**: 332–339.

Yip PSF (2001) An epidemiological profile of suicides in Beijing, China. *Suicide and Life Threatening Behavior* **31**: 62–70.

Yip PSF, Callanan C, Yuen HP (2000) Urban/rural and gender differentials in suicide rates: East and West. *Journal of Affective Disorders* **57**: 99–106.

Yip PSF, Tan RCE (1998) Suicides in Hong Kong and Singapore: a tale of two cities. *International Journal of Social Psychiatry* **44**: 267–279.

Young LT, Cooke RG, Robb JC, Levitt AJ, Joffe RT (1993) Anxious and non-anxious bipolar disorder. *Journal of Affective Disorders* **29**: 49–52.

Zalsman G, Frisch A, Bromberg M, Gelernter J, Michaelovsky E, Campino A, Erlich Z, Tyano S, Apter A, Weizman A (2001) Family-based association study of serotonin transporter promoter in suicidal adolescents: no association with suicidality but possible role in violent traits. *American Journal of Medical Genetics* **105**: 239–245.

PART III
Underlying Mechanisms

Neurobiology of Depression

Phil J. Cowen

University Department of Psychiatry, Warneford Hospital, Oxford, UK

INTRODUCTION

The aetiology of major depression is multifactorial and incompletely understood. Epidemiological research has identified several interacting risk factors for depression, including genetic inheritance, childhood adversity, neuroticism and past history of mood disorder. In people predisposed to mood disorder depression is often precipitated by stressful life events (see Kendler et al., 1992). The intimate psychological relationship between stress and depression is reflected by the involvement of common neurobiological mechanisms. In this sense depressive episodes can be seen as an idiosyncratic reaction to stress. This kind of thinking has informed much research on the pathophysiology of depression particularly with regard to the role of the hypothalamic–pituitary–adrenal (HPA) axis (see below).

There is general agreement that the clinical syndrome of major depression must be associated with characteristic neurobiological changes within the brain. However, we do not know if differing aetiologies will be associated with distinct pathophysiologies. In addition, it is unclear how far specific clinical syndromes will correlate with particular neurobiological changes.

The fact that people with depression can often make complete clinical recoveries (often without specific treatment) led to the idea that the relevant pathophysiological abnormalities might consist largely of reversible neurochemical changes. However, depression often has a poor prognosis and may become more treatment-resistant as the number of episodes increases (Greden, 2001). This has given rise to new investigations which have sought to discover whether depression may be associated with a distinct cellular and structural pathology. There is also more interest in whether some biochemical abnormalities seen in acutely depressed patients may persist into remission and recovery and may therefore represent trait markers of vulnerability to mood disorder.

Mood Disorders: Clinical Management and Research Issues. Edited by E. J. L. Griez, C. Faravelli, D. J. Nutt and J. Zohar.
©2005 John Wiley & Sons Ltd. ISBN 0 470 09426 5.

TABLE 7.1   Some 5-HT abnormalities in major depression

↓	Plasma tryptophan
↓	Prolactin response to 5-HT reuptake inhibitors
↓	Hypothermic response to 5-HT$_{1A}$ receptor agonists
↓	Growth hormone response to 5-HT$_{1D}$ agonists
↓	Cortical and raphe 5-HT$_{1A}$ receptor binding (PET)
↓	Cortical 5-HT$_{2A}$ receptor binding (PET)
↓	Brain stem 5-HT transport binding (SPET)

→ Relapse of depressive symptoms following tryptophan depletion

TABLE 7.2   Some catecholaminergic abnormalities in major depression

↓	Growth hormone response to α_2-adrenoceptor agonist
↓	Growth hormone response to D$_2$ receptor agonist
↓	Levels of HVA in CSF
	Relapse of depressive symptoms after AMPT

Pathophysiological studies in depression cover a very wide range of disciplines and methodologies. Hence any review must be selective. The present discussion will focus on areas where there is reasonable level of consensus on the presence of relevant abnormalities and where new developments have produced fresh insights. The idea that monoamine neurotransmission is abnormal in depression is an old one but supported by recent brain imaging and pharmacological challenge studies (Table 7.1 and Table 7.2). Monoamine neurotransmitters and the HPA axis play a key role in adaptation to the effects of stress and abnormal HPA activity continues to be a focus for studies of pathophysiology as well as new drug development. Finally, recent work on functional and structural brain imaging throws light on the specific brain regions that mediate key symptoms of depressive disorders. These brain regions appear to possess abnormalities in cellular architecture making it possible that depression is, in fact, associated with morphological brain abnormalities that represent a long-term risk factor for the development of recurrent illness.

MONOAMINE NEUROTRANSMITTERS

The monoamine hypothesis suggests that depressive disorder is due to an abnormality in a monoamine neurotransmitter system at one or more sites in the brain. In its early form, the hypothesis suggested a changed provision of the monoamine; more recent elaborations postulate alterations in receptors as well as in the concentrations or the turnover of the amines. Three monoamine transmitters have been implicated: serotonin (5-hydroxytryptamine; 5-HT), noradrenaline, and dopamine. To a great extent this hypothesis was derived from knowledge of the effects of antidepressant drugs on monoamine mechanisms in animals. However, the fact that increasing NA and 5-HT function can produce antidepressant effects does not mean that impaired NA and 5-HT function is necessarily involved in causing depression. Nevertheless, recent investigations in unmedicated depressed patients suggest that there are indeed changes in NA and 5-HT function in depression.

5-HT Function

Plasma Tryptophan

The synthesis of 5-HT in the brain depends on the availability of its precursor amino acid, L-tryptophan. Plasma tryptophan levels are decreased in untreated depressed patients, particularly in those with melancholic depression (Anderson et al., 1990a). Studies in healthy subjects have shown that weight loss through dieting can lower plasma tryptophan (Anderson et al., 1990b), and this factor appears to explain some, but not all, of the reduction in plasma tryptophan seen in depression. Decreases in plasma tryptophan may contribute to the impairments seen in brain 5-HT function in depressed patients but are probably not an important causal factor (Anderson et al., 1990a).

Studies of Cerebrospinal Fluid

Indirect evidence about 5-HT function in the brains of depressed patients has been sought by examining cerebrospinal fluid (CSF). Numerous studies have been carried out, but overall the data do not suggest that drug-free patients with major depression have a consistent reduction in CSF concentrations of 5-hydroxyindoleacetic acid (5-HIAA), the main metabolite of 5-HT formed in the brain. However, there is more consistent evidence that depressed patients who have made suicide attempts have low CSF 5-HIAA levels (Asberg et al., 1976).

This finding is not restricted to patients with depression. It has also been reported in, for example, patients with schizophrenia and personality disorder who have histories of aggressive behaviour directed towards themselves or other people. It has been proposed that low levels of CSF 5-HIAA, while not related specifically to depression, may be associated with a tendency of individuals to respond in an impulsive and hostile way to life difficulties (see Brown and Linnoila, 1990).

Studies of Post-mortem Brain

Measurements of 5-HT and 5-HIAA have been made in the brains of depressed patients who have died, usually by suicide. Although this is a more direct test of the monoamine hypothesis, the results are difficult to interpret for two reasons. First, the observed changes may have taken place after death. Second, the changes may have been caused before death but by factors other than the depressive disorder, for example by anoxia or by drugs used in treatment or taken to commit suicide. Overall there is little consistent evidence that depressed patients dying from natural causes or suicide have lowered brain concentrations of 5-HT or 5-HIAA (Horton, 1992).

Recently, multiple 5-HT receptors have been described in mammalian brain. There have been a number of reports that the density of brain 5-HT_{2A} receptors in certain cortical regions is increased in patients dying by suicide, particularly if violent means were used. However, there are some negative studies (Horton, 1992). Similarly there are inconsistent reports of changes in 5-HT_{1A} receptors (Matsubara et al., 1991; Lowther et al., 1997). There is rather more consensus that the density of serotonin transporters may be decreased in suicide victims (Stanley et al., 1982; Leake et al., 1991).

Neurochemical Brain Imaging Studies

Recent developments in brain imaging with selective labelled ligands has allowed assessment of certain brain 5-HT receptor subtypes in vivo. In contrast to the post-mortem studies in suicide victims, the density of 5-HT_{2A} receptor binding tends if anything to be decreased in unmedicated depressed patients (Meyer et al., 1999; Yatham et al., 2000). There is also evidence of a widespread modest decrease in 5-HT_{1A} receptor binding throughout cortical and subcortical regions, and in the raphe nuclei (Drevets et al., 1999; Sargent et al., 2000). These changes do not appear to reflect an effect of treatment and treatment with selective serotonin re-uptake inhibitors produces remarkably little effect on 5-HT_{1A} receptor binding in depressed patients. (Sargent et al., 2000). Finally there are probably reductions in brain stem 5-HT transporter sites in depressed subjects, consistent with a decrease in the density of 5-HT cell bodies (Malison et al., 1998; Willeit et al., 2000).

Neuroendocrine Tests

The functional activity of 5-HT systems in the brain has been assessed by giving a substance that stimulates 5-HT function and by measuring an endocrine response that is controlled by 5-HT pathways – usually the release of prolactin, growth hormone or cortisol. Neuroendocrine challenge tests have the advantage that they measure an aspect of brain 5-HT function. However, the 5-HT synapses involved presumably reside in the hypothalamus, which means that important changes in 5-HT pathways in other brain regions could be missed (see Cowen, 1998). A number of drugs have been used to increase brain 5-HT function for the purposes of neuroendocrine challenge.

Studies in unmedicated depressed patients have shown consistent evidence that 5-HT-mediated endocrine responses are blunted in depressed patients. The evidence is most consistent for drug challenges that increase 5-HT function via pre-synaptic mechanisms (Cowen, 1998). Thus the prolactin response to acute administration of 5-HT reuptake inhibitors is reliably blunted in depressed patients (Anderson et al., 1992; Golden et al., 1992; Kapitany et al., 1999; Bhagwagar et al., 2002). However, there is also evidence from endocrine studies that post-synaptic $5-HT_{1A}$ and $5-HT_{1D}$ receptor sensitivity may be decreased, particularly in patients with melancholic symptoms (Lesch et al., 1992; Whale et al., 2001). Certain abnormalities in 5-HT neuroendocrine responses, for example, blunted prolactin release to 5-HT reuptake inhibitor challenge, appear to persist upon clinical recovery suggesting that they are trait markers of vulnerability to depression (Bhagwagar et al., 2002) (Figure 7.1).

Hypothermic responses to $5-HT_{1A}$ receptor agonist challenge probably represent activation of $5-HT_{1A}$ autoreceptors in the raphe nuclei and these responses are blunted in melancholic depressed patients (Lesch, 1992; Cowen et al., 1994). This suggests an impaired sensitivity of $5-HT_{1A}$ autoreceptors. This would be expected to free 5-HT neurons from feedback control and therefore would not explain decreased presynaptic 5-HT function. It could represent an adaptive change attempting to facilitate 5-HT neurotransmission and a modulatory effect of cortisol has been suggested (Young et al., 1994). Certainly treatment with selective serotonin reuptake inhibitors decreases the sensitivity of $5-HT_{1A}$ autoreceptors in both animals and humans, supporting proposals that desensitization of raphe $5-HT_{1A}$

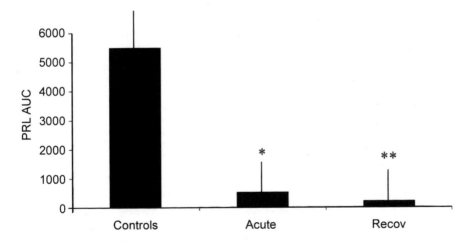

Figure 7.1   Mean ($\pm$ SEM) prolactin response to intravenous citalopram measured as area under the curve (AUC) in unmedicated acutely depressed patients, recovered depressed patients and healthy controls. Responses in both patient groups are significantly less than the controls (reproduced from Bhagwagar et al., 2002 State and trait abnormalities in serotonin function in major depression. *British Journal of Psychiatry* **180**: 24–28)

autoreceptors plays an important role in antidepressant action (Blier and de Montigny, 1994).

Tryptophan Depletion

While the findings outlined above provide strong evidence that aspects of brain 5-HT neurotransmission are abnormal in depression, they do not reveal whether these changes are central to pathophysiology or might instead represent some form of epiphenomenon. To assess this it is necessary to study the psychological consequences of lowering brain 5-HT function in healthy subjects and those at risk of mood disorder.

As mentioned above, the synthesis of brain 5-HT is dependent on the brain availability of its amino-acid precursor, L-tryptophan. It is possible to produce a transient lowering of plasma tryptophan and brain 5-HT function over a few hours by administering a mixture of amino acids that lack tryptophan. This procedure is called tryptophan depletion. Tryptophan depletion in subjects with no personal or family history of mood disorder has little measurable effect on mood and certainly does not produce significant clinical depressive symptomatology (Smith et al., 1997a). In contrast, unmedicated euthymic patients with a personal history of mood disorder undergo a rapid but temporary depressive relapse when exposed to tryptophan depletion (Smith et al., 1997b). A recent meta-analysis suggests that a number of factors predict relapse to tryptophan depletion in those at risk of mood disorder. These factors include female gender, a history of suicide attempts and recurrent illness (Booij et al., 2002).

Overall the studies with TRP depletion suggest that low brain 5-HT function is not sufficient to cause depression because tryptophan depletion fails to alter mood in those not vulnerable to mood disorder. However, in people vulnerable to mood disorder, lowering brain 5-HT function can result in clinical depressive symptomatology.

Noradrenaline Function

Metabolism and Receptors

There is no consistent evidence that brain or CSF concentrations of noradrenaline or its major metabolite 3-methoxy-4-hydroxy-phenylethylene glycol (MHPG) are altered in depressed patients (see Anand and Charney, 2000). As with 5-HT receptors, noradrenaline receptors in the brain can be divided into a number of subclasses. There is some evidence that depressed patients dying of natural causes and those who commit suicide have lowered α_1-adrenoceptor binding in some brain regions, though different studies have implicated different brain regions (Horton, 1992).

Neuroendocrine Tests

Increasing brain noradrenaline function elevates plasma concentrations of ACTH, cortisol, and growth hormone. There is fairly consistent evidence that the growth hormone response to both the noradrenaline re-uptake inhibitor desipramine and the noradrenaline receptor agonist clonidine is blunted in patients with melancholic depression (Checkley, 1992). Clonidine acts directly on post-synaptic α_2-adrenoceptors in the hypothalamus to increase plasma growth hormone, and therefore the blunted response in depressed patients suggests a decreased responsivity of these postsynaptic α_2-adrenoceptors or of mechanisms linked to them. These responses may persist after clinical recovery, suggesting that they could represent trait markers of vulnerability to depression (Mitchell et al., 1988). Other biochemical and behavioural responses to clonidine, including changes in plasma MHPG and sedation, are not altered in depressed patients, suggesting that any deficit in α_2-adrenoceptor function is fairly localized, probably to the hypothalamus (Anand and Charney, 2000).

Catecholamine Depletion

It is possible to lower the synthesis of catecholamines by inhibiting the enzyme tyrosine hydroxylase, which catalyses the conversion of the amino acid, tyrosine to L-dopa, a precursor of both noradrenaline and dopamine. The drug used to achieve this effect is α-methyl-*para*-tyrosine (AMPT). In healthy subjects AMPT produces sedation but no significant depressive symptoms. As with tryptophan depletion, however, when administered to recovered depressed patients off drug treatment it causes a striking clinical relapse in depressive symptomatology (Berman et al., 1999). This could be mediated either by diminished dopamine or noradrenaline function, or by combined inhibition of both these neurotransmitters.

These findings suggest that subjects at risk of mood disorder are vulnerable to decreases in both 5-HT and catecholamine neurotransmission. This is consistent with the clinical evidence that drugs acting selectively on noradrenaline or 5-HT pathways are effective antidepressant treatments.

Dopamine Function

The function of dopamine in depression has been less studied than that of 5-HT or noradrenaline but there are a number of reasons for thinking that dopamine neurons may be involved in the pathophysiology of the depressed state. For example, dopamine neurons in the mesolimbic system play a key role in incentive behaviour and reward, processes that are disrupted in depression, particularly melancholic states. Also antidepressant treatments in animals increase the expression of dopamine receptors in part of the mesolimbic system called the nucleus accumbens (Ainsworth et al., 1998).

As yet, there is little direct evidence that dopamine function is abnormal in depression. Nevertheless, lowered CSF levels of the dopamine metabolite homovanillic acid are found rather consistently in patients with depression. However, this has usually been associated with the clinical syndrome of motor retardation rather than depression per se (Anand and Charney, 2000). In addition, the growth hormone response to the dopamine D_2 receptor agonist, apomorphine, is probably blunted in depression, suggesting a subsensitivity of hypothalamic D_2 receptors (Ansseau et al., 1988). Finally, some brain imaging studies in depressed patients have found increased binding of dopamine D_2/D_3 receptors in striatal regions; this has been attributed to lowered presynaptic release of dopamine (see Verhoeff, 1999). It is now becoming possible to measure the binding of extra-striatal dopamine receptors in PET paradigms. Findings from such studies in depressed patients will be of great interest.

Overall these findings, taken with the effect of AMPT to cause relapse in recovered depression, suggest that impaired dopamine function may play a role in the manifestation of the depressive syndrome. Dopamine pathways might be particularly involved in the expression of symptoms such as motor retardation and anhedonia and their resolution by antidepressant drug treatment.

Monoamines and Depression

There is now good evidence that unmedicated depressed patients have abnormalities in several monoamine mechanisms. However, these abnormalities vary in extent from case to case, the changes are not large and are not sufficiently sensitive to be diagnostic.

The most convincing studies that show a key role for monoamines in the pathophysiology of depression are the tryptophan and catecholamine depletion paradigms. It is now established that in vulnerable individuals lowering of 5-HT and noradrenaline and dopamine function is sufficient to cause clinical depression. Two major questions emerge from this work.

(1) What mechanisms produce low monoamine function in depressed patients?
(2) What are the other factors that make those at risk of depression psychologically vulnerable to manipulations of monoamine function?

A likely explanation is that monoamine pathways innervate neuronal regions subserving mood regulation and that this mood-related circuitry has pre-existing abnormalities which are functionally 'revealed' by impairment of monoamine function. It is also possible that monoamine neurons themselves have trait abnormalities which compromise the regulation of neurotransmitter function under stressful conditions. There is, in fact, evidence for both these possibilities (Smith et al., 1999, 2000).

THE HPA AXIS

Plasma and Salivary Cortisol

Much research effort has been concerned with abnormalities in the control of cortisol in depressive disorders (Table 7.3). It is frequently stated that about half of patients whose depressive disorder is at least moderately severe, hypersecrete cortisol. However, this frequency of basal HPA axis hyperactivity may be apparent only in hospitalized patients (Maes et al., 1994). Increasing evidence from community samples suggests that increases in basal levels of plasma and salivary cortisol may, in fact, be rather unusual in patients with moderate depression (Strickland et al., 2002). It is, however, possible that the ratio of cortisol to DHEA might provide a better discrimination of such patients from controls (Young et al., 2002).

Dexamethasone Suppression Test

In studying depressed patients, much use has been made of the dexamethasone suppression test which suppresses cortisol levels via inhibition of corticotrophin (ACTH) release at pituitary level. This action is believed to be mediated via activation of glucocorticoid corticosteroid receptors. Again it is often stated that about 50% of depressed inpatients do not show the normal suppression of cortisol secretion induced by giving a 1 mg dose of the synthetic corticosteroid dexamethasone. However, not all cortisol hypersecretors are dexamethasone resistant and in outpatient samples rates of dexamethasone non-suppression are considerably lower.

Dexamethasone non-suppression is more common in depressed patients with melancholia, but it has not been reliably linked with any more specific psychopathological feature (Holsboer, 1992). However, abnormalities in the dexamethasone suppression test are not confined to mood disorders; they have also been reported in mania, chronic schizophrenia and dementia. This lack of diagnostic specificity

TABLE 7.3   HPA axis abnormalities in depression

↑	Basal secretion of cortisol (severe depression)
Resistance to cortisol suppressing action of dexamethasone	
↓	ACTH response to CRH
↑	ACTH/cortisol response to dexamethasone/CRH test
↑	Cortisol response to ACTH
↑	CRH level in CSF

diminished early hopes that dexamethasone non-suppression could be used as a diagnostic marker of melancholic depression. Nevertheless, dexamethasone non-suppression does predict a poorer response to placebo treatment in drug trials and a high risk of relapse in apparently recovered depressed patients (Ribeiro et al., 1993).

A number of studies have examined the effects of corticotrophin-releasing hormone (CRH) on ACTH and cortisol release in depressed patients. In general ACTH responses are blunted while cortisol responses are normal (see Dinan, 2001). The decrease in ACTH responses has been attributed to down-regulation of CRH receptors in the pituitary, presumably as a result of excessive CRH release. The preservation of cortisol responses may stem from the fact that the adrenal gland has a heightened response to ACTH in depression (see below). More recently the dexamethasone test has been combined with administration of CRH. In depressed patients, unlike controls, CRH continues to produce increases in ACTH and cortisol despite the presence of dexamethasone. This has been attributed to impaired dexamethasone feedback, perhaps due to abnormal corticosteroid receptor function (Modell et al., 1997). The combined dexamethasone/CRH test appears to have a higher rate of abnormality than the simple dexamethasone test in acutely depressed patients (Heuser et al., 1994). Moreover, subjects at genetic risk of depression who have not been ill themselves also have exaggerated ACTH and cortisol responses following CRH and dexamethasone (Holsboer et al., 1995).

Causes of HPA Axis Activity in Depression

The cause of cortisol hypersecretion in depressed patients is not clearly established. As described above, there seem to be abnormalities at various points in the regulation of the HPA axis. In addition, the adrenal gland itself appears to be enlarged and more responsive to the effect of ACTH (Dinan, 2001). Cortisol is a tropic hormone and therefore persistent hypersecretion of cortisol might explain this phenomenon.

It has been suggested that, taken together, abnormalities in cortisol regulation in depression can best be explained by hypersecretion of CRH in the hypothalamus with a resultant increase in ACTH and cortisol release (Dinan, 2001). This in turn might be attributable to impaired feedback due to decreased sensitivity of corticosteroid receptors and it is therefore of interest that many classes of antidepressant medication up-regulate corticosteroid receptors (see McQuade and Young, 2000). Another contributory factor might be increased production of arginine vasopressin (AVP) which often occurs in situations of CRH overdrive. AVP also contributes to ACTH release and would potentiate the effects of CRH in this respect (Holsboer, 1999; Dinan, 2001).

Role in Pathophysiology

In general HPA axis changes in depressed patients have been regarded as state abnormalities, that is they remit when the patient recovers. There is some evidence, however, that subtle changes in HPA axis function, for example in ACTH and cortisol responses to the dexamethasone/CRH test, may persist in recovered depressed subjects. This suggests that some vulnerable individuals may have fairly enduring abnormalities in HPA axis regulation (Modell et al., 1998). Interestingly, in experimental animals early adverse experiences produce longstanding changes in HPA axis regulation, indicating a possible neurobiological mechanism whereby childhood trauma could be translated into increased vulnerability to mood disorder (Plotsky and Meaney, 1993). Recent studies confirm that adults who were abused as children have heightened HPA axis responses to stress (Heim and Nemeroff, 2000). In addition the CRH/dexamethasone studies referred to above suggest that genetic factors might also predispose to HPA axis abnormalities (Holsboer, 1999).

In addition to its effects on cortisol secretion, CRH may play a more direct role in the aetiology of depression. It is well established that CRH has a neurotransmitter role in limbic regions of the brain where it is involved in regulating biochemical and behavioural responses to stress. Administration of CRH to animals produces changes in neuroendocrine regulation, sleep, and appetite that parallel those found in depressed patients. Furthermore, CRF levels may be increased in the CSF of depressed patients. Therefore it is possible that hypersecretion of CRH could be involved in the pathophysiology of the depressed state and non-peptide antagonists of CRH receptors may have value as antidepressant agents (see Heim and Nemeroff, 2000). Other possible approaches to the treatment of depression include glucocorticoid receptor antagonists and AVP receptor antagonists (McQuade and Young, 2000).

Taken together the data indicate that in some patients stressful life experiences may interact with a predisposition to abnormal HPA axis regulation to produce sustained HPA overactivity. In some subjects this could lead to a depressive disorder either through a direct effect of cortisol and CRH on relevant brain circuits or via impairment of monoamine function (see below). It is worth noting, however, that increased secretion of cortisol per se does not necessarily lead to depressive symptoms. For example, non-depressed carers of patients with Alzheimer's disease have increased basal levels of salivary cortisol (Da Roza Davis and Cowen, 2001) which presumably may represent an adaptive response to the stress of caring.

Cortisol, Monoamine Function and Neuronal Toxicity

Recent work has shown that corticosteroids regulate the genomic expression and function of a number of monoamine receptors in the brain. For example, it has been shown that corticosteroids can decrease the expression of postsynaptic 5-HT_{1A} receptors in the hippocampus; this finding has led to the suggestion that excessive cortisol secretion may precipitate depressive states through decreasing 5-HT neuro-transmission (Dinan et al., 1994). Experimental studies of animals have also linked excessive cortisol secretion in depression to damage to neurons in the hippocampus (see McEwen et al., 1997; McQuade and Young, 2000). Subsequently, it has been suggested that chronic cortisol hypersecretion could be associated with the cognitive impairment which may be a particular feature of chronic depression (for a review of this area see McAllister-Williams et al., 1998).

BRAIN STRUCTURE IN DEPRESSION

Changes in Brain Volume

Computerized tomography (CT) and magnetic resonance imaging (MRI) have identified a number of abnormalities in patients with major depression, particularly in those with more severe and chronic disorders (see Steffens and Krishnan, 1998). The most consistent findings are enlarged lateral ventricles, volume loss in frontal and temporal lobes, decreased hippocampal volume and decreased volume of basal ganglia structures. Although it is has been generally believed that changes in brain volume may represent long-term consequences of depression, perhaps associated with cortisol hypersecretion, more recent work indicates that decreases in hippocampal volume may, in fact, be present early in the course of the illness (Frodl et al., 2002). Such changes could therefore represent a vulnerability factor to depression and play a role in pathophysiology. The hippocampus also plays an important role in HPA axis regulation which provides an intriguing link between hippocampal dysfunction and abnormal HPA activity.

Another finding that has aroused particular interest is a decrease in grey matter volume of subgenual prefrontal cortex because this abnormality has been linked to lowered prefrontal perfusion in PET investigations and reduced glial cell numbers in post-mortem studies (Drevets et al., 1998; Ongür et al., 1998) (see below). Changes in this brain area could also represent a long-term vulnerability factor for the development of mood disorders. A general theme from imaging studies is that patients with structural abnormalities are less likely to respond to treatment.

White and Grey Matter Hyperintensities

Hyperintense MRI signals can be detected in a number of regions in both normal ageing and patients with major depression. The usual sites are in the deep white matter and subcortical grey matter. In major depression, increased deep white matter hyperintensities are associated with late onset of depressive disorder, greater illness severity and poorer treatment response, apathy, psychomotor slowness and retardation. It has been proposed that major depression with these clinical and radiological features is more likely to be of vascular origin (Steffens and Krishnan,

1998). In this situation, therefore, vascular abnormalities in brain regions relevant to mood regulation are likely to play a direct role in pathophysiology.

REGIONAL CEREBRAL BLOOD FLOW AND METABOLISM

Cerebral blood flow can be measured in a number of ways with, for example, single-photon emission tomography (SPET) or positron emission tomography (PET); the latter can also measure cerebral metabolism. Cerebral blood flow and metabolism are normally highly correlated.

Numerous studies have examined both cerebral metabolism and blood flow in groups of depressed patients. The findings have often been contradictory, and there are many methodological factors such as patient selection, drug status, and imaging techniques that may account for the discrepant findings. Nevertheless, there is some consensus that depressed patients have evidence of altered cerebral blood flow and metabolism in several regions including prefrontal cortex, anterior cingulate cortex, amygdala and thalamus and caudate nucleus (see Goodwin, 1996).

Taken together, the abnormalities in functional brain imaging in depression support a circuitry model in which mood disorders are associated with abnormal interactions between several brain regions rather than a major abnormality in a single structure. The circuits implicated involve regions of the frontal and temporal lobe as well as related areas of basal ganglia and thalamus (Drevets, 1998). Some tentative correlations between these brain regions and clinical depressive features are shown in Table 7.4.

NEUROPATHOLOGY OF DEPRESSION

There are a growing number of post-mortem neuropathological investigations of patients with bipolar disorder and major depression. Much of the focus of this work has been in prefrontal cortex and hippocampus because of structural and functional imaging studies implicating these brain regions in the pathophysiology of depression. The work is at preliminary stage but taken together the data suggest a decrease in density of glia as well the density and size of some neurons in frontal brain regions. In anterior cingulate cortex Benes et al. (2001) found a decreased density of interneurons as well as a trend towards a lower density of pyramidal neurons.

The data implicating abnormalities in GABA-ergic interneurons and gluta-matergic pyramidal cells are of interest given preliminary MRS findings of lowered cortical GABA and glutamate levels in patients with acute major depression (Sanacora et al., 2000; Auer et al., 2000). However, loss of glia could also contribute to decreased synthesis of GABA. In addition, glial cells possess several different neurotransmitter receptors and it is conceivable that lowered

TABLE 7.4   Some neuropsychological correlates of altered central perfusion in depressed patients

---

Dorsolateral and dorsomedial prefrontal cortex

- Cognitive dysfunction (particularly executive dysfunction) and cognitive slowness

Orbital and lateral prefrontal cortex

- Abnormal emotional processing
- Ruminative thinking

Anterior cingulate

- Impaired attentional processes
- Abnormal emotional processing

Amygdala

- Abnormal emotional processing
- Anxiety symptoms

Basal ganglia

- Impaired incentive behaviour
- Psychomotor disturbances

---

cortical 5-HT_{1A} receptor binding, for example, could reflect decreased glial cell density (see Harrison, 2002).

There is less evidence of consistent pathological abnormalities in other brain regions in depressed patients including the hippocampus. In bipolar disorder however, some studies have found synaptic and dendritic pathology in hippocampus. For example, Rosoklija et al. (2000) found decreased arborization of apical dendrites and reduced density of spines on subicular pyramidal neurons. Neuropathological studies of the raphe nuclei are clearly of great interest but the current data are contradictory (see Harrison, 2002).

NEUROTROPIC FACTORS IN DEPRESSION

There is growing interest in the possible role of neurotropic factors in the pathophysiology of depression and the actions of antidepressant drugs. Within the family of neurotrophic factors, brain-derived neurotropic factor (BDNF) is the most widely distributed and abundant in the brain. Neurotropic factors play a key role in neuronal differentiation and development but in addition are required for the survival and function of neurons in the adult brain (see Duman et al., 2000).

Stress and corticosteroid treatment both result in decreased expression of BDNF in hippocampus in granular cells and pyramidal cells in CA1 and CA3 regions. Down-regulation of BDNF could contribute to the stress-induced atrophy of CA3 apical dendrites seen in rodents and non-human primates and possibly in patients with mood disorders (see above). Interestingly treatment with antidepressant medications increases BDNF expression in hippocampus and also blocks stress-induced BDNF down-regulation (Duman et al., 1997).

These findings have given rise to a neurotropic hypothesis of depression in which stress leads to decreased production of neurotrophins which in turn results in depressive symptomatology, particularly in those with pre-existing impairment of hippocampal function. Impaired hippocampal function could lead to some of the cognitive impairments seen in depression as well as contributing to abnormal HPA axis activity (Duman et al., 1997, 2000).

CONCLUSIONS

The predisposition to depressive disorders has important genetic determinants. The pathophysiological level at which genetic factors operate is not known. It could be via effects on the regulation of monoamine neurotransmitters or through more remote factors such as temperament, the liability to experience life events and the psychobiological response to them. Adverse early experience such as parental discord or abuse of various kinds may also play a part in shaping features of personality which in turn determine whether, in adult life, certain events are experienced as stressful. In addition early experiences could programme the HPA axis to respond to stress in a way that might predispose to the development of mood disorder.

Major depression is commonly precipitated by stressful life events. Various biochemical theories can be used to explain how life stress and difficulty could be translated into the neurochemical changes that characterize depressive disorders. An abnormal HPA axis response to stress, particularly in more severe depressive states, seems likely to be involved in the pathophysiology of depression. Monoamine neurotransmitters are also involved in regulating responses to stress and in modifying behaviours known to be altered in mood disorders. It seems likely that both external events and a genetic predisposition bring about the changes in HPA axis activity and brain monoamine function that are seen in depressed patients. In predisposed subjects reduction in monoamine neurotransmission can bring about clinical symptomatology. Depressive states are associated with altered cerebral activity particularly in frontal cortex. In some patients, particularly those with recurrent illness, there is evidence for underlying neuropathological changes which probably act as a further predisposing factor (for a simplified model see Figure 7.2).

Major depression is a disorder with complex, environmental, and interpersonal determinants. These factors do not interact in a simple additive manner but modify each other in direct and indirect ways (Kendler et al., 1993). This formulation suggests that depressive states may involve a number of different pathophysiologies which could account for the common clinical experience that several different kinds of treatment are necessary to treat the broad range of patients who meet operational criteria for major depression.

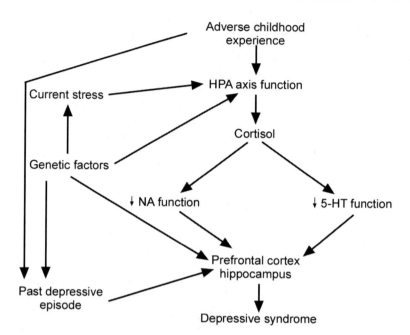

Figure 7.2 Simplified neurobiological model of the pathophysiology of major depression. Adverse childhood experience has enduring effects on HPA axis function which is further modified by stressful life events (the susceptibility to which is partly influenced by genetic factors). Abnormalities in cortisol secretion decrease monoamine function which leads to clinical depression in the setting of developmental and acquired abnormalities in prefrontal and hippocampal circuitry

ACKNOWLEDGEMENT

The work of the author is supported by the Medical Research Council.

REFERENCES

Ainsworth K, Smith SE, Zetterström TSC, Pei Q, Franklin M, Sharp T (1998) Effect of anti-depressant drugs on dopamine D_1 and D_2 receptor expression and dopamine release in the nucleus accumbens of the rat. *Psychopharmacology* **140**: 470–477.

Anand A, Charney DS (2000) Norepinephrine dysfunction in depression. *Journal of Clinical Psychiatry* **61**(Suppl 10): 16–24.

Anderson IM, Parry-Billings M, Newsholme EA, Poortmans JR, Cowen PJ (1990a) Decreased plasma tryptophan concentration in major depression: relationship to melancholia and weight loss. *Journal of Affective Disorders* **20**: 185–191.

Anderson IM, Parry-Billings M, Newsholme EA, Poortmans JR, Cowen PJ (1990b) Dieting reduces plasma tryptophan and alters brain 5-HT function in women. *Psychological Medicine* **20**: 785–791.

Anderson IM, Ware CJ, da Roza Davis JM, Cowen PJ (1992) Decreased 5-HT-mediated prolactin release in major depression. *British Journal of Psychiatry* **160**: 372–378.

Ansseau M, Vonfrenckel L, Cerfontaine R (1988) Blunted response of growth hormone to clonidine and apomorphine in endogenous depression. *British Journal of Psychiatry* **153**: 65–71.

Asberg M, Traskman L, Thoren P (1976) 5-HIAA in the cerebrospinal fluid: a biochemical suicide predictor. *Archives of General Psychiatry* **33**: 1193–1197.

Auer DP, Pütz B, Kraft E, Lipinski B, Schill J, Holsboer F (2000) Reduced glutamate in the anterior cingulate cortex in depression: an *in vivo* proton magnetic resonance spectroscopy study. *Biological Psychiatry* **47**: 305–313.

Benes FM, Vincent SL, Todtenkopf M (2001) The density of pyramidal and nonpyramidal neurons in anterior cingulate cortex of schizophrenic and bipolar subjects. *Biological Psychiatry* **50**: 395–406.

Berman RM, Narsimhan M, Miller HL, Anand A, Cappiello A, Oren DA, Heninger FR, Charney DS (1999) Transient depressive relapse induced by catecholamine depletion: potential phenotypic vulnerability marker. *Archives of General Psychiatry* **56**: 395–403.

Bhagwagar Z, Whale R, Cowen PJ (2002) State and trait abnormalities in serotonin function in major depression. *British Journal of Psychiatry* **180**: 24–28.

Blier P, de Montigny C (1994) Current advances and trends in the treatment of depression. *Trends in Pharmacological Sciences* **15**: 220–226.

Booij L, Van der Does W, Bankelfat C, Bremner JD, Cowen PJ, Fava M, Gillin C, Leyton M, Moore P, Smith KA, Van der Kloot WA (2002) Predictors of mood response to acute tryptophan depletion: a reanalysis. *Neuropsychopharmacology* (in press).

Brown GL, Linnoila MI (1990) CSF serotonin metabolite (5-HIAA) studies in depression, impulsivity, and violence. *Journal of Clinical Psychiatry* **51** (Suppl 4): 31–41.

Checkley SA (1992) Neuroendocrinology. In Paykel ES (ed) *Handbook of Affective Disorders*. Edinburgh: Churchill Livingstone, pp. 255–266.

Cowen PJ (1998) Neuroendocrine challenge tests: what can we learn from them? In Van de Kar LD (ed) *Methods in Neuroendocrinology.* Boca Raton, FL: CRC Press, pp. 205–223.

Cowen PJ, Power AC, Ware CJ, Anderson IM (1994) 5-HT$_{1A}$ receptor sensitivity in major depression: a neuroendocrine study with buspirone. *British Journal of Psychiatry* **164**: 372–379.

Da Roza Davis JM, Cowen PJ (2001) Biochemical stress of caring. *Psychological Medicine* **31**: 1475–1478.

Dinan TG (1994) Glucocorticoids and the genesis of depressive illness: a psychobiological model. *British Journal of Psychiatry* **146**: 365–371.

Dinan TG (2001) The hypothalamic–pituitary–adrenal axis in antidepressant action. In Leonard BE (ed) *Antidepressants*. Basel: Birkhäuser, pp. 83–94.

Drevets WC (1998) Functional neuroimaging studies of depression: the anatomy of melancholia. *Annual Review of Medicine* **49**: 341–361.

Drevets WC, Ongur D, Price JL (1998) Neuroimaging abnormalities in the subgenual prefrontal cortex: implications for the pathophysiology of familial mood disorders. *Molecular Psychiatry* **3**: 220–226.

Drevets WC, Frank E, Price JC, Kupfer DJ, Holt D, Greer PJ, Huang H, Gautier C, Mathis C (1999) PET imaging of serotonin 1A receptor binding in depression. *Biological Psychiatry* **46**: 1375–1387.

Duman RS, Heninger GR, Nestler EJ (1997) A molecular and cellular theory of depression. *Archives of General Psychiatry* **54**: 597–606.

Duman RS, Malberg J, Nakagawa S, D'Sa C (2000) Neuronal plasticity and survival in mood disorders. *Biological Psychiatry* **48**: 732–739.

Frodl T, Meisenzahl EM, Zetzsche T, Born C, Groll C, Jäger M, Leinsinger G, Bottlender R, Hahn K, Möller H-J (2002) Hippocampal changes in patients with a first episode of major depression. *American Journal of Psychiatry* **159**: 1112–1118.

Golden RN, Ekstrom D, Brown TM, Ruegg R, Evans DL, Haggerty JJ Jr, Garbutt JC, Pedersen CA, Mason GA, Browne J, et al. (1992) Neuroendocrine effects of intravenous clomipramine in depressed patients and healthy subjects. *American Journal of Psychiatry* **149**: 1168–1175.

Goodwin GM (1996) Functional imaging, affective disorder and dementia. *British Medical Bulletin* **51**: 495–512.

Greden JF (2001) The burden of recurrent depression: causes, consequences, and future prospects. *Journal of Clinical Psychiatry* **62** (Suppl 22): 5–9.

Harrison PJ (2002) The neuropathology of primary mood disorder. *Brain* **125**: 1428–1449.

Helm C, Nemeroff CB (2000) The impact of early adverse experiences on brain systems involved in the pathophysiology of anxiety and affective disorders. *Biological Psychiatry* **46**: 1509–1522.

Heuser I, Yassouridis A, Holsboer F (1994) The combined dexamethasone/CRH test: a refined laboratory test for psychiatric disorders. *Journal of Psychiatric Research* **28**: 341–356.

Holsboer F (1992) The hypothalamic–pituitary–adrenocortical system. In Paykel ES (ed) *Handbook of Affective Disorders*. Edinburgh: Churchill Livingstone, pp. 267–287.

Holsboer F (1999) Clinical neuroendocrinology. In Charney DS, Nestler EJ, Bunney BS (eds) *Neurobiology and Mental Illness*. Oxford: Oxford University Press, pp. 149–161.

Holsboer et al. (1995) Altered hypothalamic-pituitary-adrenocortical regulation in healthy subjects at high familial risk for affective disorders. *Neuroendocrinology* **62** (4): 340–347.

Horton RW (1992) The neurochemistry of depression: evidence derived from studies of post-mortem brain tissue. *Molecular Aspects of Medicine* **13**: 191–203.

Kapitany T, Schindl M, Schindler SD, Hesselmann B, Füreder T, Barnas C, Sieghart W, Siegfried K (1999) The citalopram challenge test in patients with major depression and in healthy controls. *Psychiatry Research* **88**: 75 88.

Kendler KS, Neale MC, Kessler RC, Heath AC, Eaves LJ (1992) A population-based twin study of major depression in women: the impact of varying definitions of illness. *Archives of General Psychiatry* **49**: 257–266.

Kendler KS et al. (1993) The lifetime history of major depression in women. *Reliability of diagnosis and heritability* **50** (11): 863–870.

Leake A, Fairbairn AF, McKeith IG (1991) Studies on the serotonin uptake binding site in major depressive disorder and control post-mortem brain: neurochemical and clinical correlates. *Psychiatry Research* **39**: 155–165.

Lesch KP (1992) 5-HT$_{1A}$ receptor responsivity in anxiety disorders and depression. *Progress in Neuropsychopharmacology and Biological Psychiatry* **15**: 723–733.

Lowther S, De Paermentier F, Cheetham SC, Crompton MR, Katona CLE, Horton RW (1997) 5-HT$_{1A}$ recepter binding sites in post-mortem brain samples from depressed suicides and controls. *Journal of Affective Disorders* **42**: 199–207.

Maes M, Calabrese J, Meltzer HY (1994) The relevance of the in- versus outpatient status for studies on HPA-axis in depression: spontaneous hypercortisolism is a feature of major depressed inpatients and not of major depression per se. *Progress in Neuropsychopharmacology and Biological Psychiatry* **18**: 503–517.

Malison RT et al. (1998) Reduced brain serotonin transporter availability in major depression as measured by [123I]-2beta-carbomethoxy-3 beta-(4-iodophenyl) tropane and single photon emission computed tomography. **44** (11): 1090–1098.

Matsubara S, Arora RC, Meltzer HY (1991) Serotonergic measures in suicide brain: 5-HT$_{1A}$ binding sites in frontal cortex of suicide victims. *Journal of Neural Transmission* **85**: 181–194.

McAllister-Williams RH, Ferrier IN, Young AH (1998) Mood and neuropsychological function in depression: the role of corticosteroids and serotonin. *Psychological Medicine* **28**: 573–584.

McEwen BS, Biron CA, Brunson KW, Bulloch K, Chambers WH, Dhabhar FS, Goldfarb RH, Kitson RP, Miller AH, Spencer RL, Weiss JM (1997) The role of adrenocorticoids as modulators of immune function in health and disease: neural, endocrine and immune interactions. *Brain Research* **23**: 79–133.

McQuade R, Young AH (2000) Future therapeutic targets in mood disorders: the glucocorticoid receptor. *British Journal of Psychiatry* **177**: 390–395.

Meyer JH, Kapur S, Houle S, DaSilva J, Owczarek B, Brown GM, Wilson AA, Kennedy SH (1999) Prefrontal cortex 5-HT$_2$ receptors in depression: an [^{18}F]Setoperone PET imaging study. *American Journal of Psychiatry* **156**: 1029–1034.

Mitchell PB, Bearn JA, Corn TH, Checkley SA (1988) Growth hormone response to clonidine after recovery in patients with endogenous depression. *British Journal of Psychiatry* **152**: 34–38.

Modell S, Yassouridis A, Huber J, Holsboer F (1997) Corticosteroid receptor function is decreased in depressed patients. *Neuroendocrinology* **65**: 216–222.

Modell S, Lauer CJ, Schreiber W, Huber J, Krieg J-C, Holsboer F (1998) Hormonal response pattern in the combined DEX–CRH test is stable over time in subjects at high familial risk for affective disorders. *Neuropsychopharmacology* **18**: 253–262.

Öngür D, Drevets WC, Price JL (1998) Glial reduction in the subgenual prefrontal cortex in mood disorders. *Proceedings of the National Academy of Sciences of the United States of America* **95**: 13 290–13 295.

Plotsky PM, Meaney MJ (1993) Early post-natal experience alters hypothalamic corticotropin-releasing factor (CRF) mRNA median eminence CRF content and stress-induced release in adult rats. *Molecular Brain Research* **18**: 195–200.

Ribeiro SCM, Tandon R, Grunhaus L, Greden JF (1993) The DST as a predictor of outcome in depression: a meta-analysis. *American Journal of Psychiatry* **150**: 1618–1629.

Rosoklija G, Toomayan G, Ellis SP, Keilp A, Mann JJ, Latov N, Hays AP, Dwork AJ (2000) Structural abnormalities of subicular dendrites in subjects with schizophrenia and mood disorders: preliminary findings. *Archives of General Psychiatry* **57**: 349–356.

Sanacora G, Mason GF, Krystal JH (2000) Impairment of GABAergic transmission in depression: new insights from neuroimaging studies. *Critical Reviews in Neurobiology* **14**: 23–45.

Sargent PA, Kjaer KH, Bench CJ, Rabiner EA, Messa C, Meyer J, Gunn RN, Grasby PM, Cowen PJ (2000) Brain serotonin$_{1A}$ receptor binding measured by positron emission tomography with [^{11}C] WAY-100635: effects of depression and antidepressant treatment. *Archives of General Psychiatry* **57**: 174–180.

Smith KA, Clifford EM, Hockney RA, Clark DM, Cowen PJ (1997a) Effect of tryptophan depletion on mood in male and female volunteers: a pilot study. *Human Psychopharmacology* **12**: 111–117.

Smith KA, Fairburn CG, Cowen PJ (1997b) Relapse of depression after rapid depletion of trypotophan. *Lancet* **349**: 915–919.

Smith KA, Morris JS, Friston KJ, Cowen PJ, Dolan RJ (1999) Brain mechanisms associated with depressive relapse and associated cognitive impairment following acute tryptophan depletion. *British Journal of Psychiatry* **174**: 525–529.

Smith KA, Williams C, Cowen PJ (2000) Impaired regulation of brain serotonin function during dieting in women recovered from depression. *British Journal of Psychiatry* **176**: 72–75.

Stanley M et al. (1982) Tritiated imipramine binding sites are decreased in the frontal cortex of suicides. 216(4552): 1337–1339.

Stanley M, Mann JJ (1983) Increased serotonin-2 binding sites in frontal cortex of suicide victims. *Lancet* **1**: 214–216.

Steffens DC, Krishnan KRR (1998) Structural neuroimaging and mood disorders: recent findings, implications for classification, and future directions. *Biological Psychiatry* **43**: 705–712.

Strickland PL, Deakin JFW, Percival C, Gater RA, Goldberg DP (2002) The bio-social origins of depression in the community: interactions between social adversity, cortisol and serotonin neurotransmission. *British Journal of Psychiatry* **180**: 168–173.

Verhoeff NPLG (1999) Radiotracer imaging of dopaminergic transmission in neuropsychiatric disorders. *Psychopharmacology* **147**: 217–249.

Whale R, Clifford EM, Bhagwagar Z, Cowen PJ (2001) Decreased sensitivity of 5-HT$_{1D}$ receptors in melancholic depression. *British Journal of Psychiatry* **178**: 454–457.

Willeit M, Praschak-Rieder N, Neurmeister A, Pirker W, Asenbaum S, Vitouch O, Tauscher J, Hilger E, Stastny J, Brucke T, Kasper S (2000) [123I]-beta-CIT SPECT imaging shows reduced brain serotonin transporter availability in drug-free depressed patients with seasonal affective disorder. *Biological Psychiatry* **47**: 482–489.

Yatham LN, Liddle PF, Shiah IS, Scarrow G, Lam RW, Adam MJ, Zis AP, Ruth TJ (2000) Brain serotonin 2 receptors in major depression: a positron emission tomography study. *Archives of General Psychiatry* **57**: 850–858.

Young AH, Sharpley AL, Campling GM, Hockney RA, Cowen PJ (1994) Effects of hydrocortisone on brain 5-HYT function and sleep. *Journal of Affective Disorders* **32**: 139–146.

Young AH, Gallagher P, Porter RJ (2002) Elevation of the cortisol-dehydroepiandrosterone ratio in drug-free depressed patients. *American Journal of Psychiatry* **159**: 1237–1239.

8

Stress and Depression: the Inflammatory Hypothesis

Dirk van West[1], Gunter Kenis[2] and Michael Maes[2,3]

[1]*University of Antwerp, Antwerp, Belgium*
[2]*University of Maastricht, Maastricht, The Netherlands*
[3]*Vanderbilt University, Nashville, USA*

INTRODUCTION

Current models concerning the biological pathophysiology of depression emphasize the role of brain monoaminergic neurotransmitters, such as serotonin (5-HT) and catecholamines, and the hypothalamic–pituitary–adrenal (HPA)-axis. However, over the last number of years a large body of evidence suggests that major depression is associated with activation of the inflammatory response system (IRS) (Connor and Leonard 1998; Holden et al., 1997; Maes 1993, 1995, 1997; Maes and Smith 1997; Maier and Watkins 1995). The hallmarks are in vivo stimulation of some aspects of cell-mediated immunity, the presence of an acute phase (AP) response and increased production of proinflammatory cytokines.

CYTOKINES AND THE IMMUNE RESPONSE

Cells of the Immune System

In this chapter, several lines of evidence for an activation of the IRS in major depression are discussed. A brief review of the most important cells and signalling molecules of the immune system is therefore appropriate.

The major part of the immune system comprises circulating leucocytes (white blood cells). The most important are monocytes, T- and B-lymphocytes (T- and B-cells), neutrophils, and natural killer (NK) cells. Monocytes recognize invading microorganisms and take them up via phagocytosis. Monocytes degrade the microorganisms in small peptides that bind with endogenous major

Mood Disorders: Clinical Management and Research Issues. Edited by E. J. L. Griez, C. Faravelli, D. J. Nutt and J. Zohar.
©2005 John Wiley & Sons Ltd. ISBN 0 470 09426 5.

histocompatibility class II (MHC-II) proteins. This complex is expressed at the cell membrane in such a way that the peptides from the microorganism are presented to T- and B-lymphocytes. Besides monocytes, also macrophages (which are derived from blood-borne monocytes and reside in tissue) and dendritic cells (present in lymph nodes, but not derived from monocytes) express foreign peptide complexes and collectively they are termed antigen presenting cells (APCs). Neutrophils are highly phagocytic cells that are attracted to the site of infection, where they phagocytose present microbes and/or apoptotic or necrotic cells. NK cells primarily destroy infected and malignant cells. Since the abovementioned cell types form the first line of defence against invading organisms, they are part of the innate immune system.

On the other hand, lymphocytes are the cells of the acquired immune system. Whereas monocytes, macrophages and neutrophils recognize conserved molecules on microbes, lymphocytes express specialized receptors that interact with the peptide/MHC-II complex on APCs. This interaction activates only those lymphocytes that bear the respective receptor that recognizes this complex. For B-lymphocytes this recognition is established through a membrane-bound antibody of the IgD type. Upon interaction with the APC, the B-cell is stimulated to proliferate and differentiate into an antibody-producing plasma cell. These antibodies then opsonize the respective microbes, which facilitates phagocytosis by phagocytic cells. Two major sets of T-lymphocytes can be distinguished: T-helper (Th-) and cytotoxic T (Tc-) cells. Both have a T-cell receptor that (as antibodies from B-cells) recognize specific peptide sequences in conjunction with MHC-II. Activated Th-cells secrete certain molecules (cytokines) that regulate the activity of other immunocompetent cells. Accordingly they are very important regulators of the immune response. Tc-cells mainly destroy cells infected with viruses or intracellular bacteria.

Lymphocyte subsets can be characterized ex vivo by specific molecules at the cell surface. Th-cells express CD4, Tc-cells CD8, B-cells CD19, and activated T-cells express CD25. In this way, percentage and number of Th-, Tc-, B- and activated T-cells can be determined. For more detailed information concerning the different cell types of the immune system, see Delves and Roitt (2000).

Cytokines

The concerted action of all the immune cells requires tight regulation and communication. This is established by two means: cell–cell contact and the production and secretion of soluble signalling molecules called cytokines. Although both are mutually important, the latter are of great interest for depression research, since cytokines can be measured in blood and are indicative for the actual activity of the immune response. Cytokines are small (15 to 44 kD) glycoproteins, primarily secreted by immune cells, but also endothelial, epithelial, and neuronal cells can produce them. They interact with a specific membrane-bound receptor on target cells. Given the large number of known cytokines (there are probably many more to be discovered) and the diverse functions attributed to each of them, classification of cytokines is still obscure. Nevertheless, when examining systemic activity of the immune system in depressed patients, differentiation into two major groups is justified, namely proinflammatory and antiinflammatory cytokines. Proinflammatory cytokines are mainly produced by activated immune cells and stimulate others, and, thereby, enhance inflammatory reactions. Antiinflammatory cytokines, on the other hand, tend to inhibit activated cells and temper inflammatory responses.

Monocytes and macrophages, activated by the recognition of pathogens, produce a diverse array of proinflammatory cytokines such as interleukin-1 (IL-1), tumour necrosis factor-α (TNFα), IL-6 and IL-12. IL-1 and TNFα promote inflammatory reactions, i.e. they stimulate other monocytes/macrophages and neutrophils to migrate to the site of infection and to phagocytosis. IL-6 activates lymphocytes and induces B-cells to differentiate to antibody producing plasma cells. After the initial activation, monocytes/macrophages also produce antiinflammatory cytokines or proteins such as IL-10 and IL-1 receptor antagonist (IL-1RA). IL-10 is a major deactivator of activated monocytes/macrophages, lymphocytes and neutrophils, and directly inhibits proinflammatory cytokine production. IL-1RA binds the IL-1 receptor and blocks the action of IL-1.

Thus, the major monocytic proinflammatory cytokines are IL-1, TNFα and IL-6 and are as such indicative for an activation of the monocytic arm of the immune system.

Activated T-lymphocytes can be divided into two major groups according to the cytokines they produce, namely T-helper-1 (Th1-) and Th2-cells. Th1-cells mainly produce interferon-γ (IFNγ), IL-2 and TNFβ; Th2-cells produce IL-4, IL-5, and IL-10. These cytokines have differential functions, i.e. Th1 cytokines stimulate cell-mediated immunity (CMI) whereas Th2 cytokines promote humoral immunity. CMI is characterized by the activation of monocytes/macrophages, neutrophils, Tc-cells and the stimulation of B-cells to produce opsonizing antibodies (thus facilitating phagocytic activity). For example, IFNγ (produced by Th1-cells) stimulates macrophages to phagocytosis; IL-2 further stimulates Th1-cells and induces Tc-cells to cytotoxic activity. On the other hand, IL-4 and IL-5 from Th2-cells mainly stimulate B-cells to produce nonopsonizing antibodies like IgE, and activate eosinophils, basophils and mast cells, which release several allergic mediators. In addition, Th1- and Th2- responses are mutually exclusive, i.e. IFNγ inhibits Th2-cells, whereas IL-4 and IL-10 inhibit Th1-cells. This results in a polarization of the phenotype of the immune response. This phenotype is determined by the kind of microbial antigen and the micro-environment at the time of immune activation. For more information on Th1/Th2-responses and the accompanying cytokines, see Abbas et al. (1996).

It is clear that the concepts pro/antiinflammatory and Th1/Th2-cytokines are more or less overlapping. Proinflammatory cytokines induce the production of Th1 cytokines which themselves have proinflammatory capacities; Th2 cytokines are antiinflammatory and inhibit Th1- and/or proinflammatory cytokine production. One exception in this respect is IL-6. It has many proinflammatory properties, but is, besides monocytes/macrophages, produced by Th2-cells. Nevertheless, IL-6 is an important activator of the inflammatory response system. A major aspect of IRS is the acute phase response, which is predominantly induced by IL-6.

As mentioned before, cytokines act through specific membrane-bound receptors. Some of these receptors can be released in a soluble form in the circulation. In most cases, they are shed from the cell membrane of activated leucocytes. For example, the soluble IL-2 receptor (sIL-2R) is shed from activated T-cells. So, increased levels of sIL-2R indicate ongoing T-cell activation. Soluble cytokine receptors usually act as antagonists, since they prevent the respective cytokine from binding with its receptor on the target cell. Again, IL-6 is an exception to this rule. The IL-6/ sIL-6R complex in serum can bind to gp130, a membrane-bound molecule that mediates IL-6 signalling. Therefore, sIL-6R can enhance the biological activity of circulating IL-6.

Direct Indicators of IRS Activation in Depression

Indicators of IRS activation in major depression are confirmed findings of increased numbers of leucocytes, monocytes, neutrophils and activated T-lymphocytes, and increased secretion of neopterin and prostaglandins. Flow-cytometry shows an increased $CD4^+/CD8^+$ T cell ratio and increased numbers of activated T cells, such as $CD25^+$ and $HLA-DR^+$ T cells, in depression (Maes 1997; Deger et al., 1996; Maes et al., 1992a, 1993a; Seidel et al., 1996). Increased concentrations of the soluble interleukin-2-receptor (sIL-2R) also point toward T-cell activation (Maes et al., 1995a). Other reports include increased concentrations of prostaglandin E2 (PGE2) in serum, cerebrospinal fluid (CSF) and mitogen-stimulated culture supernatant (Calabrese et al., 1986; Lieb and Karmali 1983; Linnoila et al., 1983; Song et al., 1998), and increased serum or urine secretion of neopterin (Bonaccorso et al., 1998; Duch et al., 1984; Dunbar et al., 1992; Maes et al., 1994a).

Indicators of an acute phase response in major depression are the confirmed findings on changes in serum concentrations of positive and negative acute phase proteins (APPs). For example, major depression is characterized by increased serum levels of positive APPs, such as haptoglobin (Hp), α1-antitrypsin, caeruloplasmin, α1-acid glycoprotein, C-reactive protein, haemopexin and α1-antichymotrypsin; and by a downregulation of the synthesis of negative AP (visceral proteins), such as albumin (Alb), retinol-binding protein (RBP) and transferrin (Tf) (Maes et al., 1992b, 1992c, 1994b, 1995b, 1997a; Song et al., 1994; Swartz 1990; Sluzewska et al., 1996) (Table 8.1).

In depression, there are also confirmed findings of increased in vivo secretion of proinflammatory cytokines, such as IL-6 and IL-8 (Song et al., 1998; Berk et al., 1997; Frommberger et al., 1997; Sluzewska et al., 1995) and increased mitogen-induced production of proinflammatory cytokines, such as IL-1β, IL-6 and IFNγ

TABLE 8.1 The acute phase response in major depressed patients: serum protein concentrations. This table shows the increase and/or decrease in serum protein concentrations of depressed patients compared with normal control values

	Increase positive APP	Decrease negative APP
Maes et al. (1992c)		transferrin albumin
Maes et al. (1997a)	α1-antitrypsin haptoglobin caeruloplasmin	retinol-binding protein
Maes et al. (1992b)		albumin transferrin
Swartz (1990)		albumin
Song et al. (1994)	haptoglobin α1-antitrypsin	albumin
Sluzewska et al. (1996)	α1-acid glycoprotein	

(Maes et al., 1994a; Sluzewska et al., 1995; Maes et al., 1991, 1993b, 1993c; Seidel et al., 1995). Since proinflammatory cytokines induce an immune and acute phase response and since we have found significant and positive correlations between cytokine production, e.g. IL-6, and indicators of immune activation, e.g. increased numbers of peripheral blood mononuclear cells (PBMC) and acute phase proteins, we have suggested that IRS activation in depression is caused by an increased production of the proinflammatory cytokines, IL-1β, IL-6 and IFNγ (Maes 1993, 1995, 1997; Maes et al., 1992a, 1993a).

INDIRECT INDICATORS OF IRS ACTIVATION IN MAJOR DEPRESSION

Zinc and Depression

There are two factors which can explain lower serum zinc in depression. First, because IRS activation results in decreased serum Alb concentrations and Alb is the major zinc-binding protein, there is potentially less zinc-binding protein available, which could in part explain lower serum zinc (Goldblum et al., 1987). However, we found that serum Alb and diagnostic classification had additive effects and independently of each other explained an important part of the variance in serum zinc. Second, lowered serum zinc during IRS activation may be secondary to sequestration of the intracellular heavy metal binding protein metallothionein in the liver, which, in turn, may be related to an increased production of the proinflammatory cytokines, IL-1 and IL-6 (Cousins and Leinart 1998; Van Miert et al., 1990).

Alterations in the Erythrocyte and Depression

It has been shown that patients with major depression have significantly lower serum iron (Fe) and transferrin (Tf), and a significantly lower number of red blood cells (RBC), lower haematocrit (Htc) and haemoglobin (Hb), and a significantly increased number of reticulocytes than normal controls (Maes et al., 1996a; Vandoolaeghe et al., 1999). We observed that serum Fe and Tf were significantly related to other well-established inflammatory markers of major depression, e.g. serum Fe was significantly related to serum Alb and zinc (positively) and to the $\alpha 1$-globulin fraction (negatively); and serum Tf was significantly related to serum Alb and zinc. Significant relationships were reported between erythron variables and indicators of IRS activation. For example, there are significant and positive correlations between serum zinc and number of RBC, Htc and Hb (all positive), and between serum Alb and RBC, Htc and Hb (all positive). There are also significant correlations between serum zinc and Fe and serum Tf (positive), serum Alb and Fe (positive), serum Alb and Tf (positive) and the α_1-globulin fraction and Fe (negative). Finally, there were significant and positive correlations between the number of reticulocytes and number of leucocytes and neutrophils and the α_1-globulin fraction (Maes et al., 1996a; Vandoolaeghe et al., 1999).

Fatty Acids and Depression

Other hallmarks of IRS activation are lower serum total cholesterol, high-density-lipoprotein cholesterol (HDL-C), a lower esterified cholesterol : total cholesterol ratio, decreased activity of lecithin : cholesterol acyltransferase (LCAT) and specific changes in polyunsaturated fatty acids (PUFAs). There is now evidence that alterations in fatty acid metabolism and the composition of phospholipids in serum and membranes are involved in the pathophysiology of major depression (Horrobin 1990; Smith 1991; Maes et al., 1994c, 1996b, 1997b; Hibbeln and Salem 1995; Maes and Smith 1998; Peet et al., 1998). Some authors (Morgan et al., 1993; Glueck et al., 1994), but not all authors (Swartz 1990; McCallum et al., 1994) reported an association between lower serum total cholesterol and major depression. Prevention trials designed to lower serum cholesterol levels by diet, drugs or both were shown to increase the number of deaths due to suicide (Maes et al., 1997b). It was shown that men with low cholesterol or serum HDL-C were more likely to have ever made a medically serious suicide attempt (Maes et al., 1997b). Depressed patients exhibit significantly reduced esterified cholesterol and lowered HDL-C and HDL-C/total cholesterol ratios (Maes et al., 1994c, 1997b). These results suggest an abnormal intake and/or metabolism of fatty acids and a decreased formation of cholesteryl esters in major depression (Maes et al., 1997b). The latter phenomenon may point toward decreased activity of LCAT, since most of the cholesteryl esters in man are formed in serum under the activity of LCAT, which reacts preferentially with free cholesterol of the HDL particles. Since in depression, lower serum HDL-C is related to indicators of IRS activation, such as $CD4^+/CD8^+$ T cell ratio (negative), and serum Zn and Alb (both positively), we have hypothesized that the changes in HDL-C may be secondary to IRS activation.

PUFAs have important effects on inflammatory processes since they are precursors of eicosanoids (Figure 8.1) ($C20:4\omega6$ or arachidonic acid is the most abundant eicosanoid precursor in people consuming a Western diet) and can affect eicosanoid and cytokine formation. It has been shown that an imbalance of $\omega6$ to $\omega3$ PUFAs may lead to an overproduction of cytokines (Endres 1993). Supplements of linoleic ($C18:2\omega6$) oil increase IL-1 and TNFα secretion (Meydani et al., 1991; Soyland et al., 1994). Recently, it has been shown that depressed patients show alterations in the $\omega6/\omega3$ ratio. Our laboratory was the first to report that depressed patients show an increased $C20:4\omega6/C20:4\omega3$ ratio in serum phospholipids and cholesteryl esters and significantly decreased total $\omega3$, $C18:3\omega3$ and $C20:5\omega3$ fractions in serum cholesteryl esters (Maes et al., 1996b). Adams et al. (1996) detected a significant positive relationship between severity of illness and the $C20:4\omega6/C20:5\omega3$ ratio and the imbalance in $\omega6/\omega3$ PUFAs in major depression may be related to the increased production of proinflammatory cytokines and eicosanoids in that illness (Maes et al., 1996b; Maes and Smith (1998). Most importantly, there were significant and positive correlations between serum Zn and $C20:5\omega3$ and $C22:6\omega3$ fractions in phospholipids; and significant inverse correlations between serum Zn and the $\omega6/\omega3$, $C20:4\omega6/C20:5\omega3$, and $C22:5\omega6/C22.6\omega3$ ratios in phospholipids (Maes et al., 2000). In the rodent, lowered intake of Zn does not affect food intake or weight gain but reduces whole-body accumulation of desaturated and elongated products of linoleic acid ($C18:2\omega6$) and α-linolenic acid ($C18:3\omega3$) (Cunnane et al., 1993). Desaturase enzymes require Zn as cofactor (Russo et al., 1997). Thus, depletion of long-chain $\omega3$ PUFAs in depression could be related to lower serum Zn, which, in turn is an indicator of IRS activation in that illness. The results suggest that (i) there is a metabolic disorder in the elongation and desaturation of fatty acids; and (ii) the fatty acid alterations in depression are related to IRS activation in that illness.

NEUROENDOCRINE DISORDERS IN MAJOR DEPRESSION AND IRS ACTIVATION

Major depression is accompanied by hypothalamic–pituitary–adrenal (HPA) axis hyperactivity, hypothalamic–pituitary–thyroid (HPT) axis alterations, such as lower basal TSH concentrations, and serotonergic disturbances. The most consistently reported signs of HPA-axis hyperactivity in major depression are

	ω6 series	ω3 series	
18 : 2ω6	Linolenic acid (LA)	Alpha linolenic acid (α-LNA)	18 : 3ω3
↓			↓
	Delta-6-desaturation		
18 : 3ω6	Gamma-linolenic acid (GLA)	*Stearidonic acid*	18 : 4ω3
↓			↓
	Elongation 20 : 3ω6		
20 : 3ω6	Dihomogammalinolenic	*Eicosatetraenoic acid*	20 : 4ω3
↓			↓
	Delta-5-desaturation		
20 : 4ω6	Arachidonic acid (AA)	Eicosapentaenoic acid (EPA)	120 : 5ω3
↓			↓
	Elongation		
20 : 4ω6	Adrenic acid	Docosapentaenoic acid	22 : 5ω3
↓			↓
	Delta-4-desaturation		
22 : 5ω6	Docosapentaenoic acid (DPA)	Docosahexaenoic acid (DHA)	22 : 6ω3

Figure 8.1 An outline of the metabolism of ω3 and ω6 essential fatty acids

endogenous hypercortisolaemia and the failure to suppress plasma cortisol with the 1-mg dexamethasone suppression test (DST) (Maes et al., 1993b). The most consistent sign of HPT axis dysfunction in depression is lower basal TSH. There is evidence that disorders in the central and peripheral neurotransmission of serotonin (5-HT) are implicated in the pathogenesis or pathophysiology of major depression (Maes and Meltzer 1995). Therefore, we have hypothesized that, if major depression is indeed characterized by IRS activation, the glucocorticoid resistance in depression, lower serum basal TSH concentrations and lower availability of tryptophan to the brain may be related to indicators of IRS activation. In accordance with this hypothesis we found the following. (i) In depressed patients, there is a significant positive correlation between IL-1β production and post-DST cortisol values, and a significant positive correlation between baseline plasma cortisol and IL-6 concentrations (Maes et al., 1993b,c). (ii) In depression, basal TSH was significantly and negatively related to haptoglobin values, whereas in normal controls a trend toward a positive correlation between both factors was found. (iii) Lower availability of plasma tryptophan to the brain was significantly correlated to serum IL-6, serum haptoglobin, the α2 globulin fractions, neopterin and the CD4$^+$/CD8$^+$ T cell ratio (inversely) and to serum Alb, Fe, Tf and zinc (all positively) (Maes et al., 1994d, 1997c).

CYTOKINES AND THE AETIOLOGY OF MAJOR DEPRESSION

Proinflammatory Cytokines Induce Depression-like Effects

Another question is whether – besides the possible role of proinflammatory cytokines in generating the IRS response and neuroendocrine changes in major depression – hypersecretion of these cytokines may contribute to the aetiology of major depression. It has been suggested that increased production of pro-inflammatory cytokines may play a role in the aetiopathology and symptomatology of depression (Maes 1997; Smith 1991). Acute or repeated administration of LPS, IL-1 and IL-6 to the rodent may induce 'sickness behaviour', a symptom complex characterized by anorexia, weight loss, sleep disorders, suppression of social, locomotor and exploratory behaviour and anhedonia, all key symptoms of major depression (Maier and Watkins 1995). Both IL-1β and tumour necrosis factor-alpha (TNFα) induced 'anxiogenic-like' effects on the elevated plus maze, whereas interleukin-2 and interleukin-6 did not (Connor and Leonard 1998). Administration of interferons, including IFNγ, results in behavioural effects and mood alterations, similar to those observed in major depression, such as anhedonia, anorexia, weight loss, anxiety, social withdrawal, psychomotor retardation, anergy, irritability, sleep disturbances and malaise (Smith 1991; Gutterman et al., 1982).

In major depression, we found significant relationships between indicators of IRS activation and the vegetative symptoms of depression. (i) Serum Alb (negatively) or the α1 and α2 globulin fractions (positively) were significantly related to psycho-motor retardation, anorexia and middle insomnia. (ii) Serum zinc was significantly and inversely related to psychomotor retardation. (iii) Plasma hapto-globin concentrations were significantly and positively related to psychomotor retardation, anorexia, weight loss, anergy, loss of interest and middle insomnia (Maes et al., 1993d). It should be underscored that no significant correlations were found between the affective (e.g. depressed mood, a distinct quality of mood, nonreactivity) and cognitive (e.g. feelings of guilt, suicidal ideation) symptoms of depression and any of the IRS activation indicators in depression. Therefore, we have hypothesized that the somatic dimension of major depression may, in fact, be related to IRS activation, through hypersecretion of proinflammatory cytokines (Maes et al., 1993d).

External Stress, Cytokines and the Aetiology of Depression

External Stressors and Cytokines in Animals

Rats exposed to electric footshock, physical restraint or a conditioned, aversive stimulus have increased concentrations of plasma IL-6 (Zhou et al., 1993). Restraint stress significantly enhances the expression of IL-6 mRNA and reduces that of the IL-6R mRNA in the midbrain (Shizuya et al., 1997). Immobilization stress increases plasma IL-6 levels, while the peak levels of stress-induced plasma IL-6 in the animals immobilized for 120 min are significantly higher than those in the animals subjected to 30 min stress (Takaki et al., 1994). In the rodent, immobiliza-tion stress increases IL-1 mRNA expression in the hypothalamus only (Minami et al., 1991). In Wistar rats, an eight-week exposure to mild, unpredictable stress induces a depression-like state with an increased capacity of splenocytes to produce IL-1 and IL-2 (Kubera et al., 1996).

It has been hypothesized that IRS activation with increased production of proinflammatory cytokines, such as IL-1, may have a central role in the stress responses (Shintani et al., 1995). In conclusion, there is strong evidence that external stressors increase the production rate of the proinflammatory cytokines IL-1 and IL-6 in animals.

External Stressors and Cytokines in Humans

Dobbin et al. (1991) found that academic stress reduces the mitogen-induced lymphoproliferative responses and the production of IFNγ in students, but at the same time significantly increases IL-β production. These authors concluded that psychological stress in humans may have different effects on different cell populations by enhancing responses of monocytes and depressing those of lymphocytes (Dobbin et al., 1991). In another study, the induction of mild negative emotional changes caused an increase in TNFα, a decrease in IL-2 and IL-3, with no changes in IL-1β and IL-6 (Mittwoch-Jaffe et al., 1995). Recently, we found that academic examination stress in university students significantly increases the stimulated production of proinflammatory cytokines, such as IL-6, TNFα and IFNγ, and of the negative immunoregulatory cytokine IL-10 (Maes et al., 1998a). Most importantly, students with a high stress perception (as measured by the Perceived Stress Scale) during the examination period have a significantly higher production of TNFα, IFNγ and IL-6 than students with lower stress perception. The stress-induced changes in perceived stress are significantly and positively related to the stress-induced production of TNFα, IFNγ and IL-6, suggesting that the stress-induced production of these cytokines is sensitive to graded differences in the perception of stressor severity.

It has been shown that the ratio of IFNγ production to IL-10 production in culture supernatant is of critical importance in determining the capacity of supernatants to activate or inhibit monocytic and T-lymphocytic functions (Maes et al., 1999). We found that the response to external (psychological) stress in humans consists of two different profiles of cytokine production, i.e. a first characterized by an increased IFNγ/IL-10 ratio, attributable to a higher IFNγ than IL-10 response (labelled IFNγ reactors) and a second characterized by a lowered IFNγ/IL-10 ratio, attributable to a higher IL-10 than IFNγ response (labelled IL-10 reactors). IFNγ reactors, but not IL-10 reactors, show a significantly increased stimulated production of other proinflammatory cytokines, i.e. TNFα and IL-6, and of serum IL-1RA, sCD8 and IgA, IgG and IgM concentrations. Thus, the external stress responsivity entails either a predominant proinflammatory cytokine response or a negative immunoregulatory cytokine response. IFNγ reactors, but not IL-10 reactors, show significant stress-induced increases in anxiety and depression ratings, suggesting that a proinflammatory response and a lower stress-induced production of the negative immunoregulatory cytokine IL-10 appears to be accompanied by increased stress-induced anxiety and depression.

The above findings in animals and humans may suggest that proinflammatory cytokines are involved in the stress response and that external stressors are perceived by the immune system and, through secretion of proinflammatory and negative immunoregulatory, take part in an integrated psychoneuroendocrine homeostatic response. The discovery that psychological stress in humans can alter the equilibrium between proinflammatory and negative immunoregulatory cytokines has important implications for human psychopathology. Indeed, since major depression may be induced by external stressors (negative life events and early life stressors) and since external stressors induce an inflammatory response in some subjects (i.e. those with increased anxiety and depression ratings), we have hypothesized that psychological stress-induced hyperproduction of proinflammatory cytokines may play a role in the aetiopathology of major depression (Maes et al., 1999).

Internal Stress, Cytokines and the Aetiology of Depression

Important epidemiological features of major depression are the higher incidence of major depression in the medically ill or in 'organic' conditions (i.e. mood disorders due to a general medical condition) and in women, and the increasing rates of depression this century. The IRS activation model is consistent with each feature.

The high occurrence of major depression in the medically ill is clearly consistent with the IRS activation model of depression (Maes 1997; Maes et al., 1997b). Indeed, medical illnesses involving IRS activation, such as infectious (e.g. herpes virus, HIV, Borna virus, influenza) and non-infectious disorders (e.g. autoimmune disorders, multiple sclerosis, Alzheimer's disease), exhibit an increased incidence of depression. Moreover, conditions that are accompanied by an enhanced production of cytokines, e.g. postpartum period, stroke and myocardial infarction are often accompanied by depressive symptoms or major depression. Thus, autoimmune-, postnatal-, inflammation- and stroke-induced cytokine hyperproduction provides a reasonable mechanism to account for the higher rates of depression linked with these conditions.

The elevated rate of depression in women is consistent with the greater immune responsivity in females and the immune activating effects of sex hormones (Ahmed et al., 1985; Knapp et al., 1992). Indeed, it is known that immune responsiveness is greater in women than in men and that sex hormones can alter immune responses (Ahmed et al., 1985). For example, female sex hormones modulate maturation of lymphocytes in the lymphoid tissues, regulate leucocyte entry into peripheral tissues, alter immune cell membrane composition, augment leucocyte adhesion, enhance proliferation of lymphocytes in response to mitogenic stimuli and increase IL-1 production by mononuclear cells (Athreya et al., 1993). We found that female students who are taking monophasic contraceptive drugs had significantly greater stress-induced response in the number of leucocytes, neutrophils, and B cells than females not taking contraceptives and than male students, suggesting that ethinyl-oestradiol and/or derivates of progesterone may increase the immune responsiveness to psychological stress (Maes and Smith 1998).

Also the increased rate of major depression since 1913 may be explained by the IRS model of depression. This increased incidence parallels the increasing ratio of ω6 to ω3 fatty acids in Western diets during the twentieth century (Smith 1991). This results in high levels of ω6 PUFAs in tissues and low levels of long-chain ω3 PUFAs in serum and membranes of the Western population. As explained above, a high dietary ω6/ω3 fatty acid ratio may increase the secretion of proinflammatory cyto-kines (Maes et al., 1996b). It has also been suggested that the increased ω6/ω3 PUFA ratio may have contributed to an increased incidence of cardiovascular and inflammatory disorders (Smith 1991).

ANTIDEPRESSANT TREATMENTS, CYTOKINES AND DEPRESSION

In Vivo Effects of Antidepressants

If increased production of proinflammatory cytokines is at all involved in the aetiology of depression one would expect that the various antidepressive treatments had negative immunoregulatory effects. It is generally believed that tricyclic anti-depressants have immunosuppressive effects ex vivo as well as in vivo (Miller and Lackner 1989). Subchronic treatment with fluoxetine, a selective 5-HT re-uptake inhibitor (SSRI), normalizes the initially increased serum IL-6 concentrations in depressed patients (Sluzewska et al., 1995). Subchronic treatment with tricyclic anti-depressants and fluoxetine is able to suppress the acute phase response in major depression (Maes et al., 1997a). The above results show that, in vivo, antidepressants have antiinflammatory effects through down-regulation of proinflammatory cyto-kines and up-regulation of the negative immunoregulatory cytokines/receptor antagonists, IL-10 and the IL-1RA.

In Vitro Effects of Antidepressants

In vitro it has been shown that antidepressants, such as clomipramine, imipramine and citalopram significantly suppress the secretion of IL-1β and TNFα by stimu-lated monocytes (Xia et al., 1996). Our laboratory found that clomipramine, sertraline and trazodone, at concentrations in the range of the therapeutic plasma concentrations achieved during clinical treatment, had a significant suppressive effect on the IFNγ/IL-10 ratio, which was attributable to a suppression of the stimu-lated production of IFNγ and a significant stimulatory effect on IL-10 production

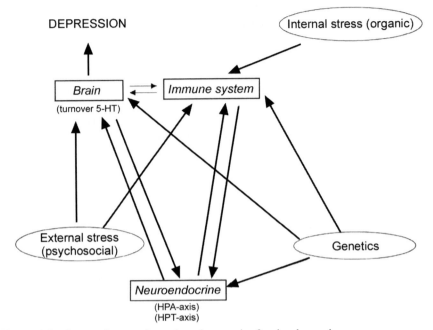

Figure 8.2 Interactions on the aetiopathogenesis of major depression

(Maes et al., 1998b). The exact mechanism by which antidepressive agents from such different classes exert their activity on cytokine production are still unknown. These effects might be mediated by serotonergic mechanisms. T-lymphocytes express 5-HT receptors, such as 5-HT1A and 5-HT2A/2C receptors, as well as a high-affinity 5-HT transporter. Macrophages have a specific active 5-HT uptake system similar in affinity to that of platelets (Jackson et al., 1988). There are now some reports that depletion of intracellular 5-HT stores, increased extracellular 5-HT and/or 5-HT2A/2C receptor blockade may result in negative immunoregulatory effects (Young and Mathews 1995). Thus, part of the immune effects of SSRIs, tricyclic and heterocyclic antidepressants may be explained by their serotonergic activities, such as depletion of intracellular 5-HT stores, increased extracellular 5-HT and/or 5-HT2A/2C receptor blockade (Maes et al., 1998b).

CONCLUSIONS

Major depression is accompanied by various direct and indirect indicators of a moderate activation of the IRS. Increased production of proinflammatory cytokines, such as IL-1, IL-6 and IFNγ, may play a crucial role in the immune and acute phase response in depression. Lower serum Zn, changes in the erythron, lower serum HDL-C, and depletion of ω3 PUFAs are indirect indicators of IRS activation of depression. The reciprocal relationships between IRS activation and HPA-axis hyperactivity, alterations in HPT-axis function and the availability of 5-HT and the HPA axis is an integral component of depression. The IRS activation model of depression provides an explanation for the psychosocial (external stress) as well as organic (internal stress) aetiology of major depression (Figure 8.2). Antidepressive treatments with various antidepressive agents, such as SSRIs and tricyclic and heterocyclic antidepressants, have in vivo and in vitro negative immunoregulatory effects, suggesting that their antidepressant efficacy may be attributable, in part, to their immune effects.

REFERENCES

Abbas AK, Murphy KM, Sher A (1996). Functional diversity of helper T lymphocytes. *Nature* **383**: 787–793.

Adams PB, Lawson S, Sanigorski A, Sinclair AJ (1996) Arachidonic acid to eicosapentaenoic acid ratio in blood correlates positively with clinical symptoms of depression. *Lipids* **31**: S157–S161.

Ahmed SA, Penhale WJ, Talal N (1985) Sex hormones, immune responses, and autoimmune diseases. *Am J Pathol* **21**: 531–551.

Athreya BH, Pletcher J, Zulian F, Weinier DB, Wiliams WV (1993) Subset-specific effects of sex hormones and pituitary gonadotropins on human lymphocyte proliferation in vitro. *Clin Immunol Immunopathol* **66**: 201–211.

Berk M, Wadee AA, Kuschke RH, O'Neill-Kerr A (1997) Acute phase proteins in major depression. *J Psychosom Res* **43**: 529–534.

Bonaccorso S, Lin A, Verkerk R, Van Hunsel F, Libbrecht I, Scharpé S, et al. (1998) Immune markers in fibromyalgia: comparison with major depressed patients and normal volunteers. *J Affect Disord* **48**: 75–82.

Calabrese JR, Skwerer RG, Barna B, Gulledge AD, Valenzuela R, Butkus A, et al. (1986) Depression, immunocompetence, and prostaglandins of the E series. *Psychiatry Res* **17**: 41–47.

Connor TJ, Leonard BE (1998) Depression, stress and immunological activation: the role of cytokines in depressive disorders. *Life Sci* **62**: 583–606.

Cousins RJ, Leinart AS (1998) Tissue-specific regulation of zinc metabolism and metallothionein genes by interleukin-1. *FASEB J* **2**: 2884–2890.

Cunnane SC, Yang J, Chen ZY (1993) Low zinc intake increases apparent oxidation of linoleic and alpha-linolenic acids in the pregnant rat. *Can J Physiol Pharmacol* **71**: 205–210.

Deger O, Bekaroglu M, Orem A, Orem S, Uluutku N, Soylu C (1996) Polymorphonuclear (PMN) elastase levels in depressive disorders. *Biol Psychiatry* **39**: 357–363.

Delves PJ, Roitt IM (2000) The immune system. First of two parts. *N Engl J Med* **343**: 37–49.

Dobbin JP, Harth M, McCain GA, Martin RA, Cousin K (1991) Cytokine production and lymphocyte transformation during stress. *Brain, Beh Imm* **5**: 339–348.

Duch DS, Woolf JH, Nichol CA, Davidson JR, Garbutt JC (1984) Urinary excretion of biopterin and neopterin in psychiatric disorders. *Psychiatry Res* **11**: 83–89.

Dunbar PR, Hill J, Neale TJ, Mellsop GW (1992) Neopterin measurement provides evidence of altered cell-mediated immunity in patients with depression, but not with schizophrenia. *Psychol Med* **22**: 1051–1057.

Endres S (1993) Messengers and mediators: interactions among lipids, eicosanoids and cyto-kines. *Am J Clin Nutr* **57**: 798–800.

Frommberger UH, Bauer J, Haselbauer P, Fraulin A, Riemann D, Berger M (1997) Inter-leukin-6-(IL-6) plasma levels in depression and schizophrenia: comparison between the acute state and after remission. *Eur Arch Psychiatr Clin Neurosci* **247**: 228–233.

Glueck CJ, Tieger M, Kunkel R, Hamer T, Tracy T, Speirs J (1994) Hypocholesterolemia and affective disorders. *Am J Med Sci* **308**: 218–225.

Goldblum SE, Cohen DA, Jay M, McClain CJ (1987) Interleukin 1-induced depression of iron and zinc: role of granulocytes and lactoferrin. *Am J Physiol* **252**: 27–32.

Gutterman JU, Fein S, Quesda J (1982) Recombinant leukocyte A interferon: pharmacoki-netics, single dose tolerance and biologic effects in cancer patients. *Ann Intern Med* **96**: 549–556.

Hibbeln JR, Salem N (1995) Dietary polyunsaturated fatty acids and depression: when cholesterol does not satisfy. *Am J Clin Nutr* **62**: 1–9.

Holden RJ, Pakula IS, Mooney PA (1997) A neuroimmunological model of schizophrenia and major depression: a review. *Hum Psychopharmacol* **12**: 177–201.

Horrobin DF (1990) Essential fatty acids, psychiatric disorders and neuropathies. In Horrobin DF (ed) *Omega-6 Essential Fatty Acids: Pathophysiology and Roles in Clinical Medicine*. New York: Wiley-Liss, pp. 305–320.

Jackson JC, Walker R, Brooks WH, Roszman TL (1988) Specific uptake of serotonin by murin macrophages. *Life Sci* **42**: 641–650.

Knapp PH, Levy EM, Giorgi RG, Black PH, Fox BH, Heeren TC (1992) Short-term immu-nological effects of induced emotion. *Psychosom Med* **54**: 133–148.

Kubera M, Symbirtsev A, Basta-Kaim A, Borycz J, Roman A, Papp M (1996) Effect of chronic treatment with imipramine on interleukin 1 and interleukin 2 production by splenocytes obtained from rats subjected to a chronic mild stress model of depression. *Polish J Pharmacol* **48**: 503–506.

Lieb J, Karmali R (1983) Elevated levels of prostaglandin E2 and thromboxane B2 in depres-sion. *Prostaglandins and Leukotrienes in Medicine* **10**: 361–368.

Linnoila M, Whorton R, Rubinow DR, Cowdry RW, Ninan PT, Waters RN (1983) CSF pros-taglandin levels in depressed and schizophrenic patients. *Arch Gen Psychiatry* **40**: 405–406.

Maes M (1993) Acute phase protein alterations in major depression: a review. *Rev Neurosci* **4**: 407–416.

Maes M (1995) The interleukin hypothesis of major depression. *Prog Neuro-Psychopharmacol Biol Psychiatry* **19**: 11–38.

Maes M (1997) The immune pathophysiology of major depression. In: Honig A, van Praag HM (eds) *Depression: Neurobiological, Psychopathological and Therapeutic Advances*. Chichester: John Wiley, pp. 197–215.

Maes M, Meltzer HYM (1995) The serotonin hypothesis of major depression. In Bloom F, Kupher D (eds) *Psychopharmacology: The Fourth Generation of Progress*. New York: Raven Press, pp. 933–944.

Maes M, Smith R (1997) Immune activation and major depression: a hypothesis. *Psychiatry, Curr Med Lit Psychiatry, Roy Soc Med* **9**: 3–6.

Maes M, Smith R (1998) Fatty acids, cytokines and major depression. *Biol Psychiatry* **43**: 319–320.

Maes M, Bosmans E, Suy E, Vandervorst C, Dejonckheere C, Minner B, et al. (1991) Depres-sion-related disturbances in mitogen-induced lymphocyte responses, interleukin-1ß, and soluble interleukin-2-receptor production. *Acta Psychiatr Scand* **84**: 379–386.

Maes M, Lambrechts J, Bosmans E, Jacobs J, Suy E, Vandervorst C, et al. (1992a) Evidence for a systemic immune activation during depression: results of leukocyte enumeration by flow cytometry in conjunction with monoclonal antibody staining. *Psychol Med* **22**: 45–53.

Maes M, Scharpé S, Bosmans E, Vandewoude M, Suy E, Uyttenbroek W, et al. (1992b) Disturbances in acute phase plasma proteins during melancholia: additional evidence for the presence of an inflammatory process during that illness. *Prog Neuropsychopharmacol Biol Psychiatry* **16**: 501–515.

Maes M, Scharpé S, Van Grootel L, Uyttenbroeck W, Cooreman W, Cosyns P, et al. (1992c) Higher αl-antitrypsin, haptoglobin, ceruloplasmin and lower retinol binding protein plasma levels during depression: further evidence for the existence of an inflammatory response during that illness. *J Affect Disord* **24**: 183–192.

Maes M, Scharpé S, Meltzer HY, Cosyns P (1993a) Relationships between increased hapto-globin plasma levels and activity of cell-mediated immunity. *Biol Psychiatry* **34**: 690–701.

Maes M, Bosmans E, Meltzer HY, Scharpe S, Suy E (1993b) Interleukin-1ß: a putative mediator of HPA-axis hyperactivity in major depression? *Am J Psychiatry* **150**: 1189–1193.

Maes M, Scharpé S, Meltzer HY, Bosmans E, Suy E, Minner B, et al. (1993c) Relationships between interleukin-6 activity, acute phase proteins and HPA-axis function in severe depression. *Psychiatr Res* **49**: 11–27.

Maes M, Meltzer HY, Scharpé S, Uyttenbroeck W, Cooremans W, Suy E (1993d) Psycho-motor retardation, anorexia, weight loss, sleep disturbances and loss of energy: psychopathological correlates of hyperhaptoglobinemia during major depression. *Psychiatr Res* **47**: 229–241.

Maes M, Scharpe S, Meltzer HY, Okayli G, D'Hondt P, Cosyns P (1994a) Increased neop-terin and interferon gamma secretion and lower L-tryptophan levels in major depression: further evidence for immune activation in severe depression. *Psychiatr Res* **54**: 143–160.

Maes M, De Langhe J, Scharpé S, Meltzer HY, Cosyns P, Suy E, et al. (1994b) Haptoglobin phenotypes and gene frequencies in unipolar major depression. *Am J Psychiatry* **151**: 112–116.

Maes M, Delanghe J, Meltzer HY, D, Hondt P, Cosyns P (1994c) Lower degree of esterifica-tion of serum cholesterol in depression: relevance for depression and suicide research. *Acta Psychiatr Scand* **90**: 252–258.

Maes M, Scharpe S, Cosyns P, Meltzer HY (1994d) Relationships between basal hypotha-lamic-pituitary-thyroid axis activity and plasma haptoglobin levels in depression. *J Psychiatr Res* **28**: 123–134.

Maes M, Meltzer HY, Bosmans E, Bergmans R, Vandoolaeghe E, Ranjan, et al. (1995a) Increased plasma concentrations of interleukin-6, soluble interleukin-6, soluble inter-leukin-2 and transferrin receptor in major depression. *J Affec Disord* **34**: 301–309.

Maes M, Scharpe S, Neels H, Wauters A, Van Gastel A, Cosyns P (1995b) Total serum protein and serum protein fractions in major depression. *J Affect Disord* **34**: 61–69.

Maes M, Van de Vyvere J, Vandoolaeghe E, Bril T, Demedts P, Wauters A, et al. (1996a) Alterations in iron metabolism and the erythron in major depression: further evidence for a chronic inflammatory process. *J Affect Disord* **40**: 23–33.

Maes M, Smith R, Christophe A, Cosyns A, Desnyder R, Meltzer HY (1996b) Fatty acid composition in major depression: decreased ω3 fractions in cholesteryl esters and increased c20:4ω6/c20:5ω3 ratio in cholesteryl esters and phospholipids. *J Affect Disord* **38**: 35–46.

Maes M, Delanghe J, Ranjan R, Meltzer HY, Desnyder R, Cooreman W, et al. (1997a) The acute phase protein response in schizophrenia, mania and major depression: effects of psychotropic drugs. *Psychiatry Res* **66**: 1–11.

Maes M, Smith R, Christophe A, Vandoolaeghe E, Van Gastel A, Neels H, et al. (1997b) Lower serum high density lipoprotein cholesterol (HDL-C) in major depression and in depressed men with serious suicidal attempts: relationships to immune-inflammatory markers. *Acta Psychiatr Scand* **95**: 212–221.

Maes M, Verkerk R, Vandoolaeghe E, Van Hunsel F, Neels H, Wauters A, et al. (1997c) Serotonin-immune interactions in major depression: lower serum tryptophan as a marker of an immune-inflammatory response. *Eur Arch Gen Psychiatry Clin Neurosci* **247**: 154–161.

Maes M, Song C, Lin A, Gabriels L, De Jongh R, Van Gastel A (1998a) The effects of psychological stress on humans: increased production of proinflammatory cytokines and a Th-1-like response in stress-induced anxiety. *Cytokine* **10**: 313–318.

Maes M, Song C, Lin A, Bonaccorso S, Scharpe S, Kenis G, et al. (1998b) Negative immunoregulatory effects of antidepressants: inhibition of interferon-gamma and stimulation of interleukin-10 secretion. *Neuropsychopharmacology* **20**: 370–379.

Maes M, Song C, Lin A, De Jongh R, Kenis G, Bosmans E, et al. (1999) Immune and clinical correlates of psychological stress-induced production of interferon-gamma and IL-10 in humans. In Plotnikoff NP (ed) *Cytokines, Stress and Immunity.* Boca Raton, FL: CRC-Press, pp. 31–51.

Maes M, Christophe A, Bosmans E, Lin A, Neels H (2000) In humans, serum polyunsaturated fatty acid levels predict the response of proinflammatory cytokines to psychological stress. *Biol Psychiatry* **47**: 910–920.

Maier SF, Watkins LR (1995) Intracerebroventricular interleukin-1 receptor antagonist blocks the enhancement of fear conditioning and interference with escape produced by inescapable shock. *Brain Res* **695**: 279–282.

McCallum J, Simons L, Simons J, Friedlander Y (1994) Low serum cholesterol is not associated with depression in the elderly: data from an Australian community study. *Aust NZ J Med* **24**: 561–564.

Meydani SN, Endres S, Woods MM (1991) Oral (ω3) fatty acid supplementation suppresses cytokine production and lymphocyte proliferation: comparison between young and older women. *J Nutr* **121**: 547–555.

Miller AH, Lackner C (1989) Tricyclic antidepressants and immunity. In Miller H (ed) *Depressive Disorders and Immunity.* Washington, DC: American Psychiatric Press, pp. 85–104.

Minami M, Kuraishi Y, Yamaguchi T, Nakai S, Hirai Y, Satoh M (1991) Immobilization stress induces interleukin-1 beta mRNA in the rat hypothalamus. *Neurosci Lett* **123**: 254–256.

Mittwoch-Jaffe T, Shalit F, Srendi B, Yehuda S (1995) Modification of cytokine secretion following mild emotional stimuli. *Neuroreport* **27**: 789–792.

Morgan RE, Palinkas LA, Barrett-Connor EL, Wingard DL (1993) Plasma cholesterol and depressive symptoms in older men. *Lancet* **341**: 75–79.

Peet M, Murphy B, Shay, J., Horrobin, D (1998) Depletion of omega-3 fatty acid levels in red blood cell membranes of depressive patients. *Biol Psychiatry* **43**: 315–319.

Russo C, Olivieri O, Girelli D, Guarini P, Pasquallini R, Azzini M, et al. (1997) Increased membrane ratios of metabolite to precursor fatty acid in essential hypertension. *Hypertension* **29**: 1058–1063.

Seidel A, Arolt V, Hunstiger M, Rink L, Behnisch A, Kirchner H (1995) Cytokine production and serum proteins in depression. *Scand J Immunol* **41**: 534–538.

Seidel A, Arolt V, Hunstiger M, Rink L, Behnisch A, Kirchner H (1996) Major depressive disorder is associated with elevated monocyte counts. *Acta Psychiatr Scand* **94**: 198–204.

Shintani F, Nakaki T, Kanba S, Kato R, Asai M (1995) Role of interleukin-1 in stress responses. *Mol Neurobiol* **10**: 47–71.

Shizuya K, Komori T, Fujiwara R, Miyahara S, Ohmori M, Nomura J (1997) The influence of restraint stress on the expression of mRNA for IL-6 and the IL-6 receptor in the hypothalamus and midbrain of the rat. *Life Sci* **61**, PL.

Sluzewska A, Rybakowski JK, Laciak M, Mackiewicz A, Sobieska M, Wiktorowiz K (1995) Interleukin-6 serum levels in depressed patients before and after treatment with fluoxetine. *Ann NY Acad Sci* **762**: 474–476.

Sluzewska A, Rybakowski JK, Sobieska M, Wiktorowicz K (1996) Concentration and micro-heterogeneity glycophorms of alpha-1-acid glycoprotein in major depressive disorder. *J Affect Disord* **39**: 149–155.

Smith RS (1991) The macrophage theory of depression. *Med Hypoth* **35**: 298–306.

Song C, Dinan T, Leonard BE (1994) Changes in immunoglobulin, complement and acute phase protein levels in the depressed patients and normal controls. *J Affect Disord* **30**: 283–288.

Song C, Lin A, Bonaccorso S, Heide C, Verkerk R, Kenis G, et al. (1998) The inflammatory response system and the availability of tryptophan to the brain of patients with major depression and sleep disorders. *J Affect Disord* **49**: 211–219.

Soyland E, Lea T, Sandstad B, Drevon A (1994) Dietary supplementation with very long-chain $\omega3$ fatty acids in man decreases expression of the interleukin-2-receptor (CD25) on mitogen-stimulated lymphocytes from patients with inflammatory skin diseases. *Eur J Clin Invest* **24**: 236–242.

Swartz CM (1990) Albumin decrement in depression and cholesterol decrement in mania. *J Affect Disord* **19**: 173–176.

Takaki A, Huang QH, Somogyvari-Vigh A, Arimura A (1994) Immobilization stress may increase plasma interleukin-6 via central and peripheral catecholamines. *Neuroimmunomodulation* **1**: 335–342.

Vandoolaeghe E, DeVos N, DeSchouwer P, Neels H, Maes M (1999) Lower number of red blood cells, hematocrit and hemoglobin in major depression: effects of antidepressants. *Hum Psychopharmacol* **43**: 45–55.

Van Miert AS, Van Duin CT, Wensing T (1990) Fever and changes in plasma zinc and iron concentrations in the goat. The effects of interferon inducers and recombinant IFN-alpha 2a. *J Comp Pathol* **103**: 289–300.

Xia Z, DePierre JW, Nassberger L (1996) Tricyclic antidepressants inhibit IL-6, IL-1β and TNF-α release in human blood monocytes and IL-2 and interferon-γ in T cells. *Immunopharmacology* **34**: 27–37.

Young MR, Mathews JP (1995) Serotonin regulation of T cell subpopulations and of macrophage accessory function. *Immunology* **84**: 148–152.

Zhou D, Kusnecov AW, Shurin MR, DePaoli M, Rabin BS (1993) Exposure to physical and psychological stressors elevates plasma interleukin 6: relationship to the activation of hypothalamic-pituitary-adrenal axis. *Endocrinology* **133**: 2523–2530.

9

Brain Imaging in Affective Disorders

Andrea L. Malizia

University of Bristol, UK

INTRODUCTION

In vivo neuroimaging in man has been increasingly used as a research tool to help us understand the neurochemistry and brain circuits of psychiatric conditions. This is predicated on the notion that the final common pathway of the expression of psychic phenomena is dictated by the summed output of specific and separate regional brain activity at the time that these phenomena are experienced. Thus tools that allow the description of brain circuits and chemistry associated with the expression of symptoms and emotions could be considered to be the most valid and appropriate type of investigation to unravel the anatomy, pharmacology and physiology of anxiety disorders.

This strategy has been used for many years in experimental animals with exquisite detail and has generated a considerable body of knowledge related to, for instance, the neuroanatomical and neurochemical changes that map anxiety conditioning and innate fear (LeDoux, 2000; Davis et al., 1994, 1999). Such knowledge, derived from animal experiments has provided a basis for the understanding of human emotions and its disorders. However, it is probably unreasonable to assume that the neural substrate of emotion and its disorders varies little between mammal species. Thus, it is unlikely that animal experimental paradigms alone would ever provide a robust understanding of emotion and its disorders in man. This is due to three principal factors:

- *Species difference* – while the building blocks of the human central nervous system are shared with other animals, the human brain is very different in size and in the relative contribution of the frontal lobes. The frontal lobes account for about one half of the human brain and this is disproportionate to all other species including primates that are closest to us in terms of phylogeny. There is a great deal of evidence which demonstrates that parts of the frontal lobe

Mood Disorders: Clinical Management and Research Issues. Edited by E. J. L. Griez, C. Faravelli, D. J. Nutt and J. Zohar.
©2005 John Wiley & Sons Ltd. ISBN 0 470 09426 5.

such as the dorso-lateral prefrontal cortex and the orbito-frontal cortex greatly contribute to human cognitive and emotional processes and these areas have extensive direct and indirect connections to all other parts of the human brain. It is hence not conceivable that a thorough understanding will be possible without elucidating the necessary, unique and modulatory inputs that these areas have on human anxiety.

- *Individual differences* – it is quite clear from animal experimentation that individual diversity such as genetic differences in colonies bred for contrasting characteristics (e.g. Maudsley reactive and non-reactive rats), variations in individual housing, disparity in early life events (such as repeated brief maternal separation) and insults during the intrauterine period, lead to unequal affective responses and to dissimilarities in pharmacological sensitivity. Similar factors also apply to humans and are probably not easily mapped between animals and man because of the influence of genetic heterogeneity, species specific appetitive behaviours and untranslatable human events such as child abuse, interpersonal and family strife and personal meaning of life events amongst many others.
- *Many of the characteristics of anxiety and affective disorders cannot be replicated in animal models* – for example spontaneous persistent and maladaptive mood cycling cannot, to date, be induced in experimental animals.

Therefore it is entirely appropriate that the recently matured tools of brain imaging such as positron emission tomography (PET) and magnetic resonance imaging (MRI) should be used to aid us understand human brain function in diseases that have a very high economic and personal burden worldwide. These neuroimaging techniques can provide charts of grey and white matter distribution and tracts as well as maps of receptor, enzyme, neurotransmitter and transporter density and metabolic activity in the human brain with a spatial resolution of the order of 4–10 mm. This information provides a unique opportunity of linking specific brain structures, regional neuropharmacology and observable behavioural or cognitive outputs in a manner that has not been possible up to recently. In order to understand the challenges in interpreting the results of these studies readers will have to be conversant with imaging methods. Thus this chapter first reviews briefly the imaging techniques that are available, their maturity, advantages and disadvantages. The second part of the chapter provides a short overview of the work carried out in anxiety and the third part an overview of imaging in affective disorders, especially using nuclear medicine techniques. This field of scientific research evolves very rapidly, therefore any chapter is likely to be soon out of date. However, the student can gain more lasting knowledge by acquiring a thorough understanding of the methodology and of the epistemology of these experiments and the discussions related to current data can be taken as a starting point for future knowledge.

PRINCIPLES OF HUMAN IMAGING

An understanding of the mechanisms of data acquisition in imaging is essential, in order to make sense of imaging studies. This section introduces the principal concepts for such an interpretation, focusing on X-ray computed tomography (CT), positron emission tomography (PET), single photon emission computed tomography (SPECT), various applications of magnetic resonance imaging (MRI) such as functional MRI (fMRI), MR spectroscopy and diffusion tensor imaging (DTI). The electrical recording and electrical averaging techniques such as electroencephalography (EEG), computed multi-array EEG and magnetoencephalography (MEG) will not be discussed here. EEG has been in existence for 50 or so years during which it has provided some leads; it has, however, not lived up to its initial promise and a comparison between EEG and the imaging modalities here discussed will be made in the concluding parts of the chapter. Dense EEG mapping and MEG are less mature techniques, so there is, to date, little volume of evidence. However, it is likely that, in combination with the techniques discussed in this section, they will provide very useful information by adding temporal resolution not possible with the tools here described that, instead, have good spatial resolution.

Anatomical Imaging

Anatomical images of the human brain can be produced by the use CT or of MRI. CT maps the tomographic attenuation of X-rays which are transmitted through the head in the camera. MRI uses a number of steps:

- a powerful magnetic field aligns all magnetic nuclei (in most cases water) parallel or antiparallel to the magnetic field,
- these molecules are excited by radiofrequency pulse protocols which are spatially varied in order to provide spatial resolution,
- radio waves are turned off,
- signals are emitted from the brain,
- signals are received, recorded and reconstructed to obtain a map, spectrum or picture.

MRI has superseded CT for structural brain imaging as MRI provides better resolution and contrast of soft tissues and, by varying the parameters of acquisition, can reveal white matter lesions and areas of altered signal intensity which reflect nonspecific pathology. Further, MRI does not employ ionizing radiation and its use is therefore not restricted by radiation dose considerations. Many studies have been carried out with these techniques to assess volumetric changes in patients' brain structures as compared with healthy controls. Volumetric studies ought to have large numbers, ought to employ automatic parcellation in order to avoid observer bias and need careful matching of variables such as age, sex, handedness, intellectual ability and level of education in order to avoid intrinsic biases. Further, it is important that control sample scanning should be temporally interleaved with scans for the patient group in order to avoid bias effects from machine parameter drift. Most of the studies published fail to meet these very stringent criteria.

More recently it has been possible to image white matter tracts with diffusion tensor imaging, this form of imaging uses MRI to produce pictures of water molecule alignment in the three separate spatial axes, thus allowing visualization of myelinated axonal direction. This will provide information about the physical connectivity of various areas of the brain and may be important in determining whether particular patient groups have abnormal connections. Further, it will be of use in exploring connections between activated areas in the brain (see below – fMRI).

Paradoxically, many of the techniques that were developed to investigate neuro-receptor density can also provide information on brain shrinkage or abnormal grey matter in brain areas. This is because a decrease or a change in neuronal density will also result in a decrease or change in total receptor density unless the whole brain matrix also shrinks proportionally. It is therefore important, especially when head injury or alcohol or substance abuse are likely to be involved, that neuroreceptor studies should involve some anatomical imaging in order to control for the possibility of this shrinkage. This is also particularly the case for structures like the hippo-campus that are vulnerable to shrinkage secondary to variations in stress hormones.

Functional Imaging

Physiological and neurochemical images of brain processing can be obtained by the use of nuclear medicine techniques such PET and SPECT. These involve the recording of signals emitted by a radiolabelled compound which has been adminis-tered to the subject. The observed tomographic signal represents the total radioactive counts from a particular region and, thus, is the sum of radioactivity from parent compound and metabolites (if present) both in blood and the various tissue compartments. PET and SPECT are used either to generate surrogate maps of brain activity associated with particular tasks or conditions or to measure neuro-chemical parameters such as receptor, transporter or enzyme density (see Table 9.1 for a list of commonly used PET tracers).

Neuronal populations engaged by mental processes use energy. This consumption can usually be imaged directly by administering radiolabelled glucose or glucose analogues or indirectly by imaging increased blood flow or perfusion to the region. This is because local blood flow is, usually, tightly coupled to variations in local oxygen requirements in the brain. Regional metabolism or blood flow maps thus produced represent changes in energy requirements at synaptic sites as synaptic neurotransmitter release and uptake is linked with the greatest proportion of brain energy expenditure. There is a debate on whether the location of the bulk of aerobic metabolism is in the neuron or the surrounding glia; this debate, however, is un-likely to influence mapping from imaging as the synapses and supporting glia are

TABLE 9.1   Some radioligands used for the investigation of anxiety and affective disorders

Name of ligand	Label	Type of ligand	Measures
Raclopride	C-11	Dopamine D_2 receptors antagonist	Dopamine D_2 receptors
IBZM	I-123	Dopamine D_2 receptors antagonist	Dopamine D_2 receptors
Flumazenil	C-11	Central benzodiazepine site antagonist (alpha 1,2,3,5)	Central benzodiazepine sites
Iomazenil	I-123	Central benzodiazepine site ?partial antagonist (alpha 1,2,3,5)	Central benzodiazepine sites
NNC 13-8241	I-123	Central benzodiazepine site ?partial antagonist (alpha 1,2,3,5)	
Diprenorphine	C-11	Opiate antagonist	Opiate receptors (μ, κ, δ)
DOPA	F-18	Dopamine precursor	DOPA transport into presynaptic terminal
WAY 100635	C-11	5-HT_{1A} antagonist	Serotonin 5-HT_{1A} receptors
PKI 1195	C-11	Peripheral benzodiazepine receptor antagonist	CNS microglia activation
Carfentanyl	C-11	Opiate (mu) agonist	Opiate receptors (mainly μ)
Setoperone	F-18	Cortical 5-HT_2 antagonist	Serotonin 5-HT_2 receptors
N-methyl-spiperone	C-11	D_2 and 5-HT_2 antagonist	D_2 5-HT_2 receptors
RTI 55	C-11	Dopamine and serotonin transporter substrate	Dopamine transporters
Beta-CIT	I-123	Dopamine and serotonin transporter substrate	Dopamine and serotonin transporters
MDL 100907	C-11	5-HT_{2A} antagonist	Serotonin 5-HT_{2A} receptor density
Ro 15-4513	C-11	Central benzodiazepine site antagonist (more selective for alpha-5)	Alpha-5 central benzodiazepine density (mainly)
Deprenyl	C-11	Monoamine oxidase B inhibitor	Monoamine B availability and glial density
DASB	C-11	Serotonin reuptake substrate	Serotonin reuptake sites

co-localized within the resolution of the techniques (Magistretti and Pellerin, 1999). Blood flow maps can also be influenced globally by changes in CO_2 concentrations and regionally by neurotransmitters (noradrenaline, acetylcholine, serotonin and a number of peptides) released in nerve endings that act on the cerebral vasculature.

The maps thus produced represent the summation of synaptic activity over hundreds of thousands of synapses. This is one of the factors which can lead to seemingly paradoxical effects. For instance, increasing inhibitory GABAergic activity in 'activated' cortex results in a decrease in local cerebral blood flow despite the increased synaptic work at inhibitory synapses; this occurs because this signal is overwhelmed by the decreased metabolism in excitatory neuron synapses (Roland and Friberg, 1988). However both increases and decreases in metabolism can be observed by increasing GABAergic input to resting cortex or to other areas of the brain where the balance between excitatory and inhibitory cells may be different (Peyron et al., 1994; Tagamets and Horwitz, 2001). This is despite the fact that GABAergic uptake processes are not associated with significant metabolic costs

(Chatton et al., 2003). Further, since the observed changes are in the synaptic fields rather than the cell bodies, the greatest activation may be in locations distal to the ones suggested by electrophysiology or lesion experiments. Finally, in the investigation of anxiety and anxiety disorders, the net result can be affected by other factors such as changes in respiration, noradrenergic activity, timing and complexity of task and of image acquisition (Mathew et al., 1997; Malizia, 1999) so that the valence of perfusion change may change according to paradigm and timing of scans but still involving the same nodal brain structures.

Fluorine labelled deoxyglucose ([18]FDG) and [^{11}C] labelled glucose have been used with PET for direct measure of glucose metabolism. [18]FDG has been used in preference as it accumulates in cells proportionally to the glucose transport rates and is not further metabolized (unlike [^{11}C] glucose). This feature results in less complex mathematical modelling in order to interpret the tomographic data and has been preferred as a method despite the fact that the transport and metabolic rate constants for fluorodeoxyglucose are different from pure glucose. [18]FDG produces a map of summed glucose transport into the cells dominated by activity over a period of approximately 30 minutes, 20 minutes after its intravenous injection. Therefore, it provides a map of energy consumption by any particular brain state that can be maintained for tens of minutes. Although only one or two scans per individual can be produced, the count statistics are very favourable and robust comparisons can be obtained with groups of 10–12 individuals per arm.

Blood flow (or more precisely perfusion) can be measured with PET using oxygen [^{15}O] labelled injected water or inhaled $C^{15}O_2$ (converted to water in the lung capillaries). [133]Xe (an inert gas which is fully diffusible) and ^{99}Tc-HMPAO (a ligand which is freely diffusible across the blood–brain barrier but gets trapped intracellularly by the changes in pH) have been used with SPECT for the same purposes. Oxygen PET maps perfusion over a period of up to two minutes post injection, with most of the information being acquired in the first 60 seconds. The amount of radioactivity administered to produce good images with contemporary PET cameras allows up to 12–16 scans to be performed in a single individual at 8–10 minutes interval. Thus repeated 'activation' experiments can be performed where statistically significant changes in regional radioactivity are interpreted as mapping the cerebral regions associated with particular tasks. Usually these studies have employed 10–20 subjects thus producing 50–150 scans per specific experimental task. This technique has been very successful in delineating areas of the brain involved in particular motor, sensory, language, affective and memory tasks.

[133]Xe is a breathed in, freely diffusible inert gas used in the original non-tomographic studies which measured brain metabolism. It has been employed tomographically by some investigators to quantify cerebral blood flow with SPECT. ^{99}Tc-HMPAO produces a 'stationary' picture of cerebral blood flow over a period of two minutes after injection which, because of the slow decay of ^{99}Tc, can be imaged for some hours. This has been particularly useful when it has been advantageous to inject patients at sites (e.g. a ward) away from the camera in order to record transient events such as hallucinations. The technique, however, exposes subjects to

large amounts of radiation as SPECT is poorly sensitive. Its use in research should therefore be restricted to the study of such transient events.

Much of the activation work, pioneered with nuclear medicine techniques, has been expanded using functional MRI (fMRI). fMRI images changes in deoxyhae-moglobin/oxyhaemoglobin associated with increased or decreased oxygen consumption. As metabolic demands increase, there is an overcompensation in the amount of oxyhaemoglobin delivered to a particular brain area and this generates the change in signal. Some technical issues have not been fully resolved, such as susceptibility artefacts causing loss of signal at tissue interfaces such as the ventral orbito-frontal cortex. However, the advantages of the absence of ionizing radiation and better spatial and temporal resolution are so great that many research centres have enthusiastically embarked on research protocols with this technique. MRI scanners are like tunnels and can generate considerable anticipatory anxiety. Some patient populations such as people with anxiety disorders find it difficult to tolerate. This adds a further potentially uncontrollable dimension to the experimental procedure that needs to be taken into account. The use of fMR has been very successful in generating data that examines changes in the role of specific brain structures in the processing of particular stimuli and in observing the change in connectivity between brain structures that is induced by psychopathology or pharmacological intervention.

Magnetic resonance spectroscopy (MRS) can also be used to produce spectra associated with particular compounds in the brain. In this sense it is a form of func-tional imaging and it produces information on the regional presence and concentration of chemicals of interest such as lactate, glutamate and GABA. Further, analysis of the ratio of N-acetyl aspartate to other compounds such as crea-tinine and choline is an index of neuronal integrity. This technique is being increasingly used to quantify regional neuronal loss.

PET and SPECT have also been used to image pharmacokinetic parameters related to receptors, transporters, enzymes and transmitters. Ligands appropriate for the system under study are labelled with radiation emitting nuclei to produce maps of their brain distribution after injection. PET is far more versatile than SPECT for this purpose as it usually labels nuclei such as carbon that are universal in molecules with biological activity. However, finding compounds which have the ideal characteristics (e.g. very selective receptor/transporter binding, low non-specific binding, easily cross the blood–brain barrier, no lipophyllic metabolites, rapid brain–blood equilibration, no physiological action) and which can be radiola-belled is extremely expensive in terms of time and resources. In addition, with single scan protocols B_{max} and K_d cannot be separated and the pharmacokinetic para-meters may also include tissue delivery effects and non-specific binding. Whenever semi-quantitative methods are applied (as most often in SPECT) errors may also arise by scanning too early after injection or by the inappropriate use of reference or comparison regions (Olsson and Farde et al., 2001). This results in either the data being heavily influenced by delivery to the brain rather than binding to the receptors, or in inappropriate conclusions based on data from brain areas where a secular equi-librium at the receptor site has not been reached. These methodological problems accompanied by unsophisticated experimental design, characteristic of new technology, have resulted in a relatively small number of adequate radioligand studies in the current brain research literature. Indeed, so far, very few centres worldwide have been able to meet the methodological challenges intrinsic to the techniques. These problems are likely to subside as researchers become more experienced in imaging methodology. An additional exciting development is that both SPET and PET may also be used to detect the endogenous release of neurotransmitters, thus allowing the study of functional neurochemistry in vivo in man, which would parallel in vivo microdialysis in animals (reviewed in Laruelle and Huang, 2001).

NEUROIMAGING RESEARCH IN ANXIETY DISORDERS

Anxiety is an emotion that allows man to prepare for and to deal with potential or actual threat. This is achieved by the induction of physiological and psychological changes that help maximize available resources. However, inappropriate or excessive anxiety incapacitates people, with considerable effects on their work, family and health. Inappropriate or excessive anxiety can present itself to physicians in a number of ways, including severe physical symptoms or comorbidity with existing medical conditions. In psychiatry, debilitating anxiety can present in three types of syndrome:

- anxiety disorders,
- anxiety symptoms that are commonly experienced as part of the illness in syndromes such as major depressive disorder and drug withdrawal,
- severe anxiety experienced either as a consequence of other psychiatric phenomena, as in reactions to the experience of hallucinations or as a possible but not very frequent part of a syndrome as in degenerative disorders such as the dementias.

This section of the chapter reviews findings in the anxiety disorders. The aetiology of these disorders comprises genetic and environmental factors that change brain chemistry and hormonal responses so as to predispose individuals to pathological reactions to anxiety provocation. Because of the interaction between genetic predisposition and environmental triggers, brain imaging has a particularly important role in unravelling aetiology and therapeutic action. This is because genetic factors on their own (e.g. a specific polymorphism) explain only a small part of the variance and therefore measuring the effects of nature plus nurture on current functional expression of brain proteins and circuits through functional imaging is very pertinent to reaching an understanding of these disorders. Anxiety disorders include generalized anxiety disorder, panic disorder, social anxiety disorder and specific phobias, where anxiety is the defining feature of the syndrome, and obsessive-compulsive disorder and post-traumatic stress disorder where anxiety is an important but not unique part of the definition and presentation.

Obsessive-Compulsive Disorder

Obsessive-compulsive disorder (OCD) is a disorder characterized by intrusive repetitive thoughts or actions that the patient is unable to control. These thoughts or actions are acknowledged as coming from the person themselves (unlike delusions and hallucinations in psychoses). They generate distress and if the person tries to resist them (as in trying to stop the washing of hands thought of as being dirty even though known to be clean) there is a surge of severe anxiety. It can be argued that at least two mechanisms are in operation here – one is a repetition/checking mechanism and the other is anxiety experience. About 1% of the population develops non-comorbid OCD; it often starts in early adulthood, although some patients experience it later on in life, usually in the context of a depressive disorder. Main treatments are serotonin reuptake inhibitors and behaviour therapy. These can achieve a response in up to 60–70% of patients.

Structural Imaging

After early reports (Behar et al., 1984) of increased ventricle to brain ratio (VBR, a non-specific measure of decreased brain parenchyma) in patients with OCD using X-ray CT, the first observation of specifically reduced caudate nucleus volume was reported by Luxenberg et al. in 1988. This study also used X-ray CT and a rather small sample of 10 male patients with severe OCD and 10 controls. The use of severely affected individuals may have provided a cleaner sample which emphasizes biological differences but results in reduced confidence in generalizing the results. Since then the results of volumetric studies have been somewhat contradictory with one study (Scarone et al., 1992) showing an increased right caudate volume, four showing no differences (Aylward et al., 1996; Jenike et al., 1996; Stein et al., 1997a; Bartha et al., 1998) and two showing a decrease in striatal volume (Robinson et al., 1995; Rosenberg et al., 1997). Factors affecting the presence or absence of reductions in caudate volume that are detectable by MRI seem to include gender (females show fewer differences), age of onset (earlier onset is more likely to be associated with volumetric reductions) and presence of soft neurological signs. These papers are complemented by MR spectroscopy studies that have demonstrated reduced NAA in caudate nuclei (Ebert et al., 1997; Bartha et al., 1998). Taken altogether the data suggests that synaptic integrity in the basal ganglia may be affected early on and that measurable changes in volume may be detectable only later in the disease.

Other reported differences include an increase in lobar white matter (Jenike et al., 1996), decreases in orbito-frontal grey matter and amygdala volume (Szesko et al., 1999), increased T1 relaxation time in the orbito-frontal cortex (Garber et al., 1989) and an abolition of amygdala-hippocampal left to right asymmetry (Szesko et al., 1999). In addition studies in paediatric OCD have demonstrated an increase in myelinated callosal fibres (Rosenberg et al., 1997) and a decrease in thalamic volume (Rosenberg et al., 2000), although the latter may be indicative of the effects of paroxetine treatment (Rosenberg et al., 2000).

Functional Imaging

OCD is the anxiety disorder in which imaging has contributed most to an understanding of the circuits associated with the condition and where predictors of treatment response are emerging. Abnormal metabolism in the orbito-frontal cortex, in the anterior cingulate and in the basal ganglia is the most consistent piece of evidence. Most such studies show hypermetabolism when compared with controls in these structures, although some show significant decreases in resting metabolism. These same areas that have abnormal glucose metabolism or blood flow both at rest show activation on symptom provocation. Successful treatment, whether psychological, pharmacological or neurosurgical reverses these abnormalities. Little progress has been made on the pharmacological imaging of this disorder with only two published studies that investigate serotonin transporter density, although further investigations of the serotonergic system are in progress.

Resting Metabolism and Symptom Provocation Studies

In OCD the main resting metabolic changes have been observed in the orbito-frontal cortex, the anterior cingulate and the caudate nucleus (see Table 9.2). The area most often involved is the orbito-frontal cortex where the majority of studies find an increase in resting metabolism. However, interestingly, studies that utilize HMPAO SPECT rather than FDG PET find a decrease in this region. This apparent contradiction is not unique to OCD, as will become apparent later in the chapter. This is because the significance of increases or decreases in metabolism or blood flow is not as unambiguous as it first appears. For instance hypermetabolism, indicating greater neuronal activity, may be followed by hypometabolism, indicating subsequent neuronal damage, or difficulty in engaging a particular brain area in processing (hypometabolism) can ultimately result in a greater recruitment of parallel local networks (hypermetabolism) and so on. Hence, for the time being, the observation of significant changes in a particular area, regardless of polarity, may be more robust in helping to identify the likely networks engaged in pathological processes.

Significant differences in thalamic, caudate and other frontal metabolism are also reported in about half the studies, but the polarity of the change is as much for decreases as for increases in metabolism. Additional areas include the parietal cortex and the cerebellum. It is of interest to note that, in comparison with controls, significant increases in resting anterior cingulate activity, in OCD patients, is always accompanied by increases in orbito-frontal activity while the same is not true of thalamic metabolism.

Historically, these findings were the first to provide evidence for a putative involvement of sub-cortical structures in the generation of psychopathology and involvement of the basal ganglia was of particular significance as they are part of cortico-striatal loops (Alexander et al., 1990). These loops have an influence on

TABLE 9.2   Resting metabolic studies of OCD. 0 = no difference found; + = increase in metabolism compared with controls; − = decrease in metabolism. OF = orbito-frontal cortex; CN = caudate nucleus; ACC = anterior cingulate cortex; Rx = treatment

Author et al.	Year	Method	OF	ACC	Other frontal	CN	Other	Notes
Mindus	1986	^{11}C glucose	+	0	0	−		Rx-resistant
Baxter	1987	FDG	+	0	0	+		
Baxter	1988	FDG	+	0	0	+		
Nordhal	1989	FDG	+	+	0	0		
Swedo	1989	FDG	+	+	+	0		
Martinot	1990	FDG	0	0	−	−		Some on Rx
Machlin	1991	HMPAO	0	0	+	0		
Sawle	1991	H_2O	+	0	+	0		
Rubin	1991	Xenon	0	0	0	0		
Rubin	1991	HMPAO	+	0	+	−	+parietal	
Perani	1995	FDG	+	+	0	0	+thalamus	
Lucey	1995	HMPAO	−	0	−	−	−thalamus −parietal	
Busatto	2000	HMPAO	−	−	0	0	+cerebellum	
Busatto	2001	HMPAO	−	−	0	0	+cerebellum	Early and late onset
Alptekin	2001	HMPAO	+	0	+	0	+thalamus	
Kwon	2003	FDG	+	0	0	0	−parietal	

thalamic gating of peripheral sensory signals. However, sceptics pointed out that results from resting metabolic studies may not be relevant in mapping the neural correlates of primarily phasic rather than tonic psychopathology. This issue was addressed by 'activation experiments' in which exposure of OCD patients to feared objects generated increases in local perfusion consistent with the reported observations of abnormal resting metabolism. The changes in blood flow were compared with rest or with an appropriate control tasks. Study design was either categorical (subtraction techniques) or correlational whereby the changes in blood flow across the scans are related to changes in symptom scores.

The first categorical study in this area was performed by Rauch's group (1994) using $C^{15}O_2$ PET. They found increases in the right caudate, bilaterally in the orbito-frontal cortex and in the anterior cingulate cortex with stimulus presentation. These findings were echoed in a correlation study of four patients using $H_2^{15}O_2$ PET (McGuire et al., 1994) where symptom severity correlated with increases in cerebral perfusion in the right inferior frontal gyrus, the caudate nuclei, putamen and globus pallidus, the thalamus, the left hippocampus and the posterior cingulate. Since then orbito-frontal cortical activation has been confirmed in another nuclear medicine study (Cottraux et al., 1996). The latter controlled for some of the comparisons and reported that the characteristics of OCD patients were:

- the activation of the caudate nuclei by neutral auditory stimulation,
- and an increased correlation between superior temporal and orbito-frontal activity, both of which were absent in control subjects.

Other studies (Horwitz et al., 1991) have reported an increased correlation in metabolism between anterior structures (orbito-frontal cortex, caudate nuclei, anterior limbic cortex) that is reversed by successful treatment (Azari et al., 1993; Brody et al., 1998). This is in keeping with the pattern emerging from other treatment studies (Table 9.3) where a reversal (in most cases a decrease) in orbito-frontal and caudate metabolism, of the baseline abnormality is associated with treatment response. These decreases are across all treatment modalities including behaviour therapy, pharmacotherapy and neurosurgery. Where this has been documented, smaller magnitude of baseline abnormalities in the above areas, especially the orbito-frontal cortex, is associated with better outcome. One study (Brody et al., 1998) proposed that basal abnormality patterns can predict differential response to behaviour therapy or pharmacological treatment. This study argues that good response to medication is, as in the other studies, associated with lower resting metabolism in orbito-frontal cortex; however, better response to behaviour therapy is related to higher resting metabolism in the orbito-frontal cortex. These findings have, to some extent, been confirmed by Rauch et al. (2002) who have reported that lower perfusion values in the orbito-frontal cortex and higher perfusion values in the posterior cingulate predicted better response to fluvoxamine (an SSRI) regardless of whether the imaging data had been acquired during rest or symptom provocation. This group has also demonstrated that good response to anterior cingulotomy (neurosurgery) in cases of treatment-resistant OCD, is also associated with higher posterior cingulate metabolism pretreatment (Rauch et al., 2001). These findings are intriguing and their robustness will have to be ascertained. However, if differential treatment efficacy can be predicted by pretreatment brain function correlates, brain imaging will have achieved a significant milestone.

Another line of enquiry which is likely to produce useful leads on patterns of brain processing in psychiatric disorders in general and in OCD in particular is the exploration of changes in task-related activations when compared with healthy volunteers. This approach has strong theoretical appeal as it aims to dissect the influence of illness on the assembly of functional networks needed for the performance of disparate tasks. As such it may inform on how individual processing modules are affected by the disorder. Such an approach has been pioneered by Rauch and colleagues using PET (1997). They established that OCD patients do not activate the inferior striatum when performing an implicit learning task, while abnormally activating the temporal cortices, thus speaking to a dysfunctional striatum.

In Vivo Neurochemistry

Two studies have been published using [^{11}C]McN 5652 PET (Simpson et al., 2003) and beta-CIT SPECT (Pogarell et al., 2003) as measures of serotonin transporter density. The US PET study showed no difference in transporter density in the basal ganglia, thalamus, midbrain, hippocampus, amygdala and anterior cingulate between OCD patients and volunteers. The European SPET study showed reduced

BRAIN IMAGING 241

TABLE 9.3 Treatment-induced changes in brain metabolism in OCD. 0 = no difference found; + = increase in metabolism; − = decrease in metabolism. OF = orbito-frontal cortex; CN = caudate nucleus; ACC = anterior cingulate cortex; Rx = treatment; FOV = field of view

Author et al.	Year	Method	Treatment	OF	CN	ACC	Other frontal	Other	Notes
Mindus	1986	[11C]glucose	Surgery	−	0	0	0	0	Limited FOV
Baxter	1987	FDG	Trazodone	−	+	0	0	0	Comorbid?
Benkelfat	1990	FDG	Clomipramine	−	0	0	0	0	
Baxter	1992	FDG	Fluoxetine/BT	0	−	0	0	0	
Swedo	1992	FDG	Various	0	0	0	0	0	
Rubin	1995	Xe	Clomipramine	−	−	0	0	0	
Rubin	1995	HMPAO	Clomipramine	−	−	0	0	0	
Biver	1995	FDG	Surgery	−	0	0	0	−thalamus	Case report
Perani	1995	FDG	SSRI	0	0	−	0	0	
Schwartz	1996	FDG	BT	0	−	0	0	0	
Saxena	1999	FDG	Paroxetine	−	−	0	0	0	
Sachdev	2001	FDG	Surgery	−	−	−	−	−thalamus	Case report
Hoehn-Saric	2001	HMPAO	Sertraline/DMI	0	0	0	−	0	
Kim	2001	HMPAO	Surgery	−	−	0	−	0	
Hansen	2002	FDG	Paroxetine	0	−	0	0	0	
Saxena	2002	FDG	Paroxetine	−	−	0	−	−thalamus	

serotonin transporter binding in the pons in patients with OCD compared with controls. These differences could be ascribable to differences in imaging methods; however, they are more likely to be related to clinical issues such as the fact that the European sample had a number of patients who had developed OCD in childhood and also had a higher prevalence of significant depression scores. Indeed if patients with late-onset OCD were compared with controls in the Pogarell study, there were no significant differences between groups.

Panic Disorder

Panic disorder is characterized by repeated and sudden paroxysms of intense anxiety or fear that are accompanied by cardiovascular, repiratory, vestibular, gastrointestinal and skin somatic symptoms as well as catastrophic cognitions. These episodes, known as panic attacks, can occur in specific situations or can be totally unexpected, sometimes occurring during sleep. Panic attacks can lead to a severe restriction in the ability to lead an independent life and panic disorder results in decreased life expectancy through cardiovascular causes and suicide. The yearly prevalence of panic disorder is about 1% with a lifetime prevalence of about 4%. Clearly the prevalence of isolated panic attacks is much higher. Panic disorder responds to antidepressant medication (especially serotonin reuptake inhibitors), high potency benzodiazepines and cognitive-behavioural therapy; with these a response rate of about 70% is achieved.

Panic attacks can be provoked in vulnerable individuals by using a variety of probes (for example CO_2 and lactate). Therefore panic attacks were one of the first psychiatric symptoms to be studied in some detail using imaging, as experimenters used these challenges to provoke the desired state in the confines of the scanners. Initial results fitted with theories derived from animal studies of anxiety as they demonstrated hippocampal and anterior temporal poles activation with the experience of anxiety in patients with panic disorder. However, this signal was re-interpreted as a consequence of the reappraisal of the anatomical specificity of data collected on prototypical PET scanners. In these cameras it was difficult to separate temporal lobe activations from extra-cranial muscular events; the latter were responsible for the large activations observed, hence discounting the original results. These reinterpretations were quite damaging to the perception of nuclear medicine techniques in the exploration of brain correlates of psychopathology because they affirmed the concept that PET data were too noisy to allow adequate brain anatomical localization without co-registration with MRI images. Clearly this is not the case with modern scanners and high specific activity; but, for a long time, anxiety researchers had to carry out control experiments that involved teeth-clenching conditions as well as MR structural scanning in order to avoid adverse critical appraisals.

Since then studies have confirmed hippocampal metabolic asymmetry and parieto-temporal hypofunction at rest as well as anterior cingulate and orbito-frontal activation with anxiety experience as the most reproduced findings. Other major advances in understanding panic disorder have come from pharmacological imaging where abnormalities in $GABA_A$-benzodiazepine and $5\text{-}HT_{1A}$ binding have been demonstrated.

Structural Imaging

Structural imaging has been used to investigate the notion that panic disorder may be associated with temporal lobe abnormalities. The results thus far indicate that this may indeed be the case, since both an increased number of nonspecific lesions and shrinkage of the temporal lobes are documented in all the published studies. There is, however, no evidence that hippocampal volume is reduced in panic disorder in contrast to PTSD and depressive disorders.

In a study of 30 consecutive patients from their clinic with panic disorder, Ontiveros et al. (1989) compared them with 20 healthy volunteers using structural MRI. 11 patients and one control were thought to have significant abnormalities on their MRI scans mainly in the right temporal lobe (mainly areas of increased signal intensity which indicate white matter abnormalities in the medial portion of the lobe) while five patients and one control showed dilatation of the temporal horn of the lateral ventricle. Patients with the temporal lobe abnormalities were younger at onset of PD, had longer duration of illness and had more panic attacks. Applying different criteria to a similar sample of patients, the same group found that 40% of patients with PD and 10% of healthy volunteers had medial temporal structural abnormalities (Fontaine et al., 1990). The strength of these studies is that they investigated consecutive panic disorder patients who were referred to a psychiatric clinic thus avoiding some of the possible selection biases; however, the sample may not be representative as many patients with PD do not get referred to secondary care. These findings are echoed in a study of 20 panic disorder patients and 28 controls by Dantendorfer et al. (1996) which also suggests that temporal lobe abnormalities as detected with MRI are much more common in panic disorder patients than in controls (29% vs. 4%). The prevalence of these abnormalities increased to 61% if only PD patients with 'non-epileptic' EEG abnormalities were selected for comparison, while they were present in 18% of the panic disorder patients without EEG abnormalities. The authors commented that a high number of septo-hippocampal abnormalities were found. Vythilingam et al. (2000) employed volumetric MRI comparing 13 patients and 14 healthy volunteers. They found that both temporal lobes (excluding the hippocampus) were smaller in panic disorder patients even after controlling for the fact that patients have smaller brains than healthy controls. Interestingly, this was not due to the larger number of women in the panic disorder group as males and females with panic disorder have almost identical brain volumes. Further, there was no difference in hippocampal volume between patients and controls. Massana et al. (2003a, 2003b), however suggested that the posterior medial temporal lobe as well as the amygdala are smaller in patients with panic disorder.

Resting Metabolism and Symptom Provocation Studies

Panic disorder was investigated early in the development of brain imaging research because of the unambiguous definition of the disorder and because of the relative effortlessness with which panic attacks could be brought on. However, it was soon realized that it was very difficult to scan patients during a panic attack as patients would find it difficult to stay in the camera. Therefore experiments were refined by concentrating on the resting state and by separating out subgroups of patients who were sensitive to anxiogenic challenges from patients who were not. It was thought that this strategy would be likely to produce a sample of people who had resting brain metabolic abnormalities.

Three initial studies (Reiman et al., 1984, 1986, 1989) showed temporal lobe activations, amongst others. These early results were congruent with animal data and with activations provoked in healthy volunteers by fear conditioning (Reiman et al., 1984). However, later it was demonstrated that the most significant activations in conditioned fear were due to extra-cerebral signal secondary to teeth-clenching (Drevets et al., 1992a) and so all the temporal activations reported by this group at that time have to be considered cautiously. The use of modern scanners and of co-registration with anatomical images makes this sort of error difficult to repeat.

Stewart et al. (1988) used symptom provocation and [^{133}Xe] SPECT to investigate 10 patients with panic disorder and five healthy controls were compared. Scans were carried out before and after either a lactate or a saline infusion. Six patients had a panic attack and were compared with non-panickers and controls. Global hemispheric blood flow was increased post lactate infusion in non-panickers and controls. This change was greatest on the right but it did not reach statistical significance. People who experienced a panic attack did not show such a change; this was interpreted by the authors to be the result of hyperventilation that would in itself decrease blood flow. People who experienced a panic attack showed a significant increase in the occipital lobe normalized blood flow, as well as a trend for a decrease in left prefrontal blood flow with panic attacks. These data can be compared with a report by Fischer and colleagues (1998) who described an experiment in which a healthy volunteer experienced a spontaneous panic attack while within a PET scanner. Panic in this woman was associated with activations in the right ventral and medial orbitofrontal cortex. Activations reported in the genual anterior cingulate and in the right temporal cortex show stereotactic coordinates which could also be interpreted as being in the orbito-frontal cortex. In summary there is little convergence between these reports indicating that more investigations are needed to understand the pattern of brain activity during a panic attack.

A consistent pattern is also difficult to establish in the five studies which have examined basal blood flow or metabolism in panic disorder, although there is some convergence of observed decreases in resting metabolism in the parieto-temporal cortices and of lower left/right hippocampal ratios in some patients. Nordahl et al. (1990) used ^{18}FDG PET to compare 12 medication-free patients with panic disorder with 30 healthy volunteers at rest. Scanning was carried out during an auditory continuous performance task (CPT) in order to control the environmental conditions. Panic disorder patients had lower left to right hippocampal metabolic ratio, a lower metabolic rate in the left inferior parietal lobule, trends towards significant increases in the right hippocampal region, medial orbito-frontal cortex and towards significant decreases in the anterior cingulate. Anxiety measures did not correlate with metabolism in any particular area while depressed mood ratings and CPT performance correlated positively with medial orbito-frontal metabolism. The same group (Nordahl et al., 1998) successively reported on nine panic disorder patients successfully treated with imipramine and compared their resting cerebral metabolism measured with [18]FDG PET with healthy volunteers and untreated panic disorder patients. Compared with healthy volunteers, treated patients had lower L/R hippocampal and prefrontal metabolic ratios; this was not different from untreated PD patients, thus speaking to a possible trait abnormality. Lower posterior orbito-frontal metabolism was found in treated patients when compared with healthy volunteers or untreated patients and this effect was ascribed to clomipramine since it was similar to effects observed in patients treated with other tricyclic antidepressants (Benkelfat et al., 1990). Post hoc comparisons revealed that hypometabolism in the left parietal and left Rolandic areas in untreated panic disorder patients was not present in the treated group.

Malizia et al. (1997) compared resting perfusion between 11 patients with panic disorder on no medication and seven healthy controls. Patients had significant lower delivery in posterior temporal, inferior parietal and cerebellar cortex bilaterally. In patients, but not controls, the Spielberger State Anxiety Inventory administered just prior to scanning covaried positively with anterior cingulate and negatively with middle temporal and cerebellar perfusion. These observations indicate that the experience of anxiety in this group correlates with increases in blood flow in the anterior cingulate and with decreases in flow in posterior structures. De Cristofaro et al. (1993) examined nine patients with PD and five controls at rest with ^{99}Tc-HMPAO SPECT. Seven patients who were lactate sensitive and treatment naive had significantly increased asymmetry (interpreted as increased right-sided flow) in the inferior orbitofrontal cortex, increased flow in the left occipital cortex and decreased flow in the hippocampal/amygdala bilaterally. Bisaga et al. (1998) also compared the resting cerebral metabolism of six lactate-sensitive, treatment-free, female patients with panic disorder with healthy volunteers using [18]FDG PET. They reported significant decreases in metabolism in panic disorder patients in the right inferior parietal area, and the right superior temporal gyrus, with increases in metabolism in the left parahippocampal gyrus.

Three studies have been conducted using a pharmacological challenge. In these studies investigators administer an agent known to be panicogenic or to significantly affect a neurochemical system thought to be involved in the generation of anxiety. Scanning is carried out before and after administration and changes in perfusion are recorded. Yohimbine is an α_2 noradrenergic antagonist that provokes anxiety in patients with a variety of anxiety disorders. Its effects are probably mediated by blockade of autoreceptors leading to larger concentrations of intrasynaptic noradrenaline. Woods and his group (1988) used a yohimbine challenge in panic disorder patients that resulted in large decreases in HMPAO SPECT signal in the frontal cortex. The study has, however, not been described in more detail elsewhere so that conclusions are difficult to reach.

Fenfluramine increases serotonergic release and transmission. Meyer and colleagues used it as a challenge in female panic disorder patients and volunteers. The scans were timed so that panic attacks, if present, would occur while the person was not being scanned. Thus no data are available on whether fenfluramine increased anxiety or indeed whether the anxiety increases were related to changes in perfusion. The investigators found that, at rest, panic disorder patients had lower blood flow in the posterior parieto-temporal area. This area of cortex also had significant greater increases in perfusion in panic disorder patients after fenfluramine when compared with healthy volunteers. This area is coterminous with the hypometabolic areas reported by other studies in panic disorder (Nordahl et al., 1990, 1998; Malizia et al., 1997). Boshuisen et al. (2002) used pentagastrin that is an agonist at cholecystokinin-B (CCK-B) receptors in order to provoke anxiety in patients with panic disorder and controls. Interestingly the areas that were activated in patients during anticipatory anxiety (i.e. before the injection of pentagastrin) were the same areas that showed large increases and decreases in perfusion post drug administration in patients. Patients had increases in perfusion of the parahippocampal gyrus, the superior temporal lobe, the anterior cingulate gyrus, and the midbrain and decreases in the in the precentral gyrus, the amygdala, the inferior frontal gyrus, and the anterior insula.

In summary three findings of altered brain metabolism or perfusion in panic disorder are consistent:

- the presence of a left to right asymmetry in hippocampal metabolism which is mainly detected at rest, although the side which is predominant is in dispute; this probably is the manifestation of a unilateral increase in metabolism;
- parieto-temporal hypometabolism which may rectify on treatment and which is in the same location as fenfluramine activation;
- changes in anterior cingulate and orbito-frontal metabolism as in other affective or anxiety conditions.

In Vivo Neurochemistry

Receptor Binding. Psychopharmacology challenge findings (e.g. Nutt et al., 1990) implicate $GABA_A$ receptor in the pathophysiology of panic disorder. Six iomazenil SPECT studies of panic disorder have thus far been published (Schlegel et al., 1994; Kuikka et al., 1995; Kaschka et al., 1995; Tokunaga et al., 1996; Brandt et al., 1998; Bremner et al., 2000b). Schlegel et al. (1994) were the first to report decreased benzodiazepine receptor binding in panic disorder using iomazenil SPECT comparing, at 90–110 minutes post injection, 10 patients with panic disorder with

10 patients with epilepsy on carbamazepine. The decreases were significant in the occipital and frontal lobes and maximal in the temporal lobes. Kaschka et al. (1995) studied nine medicated patients with PD comorbid with depression compared with a matched group of medicated patients with dysthymia using iomazenil SPECT scans at two hours after injection. Decreases in binding were seen in the inferior temporal lobes both medially and laterally and in the inferior medial and lateral frontal cortex. These changes were already detectable at 10 minutes post injection reflecting changes dominated by delivery effects. All participants were on anti-depressants. Both these studies have inappropriate control groups and one examines patients with comorbidity. On the other hand Kuikka et al. (1995) using two different SPECT cameras studied 17 unmedicated patients with panic disorder and 17 healthy age- and sex-matched controls using iomazenil and found an increase in Iomazenil signal bilaterally in the temporal cortex and in the right middle/inferior lateral frontal gyrus. Brandt et al. (1998) also showed that patients with panic disorder have a significant increase of benzodiazepine receptor binding in the right supraorbital cortex and a trend to an increased uptake in the right temporal cortex. Both studies are, however, very likely to be contaminated by signal dependent on ligand delivery. Tokunaga (1997) followed a very rigorous scanning methodology but did not use a standard psychiatric classification, thus limiting the significance of his demonstration of global reduced benzodiazepine binding in patients with anxiety disorders. Finally Bremner et al. (2000) carried out a very careful SPECT study with robust technological methodology. Panic disorder patients had a relative decrease in benzodiazepine receptor binding in left hippo-campus and precuneus relative to controls. It was further observed that panic disorder patients who had a panic attack also had a decrease in benzodiazepine receptor binding in prefrontal cortex when compared with patients who did not have a panic attack at the time of the scan. An increase in benzodiazepine binding in the right caudate, in the occipital lobes, in the middle temporal and in the middle frontal cortex was also reported. However, although patients were drug-free at the time of the scan none of them were benzodiazepine-naive and therefore changes in receptor expression due to previous treatment cannot be excluded.

In the only fully quantitative study of benzodiazepine-naive and drug-free subjects, Malizia et al. (1998) investigated panic disorder patients with [^{11}C]fluma-zenil PET and found a 20% global decrease in binding. These changes were maximal in ventral basal ganglia, orbito-frontal and temporal cortex. One other study (Abadie et al., 1999) has examined [^{11}C]flumazenil binding. This study compared patients with a number of anxiety disorders with healthy volunteers. Measures of binding were derived by using the pons as a reference region; this method considerably increased noise and resulted in the observed global decreases in benzodiazepine binding not being statistically significant.

In summary, while there are not enough methodologically sound studies to come to firm conclusions, the weight of evidence favours the observation that benzodiaze-pine receptor binding is decreased in panic disorder. This seems to be the case for 5-HT$_{1A}$ receptors also.

[^{11}C]WAY 100635 has been available as a useful PET radioligand to investigate 5-HT$_{1A}$ receptors and Sargent et al. (2000b) demonstrated decreases in cortical and subcortical 5-HT$_{1A}$ binding in medication-free panic disorder patients when compared with controls. These decreases were also present but to a much lesser extent when comparing panic disorder patients on SSRI treatment with controls, this effect being maximal in amygdala, temporal lobe and orbitofrontal cortex. The samples were from different patients but they suggest that the decrement in 5-HT$_{1A}$ binding is at least partially reversible by successful treatment in panic disorder – in contrast to major depressive disorder where the deficit seems not to be reversed. Neumeister et al. (2004) have also found decreased binding of WAY 100635 in the cingulate cortex and raphe in untreated panic disorder patients, although their sample included patients who also had major depressive disorder. Findings of an inverse correlation between 5-HT$_{1A}$ binding and anxious personality (Tauscher et al., 2001) is of great interest, as it may indicate that low 5-HT$_{1A}$ receptor density predisposes to anxiety in man. Further, reduced binding at benzodiazepine and 5-HT$_{1A}$ receptors may share a common aetiology, as demonstrated in the 5-HT$_{1A}$ knockout mice (Sibille et al., 2000).

In summary two main findings emerge from the nuclear medicine receptor imaging experiments in panic disorder although these conclusions are based on only a few experiments:

- there is reduced benzodiazepine binding in benzodiazepine-naive panic disorder patients;
- panic disorder patients also show reduced 5-HT$_{1A}$ binding that may be reversible by successful pharmacological treatment.

Post-traumatic Stress Disorder

Post-traumatic stress disorder (PTSD) is a condition that emerges three to six months after the occurrence of a threatening life event whereby the subject thought that his life or his physical integrity was at serious risk. For many sufferers the development of the disorder follows repeated exposure to such events. While increased anxiety and decreases in sleep are common in the immediate aftermath of a major trauma, these symptoms tend to subside in a few weeks in people who do not develop the disorder. Patients who develop PTSD, however, find that, rather than subsiding, the symptoms become worse. Patients suffer with reduced sleep, nightmares, severe irritability, changes in personality, flashbacks where the patient re-experiences the events as if being there, occasionally having pseudo-hallucinations. Further, they experience increased and unbearable startle responses, panic attacks, feelings of emotional flattening, of impending doom and of life being foreshortened and not worth living. PTSD is often accompanied by severe social maladjustment and by alcohol and substance abuse as patients try to self-medicate to decrease arousal and emotional turmoil.

Anatomical Imaging

PTSD is a condition which by definition occurs after an unusually severe stressful event. Acute stress is known to result in a physiological response which is mediated by ascending monoaminergic systems (noradrenaline, dopamine and serotonin) in the short term and by the hypothalamic–pituitary–adrenal axis in the longer term whereby stress results in increased glucocorticoid (GC) concentration in plasma and brain. Recently, much attention has been devoted to the noxious effects of increased GC on neurons (Sapolsky, 1996), particularly in the hippocampus where it is thought that persistently high GC concentrations induce reversible atrophy of the dendritic spines. This process is followed by neurotoxicity where, over the course of months, high GC concentrations kill hippocampal neurons. These observations lead to the conclusion that prolonged periods of stress, leading to increased GC concentration, result in hippocampal atrophy in man, a theory supported by findings in depression (which is accompanied by HPA-axis abnormalities in many patients) where atrophy is correlated with total period of illness (Sheline et al., 1999).

In PTSD severe stress is experienced repeatedly over a period of months, first because of the incident itself and then through the re-experience of the traumatic events which causes considerable distress. It should therefore follow that a reduction in hippocampal volume should be observed in patients with this condition and that the greatest damage should be seen in patients with the longest history of PTSD. Five MRI studies of adult PTSD patients have been performed that have used volumetric MRI with manual segmentation of the hippocampus (Gurvits et al., 1996; Stein et al., 1997; Bremner et al., 1995, 1997; 2003). Each study had a different criterion for definition of the hippocampus since some investigators prefer to measure a clearly defined portion (e.g. middle) rather than increasing noise by including areas with poor boundary definition.

On the whole, all studies report a decrease in hippocampal volume that is small except for Gurvits et al. (1996). However, a firm conclusion from these studies is made difficult by the usual problem of the unlikely reporting in the literature of small negative studies. In addition, as in all PTSD studies, interpretation is made more difficult by considerable clinical methodological problems such as psychiatric comorbidity, substance and alcohol abuse. Some of these MR investigations attempted to minimize these problems by careful matching and the use of multiple linear regression; however, the direct effect of these factors cannot be categorically excluded. Finally, imaging confounds such as cohort sequence in scanning (i.e. patients' group and controls' group being scanned at different times) can cause artefact which would result in the reported differences. This can be due to scanner drift, producing a significant bias in the grey values of the image. This potential problem is only reported in one paper (Gurvits et al., 1996) but should be explicitly excluded. Despite the above limitations, the consistent reported picture is of reduced hippocampal volume in patients with PTSD which may be associated to clinically important variables such as severity of exposure, severity of dissociation or Wechsler memory score.

The observation of mild hippocampal atrophy is supported by the only published magnetic resonance spectroscopy study (Freeman et al., 1998). This study shows significantly reduced NAA/Cr (*N*-acetyl aspartate/creatinine) proton MRS ratios (an index of neuronal damage) in the right medial temporal lobe and significant reduction in Cho/Cr (choline/creatinine) ratios (possibly an index of white matter damage) in the left medial temporal lobe in 21 veterans with PTSD compared with eight control veterans.

What Is the Significance and Mechanism of Hippocampal Damage in PTSD?. The significance of a decrease in hippocampal volume is difficult to interpret on its own as it may be a predisposing factor to developing PTSD rather than a consequence of the trauma. Mild hippocampal atrophy as a predisposing factor to PTSD is, however, less likely than originally postulated as Bonne et al. (2001) demonstrated that trauma victims who develop PTSD do not have smaller hippocampi than trauma victims who do not develop PTSD. In this study trauma victims had MRI and psychometry at one week and six months after the trauma.

So, if the hippocampal changes are secondary to the trauma, it would be important to determine the mediating factor. This is unlikely to be a plain increase in GC as PTSD patients have been demonstrated to have normal or low cortisol levels in the blood and a hyper-responsive pituitary (Yehuda et al., 1996). A case can be made that GC receptor sensitivity precipitates neuronal and in this case hippocampal neurons in PTSD would have hypersensitive GC receptors. It is difficult, however, to reconcile this concept with the human depression findings without invoking the contribution of other possible mediating factors (e.g. noradrenaline release (Petty et al., 1994)).

Whatever the mechanism, a recent study demonstrates that pharmacological treatment is likely to reverse the atrophy and that therefore the latter is likely to be an index of dendritic health. Vermetten et al. (2003) have demonstrated that after 9–12 months treatment with paroxetine, symptomatic improvement is accompanied by a bilateral 4–5% increase in hippocampal volume and a 30% increase in Wechsler memory scales subtest. These very exciting results, if confirmed, suggest that treatment not only reverses symptoms but has neurotrophic effects.

Lateralization of Hippocampal Damage and PTSD. The evidence so far suggests that if lateralization is indeed present, then patients with adult onset PTSD have smaller right hippocampi and patients with childhood onset PTSD have smaller left hippocampi. It is likely that lateralization is an artefact of the small sample sizes. However, if these data were to be robustly replicated, the implication would be that patients with PTSD from childhood experiences or PTSD from adult trauma have smaller hippocampi in a side by condition interaction where adult PTSD relates to right atrophy and childhood PTSD to left atrophy. The mechanism may be related to differences in brain connectivity between the adults and children.

Resting Metabolism and Symptom Provocation Studies

Activation studies have involved the subtraction of relative regional blood flow between a resting or control condition and an activation condition congruent with the trauma. In many of these other controls were also included in order to estimate whether the changes in cerebral blood flow were specific to PTSD or a general response to highly arousing stimuli in people subjected to trauma.

The psychiatry imaging group at Massachusetts General Hospital in Boston has performed the most comprehensive set of studies using $C^{15}O_2$ positron emission tomography. 31 patients were studied in total, one study being completely on childhood sexual abuse victims and one in war veterans. In all the studies the exposure to the trauma-related stimuli (either autobiographical memories or imagery/perception of trauma scenes) produced an increase in emotional cognitions and physiological signs of increased arousal; these changes were far greater in magnitude in PTSD patients than controls. Two studies (Rauch et al., 1996; Shin et al., 1999) employed autobiographical scripts to induce emotion. In these experiments the resting condition is listening to a script of neutral autobiographical memories while the activated condition consists of listening to a script of memories of the traumatic event. Both studies showed a similar pattern of increased blood flow in the anterior cingulate, anterior insula, orbito-frontal cortex, and anterior temporal pole. Decreases in blood flow were observed in the left inferior frontal cortex. Anterior cingulate and anterior insula activations were thought to be nonspecific as they were induced by the experience of strongly emotionally laden memories irrespective of having developed PTSD. Volunteers re-experiencing traumatic events (but who had not developed PTSD) also had similar magnitudes or larger activations than PTSD patients in these areas. Orbito-frontal and anterior temporal activations were larger in PTSD patients but not unique to the patient group, suggesting a quantitative rather than qualitative difference in the circuits linked to emotional responses to trauma memories. The left inferior frontal decreases were present only in the PTSD patients and could therefore represent a specific pathological response. Another study (Shin et al., 1997) compared the activations produced by perception or imagery of war scenes with either negative or neutral stimuli. The study selected war veterans with and without PTSD. The pattern of regional blood flow change differed according to the modality of the subtraction paradigm employed and the only common pattern that emerged was of cingulate increases (albeit in very different loci) and of left inferior frontal decreases.

The fact that anterior cingulate increases were much more prominent in control trauma victims lead the Boston group to postulate that PTSD patients did not activate the anterior cingulate in response to emotional stimuli. This notion was tested in a study by Shin et al. (2001) who demonstrated, using fMRI, that PTSD patients did not activate the anterior cingulate when performing an emotional Stroop task.

In this context Lanius et al. (2001) demonstrated that on recall of traumatic events, PTSD subjects activate the anterior cingulate more than controls; however, the spatial extent of this activation is more limited and therefore it is possible that it would only be picked up at higher field strengths.

One of the contemporary paradigms of choice that has evolved from previous experiments is related to testing the functionality of particular brain areas in response to specific tasks. In this context Rauch et al. (2000) demonstrated that on presentation of masked faces with emotional expression, patients with PTSD activate the amygdala more than controls suggesting a hyper-reactivity of these subjects to novel threatening stimuli.

Other activation studies contribute to current knowledge. One study documented a failure of parietal activation with an attentional task in PTSD patients when compared with controls (Semple et al., 1996) but little can be concluded from this study as the performance was also impaired; thus the difference in activation may be due to the subjects not performing the task equally well. One employed a similar strategy to the Boston group by investigating victims of childhood sexual abuse with and without PTSD using autobiographical scripts of trauma minus neutral scripts (Bremner, 1999). This study showed a completely different pattern of regional blood flow change compared with the Boston group with increases in perfusion in posterior insula, posterior cingulate, superior and middle frontal gyri and motor cortex and decreases in perfusion in inferior temporal, supramarginal and fusiform gyri in PTSD compared with controls. In seemingly common areas the changes differ either by exact location (e.g. increases in the posterior rather than anterior insula) or by valence (decreases rather than increases in anterior cingulate).

Two other studies are from the same group. One study set out to test the hypothesis of an increase in medial prefrontal blood flow in PTSD victims (medial prefrontal cortex is involved in extinction and had been activated in previous studies by the same group) when compared with healthy controls or veterans while listening to combat sounds compared with white noise (Zubieta et al., 1999) and indeed found such an increase. The other (Liberzon et al., 1999) described an increase in anterior cingulate perfusion with exposure to combat sounds irrespective of diagnosis as well as increases in left amygdala and a decrease in retrosplenial cortex particular to patients with PTSD. This same group also described the changes in brain metabolism in one patient observed during a flashback which occurred by chance during an HMPAO SPECT study (Liberzon et al., 1997). In this paradigm the images obtained by scanning represent the sum of the regional brain blood flow occurring in the first few minutes after injection of the ligand when, having listened to a tape of combat sounds, the subject experienced feeling 'back in Vietnam' and extreme distress. The scan demonstrated an alteration in perfusion ratio between the thalamus and the cortex so that during the flashback the ratio of thalamic/cortical-basal ganglia metabolism was increased by 15%. This change in cortico-thalamic ratio could not be explained by changes due to hyperventilation and the authors interpreted it as representing a dissociative change in state of consciousness. Osuch et al. (2001) also found positive correlations between the intensity of flashbacks and perfusion in the brainstem, lingula, bilateral insula, right putamen and left hippocampal and perihippocampal, somatosensory and cerebellar regions, while negative correlations were observed in bilateral dorsolateral prefrontal, right fusiform and right medial temporal cortices. On the other hand Pissiota et al. (2002) found that the experience of symptoms was linked with increases in the pons, amygdala, sensory motor areas and the cerebellum.

While dorsolateral and medial prefrontal decreases and limbic increases are seen in some studies, it is difficult to subscribe to a consistent picture emerging from the imaging studies thus far conducted in PTSD. In particular the total dissonance of two studies which at face value are very similar (Shin et al., 1999; Bremner et al., 1999) could be a cause for concern. Because of the differences in the laboratories, of the detail of the paradigms employed and of the relatively small number of subjects it is perhaps not surprising that differences are as striking as the similarities. Thus it can be concluded that large studies employing comparable techniques in different laboratories are needed in order to generate robust analyses of a generalizable nature. This conclusion may be more pertinent to PTSD than other psychiatric groups because of the heterogeneity of the pathogenesis and comorbidity. Much of this work will be carried out using MR techniques in future.

In Vivo Neurochemistry

The Yale group (Bremner et al., 2000a) investigated Vietnam veterans with PTSD using iomazenil SPECT and found that there was a significant decrease in the volume of distribution of benzodiazepine $GABA_A$ receptors in the frontal cortex. The authors argue that, despite the lack of human pharmacological data to indicate that GABA receptors are dysfunctional in PTSD, this finding is consistent with the preclinical observations which suggest that exposure to chronic stress decreases benzodiazepine binding maximally in the frontal cortex (Weizman et al., 1989). This finding may be of particular significance as this area is involved in extinction of conditioned responses, thus misfunction of local inhibitory circuits could be either a consequence or a predispositon to developing inappropriate responses to trauma. Another investigation by the Yale group (Bremner et al., 1997) examined the differences in regional metabolic rate after the administration of yohimbine to patients with PTSD and healthy volunteers. Yohimbine is an $\alpha 2$ noradrenergic antagonist which increases noradrenaline release by blocking the presynaptic autoreceptors. The study employed ^{18}FDG PET as the measure of metabolism. The metabolic effects of noradrenaline are inhibitory on postsynaptic neurons; however the overall metabolic effects for a cortical volume depend on the extent of noradrenergic activation. Low levels of noradrenaline release are postulated to increase regional metabolism through an increase in local synaptic work that is responsible for a large proportion of the local metabolic requirements. At higher levels of noradrenergic activity (as seen with presynaptic blockade), however, a net decrease in local metabolism is observed. This occurs, presumably, because the reduction in the number of active local interneurons becomes predominant in comparison to the increased synaptic transmiston at noradrenergic synapses. Although noradrenergic modulation affects vascular responsivity, this can be corrected for in [18]FDG PET and is therefore not a confounding factor. This study demonstrated that yohimbine generates a global small increase in grey matter metabolism in healthy volunteers consistent with a small increase in noradrenaline release, while patients with PTSD responded with a moderate global decrease in grey matter metabolism, that was maximal in the orbito-frontal cortex and significant in the prefrontal, parietal and temporal cortices. Significant behavioural activation occurred in PTSD patients but not in volunteers. The authors interpreted this observation as evidence of increased sensitivity to the noradrenergic releasing properties of yohimbine in PTSD, which is in line with their previous pharmacological observations in this patient group.

Social Anxiety Disorder (Social Phobia)

Social anxiety disorder has been recognized as a psychiatric disorder with important personal consequences only in the last 10 or so years. Its lifetime prevalence has been estimated to be over 10% but only 5% of patients with this disorder seek treatment. The disorder is characterized by excessive fear of public scrutiny in situations that normally do not arouse anxiety such as eating in public, entering in a public place or even standing in a queue or filling up the car with petrol at a petrol pump. In these situations patients experience somatic and cognitive symptoms of anxiety and seek to escape the situation. Blushing and upper chest and facial flushing are commonly described and these lead to panic-like feelings as patients believe that these signs can be seen by others thus increasing the chance of being scrutinized. This description relates to generalized social anxiety disorder. Some people experience specific or circumscribed social anxiety disorder whereby they experience anxiety only in some situations such as public performance. This latter picture is probably on a continuum with performance anxiety that many people experience but can have deleterious consequences when the person depends on public performance for his living. For many, social anxiety disorder starts in childhood and has a chronic course; most people do not present for treatment until their late twenties or early thirties.

Structural Imaging

Only one volumetric study using MRI has reported on the comparison of anatomical brain structures between healthy volunteers and patients. Potts et al. (1994) using a 1.5 tesla camera showed that there were no differences in brain structure volumes; however the age-related decrease in putamen volume was more marked in patients with the disorder than in healthy controls. This reduction was not correlated to symptom severity but is of interest given the changes in dopaminergic function reported below.

Functional Imaging

The first study that compared resting metabolism between healthy volunteers and controls used HMPAO SPECT with a single-headed rotating gamma camera and showed no difference between 11 patients and 11 controls (Stein and Leslie, 1996). Since then a treatment study by Van der Linden et al. (2000) using the same technique, showed that an eight-week course of citalopram reduced metabolism in the left temporal and frontal cortices and the left cingulum. This reduction was not observed in non-responders who had higher baseline metabolism in these regions when compared with responders. There was no healthy volunteer group in this study.

Activation Studies

Two groups have examined whole brain changes in blood flow with anxiety provocation in patients with social anxiety disorder using $H_2^{15}O$ PET. Tillfors et al. (2001) compared 18 patients with social phobia with six healthy volunteers during the private or public performance of a prepared 2.5 minutes speech about a travel experience or a holiday. When the public performance was subtracted with the private performance, patients with social phobia (who experienced significant changes in anxiety ratings and psychophysiological measures) showed significant relative increases in the right amygdala and relative decreases in the right and left insula, right and left retrosplenial cortex, right and left perirhinal cortex, right temporal pole, right secondary visual cortex and right parietal cortex. Significant activation in all these areas was demonstrated on the basis of predictions made by analysis of previous imaging studies in anxiety disorders.

Malizia (2001) investigated seven patients with social phobia using an autobiographical scripts paradigm; there was no comparison with healthy volunteers. In this, scans acquired during listening to different autobiographical scripts of recent social anxiety and positive affect generating events, were compared. During the anxiogenic scripts, self-reported and psychophysiological measures of anxiety were increased and blood flow increases were noted in the right anterior insula, right anterior prefrontal cortex, left thalamus, left anterior cingulate and decreases in the left amygdala with a trend for decrease in the right amygdala.

Direct comparison of the two studies is difficult because of the different methods employed, the different thresholds accepted for significance ($z = 2.6$ in Uppsala and $z = 3.1$ in Bristol) and the lack of a comparison with healthy volunteers in the second study. However, alterations in essential limbic structures such as the amygdala and anterior insula were present in both studies, albeit in a reciprocal fashion in terms of direction of change. The amygdala was also implicated in two other studies which employed fMRI to test specific hypotheses about brain processing in social phobia. Birbaumer et al. (1998) elegantly demonstrated that patients with social phobia activate the amygdala when exposed to slides of neutral faces while controls do not. The same group also demonstrated (Schneider et al., 1999) that these differences are exacerbated when neutral faces are paired with a negative odour thus becoming a conditioned negative stimulus. In this experiment, controls decreased perfusion in the amygdala in the presence of the conditioned stimulus while patients with social phobia increased it; no significant statistical differences were, however, observed in the habituation or extinction phases.

All these experiments seem to indicate that the amygdala is an essential part of the malfunctioning networks in social anxiety disorder and confirm that the exact direction of perfusion change is changeable according to the paradigm used.

In Vivo Neurochemistry

Dopaminergic underactivity and social anxiety have been postulated to be related from animal models, human diseases such as Parkinson's and the effects of dopamine modulating agents (reviewed in Bell et al., 1999). Two studies have provided evidence for dopaminergic dysfunction in social phobia by measuring the density of dopamine transporters and D_2 (mainly postsynaptic) receptors in the basal ganglia of patients with this condition and controls, using SPET. The first study, using [^{123}I]beta-CIT, demonstrated that 11 Finnish social phobia patients had decreasd binding potential for the dopamine transporter in the striatum. This has been followed by a study by Schneier et al. (2000) who have demonstrated that 10 New York patients with social phobia had lower D_2 binding potential than controls. These data suggest three possibilities:

- Down regulation of both sites as a trait associated with possible dopaminergic hypofunction.
- Increased dopaminergic tonic release, which would decrease the proportion of sites available for radioligand binding.
- Mild atrophy of the basal ganglia.

Spectroscopy

Two studies (Davidson et al., 1993; Tupler et al., 1997) have examined creatine, NAA, choline and myoinositol spectra in patients with social anxiety disorder. The measures have all been relative and the second study allowed separation of cortical and subcortical grey and white matter. The authors find a number of significant differences in spectra between patients and controls which they interpret as cortical increases in myoinositol and choline concentrations in patients that were not altered by eight weeks' treatment with benzodiazepines. The biological significance of these altered signals is, however, uncertain. Thus these findings do not, as yet, contribute to a biological understanding of this disorder.

Generalized Anxiety Disorder

Generalized anxiety disorder has been little studied with imaging. This is in keeping with the fact that there is a dearth of biological investigations in this disorder, possibly because its pure form does not come to the attention of secondary services and therefore recruiting into laboratory-based studies is additionally difficult. No conclusion can be drawn from any of the published studies in anxiety disorders, except that benzodiazepines reduce global and regional brain metabolism in a manner similar to healthy volunteers. The nonspecific effects of benzodiazepines are larger than any specific ones related to decreased anxiety.

Three studies have investigated the effect of benzodiazepines in GAD (Buchs-baum et al., 1987; Wu et al., 1991; Mathew and Wilson, 1991). In all three studies the administration of diazepam resulted in decreases in global and regional metabolism which was greatest in the areas with the greatest density of benzodiazepine binding sites. Changes in anxiety score on benzodiazepines did not correlate with any of the regional changes, while changes in anxiety score during placebo administration correlated with reductions in limbic and basal ganglia metabolism. Wu et al. (1991) also observed that GAD patients did not exhibit the usual left to right asymmetry in hippocampal metabolism.

Two further studies contribute to the meagre information available for this disorder. Tiihonen et al. (1997b) demonstrated a significant decrease in left temporal pole benzodiazepine binding using [^{123}I]NNC 13-8241 SPET. This was accompanied by a decrease in variability in binding (as assessed by fractal analysis) which the authors interpreted as being pathological. More recently larger bilateral amygdala volumes have been described with MRI in children with generalized anxiety disorder when compared with controls (De Bellis et al., 2000).

Specific Phobias

Initial studies showed no change in perfusion with exposure to feared objects (Mountz et al., 1989); however this was probably due to technical limitations as Rauch et al. (1995) demonstrated increases in perfusion of the anterior cingulate, insula, anterior temporal and somatosensory cortex, posterior medial orbito-frontal cortex and thalamus when subtracting control condition from exposure to feared objects; these findings are consistent with the idea that all anxiety disorders would share some common activations related to the experience of this emotion. O'Carroll et al. (1993), however, using SPECT reported decreased HMPAO uptake in the occipital cortex while patients with specific phobias listened to a four-minute recording recounting exposure to phobic stimulus when this was compared with a relaxation tape; the findings may be related to the visual salience of the imagined stimuli but no activations in common anxiety-related brain areas were reported, possibly because of the low statistical power of the technique. No other studies have been conducted since these three have been reported.

Commonalities among Anxiety Disorders

There are three groups who have done similar anxiety provocation studies in more than one group of volunteers. Rauch and colleagues (Rauch et al., 1993, 1995, 1996) in Boston have studied patients with obsessive-compulsive disorder, with simple phobia and with post-traumatic stress disorder and have subsequently reported a formal comparison (Rauch et al., 1997). Fredrikson and colleagues (Tillfors et al., 2001) have investigated two separate groups of patients with simple phobia, a group with social anxiety disorder and a group of bank clerks re-experiencing a robbery as well as the neural networks of conditioning by pairing a snake video with the delivery of electric shocks to the hand. This group published a comparison between the phobic provocation and the re-experience of the bank robbery, but without formal statistical comparison. Malizia and colleagues (Malizia, 2001) have examined patients with social phobia and healthy volunteers taking part in a conditioned anticipatory anxiety paradigm and conducted a formal comparison of these groups.

Altogether, these data have to be interpreted in the light of comparative findings in studies of anxiety provocation in healthy volunteers (Benkelfat et al., 1995; Malizia, 2001; Servan-Schreiber et al., 1998; Chua et al., 1999; Javanmard et al., 1999; Simpson et al., 2001). In general two sets of areas seem to be activated in anxiety and anxiety disorders whether at rest or after a challenge. The first set comprises the supragenual anterior cingulate, the orbito-frontal cortex, the insulae, the cerebellum, a pontine locus variously described as superior colliculi or PAG and often, but not always, medial temporal structures (amygdala, parahippocampal gyrus) especially on the left. All these (except the cerebellum) are areas which are directly involved with the evaluation of noxious stimuli and which produce autonomic responses when stimulated. In essence they may represent the essential circuits of the anxiety responses. The surprising element here is the activation of the cerebellum which speaks to its hitherto unsuspected involvement in processes which do not have a primary motor component. This finding is not specific to anxiety as it has been observed in cognitive manipulations where movement components have been controlled for (e.g. Kim et al., 1994).

The second set of activations represents areas of sensory or polymodal association cortices which may represent the processing of relevant anxiogenic stimuli or their imagery.

Other activations seem to be congruent with particular aspects of the anxiety disorder; so basal ganglia activation fits well with the theory of cortico-striatal involvement in the obsessive-compulsive aspects of this disorder (Saxena and Rauch, 2000), amygdala is consistently involved in studies of social anxiety disorder and decreased activations in the inferior frontal lobes in PTSD.

Overall this set of data has to be considered as pilot data to be used to guide hypothesis generation. This is because a direct comparison (and therefore an assessment of the robustness of the findings) is not possible as paradigms, technology, analysis and reporting were very different between the different centres.

Brain Imaging and Anxiety Disorders: Conclusions

The impact of the last 10 years of imaging on the understanding of anxiety disorders is difficult to assess. This is not because there has been a shortage of findings but because, as the studies have informed contemporary thinking, it is difficult to retrace a time when these data were not available.

In general the main findings are:

- Anxiety experience, whether 'healthy' or pathological, whether behaviourally or pharmacologically induced, provokes regional brain metabolic changes that can be mapped. Some of these regions are consistently activated *across* anxiety disorders and conditions. Within these regions, some, such as anterior cingulate, orbito-frontal cortex, medial temporal structures and anterior insula could be predicted *a priori*. Some such as the cerebellum could not.
- Resting brain metabolism in the scanner is altered in anxiety disorders patients when compared with healthy volunteers. Areas of hyper- or hypo-metabolism often correspond to areas activated by the experience of pathological emotions as exemplified by OCD and possibly panic disorder.
- The above findings support a notion of a network in which some global processes are tapped by various tasks and local regions which are consistently by particular disease or emotional domains. For instance, while activations of the anterior cingulate cortex may be considered to be common to many activation studies in all types of cognitive domains other than emotions, orbito-frontal cortex involvement is likely to be common with other affective domains (including affective decision making) but not with many other cognitive domains. Further, increased correlations between orbito-frontal, thalamic and caudate metabolism are likely to be specific to OCD. These observations support the theory of a modular model of brain function where individual components are responsible for particular tasks but also affect and change the function of other components of the network. These ideas are discussed in detail in Malizia (1999) and Cabeza and Nyberg (2000).
- Hypotheses that specific processing dysfunction are associated with particular disorders can start to be generated and therefore tested. These patterns of dysfunction may be predictive of treatment response as early data in OCD suggest.
- Specific neurochemical abnormalities can be detected and these may inform future therapeutic developments and pharmacogenomic investigations. For example investigation of $GABA_A$ $\alpha1$, $\alpha2$ and $\psi2$ polymorphisms (if they exist in man) and selective agonists may lead to a better understanding of the pathophysiology and treatment of panic disorder.

Brain Imaging and Anxiety Disorders: the Future

The same enthusiasm now witnessed for MR and nuclear brain imaging was apparent in the early days of EEG; however, this technique failed to deliver its promise. This was due to a number of factors including poor localization and identification of the signals and large interindividual variability in signal and signal modulation. The future of brain imaging in the investigation of anxiety disorders will depend upon a number of factors, some of which have already been mentioned in the chapter:

- Standardization of technical methods, analysis techniques and experimental protocols.
- Increased signal-to-noise to allow individual subject experiments to produce maps of function.
- Involvement of large numbers of experimental subjects.
- Combination of naturalistic experiments and experiments designed to test specific aspects of brain function.
- Combining techniques with good spatial resolution with techniques which have superior temporal resolution such as magnetoencephalography (MEG).
- Production of new radioligands which will allow definition of the various neurochemical systems in health and disease.
- Combined approaches where other information, e.g. genomics, is used to select samples of patients or healthy volunteers.
- Synergy with preclinical science whereby human imaging results are used as starting hypotheses for testing in animal and in vitro models.

Many of these are being worked on at present and these efforts should result in robust and effective investigational tools.

NEUROIMAGING RESEARCH IN AFFECTIVE DISORDERS

Affective disorders are psychiatric conditions in which the main recognized disturbance comes from a persistent and abnormal variation in mood over prolonged periods of time (from weeks to months). The most common affective disorder is depression but abnormal elation leading to mania is also seen in a significant part of the population. Affect disturbances can also occur in a variety of other brain disorders such as stroke, multiple sclerosis, Parkinson's disease and hypothyroidism to name but a few. Up to 30% of people will experience at least one episode of affective disorder in their lifetime; however, a smaller number (about 4%) will experience recurrent disturbances that can lead to significant personal, economic and social disability. Hundreds of million of people worldwide suffer with these disorders that, like many other medical conditions, strongly affect the poor. For example, unipolar major depressive disorder accounts for over 4% of the total burden of disease making it the fifth leading cause of disability (WHO, 1999) and is the single leading cause of disability in people aged 16–44 in many countries (Murray and Lopez, 1997). In addition, while depressive disorders affect up to 25% of patients attending primary care, these disorders often go unrecognized and untreated.

Three main types of affective disorder are recognized; their separation is based on the fact that treatment for these three major categories is different. Major depressive disorder (also known as unipolar depression) is characterized by periods of depressed mood accompanied by lack of energy, loss of pleasure, decreased or increased sleep and appetite with accompanying variations in weight, poor concentration, changes in sex drive and menstruation, cognitive changes including worthlessness, hopelessness and helplessness. More severe cases develop notions that life is not worth living, a desire to be dead, suicidal ideation and intent. While many people will only experience one such episode in their lifetime, some have recurrent episodes. The disorder is clearly episodic. Prior to effective treatments, the median duration of an episode would be about three months and the mean six months; the distribution is strongly skewed with some people experiencing profound depression for many months and perhaps years. Up to 15% of patients with recurrent depression will be successful in eventually committing suicide. Unipolar depression is treated with antidepressants and the current consensus is that if three or more episodes occur in less than five years or if such episodes lead to significant disability, then patients should consider taking treatment for life. There is now considerable evidence that prolonged use of antidepressants prevents relapse in many such cases.

If episodes of depression are accompanied by psychotic symptoms (the presence of delusions and/or hallucinations) the condition is known as major depressive disorder with psychotic symptoms, or psychotic depression, and antidepressants alone are not sufficient – combinations of antidepressants and antipsychotics are administered for treatment to be effective.

Finally some patients experience cyclical changes in mood that can lead to episodes of inappropriate elation and overactivity accompanied by socially destructive behaviours (sexual promiscuity, excessive spending, aggression). Patients with these episodes will at some time in their life also experience depressive episodes and the balance between depression and mania depends on the individual cases. Some people experience mild mania occasionally but severe depression often; at the other end of the spectrum some have transient depression but recurrent mania that leads them to be hospitalized often. This condition, known as bipolar affective disorder, is treated mainly with mood stabilizers such as lithium, carbamazepine and sodium valproate, alone or in combination. Antipsychotics or antidepressants may be used to treat residual symptoms.

Nuclear medicine techniques have been extensively used in research in these disorders although, for obvious clinical reasons, it is very difficult to study patients who have mania at the time of investigation. This is because patients will, in general, find it very difficult to keep focus for long enough to collaborate with an imaging study. The episodic nature of the affective disorders makes them attractive for investigations of changes that occur with psychopathological state. However, centres that are technologically advanced and can, therefore perform such studies meaningfully, are co-localized with communities where the recognition and treatment of affective disorders is high and therefore it has at times proved difficult to study drug-naive patients, thus limiting some of the conclusions that can be drawn about the neuro-chemical and metabolic changes underlying the conditions.

This chapter will describe the state of play for a number of themes that have emerged from these studies. The themes that have emerged are neurochemical and related to functional anatomy (brain circuits). The major themes are changes in dopaminergic and serotonergic systems, abnormal resting brain metabolism, abnormal brain activation, metabolic predictors of response to treatment, changes in metabolism related to treatment and changes in receptor density following treatment. While nuclear medicine techniques have been essential in developing the methodology related to brain activation, functional MRI is largely supplanting them in this arena. However, nuclear medicine techniques are still essential in the measure of receptor binding, transporter density, enzyme concentration, transmitter release and intracellular messenger changes. In addition while magnetic resonance imaging techniques are emerging that allow the measure of resting brain metabolism it is unlikely that FDG PET will be supplanted for such measures in the next three to four years.

In Vivo Neurochemistry

Serotonergic System

The serotonergic system consists of very long neurons whose cell bodies are distributed in the median and dorsal raphe nuclei. These neurons project with fine or medium size fibres to widespread locations throughout the brain. While their precise function is still being researched, it is likely that changes in serotonergic tone are important in the elaboration of affective, anxiety and social information. More than 12 types of differentially distributed postsynaptic receptors have been identified and serotonin release is controlled by presynaptic homo- and hetero-receptors, by the activity of the synaptic serotonin transporters and by somatodendritic receptors situated on cell bodies in the raphe. These act as 'brakes' on the system so that their activation results in a decreased rate of firing. Serotonin (5-HT: 5-hydroxytryptamine) in the brain is synthesized from tryptophan, an essential neutral amino acid, that is transported by a specific mechanism into the brain; there are no stores of tryptophan in the brain and one of the synthetic steps is rate limiting for the synthesis of 5-HT. Serotonergic dysfunction has been thought to be implicated in depression since the 1970s, this notion being reinforced by the effectiveness of medicines that selectively act on this system (selective serotonin reuptake inhibitors (SSRIs) and 5-HT2 antagonists) in treating these disorders. There has, however, been a relative dearth of good radioligands for this system and therefore the number of relevant studies is still relatively small.

5-HT$_{1A}$ Receptors

5-HT$_{1A}$ receptors are located ubiquitously in the cortex as well as in the hippocampus, raphe and, to a lesser extent, the basal ganglia. Increased transmission through these cortical postsynaptic receptors has been hypothesized to be important in antidepressant and neurotrophic activity; this is especially so in the hippocampus where activity at these sites may reverse the neurodegenerative effects of increased cortisol commonly seen in psychiatric conditions. As previously mentioned, however, increased activity at somatodendritic receptors in the raphe is known to decrease the firing rate of serotonergic neurons thus decreasing net trafficking at cortical and hippocampal synapses; this mechanism is thought to be responsible for the time lag in response seen with antidepressants: it is thought that while each synaptic release is immediately larger following the administration of SSRIs, the net cortical serotonergic release does not increase until raphe 5-HT_{1A} receptors desensitize or down-regulate thus 'taking the brake off' the system and allowing the rate of firing to increase.

5-HT$_{1A}$ Receptors Density in Depression and its Treatment

5-HT_{1A} receptors can be measured in man by using $[^{11}\text{C}]$WAY100635 PET. Studies using this compound have demonstrated that 5-HT_{1A} binding is globally reduced in patients with unipolar and familial (bipolar or unipolar) depression (Drevets et al., 1999; Sargent et al., 2000a) being more prominent (40%) in the raphe than in temporal cortex (Drevets et al., 1999) and more pronounced in families who have a bipolar phenotype. Further, treatment with SSRIs does not alter the reduced binding (Sargent et al., 2000a) thus speaking to a trait or to a slowly changing abnormality that is perhaps linked to neuronal or glial cellular structural deficits. It is also possible that if both $B_{\max}$ and K_d change in the same direction (as would be predicted by studies in neurosurgical samples of depressed patients (Francis et al., 1993)), then a composite ratio measure such as binding potential would not detect such a change.

5-HT$_{1A}$ Receptor Occupancy by Receptor Antagonists

The notion that delays in response to antidepressants are related to the 'brake'-like action of increased activity at somatodendritic raphe 5-HT_{1A} receptors has led a number of researchers worldwide attempting to block this receptor in order to either speed up the response to antidepressants or to increase their efficacy. To this end pindolol a noradrenegic beta blocker that also binds (as a partial agonist) to 5-HT_{1A} receptors has been used in a number of open label or placebo-controlled studies in doses averaging 15 mg daily (on the basis of tolerability of this dose). Some clinical studies reported desired effects but many did not, leading to questions about the theory underpinning the studies. However, all studies were conducted without assessing occupancy at 5-HT_{1A} receptors and it is therefore possible that lack of effect would be related to insufficient occupancy. Pharmacological theory predicts that at least 60–80% occupancy needs to be achieved in order to have sufficient blockade at a receptor with considerable receptor reserve. Two groups of researchers have thus addressed this issue by measuring pindolol occupancy at 5-HT$_{1A}$ receptors. These experiments revealed that currently used pindolol doses are insufficient to achieve the required degree of blockade (Martinez et al., 2001; Rabiner et al., 2000). In addition both groups revealed that pindolol occupancy at the raphe nuclei was almost double than occupancy at cortical receptors and Rabiner and colleagues demonstrated that pure antagonists do not share this property. These results indicated that the hypothesis of improving and speeding up antidepressant effects with 5-HT$_{1A}$ blockade in the raphe has not been adequately tested in clinical studies. In addition, they have reopened debate on whether a pure antagonist would be effective in doing so, as any beneficial effects through raphe blockade will be counterbalanced by equal blockade at one of the postsynaptic sites thought to be important for antidepressant response.

5-HT$_2$ Receptors

The notion that these receptors may be of interest in depression is supported by the fact that 5-HT$_2$ antagonists (nefazodone, trazodone and mirtazapine) are effective antidepressants, although they all have other receptor or transporter binding properties that may explain their therapeutic action. In addition a number of studies have reported increases in 5-HT$_{2A}$ binding in brains of patients who have committed suicide (e.g. Mann et al., 1986). There are three PET ligands that have been used to investigate 5-HT$_2$ binding: setoperone, altanserin and ethylspiperone; ketanserin has been used for SPECT studies. All the ligands have significant drawbacks in that the ratio of specific to nonspecific binding is so low that the signal-to-noise ratio is poor; although [^{11}C]MDL 100902 would be an improvement on the above as it is a very specific ligand for cortical 5-HT$_{2A}$ receptors, no studies in depression have yet been published using it.

Studies using these ligands report either no difference (Meyer et al., 1999; Meltzer et al., 1998) or a decrease (D'haenen et al., 1992; Biver et al., 1997; Attar Levy et al., 1999; Yatham et al., 2000; Larisch et al., 2001) in 5-HT$_2$ binding in patients with depression with one study reporting an increase in 5-HT$_2$ availability after successful paroxetine (an SSRI) treatment (Zanardi et al., 2001), one showing a decrease in 5-HT$_2$ binding after desipramine (a noradrenaline reuptake inhibitor) treatment (Yatham et al., 1999) and finally, one showing age × treatment interaction in decreasing setoperone binding with paroxetine treatment (Meyer et al., 2001a) Differences in these studies may be related to differences in clinical samples and to the fact that all studies showing a decreased binding in specific brain regions (frontal being the common one) employed patients who were on treatment or who had come off treatment only two to three weeks previously. In addition all these studies have used analytical methodologies that make assumptions about reference areas in brain and therefore methodological issues may also cloud the reported results

5-HT Transporter

The 5-HT presynaptic reuptake site is blocked by most of the effective antidepressants and nuclear medicine studies have been employed to investigate the degree of occupancy that is needed for pharmacological response, how occupancy relates to plasma antidepressant levels and whether transporter densities are altered in depressive states, particularly in conjunction with transporter polymorphisms is thought to be relevant to depression. However, again, the ligands used have poor signal-to-noise ratios and it is likely that further understanding will come from the development of better ligands. Cortical binding of beta-CIT (2-beta-carbomethoxy-3-beta-(4-iodophenyl)-tropane) has been used for SPECT studies and DASB (3-amino-4-(2-dimethylaminomethyl-phenylsulfanyl)-benzonitrile) for PET studies.

The feasibility of using beta-CIT SPECT for measuring SSRI occupancy was first established by Pirker et al. (1995) in patients taking citalopram and Tauscher et al. (1999) confirmed in patients taking fluoxetine that at least 40% occupancy was achieved in clinically relevant doses. Meyer et al. (2001c) using [^{11}C]DASB confirmed that up to 80% occupancy could be achieved with 20 mg of fluoxetine or paroxetine and that paroxetine plasma concentrations of 28 ng/ml would achieve this high figure.

Two studies, one in seasonal affective disorder (Willeit et al., 2000), have reported decreased transporter binding potential in the raphe (Malison et al., 1998) and in the thalamus (Willeit et al., 2000). However, there is no evidence for a link between human in vivo transporter availability, measured by this method, and serotonin transporter promoter gene polymorphism (Willeit et al., 2001). These studies will need to be repeated in larger samples with more dependable ligands and methods; however, they offer tantalizing data to construct a theory of serotonin transporter involvement in depressive disorders. The field is also open to the study of the developmental significance of transporter density as Dahlstrom et al. (2000) found a correlation between increased transporter availability and and depression score in children and adolescents – a finding that will have to be extended as the absence of a healthy control group means that it is unclear whether the finding represents an increase in availability compared with healthy controls.

Serotonin Precursors

Tryptophan uptake can be measured using [^{11}C]alpha-methyl tryptophan and 5-HT uptake by measuring [^{11}C]5-HT uptake. The first has been reported to be higher in males than females (Nishizawa et al., 1997). The latter has been reported to be low in depression except for the medial prefrontal cortex where it may be increased (Agren et al., 1992, 1994). These results are of interest but their interpretation has to be cautious as differences in transport may not be linked to differences in rates of synthesis (Shoaf et al., 2000).

Dopaminergic System

The dopaminergic system is not thought to be primarily involved in depression. However, a number of observations make it interesting for the study of this condition. One powerful antidepressant (buproprion) possibly acts primarily as a dopamine reuptake inhibitor, depression is often associated with degenerative diseases such as Parkinson's that affect the dopaminergic system, psychomotor retardation (a feature of depression in some patients) can be reversed by the administration of L-dopa (dopamine precursor) and ECT (electroconvulsive therapy; still considered to be the most powerful treatment in depression) alters dopamine turnover in the brain. The notion of excess release of dopamine in mania is stronger with evidence of altered dopaminergic turnover and response to agents that block postsynaptic dopaminergic activity such as antipsychotic D_2 antagonists. These observations have led to a number of imaging studies of dopaminergic binding in the brain of depressed patients, partly facilitated by the ready availability of presynaptic and postsynaptic dopamine ligands. For this discussion the findings will be divided between unipolar depression and bipolar affective disorder.

Unipolar Depression

Dopamine Precursors. [^{18}F]dopa can be used to assess dopa transport into the brain. Assuming that the transport is related to the subsequent utilization of dopa for the synthesis of dopamine, two groups have found evidence for decreased dopamine turnover in depression (Agren and Reibring, 1994; Martinot et al., 2001); the groups used are small but, on the basis of careful selection of patients, authors argue that these changes are related to psychomotor retardation and are not seen in anxious depression.

Dopamine Release. Using amphetamine as a challenge agent, nuclear medicine studies can be employed to indirectly measure the intrasynaptic release of dopamine. The assumption is that decreases in postsynaptic radioligand binding (IBZM for SPECT and raclopride for PET) observed after the administration of the challenge agent are due to the large increases in intrasynaptic dopamine release subsequent to the effects of amphetamine. Using this methodology and [^{123}I]IBZM SPECT, Parsey et al. (2001) demonstrated that patients with unipolar depression were not significantly different from healthy controls in releasing dopamine after amphetamine administration. This was despite the fact that in patients the administration of dopamine had a definite euphoriant effect. This observation of course, does not necessarily imply normal dopaminergic function in depression but suggests that the system's responsivity is unaltered by the illness.

Dopamine D_2 Binding. Higher [^{123}I]IBZM binding in the striatum of patients with depression has been reported by two groups, bilaterally (D'haenen and Bossuyt,

1994) and on the right (Shah y et al., 1997). The implication of these studies if repli-cated, is that depression is accompanied by a decrease in intrasynaptic dopamine or by an up-regulation of postsynaptic D_2 receptors. One other study found similar changes but only in patients with psychomotor retardation (Ebert et al., 1996) while three other studies have not confirmed a baseline difference in binding (Ebert et al., 1994; Klimke et al., 1999; Parsey et al., 2001). The notion of decrease in dopaminergic transmission at baseline is attractive, especially in patients with psychomotor retardation, but larger and better controlled studies are needed to resolve this issue, as the weight of evidence is at present equivocal. Treatment studies cannot help us here as sleep deprivation (Ebert et al., 1994) and amitriptyline response are associated with decreased IBZM binding (speaking to an increase in dopaminergic function or down-regulation) while larger studies with paroxetine or fluoxetine responders (Klimke et al., 1999) have indicated an increase in IBZM binding (speaking to upregulation or decreased dopaminergic function). The inter-pretation of these results is complicated by the finding that raclopride binding was shown to be decreased in healthy volunteers on prolonged citalopram (an SSRI) treatment (Tiihonen et al., 1996).

Dopamine Transporter. The availability of the dopamine transporter in major depression has been described as increased by early beta-CIT SPECT studies carried out in Finland (Laasonen-Balk, 1999); however, a Canadian PET study utilizing RTI-32 (Meyer et al., 2002) describes a decrease in binding. Interestingly both groups come to the same conclusion: synaptic dopamine is decreased in depression. The Canadian group argues that patients with lowest binding potential performed best in neuropsy-chological tests of dopaminergic function and that therefore this should be seen as a compensatory down-regulation that would allow maintenance of function in the face of decreased transmission. There is, however, no clear reason for which the two results should produce diametrically opposite imaging finding, except for the fact that the influence of differences in methodology is still not well understood.

In seasonal affective disorder Neumeister et al. (2001) also reported a decrease in striatal [^{123}I]beta-CIT binding and again argued that the results indicate an adap-tive response to decreased dopaminergic efflux. Clearly better designed studies will be required to resolve these discrepancies.

Finally Meyer et al. (2002) reported that bupropion is an effective antidepressant at doses that occupy less than 20% of the transporter, thus questioning whether dopamine reuptake site inhibition is indeed the mechanism by which this drug exer-cises its antidepressant effects.

Bipolar Affective Disorder

Dopamine Precursors and Release. [^{18}F]dopa uptake was not different in a carefully conducted study of non-psychotic mood stabilizer naive manic patients compared with controls (Yatham et al., 2002b) and Anand et al. (2000) demonstrated that changes in [^{123}I]IBZM binding induced by amphetamine were not significantly different between euthymic patients with bipolar affective disorders and controls despite the fact that patients experienced greater behavioural activation in response to the challenge.

Dopamine D_2 Binding. Three studies using [^{123}I]IBZM SPECT (Anand et al., 2000), [^{11}C]n-methyl-spiperone PET (Wong et al., 1985) and [^{11}C] raclopride PET (Yatham et al., 2002a) have demonstrated that there is no significant difference in striatal D_2 receptor binding in patients who have non-psychotic bipolar affective disorder even if they are in the active manic phase of their illness. Pearlson et al. (1995) found some increase in D_2 binding in patients with mania; however, many of these had psychotic symptoms at the time of the experiment and thus may represent the effects of psychosis rather than mania.

Dopamine D_1 Binding. Suhara et al. (1992) used [^{11}C]SCH23390 to determine D_1 dopamine receptor density in 10 patients with bipolar affective disorder in different phases of illness. 9/10 had frontal cortex binding potentials that were below the control values. This may speak to a trait abnormality; however, the cortical signal for this ligand is quite small and we will have to await the development of ligands with improved signal for cortical regions before confirming this finding.

Vesicular Transporter. Monoamines are stored presynaptically in vesicles. After synthesis or synaptic reuptake the molecules are transported into these vesicles by a specific transporter (VMAT2). This process can be measured by PET using [^{11}C]DTBZ (dihydrotetrabenazine); Zubieta and colleagues (2000) demonstrated in 16 euthymic bipolar patients that there is no difference in basal ganglia vesicular transporter density between patients with bipolar affective disorder and controls.

Effects of Treatment on Precursor Transport and Postsynaptic Binding

Yatham et al. (2002b) demonstrated that although [^{18}F]dopa transport is decreased following treatment with a mood stabilizer (sodium valproate) this effect does not translate into a reduction of postsynaptic raclopride binding. These findings put together have two possible conclusions: no conclusion on turnover can be made by studying dopa transport into the brain or D_2 receptors down-regulate with successful mood stabilizer treatment. Appropriate experiments will have to be designed to test the second hypothesis since the first cannot be adequately falsified.

Noradrenergic Function

No adequate radioligands exist that allow the study of noradrenergic receptors and transporters in the brain. This is an area for obvious expansion since noradrenergic function is altered in depression and some effective antidepressants alter noradrenergic function primarily (reboxetine, mirtazapine, desipramine, nortriptyline). Melichar et al. (2001) using heart binding demonstrated that venlafaxine does not significantly bind to noradrenergic transporters in vivo in man until doses larger than 1 mg/kg are achieved. This is in keeping with preclinical data but the clinical significance of this finding will have to be confirmed by appropriate brain studies in the future.

Neurokinin Receptors

The possibility that neurokinin-1 antagonists were antidepressant opened a new field of investigation. While antagonists at these receptors are not now thought to be likely to be effective antidepressants, adequate radioligands have been developed in two or three PET centres worldwide. The release of information related to their use has been slow. [^{18}F]SPA-RQ (Hargreaves, 2002) has been identified as one of the promising ligands and the result of appropriate binding studies is awaited.

GABA

GABA is the most common inhibitory neurotransmitter in the brain and although abnormalities in its concentration and function have been investigated with other imaging modalities, there have been no nuclear medicine studies in affective disorders except for a recent report indicating a possible increase in iomazenil SPECT binding after ECT in five Finnish patients (Mervaala et al., 2001).

Brain Circuits of Depression

There have been many studies of resting metabolism (FDG PET, water PET, HMPAO SPECT) and brain activation (water PET, HMPAO SPECT) in both unipolar and bipolar affective disorders. No unifying pattern of dysfunction has emerged. The reasons for this are multiple: inhomogeneity of study populations used including factors such as recurrence, family history, previous treatments and anatomical brain abnormalities, differences in scanning methodology and analysis, weaknesses in overall study design. This may seem rather dispiriting, given the amount of resource employed. However, despite important differences a number of convergent themes are emerging. These point to the fact that particular areas of the brain seem to be intrinsically involved in affective circuits even though the polarity of metabolism or activation can be discordant in different studies. These areas seem to be involved in 'healthy' mood induction as well as pathological states, treatment on the whole leads to 'normalization' of abnormal patterns and areas affected are convergent even between such disparate therapies as interpersonal psychotherapy and neurosurgery. Since this field of investigation will be mainly advanced through the use of magnetic resonance techniques (and many studies using this technology have already been published) this section does not aim to fully review all the 50 or so major studies that have been published but will only indicate the important advances.

Important notions that have emerged from nuclear medicine studies of brain metabolism and activation in affective disorder include:

(1) Abnormal function of limbic and paralimbic structures are common in patients with affective disorders: these include most commonly the orbito-frontal cortex, the anterior cingulate and the amygdala. These abnormalities are often reversed by successful treatment.

(2) Induction of mood changes is accompanied by changes in brain metabolism in the above limbic and para-limbic structures.

(3) There are symptom-based similarities in brain dysfunction across different diagnoses; for instance decreases in dorsolateral prefrontal activity are seen both in schizophrenia and in depression with the similar symptoms of psychomotor retardation or poverty.

(4) Most studies report cortical under-perfusion or decreases in resting metabolism in cortices during pathological depression and induction of dysphoric mood.

(5) Areas activated by induction of mood changes by pharmacological means have considerable overlap with areas affected by psychological mood induction

(6) Networks activated by specific tasks are different between depressed patients and healthy controls even when differences in performance are not significant.

(7) Impaired episodic memory is associated with medial temporal lobe abnormalities.

Investigations that have generated the above statements will now be discussed grouping them by paradigm.

Mood Induction in Healthy Volunteers

Various methods have been used to induce emotion, including recalling autobiographical memories, seeing or imagining emotive events, lack of reward, attempts to solve insoluble problems, autobiographical scripts, listening to speeded-up or slowed-down music, presenting standardized facial expressions or administering mood-altering drugs.

George et al. (1995) and Ketter et al. (1996) working with the same group of investigators used sad event recall and the injection of the local anaesthetic procaine to provoke dysphoria in healthy volunteers; they observed activations in anterior paralimbic areas with considerable overlap in activations between the studies. Mayberg et al. (1999) also described increases in paralimbic perfusion and decreases in cortical perfusion that were associated with induction of sadness in healthy volunteers. Elliot et al. (1997) described activations in caudate and ventral orbito-frontal cortex by negative performance feedback in healthy volunteers and observed that patients with depression did not activate the same areas when faced with the same paradigm. This is in contrast to increases in amygdala perfusion and decreases in hippocampus that were found by Schneider et al. (1996) during dysphoria associated with attempting to solve unsolvable anagrams. It also taps into a different system than Baker et al. (1997) who observed reduced activation in orbito-frontal and dorsal anterior cingulate during a verbal fluency task after inducing sad mood by playing slowed-down music.

Baseline Abnormalities in Depression

The most consistent finding in resting studies of depressed patients has been a reduction in dorso-lateral prefrontal and dorsal cingulate signal and an increase in anterior paralimbic structures such as the orbito-frontal cortex, the subgenual cingulate and the amygdala. Some studies also describe changes in basal ganglia metabolism thus implicating fronto-thalamic basal ganglia circuits in the genesis of the disorders; temporal and parietal changes are often also described (Buchsbaum et al., 1986; Post et al., 1987; Schwartz et al., 1987; Baxter et al., 1989; Schlegel et al., 1989; Martinot et al., 1990b; Austin et al., 1992; Bench et al., 1992; Drevets et al., 1992b; Biver et al., 1994; Mayberg et al., 2000; Dunn et al., 2002; Kimbrell et al., 2002). Of particular note are the notions that there is an inverse relationship between limbic overactivity and cortical underactivity (Mayberg, 1997), that particular symptom clusters rather than syndromes are associated with specific brain patterns (Bench et al., 1992; Mayberg et al., 2002) and that an overactive amygdala is part of the system driving the orbito-frontal cortex in patients with severe primary familial depression (Drevets et al., 1992b). A lot of debate has centred around the role of the differential role of the dorsal and pregenual anterior cingulate between cognitive and emotional circuits – this will carry on being an area of focused investigation. Other observations of changes in activation include decreased emotional word activations in ventral cingulate, pulvinar and inferior frontal gyrus, increased ACC activity with sad stimuli and increased orbitofrontal activity with sad distractors.

Other data of interest relates to symptom provocation with tryptophan depletion studies where increasing levels of depression after tryptophan depletion were associated with diminished neural activity in the ventral anterior cingulate, orbito-frontal cortex and caudate nucleus regions. In addition, depressive relapse attenuated cognitive task-related activation in the anterior cingulate cortex (Smith et al., 1999). Neural activity in several 5-HT-related brain areas, e.g., dorsal raphe, habenula, septal region, amygdala, and orbito-frontal cortex, covaried significantly with plasma levels of tryptophan and ratings of depressed mood. Task-specific responses in left amygdala and left anterior cingulate were attenuated by tryptophan depletion.

Finally de Asis et al. (2001) have demonstrated that patients with depression who have memory deficits also show lowered hippocampal activity at rest and on activation.

Treatment Studies

The major finding from treatment effects on brain metabolism is that the major changes in metabolism tend to occur in structures germane to affect evaluation and that, on the whole, basal abnormalities are reversed. So for instance Mayberg et al. (2002) found that both placebo and fluoxetine responders (identified in a previous studies to differ from non-responders in the polarity of their resting pregenual cingulate metabolism (Mayberg et al., 1997)) show increases in prefrontal, anterior and posterior cingulate, frontal and parietal metabolism and decreases in subgenual cingulate, parahippocampus and thalamus. These changes result in patients' brain metabolic maps reverting to 'healthy' patterns. In addition there is the possibility of the initial pattern of activation being related to eventual treatment outcome: Davidson et al. (2003) showed that greater anterior cingulate activation with emotional stimuli at baseline predicts better treatment response with venlafaxine at eight weeks.

The notion of reverting to healthy metabolic patterns is also evident in studies that start with differing baselines. For instance Drevets et al. (2002) describe normalization of increased left amygdala metabolism with mood stabilizers. Brody et al. (2001) report decreases in ventral frontal lobe metabolism with successful treatment of 24 patients with unipolar depression with either psychotherapy or antidepressants. In this sample covarying specific symptom clusters with changes in metabolism shows an association between decreases in anterior ventral cingulate and anterior insula activity and an improvement in anxiety symptoms, while improvements in psychomotor retardation and cognitive symptoms were associated with increases in dorsal cingulate and dorso-lateral prefrontal activity respectively. Similarly Kennedy and colleagues (2001), reporting on 13 male patients before and after paroxetine treatment, noted increased metabolism in all aspects of the frontal and parietal cortex and in the dorsal anterior cingulate but reductions in pregenual anterior cingulate, bilateral insulae and right hippocampus.

While somewhat similar patterns can be seen in other treatments for depression such as buproprion (Nofzinger et al., 2001), sleep deprivation (Volk et al., 1997; Smith et al., 1999) mood stabilizers (Ketter et al., 1999) and neurosurgery (Malizia et al., 1994), electroconvulsive therapy produces a pattern of change that is counterintuitive since further cortical decreases are seen after treatment. This may be because the effects of generalized seizures override any subtler change in relative metabolism as all ECT studies (Rosenberg et al., 1988; Scott et al., 1993; Nobler et al., 1994; Henry et al., 2001; Nobler et al., 2001) that find a change associated with treatment describe decreases in various parts of the brain including the dorsal frontal cortex where most other treatments result in an increase in perfusion. Cognitive-behaviour therapy, if successful, may, however, operate through different mechanisms.

Specific treatment effects have also been seen in terms of changes in brain responsivity to particular stimuli. Sheline et al. (2001) demonstrated that the hyperreactivity to emotional faces seen in patients with depression is reversed by successful treatment with the SSRI sertraline.

Conclusion: Affective Disorders

Neuroimaging techniques have proved invaluable in the investigation of affective disorders. Despite the apparent discrepancies in the current literature, patterns are emerging from which theories can be formulated and tested. At a rather general level, the data, now permeating into popular culture, has supported the notion that psychiatric disorders are associated with changes in neurochemical function and distributed processing. It can be argued that imaging allows the investigation of the effects of both nature and nurture on brain function and that therefore it is essential to carry it out if we want to understand how genetic predisposition interacts with environmental factors and experiences to produce brain changes that are related to symptom experience.

Two main areas of investigation have been pertinent. Brain metabolism and circuitry were initially explored using nuclear medicine techniques that have been very productive; much of this work will, however, be carried on with magnetic resonance techniques. Nuclear medicine will, however, carry on being very important for the area of chemical and pharmacological investigation. Many of the advances in this have come from improvements in radiosynthesis and scanners. However, current progress is mostly impeded by the relative lack of useful radioligands that adequately describe the systems that we wish to investigate and to a lesser extent by the lack of standardization of robust protocols that would then allow comparisons between centres to be more transparent. In particular, attention will have to be paid not only to imaging methodology (including the environment of the scanner) but also to patient selection according to strict phenotypes or genotypes. All these problems will have to be grappled with if progress is to be maintained. This will require collaboration between academia, industry and health services as all possess information and skills that the others do not.

OVERALL CONCLUSION

Brain imaging is providing us with a variety of leads that would not be available from animal studies. Further, ideas generated from animal studies can be tested and extended with human brain imaging. The latter is starting to produce hypotheses that can be also further extended by appropriate preclinical studies. In this sense, one of the most exciting consequences of these techniques is to reaffirm a loop whereby human and animal experimentation inform each other, thus extending our knowledge.

A review of the current literature can be daunting because of the disparity of techniques used and the seemingly contrasting results that are generated. These effects, however, can be found with all other technologies employed to investigate human brain disorders and therefore we should be neither surprised nor disappointed. Replication and time will help in sorting out robust findings from artefacts. However, the serious student needs to invest time in understanding the technology and the methodology for this will help her greatly in formulating an early opinion of the validity of the findings.

REFERENCES

Abadie P, Boulenger JP, Benali K, Barre L, Zarifian E, Baron JC (1999) Relationships between trait and state anxiety and the central benzodiazepine receptor: a PET study. *European Journal of Neuroscience* **11**: 1470–1478.

Agren H, Reibring L (1994) PET studies of presynaptic monoamine metabolism in depressed patients and healthy volunteers. *Pharmacopsychiatry* **27**(1): 2–6.

Agren H, Reibrign L, Hartvig P, Tedroff J, Bjurling P, Lundqvist H, Langstrom B (1992) PET studies with L-[11C]5-HTP and L-[11C]dopa in brains of healthy volunteers and patients with major depression. *Clinical Neuropharmacology* **15**(Suppl 1 Pt A): 235A–236A.

Alexander GE, Crutcher MD, DeLong MR (1990) Basal ganglia-thalamocortical circuits: parallel substrates for motor, oculomotor, 'prefrontal' and 'limbic' functions. *Progress in Brain Research* **85**: 119–146.

Alptekin K, Degirmenci B, Kivircik B, Durak H, Yemez B, Derebek E, Tunca Z (2001) Tc-99m HMPAO brain perfusion SPECT in drug-free obsessive-compulsive patients without depression. *Psychiatry Research* **107**(1): 51–56.

Anand A, Verhoeff P, Seneca N, Zoghbi SS, Seibyl JP, Charney DS, Innis RB (2000) Brain SPECT imaging of amphetamine-induced dopamine release in euthymic bipolar disorder patients. *American Journal of Psychiatry* **157**(7): 1108–1114.

Attar-Levy D, Martinot JL, Blin J, Dao-Castellana MH, Crouzel C, Mazoyer B, Poirier MF, Bourdel MC, Aymard N, Syrota A, Feline A (1999) The cortical serotonin2 receptors studied with positron-emission tomography and [18-F]-setoperone during depressive illness and antidepressant treatment with clomipramine. *Biological Psychiatry* **45**(2): 180–186.

Austin MP, Dougall N, Ross M, Murray C, O'Carroll RE, Moffoot A, Ebmeier KP, Goodwin GM (1992) Single photon emission tomography with 99mTc-exametazime in major depression and the pattern of brain activity underlying the psychotic/neurotic continuum. *Journal of Affective Disorders* **26**(1): 31–43.

Aylward EH, Harris GJ, Hoehn-Saric R, Barta PE, Machlin SR, Pearlson GD (1996) Normal caudate nucleus in obsessive compulsive disorder assessed by quantitative neuro-imaging. *Archives of General Psychiatry* **53**(7): 577–574

Azari NP, Pietrini P, Horwitz B, Pettigrew KD, Leonard HL, Rapoport JL, Schapiro MB, Swedo SE (1993) Individual difference in cerebral metabolic patterns during pharmacotherapy in obsessive–compulsive disorder: a multiple regression/discriminant analysis of positron emission tomographic data. *Biological Psychiatry* **34**(11): 798–809.

Baker SC, Frith CD, Dolan RJ (1997) The interaction between mood and cognitive function studied with PET. *Psychological Medicine* **27**(3): 565–578.

Bartha R, Stein MB, Williamson PC, Drost DJ, Neufeld RW, Carr TJ, Canaran G, Densmore M, Anderson G, Siddiqui AR (1998) A short echo 1H spectroscopy and volumetric MRI study of the corpus striatum in patients with obsessive—compulsive disorder and comparison subjects. *American Journal of Psychiatry* **155**(11): 1584–1591.

Baxter LR Jr, Phelps ME, Mazziotta JC, Guze BH, Schwartz JM, Selin CE (1987) Local cerebral glucose metabolic rates in obsessive-compulsive disorder. A comparison with rates in unipolar depression and in normal controls. *Archives of General Psychiatry* **44**(3): 211–218.

Baxter LR Jr, Schwartz JM, Berman KS, Szuba MP, Guze BH, Mazziotta JC, Alazraki A, Selin CE, Ferng HK, Munford P (1992) Caudate glucose metabolic rate changes with both drug and behavior therapy for obsessive-compulsive disorder. *Archives of General Psychiatry* **49**(9): 681–689.

Baxter LR Jr, Schwartz JM, Mazziotta JC, Phelps ME, Pahl JJ, Guze BH, Fairbanks L (1988) Cerebral glucose metabolic rates in nondepressed patients with obsessive—compulsive disorder. *American Journal of Psychiatry* **145**(12): 1560–1563.

Baxter LR Jr, Schwartz JM, Phelps ME, Mazziotta JC, Guze BH, Selin CE, Gerner RH, Sumida RM (1989) Reduction of prefrontal cortex glucose metabolism common to three types of depression. *Archives of General Psychiatry* **46**(3): 243–250.

Behar D, Rapoport JL, Berg CJ, Denckla MB, Mann L, Cox C, Fedio P, Zahn T, Wolfman MG (1984) Computerized tomography and neuropsychological test measures in adolescents with obsessive-compulsive disorder. *American Journal of Psychiatry* **141**(3): 363–369.

Bell CJ, Malizia AL, Nutt DJ (1999) The neurobiology of social phobia. *European Archives of Psychiatry Clinical Neuroscience* **249**(Suppl 1): S11–S18.

Bench CJ, Friston KJ, Brown RG, Scott LC, Frackowiak RS, Dolan RJ (1992) The anatomy of melancholia — focal abnormalities of cerebral blood flow in major depression. *Psychological Medicine* **23**(3): 607–615.

Benkelfat C, Bradwejn J, Meyer E, Ellenbogen M, Milot S, Gjedde A, Evans A (1995) Functional neuroanatomy of CCK4-induced anxiety in normal healthy volunteers. *Am J Psychiatry* **152**(8): 1180–1184.

Benkelfat C, Nordahl TE, Semple WE, King AC, Murphy DL, Cohen RM (1990) Local cerebral glucose metabolic rates in obsessive-compulsive disorder. Patients treated with clomipramine. *Archives of General Psychiatry* **47**(9): 840–848.

Birbaumer N, Grodd W, Diedrich O, Klose U, Erb M, Lotze M, Schneider F, Weiss U, Flor H (1998) fMRI reveals amygdala activation to human faces in social phobics. *Neuroreport* **9**(6): 1223–1226.

Bisaga A, Katz JL, Antonini A, Wright CE, Margouleff C, Gorman JM, Eidelberg D (1998) Cerebral glucose metabolism in women with panic disorder. *American Journal of Psychiatry* **155**(9): 1178–1183.

Biver F, Goldman S, Delvenne V, Luxen A, De Maertelaer V, Hubain P, Mendlewicz J, Lostra F (1994) Frontal and parietal metabolic disturbances in unipolar depression. *Biological Psychiatry* **36**(5): 381–388.

Biver F, Goldman S, Francois A, De La Porte C, Luxen A, Gribomont B, Lostra F (1995) Changes in metabolism of cerebral glucose after stereotactic leukotomy for refractory obsessive-compulsive disorder: a case report. *Journal of Neurology, Neurosurgery and Psychiatry* **58**(4): 502–550.

Biver F, Wikler D, Lotstra F, Damhaut P, Goldman S, Mendlewicz J (1997) Serotonin 5-HT2 receptor imaging in major depression: focal changes in orbito-insular cortex. *British Journal of Psychiatry* **171**: 444–448.

Bonne O, Brandes D, Gilboa A, Gomori JM, Shenton ME, Pitman RK, Shalev AY (2001) Longitudinal MRI study of hippocampal volume in trauma survivors with PTSD. *Am J Psychiatry* **158**(8): 1248–1251.

Boshuisen ML, Ter Horst GJ, Paans AMJ, Reinders AATS, den Boer JA (2002) rCBF differences between panic disorder patients and control subjects during anticipatory anxiety and rest. *Biological Psychiatry* **52**(2): 126–135.

Brandt CA, Meller J, Keweloh L, Hoschel K, Staedt J, Munz D, Stoppe G (1998) Increased benzodiazepine receptor density in the prefrontal cortex in patients with panic disorder. *Journal of Neural Transmission* **105**(10–12): 1325–1133.

Bremner JD, Innis RB, Ng CK, Staib LH, Salomon RM, Bronen RA, Duncan J, Southwick SM, Krystal JH, Rich D, Zubal G, Dey H, Soufer R, Charney DS (1997) Positron emission tomography measurement of cerebral metabolic correlates of yohimbine administration in combat-related posttraumatic stress disorder. *Archives of General Psychiatry* **54**(3): 246–254.

Bremner JD, Innis RB, Southwick SM, Stabi L, Zoghbi S, Charney DS (2000a) Decreased benzodiazepine receptor binding in prefrontal cortex in combat-related posttraumatic stress disorder. *American Journal of Psychiatry* **157**(7): 1120–1126.

Bremner JD, Innis RB, White T, Fujita M, Silbersweig D, Goddard AW, Staib L, Stern E, Cappiello A, Woods S, Baldwin R, Charney DS (2000b) SPECT [I-123]iomazenil measurement of the benzodiazepine receptor in panic disorder. *Biological Psychiatry* **47**(2): 96–106.

Bremner JD, Narayan M, Staib LH, Southwick SM, McGlashan T, Charney DS (1999) Neural correlates of memories of childhood sexual abuse in women with and without post-traumatic stress disorder. *American Journal of Psychiatry* **156**: 1787–1795.

Bremner JD, Randall P, Scott TM, Bronen RA, Seibyl JP, Southwick SM, Delaney RC, McCarthy G, Charney DS, Innis RB (1995) MRI-based measurement of hippocampal volume in patients with combat-related posttraumatic stress disorder. *Am J Psychiatry* **152**(7): 973–981.

Bremner JD, Randall P, Vermetten E, Staib L, Bronen RA, Mazure C, Capelli S, McCarthy G, Innis RB, Charney DS (1997) Magnetic resonance imaging-based measurement of hippocampal volume in posttraumatic stress disorder related to childhood physical and sexual abuse – a preliminary report. *Biol Psychiatry* **41**(1): 23–32.

Bremner JD, Vythilingam M, Ng CK, Vermetten E, Nazeer A, Oren DA, Berman RM, Charney DS (2003) Regional brain metabolic correlates of alpha-methylparatyrosine-induced depressive symptoms: implications for the neural circuitry of depression. *JAMA* **289**(23): 3125–3134.

Brody AL, Saxena S, Schwartz JM, Stoessel PW, Maidment K, Phelps ME, Baxter LR Jr (1998) FDG-PET predictors of response to behavioral therapy versus pharmacotherapy in obsessive-compulsive disorder. *Psychiatry Research: Neuroimaging* **84**(1): 1–6.

Brody AL, Saxena S, Stoessel P, Gillies LA, Fairbanks LA, Alborzian S, Phelps ME, Huang SC, Wu HM, Ho ML, Ho MK, Au SC, Maidment K, Baxter LR Jr (2001) Regional brain metabolic changes in patients with major depression treated with either paroxetine or interpersonal therapy: preliminary findings. *Archives of General Psychiatry* **58**(7): 631–640.

Buchsbaum MS, Wu J, DeLisi LE, Holcomb H, Kessler R, Johnson J, King AC, Hazlett E, Langston K, Post RM (1986) Frontal cortex and basal ganglia metabolic rates assessed by positron emission tomography with [18F]2-deoxyglucose in affective illness. *Journal of Affective Disorders* **10**(2): 137–152.

Buchsbaum MS, Wu J, Haier R, Hazlett E, Ball R, Katz M, Sokolski K, Lagunas-Solar M, Langer D (1987) Positron emission tomography assessment of effects of benzodiazepines on regional glucose metabolic rate in patients with anxiety disorder. *Life Sciences* **40**(25): 2393–2400.

Busatto GF, Buchpiguel CA, Zamignani DR, Garrido GE, Glabus MF, Rosario-Campos MC, Castro CC, Maia A, Rocha ET, McGuire PK, Miguel EC (2001) Regional cerebral blood flow abnormalities in early-onset obsessive-compulsive disorder: an exploratory SPECT study. *Journal of the American Academy of Child and Adolescent Psychiatry* **40**(3): 347–354.

Busatto GF, Zamignani DR, Buchpiguel CA, Garrido GE, Glabus MF, Rocha ET, Maia AF, Rosario-Campos MC, Campi Castro C, Furuie SS, Gutierrez MA, McGuire PK, Miguel EC (2000) A voxel-based investigation of regional cerebral blood flow abnormalities in obsessive-compulsive disorder using single photon emission computed tomography (SPECT). *Psychiatry Research* **99**(1): 15–27.

Chatton JY, Pellerin L, Magistretti PJ (2003) GABA uptake into astrocytes is not associated with significant metabolic cost: implications for brain imaging of inhibitory transmission. *Proc Natl Acad Sci USA* **100**(21): 12 456–12 461.

Chua P, Krams M, Toni I, Passingham R, Dolan R (1999) A functional anatomy of anticipatory anxiety. *Neuroimage* **9** (6 Pt 1): 563–571.

Coryell W (1988) Panic disorder and mortality. *Psychiatric Clinics North America* **11**: 433–440.

Cottraux J, Gerard D, Cinotti L, Froment JC, Deiber MP, Le Bars D, Galy G, Millet P, Labbe C, Lavenne F, Bouvard M, Mauguiere F (1996) A controlled positron emission tomography study of obsessive and neutral auditory stimulation in obsessive-compulsive disorder with checking rituals. *Psychiatry Research* **60**(2–3): 101–112.

Crabbe JC, Wahlsten D, Dudek BC (1999) Genetics of mouse behavior: Interactions with laboratory environment. *Science* **284**: 1670–1672.

Dahlstrom M, Ahonen A, Ebeling H, Torniainen P, Heikkila J, Moilanen I (2000) Elevated hypothalamic/midbrain serotonin (monoamine) transporter availability in depressive drug-naive children and adolescents. *Molecular Psychiatry* **5**(5): 514–522.

Dantendorfer K, Prayer D, Kramer J, Amering M, Baischer W, Berger P, Schoder M, Steinberger K, Windhaber J, Imhof H, Katschnig H (1996) High frequency of EEG and MRI brain abnormalities in panic disorder. *Psychiatry Res* **68**(1): 41–53.

Davidson JR, Krishnan KR, Charles HC, Boyko O, Potts NL, Ford SM, Patterson L (1993) Magnetic resonance spectroscopy in social phobia: preliminary findings. *J Clin Psychiatry* **54** (Suppl): 19–25.

Davis M, Rainnie D, Cassell M (1994) Neurotransmission in the rat amygdala related to fear and anxiety. *Trends in Neuroscience* **17**: 208–214.

Davis M, Shi C (1999) The extended amygdala: are the central nucleus of the amygdala and the bednucleus of the stria terminalis differentially involved in fear versus anxiety? *Annals of the New York Academy of Sciences* **877**: 281–291.

de Asis JM, Stern E, Alexopoulos GS, Pan H, Van Gorp W, Blumberg H, Kalayam B, Eidelberg D, Kiosses D, Silbersweig DA (2001) Hippocampal and anterior cingulate activation deficits in patients with geriatric depression. *American Journal of Psychiatry* **158**(8): 1321–1323.

De Bellis MD, Casey BJ, Dahl RE, Birmaher B, Williamson DE, Thomas KM, Axelson DA, Frustaci K, Boring AM, Hall J, Ryan ND (2000) A pilot study of amygdala volumes in pediatric generalized anxiety disorder. *Biol Psychiatry* **48**(1): 51–57.

De Cristofaro MT, Sessarego A, Pupi A, Biondi F, Faravelli C (1993) Brain perfusion abnormalities in drug-naive, lactate-sensitive panic patients: a SPECT study. *Biological Psychiatry* **33**(7): 505–512.

D'haenen HA, Bossuyt A (1994) Dopamine D2 receptors in depression measured with single photon emission computed tomography. *Biological Psychiatry* **35**(2): 128–132.

D'haenen H, Bossuyt A, Mertens J, Bossuyt-Piron C, Gijsemans M, Kaufman L (1992) SPECT imaging of serotonin-2 receptors in depression. *Psychiatry Research* **45**(4): 227–237.

Drevets WC, Bogers W, Raichle ME (2002) Functional anatomical correlates of antidepressant drug treatment assessed using PET measures of regional glucose metabolism. *European Neuropsychopharmacology* **12**(6): 527–544.

Drevets WC, Frank E, Price JC, Kupfer DJ, Holt D, Greer PJ, Huang Y, Gautier C, Mathis C (1999) PET imaging of serotonin 1A receptor binding in depression. *Biological Psychiatry* **46**(10): 1375–1387.

Drevets WC, Videen TQ, MacLeod AK, Haller JW, Raichle ME (1992a) PET images of blood flow changes during anxiety: correction. *Science* **256**(5064): 1696.

Drevets WC, Videen TO, Price JL, Preskorn SH, Carmichael ST, Raichle ME (1992b) A functional anatomical study of unipolar depression. *Journal of Neuroscience* **12**(9): 3628–3641.

Dunn RT, Kimbrell TA, Ketter TA, Frye MA, Willis MW, Luckenbaugh DA, Post RM (2002) Principal components of the Beck Depression Inventory and regional cerebral metabolism in unipolar and bipolar depression. *Biological Psychiatry* **51**(5): 387–399.

Ebert D, Feistel H, Kaschka W, Barocka A, Pirner A (1994) Single photon emission computerized tomography assessment of cerebral dopamine D2 receptor blockade in depression before and after sleep deprivation – preliminary results. *Biological Psychiatry* **35**(11): 880–885.

Ebert D, Feistel H, Loew T, Pirner A (1996) Dopamine and depression – striatal dopamine D2 receptor SPECT before and after antidepressant therapy. *Psychopharmacology* **126**(1): 91–94.

Ebert D, Speck O, Konig A, Berger M, Hennig J, Hohagen F (1997) 1H-magnetic resonance spectroscopy in obsessive-compulsive disorder: evidence for neuronal loss in the cingulate gyrus and the right striatum. *Psychiatry Research* **74**(3): 173–176.

Elliott R, Baker SC, Rogers RD, O'Leary DA, Paykel ES, Frith CD, Dolan RJ, Sahakian BJ (1997) Prefrontal dysfunction in depressed patients performing a complex planning task: a study using positron emission tomography. *Psychological Medicine* **27**(4): 931–942.

Fischer H, Anderrson JL, Furmark T, Fredrickson M (1998) Brain correlates of an unexpected panic attack: a human positron emission tomographic study. *Neuroscience Letters* **251**(2): 137–140.

Fontaine R, Breton G, Dery R, Fontaine S, Elie R (1990) Temporal lobe abnormalities in panic disorder: an MRI study. *Biol Psychiatry* **27**(3): 304–310.

Francis PT, Pangalos MN, Stephens PH, Bartlett JR, Bridges PK, Malizia AL, Neary D, Procter AW, Thomas DJ, Bowen DM (1993) Antemortem measurements of neurotransmission: possible implications for pharmacotherapy of Alzheimer's disease and depression. *Journal of Neurology, Neurosurgery and Psychiatry* **56**(1): 80–84.

Freeman TW, Cardwell D, Karson CN, Komoroski RA (1998) In vivo proton magnetic resonance spectroscopy of the medial temporal lobes of subjects with combat-related posttraumatic stress disorder. *Magnetic Resonance in Medicine* **40**(1): 66–71.

Furmark T, Tillfors M, Marteinsdottir I, Fischer H, Pissiota A, Langstrom B, Fredrikson M (2002) Common changes in cerebral blood flow in patients with social phobia treated with citalopram or cognitive-behavioral therapy. *Archives of General Psychiatry* **49**(5): 425–433.

Garber HJ, Ananth JV, Chiu LC, Griswold VJ, Oldendorf WH (1989) Nuclear magnetic resonance study of obsessive-compulsive disorder. *American Journal of Psychiatry* **146**(8): 1001–1005.

George MS, Ketter TA, Parekh PI, Horwitz B, Herscovitch P, Post RM (1995) Brain activity during transient sadness and happiness in healthy women. *American Journal of Psychiatry* **152**(3): 341–351.

Gurvits TV, Shenton ME, Hokama H, Ohta H, Lasko NB, Gilbertson MW, Orr SP, Kikinis R, Jolesz FA, McCarley RW, Pitman RK (1996) Magnetic resonance imaging study of hippocampal volume in chronic, combat-related posttraumatic stress disorder. *Biological Psychiatry* **40**(11): 1091–1099.

Hansen ES, Hasselbalch S, Law I, Bolwig TG (2002) The caudate nucleus in obsessive-compulsive disorder. Reduced metabolism following treatment with paroxetine: a PET study. *International Journal of Neuropsychopharmacology* **5**(1): 1–10.

Hargreaves R (2002) Imaging substance P receptors (NK1) in the living human brain using positron emission tomography. *Journal of Clinical Psychiatry* **63**(Suppl 11): 18–24.

Hariri AR, Mattay VS, Tessitore A, Kolachana B, Fera F, Goldman D, Egan MF, Weinberger DR (2002) Serotonin transporter genetic variation and the response of the human amygdala. *Science* **297**(5580): 400–403.

Henry ME, Schmidt ME, Matochik JA, Stoddard EP, Potter WZ (2001) The effects of ECT on brain glucose: a pilot FDG PET study. *Journal of ECT* **17**(1): 33–40.

Hoehn-Saric R, Schlaepfer TE, Greenberg BD, McLeod DR, Pearlson GD, Wong SH (2001) Cerebral blood flow in obsessive-compulsive patients with major depression: effect of treatment with sertraline or desipramine on treatment responders and non-responders. *Psychiatry Research* **108**(2): 89–100.

Horwitz B, Swedo SE, Grady CL, Pietrini P, Schapiro MB, Rapoport JL, Rapoport SI (1991) Cerebral metabolic pattern in obsessive-compulsive disorder: altered intercorrelations between regional rates of glucose utilization. *Psychiatry Research* **40**(4): 221–237.

Javanmard M, Shlik J, Kennedy SH, Vaccarino FJ, Houle S, Bradwejn J (1999) Neuroanatomic correlates of CCK-4-induced panic attacks in healthy humans: a comparison of two time points. *Biol Psychiatry* **45**(7): 872–882.

Jenike MA, Breiter HC, Baer L, Kennedy DN, Savage CR, Olivares MJ, O'Sullivan RL, Shera DM, Rauch SL, Keuthen N, Rosen BR, Caviness VS, Filipek PA (1996) Cerebral structural abnormalities in obsessive–compulsive disorder: a quantitative morphometric magnetic resonance imaging study. *Archives of General Psychiatry* **53**(7): 625–632.

Kaschka W, Feistel H, Ebert D (1995) Reduced benzodiazepine receptor binding in panic disorders measured by iomazenil SPECT. *Journal of Psychiatric Research* **29**: 427–423.

Kennedy SH, Evans KR, Kruger S, Mayberg HS, Meyer JH, McCann S, Arifuzzman AI, Houle S, Vaccarino FJ (2001) Changes in regional brain glucose metabolism measured with positron emission tomography after paroxetine treatment of major depression. *American Journal of Psychiatry* **158**(6): 899–905.

Kessler RC, DuPont RL, Berglund P, Wittchen HU (1999) Impairment in pure and comorbid generalized anxiety disorder and major depression at 12 months in two national surveys. *American Journal of Psychiatry* **156**(12): 1915–1923.

Ketter TA, Andreason PJ, George MS, Lee C, Gill DS, Parekh PI. Willis MW, Herscovitch P, Post RM (1996) Anterior paralimbic mediation of procaine-induced emotional and psychosensory experiences. *Archives of General Psychiatry* **53**(1): 59–69.

Ketter TA, Kimbrell TA, George MS, Willis MW, Benson BE, Danielson A, Frye MA, Herscovitch P, Post RM (1999) Baseline cerebral hypermetabolism associated with carbamazepine response, and hypometabolism with nimodipine response in mood disorders. *Biological Psychiatry* **46**(10): 1364–1374.

Kim MC, Lee TK, Son BC, Choi CR, Lee C (2001) Regional cerebral blood flow changes in patients with intractable obsessive compulsive disorders treated by limbic leukotomy. *Stereotactic and Functional Neurosurgery* **76**(3–4): 249–255.

Kim SG, Ugurbil K, Strick PL (1994) Activation of a cerebellar output nucleus during cognitive processing. *Science* **265**(5174): 949–951.

Kimbrell TA, Ketter TA, George MS, Little JT, Benson BE, Willis MW, Herscovitch P, Post RM (2002) Regional cerebral glucose utilization in patients with a range of severities of unipolar depression. *Biological Psychiatry* **51**: 237–252.

Klimke A, Larisch R, Janz A, Vosberg H, Muller-Gartner HW, Gaebel W (1999) Dopamine D2 receptor binding before and after treatment of major depression measured by [123I]IBZM SPECT. *Psychiatry Research* **90**(2): 91–101.

Kuikka JT, Pitkanen A, Lepola U, Partanen K, Vainio P, Bergstrom KA, Wieler HJ, Kaiser KP, Mittelbach L, Koponen H (1995) Abnormal regional benzodiazepine receptor uptake in the prefrontal cortex in patients with panic disorder. *Nuclear Medicine Communications* **16**: 273–280.

Kwon JS, Kim JJ, Lee DW, Lee JS, Lee DS, Kim MS, Lyoo IK, Cho MJ, Lee MC (2003) Neural correlates of clinical symptoms and cognitive dysfunctions in obsessive-compulsive disorder. *Psychiatry Research* **122**(1) :37–47.

Laasonen-Balk T, Kuikka J, Viinamaki H, Husso-Saastamoinen M, Lehtonen J, Tiihonen J (1999) Striatal dopamine transporter density in major depression. *Psychopharmacology* **144**(3): 282–285.

Lanius RA, Williamson PC, Densmore M, Boksman K, Gupta MA, Neufeld RW, Gati JS, Menon RS (2001) Neural correlates of traumatic memories in posttraumatic stress disorder: a functional MRI investigation. *Am J Psychiatry* **158**(11): 1920–1922.

Larisch R, Klimke A, Mayoral F, Hamacher K, Herzog HR, Vosberg H, Tosch M, Gaebel W, Rivas F, Coenen HH, Muller-Gartner H-W (2001) Disturbance of serotonin 5-HT2 receptors in remitted patients suffering from hereditary depressive disorder. *Nuklearmedizin* **40**(4): 129–134.

Laruelle M, Huang Y (2001) Vulnerability of positron emission tomography radiotracers to endogenous competition. New insights. *Q J Nucl Med* **45**(2): 124–138.

LeDoux JE (2000) Emotion circuits in the brain. *Annual Review of Neuroscience* **23**: 155–184.

Liberzon I, Taylor SF, Amdur R, Jung TD, Chamberlain KR, Minoshima S, Koeppe RA (1999) Brain activation in PTSD in response to trauma-related stimuli. *Biological Psychiatry* **45**: 817–826.

Liberzon I, Taylor SF, Fig LM, Koeppe RA (1996–97) Alteration of corticothalamic perfusion ratios during a PTSD flashback. *Depression and Anxiety* **4**(3): 146–150.

Lucey JV, Costa DC, Blanes T, Busatto GF, Pilowsky LS, Takei N, Marks IM, Ell PJ, Kerwin RW (1995) Regional cerebral blood flow in obsessive-compulsive disordered patients at rest. Differential correlates with obsessive-compulsive and anxious-avoidant dimensions. *British Journal of Psychiatry* **167**(5): 629–634.

Luxenberg JS, Swedo SE, Flament MF, Friedland RP, Rapoport J, Rapoport SI (1988) Neuroanatomical abnormalities in obsessive-compulsive disorder detected with quantitative X-ray computed tomography. *American Journal of Psychiatry* **145**(9): 1089–1093.

Machlin SR, Harris GJ, Pearlson GD, Hoehn-Saric R, Jeffery P, Camargo EE (1991) Elevated medial-frontal cerebral blood flow in obsessive-compulsive patients: a SPECT study. *American Journal of Psychiatry* **148**(9): 1240–1242.

Magistretti PJ, Pellerin L (1999) Cellular mechanisms of brain energy metabolism and their relevance to functional brain imaging. *Philos Trans R Soc Lond B Biol Sci* **354**(1387): 1155–63.

Malison RT, Price LH, Berman R, van Dyck CH, Pelton GH, Carpenter L, Sanacora G, Owens MJ, Nemeroff CB, Rajeevan N, Baldwin RM, Seibyl JP, Innis RB, Charney DS (1998) Reduced brain serotonin transporter availability in major depression as measured by [123I]-2 beta-carbomethoxy-3 beta-(4-iodophenyl)tropane and single photon emission computed tomography. *Biological Psychiatry* **44**(11): 1090–1098.

Malizia AL (1999) What do brain imaging studies tell us about anxiety disorders? *J Psychopharmacol* **13**(4): 372–378.

Malizia AL (2001) Positron emitting ligands in the study of the clinical psychopharmacology of anxiety and anxiety disorders. MD thesis. University of Bristol.

Malizia AL, Allen S, Maisey M, Bartlett JR, Bridges PK (1994) Changes in low frontal cerebral blood flow measured with Tc-99hmpao SPECT correlate with outcome in stereotactic subcaudate tractotomy carried out for treatment resistant depression. In Zohar J, Roose SP, Nolen WA (eds) *Refractory Depression*. Chichester, UK: John Wiley, pp. 163–167.

Malizia AL, Cunningham VJ, Bell CJ, Liddle PF, Jones T, Nutt DJ (1998) Decreased brain GABA(A)-benzodiazepine receptor binding in panic disorder: preliminary results from a quantitative PET study. *Archives of General Psychiatry* **55**(8): 715–720.

Malizia AL, Cunningham VJ, Nutt DJ (1997) Flumazenil delivery changes in panic disorder at rest. *Neuroimage* **5**(4, part 2): S302.

Mann JJ, Stanley M, McBride PA, McEwen BS (1986) Increased serotonin2 and beta-adrenergic receptor binding in the frontal cortices of suicide victims. *Archives of General Psychiatry* **43**(10): 954–959.

Martinez D, Hwang DR, Mawlawi O, Kent J, Simpson N, Parsey RV, Slifstein M, Huang Y, Van Heertum R, Abi-Dargham A, Caltabiano S, Malizia A, Cowley H, Mann JJ, Laruelle M (2001) Differential occupancy of somatodendritic and postsynaptic 5-HT$_{1A}$

receptors by pindolol: a dose-occupancy study with [^{11}C]WAY100635 and positron emission tomography in humans. *Neuropsychopharmacology* **24**(3): 209–229.

Martinot JL, Allilaire JF, Mazoyer BM, Hantouche E, Huret JD, Legaut-Demare F, Deslauriers AG, Hardy P, Pappata S, Baron JC (1990a) Obsessive-compulsive disorder: a clinical, neuropsychological and positron emission tomography study. *Acta Psychiatrica Scandinavica* **82**(3): 233–242.

Martinot M-LP, Bragulat V, Artiges E, Dolle F, Hinnen F, Jouvent R, Martinot J-L (2001) Decreased presynaptic dopamine function in the left caudate of depressed patients with affective flattening and psychomotor retardation. *American Journal of Psychiatry* **158**(2): 314–316.

Martinot JL, Hardy P, Feline A, Huret JD, Mazoyer B, Attar-Levy D, Pappata S, Syrota A (1990b) Left prefrontal glucose hypometabolism in the depressed state: a confirmation. *American Journal of Psychiatry* **147**(10): 1313–1317.

Massana G, Serra-Grabulosa JM, Salgado-Pineda P, Gasto C, Junque C, Massana J, Mercader JM, Gomez B, Tobena A, Salamero M (2003a) Amygdalar atrophy in panic disorder patients detected by volumetric magnetic resonance imaging. *Neuroimage* **19**(1): 80–90.

Massana G, Serra-Grabulosa JM, Salgado-Pineda P, Gasto C, Junque C, Massana J, Mercader JM (2003b) Parahippocampal gray matter density in panic disorder: a voxel-based morphometric study. *Am J Psychiatry* **160**(3): 566–568.

Mathew RJ, Wilson WH (1991) Evaluation of the effects of diazepam and an experimental anti-anxiety drug on cerebral blood flow. *Psychiatry Research* **40**: 125–134.

Mathew RJ, Wilson WH (1997) Intracranial and extracranial blood flow during acute anxiety. *Psychiatry Res* **74**(2): 93–107.

Mayberg H (2002) Depression, II: localization of pathophysiology. *American Journal of Psychiatry* **159**(12): 1979.

Mayberg HS, Brannan SK, Mahurin RK, Jerabek PA, Brickman JS, Tekell JL, Silva JA, McGinnis S, Glass TG, Martin CC, Fox PT (1997) Cingulate function in depression: a potential predictor of treatment response. *Neuroreport* **8**(4): 1057–1061.

Mayberg HS, Brannan SK, Tekell JL, Silva JA, Mahurin RK, McGinnis S, Jerabek PA (2000) Regional metabolic effects of fluoxetine in major depression: serial changes and relationship to clinical response. *Biological Psychiatry* **48**(8): 830–843.

Mayberg HS, Liotti M, Brannan SK, McGinnis S, Mahurin RK, Jerabek PA, Silva JA, Tekell JL, Martin CC, Lancaster JL, Fox PT (1999) Reciprocal limbic-cortical function and negative mood: converging PET findings in depression and normal sadness. *American Journal of Psychiatry* **156**(5): 675–682.

McGuire PK, Bench CJ, Frith CD, Marks IM, Frackowiak RS, Dolan RJ (1994) Functional anatomy of obsessive-compulsive phenomena. *British Journal of Psychiatry* **164**: 459–468.

Melichar JK, Haida A, Rhodes C, Reynolds AH, Nutt DJ, Malizia AL (2001) Venlafaxine occupation at the noradrenaline reuptake site: in-vivo determination in healthy volunteers. *Journal of Psychopharmacology* **15**(1): 9–12.

Meltzer CC, Smith G, Price JC, Reynolds III CF, Mathis CA, Greer P, Lopresti B, Mintun MA, Pollock BG, Ben-Eliezer D, Cantwell MN, Kaye W, DeKosky ST (1998) Reduced binding of [18F]altanserin to serotonin type 2A receptors in aging: persistence of effect after partial volume correction. *Brain Research* **813**: 167–171.

Mervaala E, Kononen M, Fohr J, Husso-Saastamoinen M, Valkonen-Korhonen M, Kuikka JT, Viinamaki H, Tammi AK, Tiihonen J, Partanen J, Lehtonen J (2001) SPECT and neuropsychological performance in severe depression treated with ECT. *Journal of Affective Disorders* **66**(1): 47–58.

Messa C, Colombo C, Moresco RM, Gobbo C, Galli L, Lucignani G, Gilardi M, Rizzo G, Smeraldi E, Zanardi R, Artigas F, Fazio F (2003) 5-HT2A receptor binding is reduced in drug-naive and unchanged in SSRI-responder depressed patients compared to healthy controls: a PET study. *Psychopharmacology* **167**(1): 72–78.

Meyer JH, Goulding VS, Wilson AA, Hussey D, Christensen BK, Houle S (2002) Bupropion occupancy of the dopamine transporter is low during clinical treatment. *Psychopharmacology* **163**(1): 102–105.

Meyer JH, Kapur S, Eisfeld B, Brown GM, Houle S, DaSilva J, Wilson AA, Rafi-Tari S, Mayberg HS, Kennedy SH (2001a) The effect of paroxetine on 5-HT(2A) receptors in depression: an [(18)F]setoperone PET imaging study. *American Journal of Psychiatry* **158**(1): 78–85.

Meyer JH, Kapur S, Houle S, DaSilva J, Owczarek B, Brown GM, Wilson AA, Kennedy SH (1999) Prefrontal cortex 5-HT2 receptors in depression: an [18F]setoperone PET imaging study. *American Journal of Psychiatry* **156**(7): 1029–1034.

Meyer JH, Kruger S, Wilson AA, Christensen BK, Goulding VS, Schaffer A, Minifie C, Houle S, Hussey D, Kennedy SH (2001b) Lower dopamine transporter binding potential in striatum during depression. *Neuroreport* **12**(18): 4121–4125.

Meyer JH, Swinson R, Kennedy SH, Houle S, Brown GM. (2000) Increased left posterior parietal-temporal cortex activation after D-fenfluramine in women with panic disorder. *Psychiatry Research* **98**(3): 133–143

Meyer JH, Wilson AA, Ginovart N, Goulding V, Hussey D, Hood K, Houle S (2001c) Occupancy of serotonin transporters by paroxetine and citalopram during treatment of depression: a [(11)C]DASB PET imaging study. *American Journal of Psychiatry* **158**(11): 1843–1849.

Mindus P, Ericson K, Greitz T, Meyerson BA, Nyman H, Sjogren I (1986) Regional cerebral glucose metabolism in anxiety disorders studied with positron emission tomography before and after psychosurgical intervention. A preliminary report. *Acta Radiologica – Supplementum* **369**: 444–448.

Mountz JM, Modell JG, Wilson MW, Curtis GC, Lee MA, Schmaltz S, Kuhl DE (1989) Positron emission tomographic evaluation of cerebral blood flow during state anxiety in simple phobia. *Archives of General Psychiatry* **16**: 501–504.

Murray CJ, Lopez AD (1997) Global mortality, disability, and the contribution of risk factors: Global Burden of Disease Study. *Lancet* **349**(9063): 1436–1442.

Neumeister A, Willeit M, Praschak-Rieder N, Asenbaum S, Stastny J, Hilger E, Pirker W, Konstantinidis A, Kasper S (2001) Dopamine transporter availability in symptomatic depressed patients with seasonal affective disorder and healthy controls. *Psychological Medicine* **31**(8): 1467–1473.

Neumeister A, Bain E, Nugent AC, Carson RE, Bonne O, Luckenbaugh DA, Eckelman W, Herscovitch P, Charney DS, Drevets WC (2004) Reduced serotonin type 1A receptor binding in panic disorder. *J Neurosci* **24**(3): 589–591.

Nishizawa S, Benkelfat C, Young SN, Leyton M, Mzengeza S, de Montigny C, Blier P, Diksic M (1997) Differences between males and females in rates of serotonin synthesis in human brain. *Proceedings of the National Academy of Sciences of the United States of America* **94**(10): 5308–5313.

Nobler MS, Oquendo MA, Kegeles LS, Malone KM, Campbell CC, Sackeim HA, Mann JJ (2001) Decreased regional brain metabolism after ect. *American Journal of Psychiatry* **158**(2): 305–308.

Nobler MS, Sackeim HA, Prohovnik I, Moeller JR, Mukherjee S, Schnur DB, Prudic J, Devanand DP (1994) Regional cerebral blood flow in mood disorders, III. Treatment and clinical response. *Archives of General Psychiatry* **51**(11): 884–897.

Nofzinger EA, Berman S, Fasiczka A, Miewald JM, Meltzer CC, Price JC, Sembrat RC, Wood A, Thase ME (2001) Effects of bupropion SR on anterior paralimbic function during waking and REM sleep in depression: preliminary findings using. *Psychiatry Research* **106**(2): 95–111.

Nordahl TE, Benkelfat C, Semple WE, Gross M, King AC, Cohen RM (1989) Cerebral glucose metabolic rates in obsessive compulsive disorder. *Neuropsychopharmacology* **2**(1): 23–28.

Nordahl TE, Semple WE, Gross M, Mellman TA, Stein MB, Goyer P, King AC, Uhde TW, Cohen RM (1990) Cerebral glucose metabolic differences in patients with panic disorder. *Neuropsychopharmacology* **3**: 261–272.

Nordahl TE, Stein MB, Benkelfat C, Semple WE, Andreason P, Zametkin A, Uhde TW, Cohen RM (1998) Regional cerebral metabolic asymmetries replicated in an independent group of patients with panic disorders. *Biological Psychiatry* **44**(10): 998–1006.

Nutt DJ, Glue P, Lawson C, Wilson S (1990) Flumazenil provocation of panic attacks. *Archives of General Psychiatry* **47**: 917–925.

O'Carroll RE, Moffoot AP, van Beck M, Dougall N, Murray C, Ebmeier KP, Goodwin GM (1993) The effect of anxiety induction on the regional uptake of 99tc-exametazime in simple phobia as shown by single photon emission tomography (SPET). *Journal of Affective Disorders* **28**: 203–210.

Olsson H, Farde L (2001) Potentials and pitfalls using high affinity radioligands in PET and SPET determinations on regional drug induced D2 receptor occupancy – a simulation study based on experimental data. *Neuroimage* **14**(4): 936–945.

Ontiveros A, Fontaine R, Breton G, Elie R, Fontaine S, Dery R (1989) Correlation of severity of panic disorder and neuroanatomical changes on magnetic resonance imaging. *J Neuropsychiatry Clin Neurosci* **1**(4): 404–408.

Osuch EA, Benson B, Geraci M, Podell D, Herscovitch P, McCann UD, Post RM (2001) Regional cerebral blood flow correlated with flashback intensity in patients with posttraumatic stress disorder. *Biological Psychiatry* **50**(4): 246–253.

Parsey RV, Oquendo MA, Zea-Ponce Y, Rodenhiser J, Kegeles LS, Pratap M, Cooper TB, Van Heertum R, Mann JJ, Laruelle M (2001) Dopamine D(2) receptor availability and amphetamine-induced dopamine release in unipolar depression. *Biological Psychiatry* **50**(5): 313–322.

Pearlson GD. Wong DF. Tune LE. Ross CA. Chase GA. Links JM. Dannals RF, Wilson AA, Ravert HT, Wagner HN Jr (1995) In vivo D2 dopamine receptor density in psychotic and nonpsychotic patients with bipolar disorder. *Archives of General Psychiatry* **52**(6): 471–477.

Perani D, Colombo C, Bressi S, Bonfanti A, Grassi F, Scarone S, Bellodi L, Smeraldi E, Fazio F (1995) [18F]FDG PET study in obsessive-compulsive disorder. A clinical/metabolic correlation study after treatment. *British Journal of Psychiatry* **166**(2): 244–250.

Petty F, Chae Y, Kramer G, Jordan S, Wilson L (1994) Learned helplessness sensitizes hippocampal norepinephrine to mild restress. *Biological Psychiatry* **35**(12): 903–908.

Peyron R, Le Bars D, Cinotti L, Garcia-Larrea L, Galy G, Landais P, Millet P, Lavenne F, Froment JC, Krogsgaard-Larsen P (1994) Effects of GABAA receptors activation on brain glucose metabolism in normal subjects and temporal lobe epilepsy (TLE) patients. A positron emission tomography (PET) study. Part I: Brain glucose metabolism is increased after GABAA receptors activation. *Epilepsy Res* **19**(1): 45–54.

Pirker W, Asenbaum S, Kasper S, Walter H, Angelberger P, Koch G, Pozzera A, Deecke L, Podreka I, Brucke T (1995) beta-CIT SPECT demonstrates blockade of 5-HT-uptake sites by citalopram in the human brain in vivo. *Journal of Neural Transmission – General Section* **100**(3): 247–256.

Pissiota A, Frans O, Fernandez M, von Knorring L, Fischer H, Fredrikson M (2002) Neurofunctional correlates of posttraumatic stress disorder: a PET symptom provocation study. *European Archives of Psychiatry and Clinical Neuroscience* **252**(2): 68–75.

Pogarell O, Hamann C, Popperl G, Juckel G, Chouker M, Zaudig M, Riedel M, Moller HJ, Hegerl U, Tatsch K (2003) Elevated brain serotonin transporter availability in patients with obsessive-compulsive disorder. *Biol Psychiatry* **54**(12): 1406–1413.

Post RM, DeLisi LE, Holcomb HH, Uhde TW, Cohen R, Buchsbaum MS (1987) Glucose utilization in the temporal cortex of affectively ill patients: positron emission tomography. *Biological Psychiatry* **22**(5): 545–553.

Potts NL, Davidson JR, Krishnan KR, Doraiswamy PM (1994) Magnetic resonance imaging in social phobia. *Psychiatry Res* **52**(1): 35–42.

Rabiner EA, Gunn RN, Wilkins MR, Sargent PA, Mocaer E, Sedman E, Cowen PJ, Grasby PM (2001) Drug action at the 5-HT(1A) receptor in vivo: autoreceptor and postsynaptic receptor occupancy examined with PET and [carbonyl-(11)C]WAY-100635. *Nuclear Medicine and Biology* **27**(5): 509–513.

Rauch SL, Dougherty DD, Cosgrove GR, Cassem EH, Alpert NH, Price BH, Nierenberg AA, Mayberg HS, Baer L, Jenike MA, Fischman AJ (2001) Cerebral metabolic correlates as potential predictors of response to anterior cingulotomy for obsessive compulsive disorder. *Biological Psychiatry.*

Rauch SL, Jenike MA, Alpert NM, Baer L, Breiter HC, Savage CR, Fischman AJ (1994) Regional cerebral blood flow measured during symptom provocation in obsessive-compulsive disorder using ^{15}O-labeled CO_2 and positron emission tomography. *Archives of General Psychiatry* **51**: 62–70.

Rauch SL, Savage CR, Alpert NM, Dougherty D, Kendrick A, Currin T, Brown HD, Manzo P, Fischman AJ, Jenike MA (1997) Probing striatal function in obsessive compulsive disorder: a PET study of implicit sequence learning. *Journal of Neuropsychiatry* **9**: 568–573.

Rauch SL, Savage CR, Alpert NM, Fischman AJ, Jenike MA (1997) The functional neuroanatomy of anxiety: A study of three disorders using positron emission tomography and symptom provocation. *Biological Psychiatry* **42**(6): 446–452.

Rauch SL, Savage CR, Alpert, NM, Miguel EC, Baer L, Breiter HC, Fischman AJ, Manzo PA, Moretti C, Jenike MA (1995) A positron emission tomographic study of simple phobic symptom provocation. *Archives of General Psychiatry* **52**: 20–28.

Rauch SL, Shin LM, Dougherty DD, Alpert NM, Fischman AJ, Jenike MA (2002) Predictors of fluvoxamine response in contamination-related obsessive compulsive disorder: a PET symptom provocation study *Neuropsychopharmacology* **27**(5): 782–791.

Rauch SL, van der Kolk BA, Fisler RE, Alpert NM, Orr SP, Savage CR, Fischman AJ, Jenike MA, Pitman RK (1996) A symptom provocation study of posttraumatic stress disorder using positron emission tomography and script-driven imagery. *Archives of General Psychiatry* **53**: 380–387.

Rauch SL, Whalen PJ, Shin LM, McInerney SC, Macklin ML, Lasko NB, Orr SP, Pitman RK (2000) Exaggerated amygdala response to masked facial stimuli in posttraumatic stress disorder: a functional MRI study. *Biol Psychiatry* **47**(9): 769–776.

Reiman EM, Raichle ME, Butler FK, Herscovitch P, Robins E (1984) A focal brain abnormality in panic disorder, a severe form of anxiety. *Nature* **310**(5979): 683–685.

Reiman EM, Raichle ME, Robins E, Butler FK, Herscovitch P, Fox P, Perlmutter J (1986) The application of positron emission tomography to the study of panic disorder. *American Journal of Psychiatry* **143**: 469–477.

Reiman EM, Raichle ME, Robins E, Mintun MA, Fusselman MJ, Fox PT, Price JL, Hackman KA (1989) Neuroanatomical correlates of a lactate-induced anxiety attack. *Archives of General Psychiatry* **46**: 493–500.

Rice DP, Miller LS (1998) Health economics and cost implications of anxiety and other mental disorders in the United States. *British Journal of Psychiatry* **34**(Suppl.): 4–9.

Robinson D, Wu H, Munne RA, Ashtari M, Alvir JM, Lerner G, Doreen A, Cole K, Bogerts B (1995) Reduced caudate nucleus volume in obsessive-compulsive disorder. *Archives of General Psychiatry* **52**: 393–398.

Roland PE, Friberg L (1988) The effect of the GABA-A agonist THIP on regional cortical blood flow in humans. A new test of hemispheric dominance. *J Cereb Blood Flow Metab* **8**(3): 314–323.

Rosenberg DR, Keshavan MS, O'Hearn KM, Dick EL, Bagwell WW, Seymour AB, Montrose DM, Pierri JN, Birmaher B (1997) Frontostriatal measurement in treatment-naive children with obsessive-compulsive disorder. *Archives of General Psychiatry* **554**: 824–830.

Rosenberg DR, MacMaster FP, Keshavan MS, Fitzgerald KD, Stewart CM, Moore GJ (2000) Decrease in caudate glutamatergic concentrations in pediatric obsessive-compulsive disorder patients taking paroxetine. *Journal of the American Academy of Child and Adolescent Psychiatry* **39**(9): 1096–1103.

Rosenberg R, Vorstrup S, Andersen A, Bolwig TG. (1988) Effect of ECT on cerebral blood flow in melancholia assessed with SPECT. *Convulsive Therapy* **4**(1): 62–73

Rubin RT, Ananth J, Villanueva-Meyer J, Trajmar PG, Mena I (1995) Regional 133xenon cerebral blood flow and cerebral 99mTc-HMPAO uptake in patients with obsessive-compulsive disorder before and during treatment. *Biological Psychiatry* **38**(7): 429–437.

Rubin RT, Villanueva-Meyer J, Ananth J, Trajmar PG, Mena I (1992) Regional xenon 133 cerebral blood flow and cerebral technetium 99m HMPAO uptake in unmedicated patients with obsessive-compulsive disorder and matched normal control subjects. Determination by high-resolution single-photon emission computed tomography. *Archives of General Psychiatry* **49**(9): 695–702.

Sachdev P, Trollor J, Walker A, Wen W, Fulham M, Smith JS, Matheson J (2001) Bilateral orbitomedial leucotomy for obsessive-compulsive disorder: a single-case study using positron emission tomography. *Australian and New Zealand Journal of Psychiatry* **35**(5): 684–690.

Sapolsky RM (1996) Why stress is bad for your brain. *Science* **273**(5276): 749–750.

Sargent PA, Kjaer KH, Bench CJ, Rabiner EA, Messa C, Meyer J, Gunn RN, Grasby PM, Cowen PJ (2000a) Brain serotonin-1A receptor binding measured by positron emission tomography with [11C]WAY-100635: effects of depression and antidepressant treatment. *Archives of General Psychiatry* **57**(2): 174–180.

Sargent PA, Nash, J, Hood S, Rabiner E, Messa C, Cowen P, Nutt DJ, Grasby P (2000b) 5-HT1A receptor binding in panic disorder: comparison with depressive disorder and healthy volunteers using PET and [11C] WAY 100635. *Neuroimage* **11**(5): s189.

Sawle GV, Hymas NF, Lees AJ, Frackowiak RS (1991) Obsessional slowness. Functional studies with positron emission tomography. *Brain* **114**(Pt 5): 2191–202.

Saxena S, Brody AL, Ho ML, Alborzian S, Maidment KM, Zohrabi N, Ho MK, Huang SC, Wu HM, Baxter LR Jr (2002) Differential cerebral metabolic changes with paroxetine treatment of obsessive-compulsive disorder vs major depression. *Archives of General Psychiatry* **59**(3): 250–61.

Saxena S, Brody AL, Maidment KM, Dunkin JJ, Colgan M, Alborzian S, Phelps ME, Baxter LR Jr (1999) Localized orbitofrontal and subcortical metabolic changes and predictors of response to paroxetine treatment in obsessive-compulsive disorder. *Neuropsychopharmacology* **21**(6): 683–693.

Saxena S, Rauch SL (2000) Functional neuroimaging and the neuroanatomy of obsessive-compulsive disorder. *Psychiatr Clin North Am* **23**(3): 563–586.

Scarone S, Colombo C, Livian S, Abbruzzese M, Ronchi P, Locatelli M, Scotti G, Smeraldi E (1992) Increased right caudate nucleus size in obsessive compulsive disorder: detection with magnetic resonance imaging. *Psychiatry Research: Neuroimaging* **45**: 115–121.

Schlegel S, Aldenhoff JB, Eissner D, Lindner P, Nickel O (1989) Regional cerebral blood flow in depression: associations with psychopathology. *Journal of Affective Disorders* **17**(3): 211–218.

Schlegel S, Steinert H, Bockisch A, Hahn K, Schloesser R, Benkert O (1994) Decreased benzodiazepine receptor binding in panic disorder measured by Iomazenil SPECT. A preliminary report. *European Archives of Psychiatry Clinical Neuroscience* **244**: 49–51.

Schneider F, Gur RE, Alavi A, Seligman ME, Mozley LH, Smith RJ, Mozley PD, Gur RC (1996) Cerebral blood flow changes in limbic regions induced by unsolvable anagram tasks. *American Journal of Psychiatry* **153**(2): 206–212.

Schneider F, Weiss U, Kessler C, Muller-Gartner HW, Posse S, Salloum JB, Grodd W, Himmelmann F, Gaebel W, Birbaumer N (1999) Subcortical correlates of differential classical conditioning of aversive emotional reactions in social phobia. *Biol Psychiatry* 45(7): 863–871.

Schneier FR, Liebowitz MR, Abi-Dargham A, Zea-Ponce Y, Lin S, Laruelle M (2000) Low dopamine D(2) receptor binding potential in social phobia. *American Journal of Psychiatry* 157(3): 457–459.

Schwartz JM, Baxter LR Jr, Mazziotta JC, Gerner RH, Phelps ME (1987) The differential diagnosis of depression. Relevance of positron emission tomography studies of cerebral glucose metabolism to the bipolar–unipolar dichotomy. *JAMA* 258(10): 1368–1374.

Schwartz JM, Stoessel PW, Baxter LR Jr, Martin KM, Phelps ME (1996) Systematic changes in cerebral glucose metabolic rate after successful behavior modification treatment of obsessive-compulsive disorder. *Archives of General Psychiatry* 53(2): 109–113.

Scott AI, Dougall N, Ross M, O'Carroll RE, Riddle W, Ebmeier KP, Goodwin GM (1993) Short-term effects of electroconvulsive treatment on the uptake of 99mTc-exametazime into brain in major depression shown with single photon emission tomography. *Journal of Affective Disorders* 30(1): 27–34.

Semple WE, Goyer P, McCormick R, Morris E, Comptom B, Muswick G, Nelson D, Donovan B, Leisure G, Berridge M, et al. (1993) Preliminary report: brain blood flow using PET in patients with posttraumatic stress disorder and substance-abuse histories. *Biological Psychiatry* 34: 115–118.

Semple WE, Goyer PF, McCormick R, Compton-Toth B, Morris E, Donovan B, Muswick G, Nelson D, Garnett ML, Sharkoff J, Leisure G, Miraldi F, Schulz SC (1996) Attention and regional cerebral blood flow in posttraumatic stress disorder patients with substance abuse histories. *Psychiatry Research* 67(1): 17–28.

Shah PJ, Ogilvie AD, Goodwin GM, Ebmeier KP (1997) Clinical and psychometric correlates of dopamine D2 binding in depression. *Psychological Medicine* 27(6): 1247–1256.

Sheline YI, Sanghavi M, Mintun MA, Gado MH (1999) Depression duration but not age predicts hippocampal volume loss in medically healthy women with recurrent major depression. *Journal of Neuroscience* 19(12): 5034–5043.

Shin LM, Kosslyn SM, McNally RJ, Alpert NM, Thompson WL, Rauch SL, Macklin ML, Pitman RK (1997) Visual imagery and perception in posttraumatic stress disorder: a positron emission tomographic investigation. *Archives of General Psychiatry* 54: 233–241.

Shin LM, McNally RJ, Kosslyn SM, Thompson WL, Rauch SL, Alpert NM, Metzger LJ, Lasko NB, Orr SP, Pitman RK (1999) Regional cerebral blood flow during script-driven imagery in childhood sexual abuse-related posttraumatic stress disorder: a PET investigation. *American Journal of Psychiatry* 156: 575–584.

Shin LM, Whalen PJ, Pitman RK, Bush G, Macklin ML, Lasko NB, Orr SP, McInerney SC, Rauch SL (2001) An fMRI study of anterior cingulate function in posttraumatic stress disorder. *Biol Psychiatry* 50(12): 932–942.

Shoaf SE, Carson RE, Hommer D, Williams WA, Higley JD, Schmall B, Herscovitch P, Eckelman WC, Linnoila M (2000) The suitability of [11C]-alpha-methyl-L-tryptophan as a tracer for serotonin synthesis: studies with dual administration of [11C] and [14C] labeled tracer. *Journal of Cerebral Blood Flow and Metabolism* 20(2): 244–252.

Sibille E, Pavlides C, Benke D, Toth M (2000) Genetic inactivation of the serotonin(1A) receptor in mice results in downregulation of major GABA(A) receptor alpha subunits, reduction of GABA(A) receptor binding, and benzodiazepine-resistant anxiety. *Journal of Neuroscience* 20(8): 2758–2765.

Simpson HB, Lombardo I, Slifstein M, Huang HY, Hwang DR, Abi-Dargham A, Liebowitz MR, Laruelle M (2003) Serotonin transporters in obsessive-compulsive disorder: a positron emission tomography study with [(11)C]McN 5652. *Biol Psychiatry* 54(12): 1414–1421.

Simpson JR Jr, Drevets WC, Snyder AZ, Gusnard DA, Raichle ME (2001) Emotion-induced changes in human medial prefrontal cortex: II. During anticipatory anxiety. *Proc Natl Acad Sci USA* **98**(2): 688–693.

Smith GS, Reynolds CF, Pollock B, Derbyshire S, Nofzinger E, Dew MA, Houck PR, Milko D, Meltzer CC, Kupfer DJ (1999) Cerebral glucose metabolic response to combined total sleep deprivation and antidepressant treatment in geriatric depression. *American Journal of Psychiatry* **156**(5): 683–689

Stein MB, Koverola C, Hanna C, Torchia MG, McClarty B (1997) Hippocampal volume in women victimized by childhood sexual abuse. *Psychological Medicine* **27**: 951–960.

Stein DJ, Coetzer R, Lee M, Davids B, Bouwer C (1997a) Magnetic resonance brain imaging in women with obsessive-compulsive disorder and trichotillomania. *Psychiatry Research* **74**(3): 177–182.

Stein MB, Leslie WB (1996) A brain single photon-emission computed tomography (SPECT) study of generalized social phobia. *Biological Psychiatry* **39**(9): 825–828.

Stewart RS, Devous MD Sr, Rush AJ, Lane L, Bonte FJ (1988) Cerebral blood flow changes during sodium-lactate-induced panic attacks. *American Journal of Psychiatry* **145**(4): 442–449.

Suhara T, Nakayama K, Inoue O, Fukuda H, Shimizu M, Mori A, Tateno Y (1992) Dl dopamine receptor binding in mood disorders measured by positron emission tomography. *Psychopharmacology* **106**(1): 14–18.

Swedo SE, Pietrini P, Leonard H, Schapiro MB, Rettew DC, Goldberger EL, Rapoport SI, Rapoport JL, Grady CL, (1992) Cerebral glucose metabolism in childhood-onset obsessive-compulsive disorder. Revisualization during pharmacotherapy. *Archives of General Psychiatry* **49**(9): 690–694.

Swedo SE, Schapiro MB, Grady CL, Cheslow DL, Leonard HL, Kumar A, Friedland R, Rapoport SI, Rapoport JL (1989) Cerebral glucose metabolism in childhood-onset obsessive-compulsive disorder. *Archives of General Psychiatry* **46**(6): 518–523.

Szeszko PR, Robinson D, Alvir JM, Bilder RM, Lencz T, Ashtari M, Wu H, Bogerts B (1999) Orbital frontal and amygdala volume reductions in obsessive-compulsive disorder. *Archives of General Psychiatry* **56**(10): 913–919.

Tagamets MA, Horwitz B (2001) Interpreting PET and fMRI measures of functional neural activity: the effects of synaptic inhibition on cortical activation in human imaging studies. *Brain Res Bull* **54**(3): 267–273.

Tauscher J, Bagby RM, Javanmard M, Christensen BK, Kasper S, Kapur S (2001) Inverse relationship between serotonin 5-HT(1A) receptor binding and anxiety: a [(11)C]WAY-100635 PET investigation in healthy volunteers. *American Journal of Psychiatry* **158**(8): 1326–1328.

Tiihonen J, Kuikka J, Bergstrom K, Lepola U, Koponen H, Leinonen E (1997a) Dopamine reuptake site densities in patients with social phobia. *American Journal of Psychiatry* **154**(2): 239–242.

Tiihonen J, Kuikka J, Rasanen P, Lepola U, Koponen H, Liuska A, Lehmusvaara A, Vainio P, Kononen M, Bergstrom K, Yu M, Kinnunen I, Akerman K, Karhu J (1997b) Cerebral benzodiazepine receptor binding and distribution in generalized anxiety disorder: a fractal analysis. *Molecular Psychiatry* **2**(6): 463–471.

Tiihonen J, Kuoppamaki M, Nagren K, Bergman J, Eronen E, Syvalahti E, Hietala J (1996) Serotonergic modulation of striatal D2 dopamine receptor binding in humans measured with positron emission tomography. *Psychopharmacology* **126**(4): 277–280.

Tillfors M, Furmark T, Marteinsdottir I, Fischer H, Pissiota A, Langstrom B, Fredrikson M. (2001) Cerebral blood flow in subjects with social phobia during stressful speaking tasks: a PET study. *American Journal of Psychiatry* **158**(8): 1220–1226.

Tokunaga M, Ida I, Higuchi T, Mikuni M (1997) Alterations of benzodiazepine receptor binding potential in anxiety and somatoform disorders measured by 123I-iomazenil SPECT. *Radiation Medicine* **15**(3): 163–169.

Tupler LA, Davidson JR, Smith RD, Lazeyras F, Charles HC, Krishnan KR (1997) A repeat proton magnetic resonance spectroscopy study in social phobia. *Biol Psychiatry* **42**(6): 419–424.

Van der Linden G, van Heerden B, Warwick J, Wessels C, van Kradenburg J, Zungu-Dirwayi N, Stein DJ (2000) Functional brain imaging and pharmacotherapy in social phobia: single photon emission computed tomography before and after treatment with the selective serotonin reuptake inhibitor citalopram. *Progress in Neuropsychopharmacological and Biological Psychiatry* **24**(3): 419–438.

Vermetten E, Vythilingam M, Southwick SM, Charney DS, Bremner JD (2003) Long-term treatment with paroxetine increases verbal declarative memory and hippocampal volume in posttraumatic stress disorder. *Biol Psychiatry* **54**(7): 693–702.

Volk SA, Kaendler SH, Hertel A, Maul FD, Manoocheri R, Weber R, Georgi K, Pflug B, Hor G (1997) Can response to partial sleep deprivation in depressed patients be predicted by regional changes of cerebral blood flow? *Psychiatry Research* **75**(2): 67–74.

Vythilingam M, Anderson ER, Goddard A, Woods SW, Staib LH, Charney DS, Bremner JD (2000) Temporal lobe volume in panic disorder – a quantitative magnetic resonance imaging study. *Psychiatry Res* **99**(2): 75–82.

Weizman R, Weizman A, Kook KA, Vocci F, Deutsch SI, Paul SM. (1989) Repeated swim stress alters brain benzodiazepine receptors measured in vivo. *Journal of Pharmacology Experimental Therapy* **249**: 701–707.

WHO (2001) *World Health Report 'New Understanding, New Hope'*. Geneva: WHO. ISBN 92 4 156201 3.

Willeit M, Praschak-Rieder N, Neumeister A, Pirker W, Asenbaum S, Vitouch O, Tauscher J, Hilger E, Stastny J, Brucke T, Kasper S (2000) [123I]-beta-CIT SPECT imaging shows reduced brain serotonin transporter availability in drug-free depressed patients with seasonal affective disorder. *Biological Psychiatry* **47**(6): 482–489.

Willeit M, Stastny J, Pirker W, Praschak-Rieder N, Neumeister A, Asenbaum S, Tauscher J, Fuchs K, Sieghart W, Hornik K, Aschauer HN, Brucke T, Kasper S (2001) No evidence for in vivo regulation of midbrain serotonin transporter availability by serotonin transporter promoter gene polymorphism. *Biological Psychiatry* **50**(1): 8–12.

Wong DF, Wagner HN Jr, Pearlson G, Dannals RF, Links JM, Ravert HT, Wilson AA, Suneja S, Bjorvvinssen E, Kuhar MJ (1985) Dopamine receptor binding of C-11-3-N-methylspiperone in the caudate in schizophrenia and bipolar disorder: a preliminary report. *Psychopharmacology Bulletin* **21**(3): 595–598.

Woods SW, Koster K, Krystal JK, Smith EO, Zubal IG, Hoffer PB, Charney DS (1988) Yohimbine alters regional cerebral blood flow in panic disorder [letter]. *Lancet* **2**(8612): 678.

Wu JC, Buchsbaum MS, Hershey TG, Hazlett E, Sicotte N, Johnson JC (1991) PET in generalized anxiety disorder. *Biological Psychiatry* **29**(12): 1181–1199.

Yatham LN, Liddle PF, Dennie J, Shiah IS, Adam MJ, Lane CJ, Lam RW, Ruth TJ (1999). Decrease in brain serotonin-2 receptor binding in patients with major depression following desipramine treatment: a positron emission tomography study with fluorine-18-labeled setoperone. *Archives of General Psychiatry* **56**(8): 705–711.

Yatham LN, Liddle PF, Dennie J, Shiah IS, Adam MJ, Lane CJ, Lam RW, Ruth TJ (2000) Brain serotonin2 receptors in major depression: a positron emission tomography study. *Archives of General Psychiatry* **57**(9): 850–858.

Yatham LN, Liddle PF, Lam RW, Shiah IS, Lane C, Stoessl AJ, Sossi V, Ruth TJ (2002a) PET study of the effects of valproate on dopamine D(2) receptors in neuroleptic- and mood-stabilizer-naive patients with nonpsychotic mania. *American Journal of Psychiatry* **159**(10): 1718–1723.

Yatham LN, Liddle PF, Shiah IS, Lam RW, Ngan E, Scarrow G, Imperial M, Stoessl J, Sossi V, Ruth TJ (2002b) PET study of [(18)F]6-fluoro-L-dopa uptake in neuroleptic- and mood-stabilizer-naive first-episode nonpsychotic mania: effects of treatment with divalproex sodium. *American Journal of Psychiatry* **159**(5): 768–774.

Yehuda R, Levengood RA, Schmeidler J, Wilson S, Guo LS, Gerber D (1996) Increased pituitary activation following metyrapone administration in post traumatic stress disorder. *Psychoneuroendocrinology* **21**(1): 1–16.

Zanardi R, Artigas F, Moresco R, Colombo C, Messa C, Gobbo C, Smeraldi E, Fazio F (2001) Increased 5-Hydroxytryptamine-2 receptor binding in the frontal cortex of depressed patients responding to paroxetine treatment: a positron emission tomography scan study. *Journal of Clinical Psychopharmacology* **21**(1): 53–58.

Zubieta JK, Chinitz JA, Lombardi U, Fig LM, Cameron OG, Liberzon I (1999) Medial frontal cortex involvement in PTSD symptoms: a SPECT study. *Journal of Psychiatric Research* **33**(3): 259–264.

Zubieta JK, Huguelet P, Ohl LE, Koeppe RA, Kilbourn MR, Carr JM, Giordani BJ, Frey KA (2000) High vesicular monoamine transporter binding in asymptomatic bipolar I disorder: sex differences and cognitive correlates. *American Journal of Psychiatry* **157**(10): 1619–1628.

PART IV
Treatment

10

The Treatment of Depression

Anthony S. Hale

University of Kent, Canterbury, UK

This chapter aims to cover commonly used treatments for unipolar depressive episodes and for the depressive phase of bipolar affective disorder.

UNIPOLAR DEPRESSION

The treatment of depression has changed fundamentally in recent years. In many countries, the first-line treatment of depression utilizes talking therapies, with anti-depressant medication offered as a second-line treatment. This has been understood as in part reflecting a generally held lay belief in the causation of depression by trauma and circumstance, and in part because of reluctance to use antidepressant drugs because of their toxicity in overdose and side-effect profile.

In the UK, an opinion poll was conducted at the beginning and end of a five-year public education campaign. Interviewing the public, including recovered depres-sives and their relatives, it asked what treatments people would feel they might want if they were ever to become depressed again (Priest et al., 1996; Paykel et al., 1998). Over 90% of people in both surveys were clear that they would not want antidepressant drugs at all, but would prefer talking therapy. Only 17% of people thought drugs were ever indicated and most believed they would benefit most from counselling. The reasons given for this included the side effects of the drugs; the idea that drug therapy was second best and a cheap substitute for 'proper' talking therapy which would somehow cure rather than suppress symptoms; a belief in the addictive potential of antidepressants (78% said so explicitly); and non-acceptance of the medical model of depression and its treatment. Less than half of the sample believed that antidepressants would work at all.

The range of antidepressant drugs available has expanded greatly since the 1970s, when only older tricyclic antidepressants (TCAs) and monoamine oxidase inhibitors (MAOIs) were available. More adrenergically selective tricyclic anti-depressants were developed such as lofepramine, desipramine and nortriptyline. These drugs offered an improved side-effect profile, primarily through having

Mood Disorders: Clinical Management and Research Issues. Edited by E. J. L. Griez, C. Faravelli, D. J. Nutt and J. Zohar.
©2005 John Wiley & Sons Ltd. ISBN 0 470 09426 5.

fewer anticholinergic side effects. Mianserin offered an improved toxicity profile, allowing outpatient treatment without the risks of overdose, but there were some doubts about efficacy at the doses commonly used. The 1980s saw a revolution with the introduction of the selective serotonin reuptake inhibitors (SSRIs), the first 'designer' antidepressants. These were hugely successful because of much improved side-effect profiles and simple dosing regimes, overcoming previous widespread reluctance to prescribe effective doses. This produced a backlash from the psychotherapy lobby, who saw their livelihood under threat from acceptable and effective drug treatments (Kramer, 1993; Breggin, 1991). The 1990s saw further expansion of the range of antidepressants available, with the launch of a more selective MAOI, moclobemide; of a dual serotonin and noradrenaline selective reuptake inhibitor (venlafaxine); of an SSRI with additional serotonin antagonist properties (nefazadone); of a mixed presynaptic alpha-2 and serotonin antagonist (mirtazepine); and of an even more selective noradrenaline reuptake inhibitor (reboxetine). All these drugs were antidepressants with efficacy comparable to the older TCAs, but with different side-effect and toxicity profiles (Mason et al., 2000; Nelson, 1997) conferred by their binding and reuptake profiles (Hale, 1997). However, despite these advances, side effects remain, albeit somewhat different, and proof of the better public acceptance of these newer drugs remains somewhat elusive.

The acceptability of antidepressants as first-line treatment depends on the alternative treatments on offer. Whether such alternatives are effective and hence are valid choices depends on the type and severity of depression. There has been a growing understanding of the differential response of different subpopulations of depressives to treatments. At the milder end of depression common in primary care, the older TCAs were no more effective than placebo (Paykel et al., 1987 et al: Stewart et al., 1992a). However, this was at variance with a belief in primary care that these drugs were effective, but at smaller doses than that which psychiatrists considered the minimum effective dose, 125–150 mg of TCAs (Quitkin, 1985; Bridges, 1983). This suggested that, with less severe depression, the side effects might be less tolerable than the underlying depression, leading to poor concordance with treatment. There are some suggestions that the SSRIs may be effective even in less severe depression (Dunlop et al., 1990; Pande and Sayler, 1993), perhaps because of improved tolerability and hence improved adherence.

A recent meta-analysis of the treatment of depression in primary care (Mulrow et al., 2000), however, found comparable response rates for SSRIs and TCAs (63% vs 60%) compared with 35% for placebo. The response rate for milder depression may, as in major depression, depend on the subtype of depression. In atypical depressive patients with low initial Hamilton Depression Rating Scale (HDRS) scores, Stewart et al. (1992b) showed response to phenelzine in 83% of cases, whilst 60% responded to imipramine and 33% to placebo. In patients with medium and high HDRS scores, the ratio of responders was similar across treatment groups, but the absolute percentages lower. Among the 140 patients who had low pretreatment HDRS scores, 19% of those patients given placebo, 25% of those given imipramine, and 34% of those given phenelzine, responded to treatment. Each of the antidepressants was superior to placebo. Similar findings applied to the patients with medium and high HDRS, except that the rates of placebo response were lower (29% and 10%, respectively).

Many primary care patients presenting with 'depression' may not suffer with major depressive disorder as defined by DSM-IV. For more severe major depression, there is evidence for counselling being ineffective (King et al., 1994; Friedli et al., 1997; Harvey et al., 1998). For less severe major and non-major depression, primary care talking therapies such as counselling may be effective treatment. A recent primary care study randomized patients with major depression to antidepressants or counselling, with additional non-randomized arms allowing patient preference (Chilvers et al., 2001). Generic counselling and antidepressants were reported as equally effective at 12 months, but the antidepressants were 50% faster in onset of action (two vs. three months). The authors noted that patients preferring counselling were less severely depressed than the randomized patients or those preferring antidepressants. Whether or not patients chose, or were randomized to, antidepressants made no difference to outcome, but patients who chose counselling did better than those randomized to it. While there was apparently no difference in final depression severity (Beck) score between the randomized groups, of patients assessed at one year, significantly more (53%) of patients in the counselling group still fulfilled RDC criteria for current major depression compared with 19% in the antidepressant group ($p = 0.07$). Whether this represented a lower rate of complete remission or a higher relapse rate is unclear. This study casts doubt on the completeness of recovery when primary care depression is treated with counselling.

Treatment Guidelines for Unipolar Depression

A variety of treatment guidelines and treatment algorithms have been produced for depression, such as the American Psychiatric Association Guidelines (American Psychiatric Association, 2000), Canadian Guidelines (Kennedy et al., 2001) and British Association of Psychopharmacology Guidelines (Anderson et al., 2000). They all offer similar advice. Antidepressants are seen as the first-line treatment for major depression, irrespective of environmental factors, but with benefit uncertain at the mildest severity, in keeping with the findings described above. Depression-specific psychological treatments are seen as an alternative for mild to moderate depression but not for more severe depression, where they are clearly inferior to antidepressants. Combined pharmacological/depression-specific psychological treatment is not considered first-line treatment (because of limited availability) but may be considered for more severely ill patients or partial responders. For milder depression, antidepressants are not generally advocated immediately, but education, support and simple problem solving are recommended, with monitoring for persistence or development of major depression, when a trial of antidepressants is suggested. For patients requesting alternative treatment, St John's wort, bibliotherapy and exercise are suggested. Guidelines include advice on different treatments indicated for subtypes of depression. NICE (2004) have recently reviewed guidelines and performed new meta-analyses of all treatments for major depression and its subtypes, at differing levels of severity. For initial presentation in primary care, they recommend a strategy of 'watchful waiting' followed by counselling, to account for the difficulty in differentiating a depressive episode from an acute situational disturbance in that setting.

Major Depressive Subtypes

The rest of this chapter will describe treatment for major depressive episodes or for the depressive phase of bipolar illness. However, there is some evidence for differential responses to various treatments in different subtypes of depression.

Melancholic Major Depression

For the melancholic subtype of major depression, adequate doses of TCAs and SSRIs (Roose et al., 1994; Perry, 1996), venlafaxine (Benkert et al., 1996), and nefazodone (Feighner et al., 1998), together with electroconvulsive therapy (ECT) (Peselow et al., 1992), are strongly supported by available evidence. Parker et al. (1999, 2001) provide support for doubts that the SSRIs are as effective as older drugs in melancholics.

Psychotic Depression

The prevalence of psychotic depression has been shown to be 0.4% (95% CI 0.35–0.54%), and the prevalence of a current major depressive episode without psychotic features was 2.0% (95% CI = 1.9–2.1%), with higher rates of psychosis in women than in men (Ohayon and Schatzberg, 2002). In all, 18.5% of the subjects who fulfilled the criteria for a major depressive episode had psychotic features. Treatment strategies for psychotic depression are reviewed by Wheeler Vega et al. (2000) and Rothschild (2003). These include: (1) combined antidepressant and antipsychotic therapy with TCAs and typical antipsychotic; (2) ECT; (3) amoxapine; (4) SSRIs, alone and in combination; (5) several atypical antipsychotics, alone and in combination; (6) mood stabilizers and anticonvulsants. The evidence base is not robust, but ECT or TCA/SSRI antidepressants with an antipsychotic are indicated (Spiker et al., 1985; Parker et al., 1992; Rothschild et al., 1996). A meta-analysis by NICE (2004) has shown a trend in favour of better outcome for antidepressant/antipsychotic combinations compared to antidepressants alone, but this is only significant for amitriptyline–perphenizine on mean change endpoint analysis

(-0.69 CI -1.38 to -0.01) and not significant for other combinations, while there were no differences in remission status.

Rothschild and Duval (2003) show that withdrawal of the antipsychotic after four months leads to relapse and it is necessary to continue with both drugs. It is unclear for how long this is necessary but current recommendations suggest a minimum of one year, based on Aronson et al. (1988). Psychotic depression had only a 30% to 40% response rate to TCAs in several trials but may have a 70% response rate to the tetracyclic amoxapine (Anton and Sexauer, 1983). However, its metabolite is a neuroleptic that may cause tardive dyskinesia. The growing use of both SSRIs and atypical antipsychotics has led to a growing popularity of their use in combination for this indication, with some preliminary supportive evidence both for clozapine (Ranjan and Meltzer, 1996) and other atypical antipsychotics (Rothschild et al., 1999; Miodownik and Lerner, 2000). Shelton et al. (2001) reports a marked antidepressant response in patients with treatment-refractory non-psychotic unipolar depression treated with an olanzapine and fluoxetine combination (OFC). Corya et al. (2003) demonstrates a sustained improvement in a 73-week open label study of 560 treatment-resistant major depressives. Given the efficacy demonstrated in these two studies, it is likely that OFC will be widely used in psychotic depression. The use of glucocorticoid antagonists have been studied in depression due to the elevated glucocorticoid activity in depression. Mifepristone has recently been shown to reduce the psychotic sysmptoms of psychotic depression in a double-blind RCT using 600-mg daily versus placebo (Schatzberg et al., 2004). It produced a 30% improvement in total score and a 50% improvement in positive psychotic symptoms on the BPRS.

Atypical Depression

For atypical depression, phenelzine and imipramine (Liebowitz et al., 1988), and perhaps some SSRIs (Pande et al., 1996; Stratta et al., 1991) and moclobemide (Lonnqvist et al., 1994; Tiller et al., 1989; Sogaard et al., 1999) have an evidence base. The use of the older MAOIs as a first-line treatment is limited by dietary restrictions.

Depression with Predominant Anxiety

For this subtype, most modern antidepressants are indicated but TCAs are poorly tolerated (Stahl, 1993; Prescorn and Fast, 1993; Ravindran et al., 1997).

Seasonal Affective Disorder (SAD)

Light therapy, SSRIs and perhaps moclobemide or L-tryptophan, are advised for seasonal affective disorder (Lam et al., 1995; Eastman et al., 1998).

Dysthymia

Thase et al. (1996) compared sertraline, imipramine and placebo in dysthymia and showed similar responder and remission rates for both active treatments. In female patients, sertraline was more effective than imipramine. Vanelle et al. (1997) compared fluoxetine 20 mg and placebo in dysthymia, re-randomizing fluoxetine non-responders to either 20 or 40 mg fluoxetine. Fluoxetine produced significantly more remission, and fluoxetine patients stayed well during a six-month follow-up. Significantly more initial non-responders responded when the dose of fluoxetine was increased to 40 mg compared with those who remained on 20 mg daily. Lecrubier et al. (1997) showed dysthymic patients to respond to both imipramine and amisulpride significantly more often than placebo. Dunner et al. (1996) compared CBT and fluoxetine in treatment of dysthymia. They found CBT the 'more desired treatment' (more patients accepted randomization), but no difference in efficacy. Ravindran et al. (1999) compared the efficacy of sertraline and group CBT, alone and in combination, in a placebo controlled double-blind study of dysthymia. Sertraline but not group CBT was significantly more effective than placebo at reducing depression scores. CBT was able to augment the improvement in functional impairment produced by sertraline, but was not effective when combined with placebo.

Complicated Bereavement

This subtype should be treated as major depression after two months of support, with hypnotics if needed, if there are after that time persistent features of guilt, preoccupation, worthlessness, suicidal thoughts (Zisook and Shuchter 1993; Rosenzweig et al., 1996).

Adjustment Disorder

This subtype should be treated with support and, if needed, symptomatic relief (Uhlenhuth et al., 1999) although Jones et al. (1999) found it difficult to differentiate from other non-major depression in terms of treatment response.

Minor Depression

The evidence base suggests that, for minor depression, in the absence of transition to major depression, the role of pharmacotherapy is unclear (Stewart et al., 1992b), although antidepressant repose is seen more often and is more persistent than with dysthymia (Oxman et al., 2001). Where severity is less than 13 on a 17-item Hamilton Depression Rating Scale, there is little evidence of any antidepressant being superior to placebo.

Mixed Anxiety and Depression

All antidepressants alleviate symptoms but there are few adequate studies. Rausch et al. (2001) have suggested that the therapeutic effect of SSRI treatment can be linked to the magnitude and time-course of 5-HT transport inhibition effected with fluvoxamine, a drug that seems to have an anti-anxiety effect of the same magnitude as its effect on depression. Effective treatments might thus include SSRIs and venlafaxine (Perugi et al., 2002).

Brief Recurrent Depression

There is no useful evidence base on the treatment and the benefits of SSRIs (Stamenkovic et al., 2001) and mirtazepine (Stamenkovic et al., 1998) remain unproven. The former study suggests that fluoxetine may decrease the frequency but not the duration or severity of depressive episodes. There is some anecdotal evidence for benefit with lithium (Corominas et al., 1998).

Premenstrual Dysphoric Disorder

SSRIs and venlafaxine may be more useful in depression associated with this disorder than TCAs (Yonkers, 1997; Freeman et al., 1999, 2001). There is some evidence that SSRIs given only during the luteal phase may be as effective as continuous treatment (Halbreich and Smoller, 1997). Pearlstein (2002) reviews 12 RCTs and finds that fluoxetine, sertraline, paroxetine and citalopram have reported positive efficacy, with less clear results for fluvoxamine. Drugs which enhance serotonin seem to improve premenstrual irritability and dysphoria rapidly, suggesting a different mechanism of action than in the treatment of depression.

Primary Care Depressive Subtypes

Recent epidemiological work on primary care depression (Tylee et al., 1999) suggests subtypes which have only partial overlap with subtypes recognized in psychiatry. The significance of these newly proposed primary care subtypes for treatment response remains to be investigated.

Response versus Remission

There has been much debate over recent years concerning the nature of a clinically meaningful change with antidepressant treatment. Historically, efficacy has been assessed by comparison of mean change from a baseline severity score compared between treatment groups. More recently, emphasis has been placed on the achievement of response to treatment, usually defined as a 50% reduction in baseline score on the scale used. Patients starting treatment with a high baseline score may be 'responders' but still have a significant symptom load – for example, a 50% reduction from the maximum score on the Hamilton Depression Rating Scale (HDRS) of 56 will still score 28, in the severe depression range. More usually, 'responders' in a drug trial will have residual post-treatment scores of 8–12 points (Nierenberg and Wright, 1999). What is full remission from depression? Thase et al. (2002) have shown a relative lack of overlap between HDRS score distribution between healthy controls and major depressives between scores of 6.5 and 11.5. A generally accepted cutoff point of $\leqslant 7$ on the 17-item HDRS has been developing, regardless of baseline score (Fawcett and Barkin, 1997). This is associated with lower subsequent relapse rate rather than higher cutoff points (Thase et al., 1992; Paykel et al., 1995). Fawcett and Barkin show however, that only about 63% of patients treated with antidepressants in clinical trials are even responders, and O'Reardon and Amsterdam (1998) show that only one-third of treated patients achieve remission. Unremitted patients have poorer social and physical functioning (Doraiswamy et al., 2001; Miller et al., 1998).

Chronic Unipolar Depression

Chronic major depression is defined as persistent depressive symptoms for two or more years, with protracted episodes or incomplete remission between episodes (Rush and Trivedi, 1995). Chronic depressive cohorts are often confounded by cases of dysthymia and of double depression. Scott et al. (1992) showed chronicity to be predicted by premorbid neuroticism and by the interval between onset and the receipt of effective treatment. In the USA 50–60% of chronically depressed patients presenting for drug therapy have received only counselling or psychotherapy and are significantly more likely to have received talking therapy than previous drug treatment (Shelton et al., 1997).

Once present, chronic depression responds to the usual antidepressant treatments, but slowly and with reduced efficacy (Keller et al., 1998a). Kocsis et al. (1988) noted that antidepressant medication was moderately effective for many chronic depressions (51% response rate despite high dose desipramine), which had previously been untreated or undertreated, 'presumably related to misdiagnosis'. Maintenance treatment of successfully treated chronic depressives has also been shown to be effective (Kocsis et al., 1996). Keller et al. (2000) show equivalent efficacy for the antidepressant nefazodone and for CBT in the treatment of chronic depression (response rates 55% and 52% respectively), but a significantly higher response rate when the two treatments are combined (85%).

Trivedi and Kleiber (2001) describe an algorithm with progressive stages in the treatment of chronic depression. Monotherapy with an SSRI, nefazodone, bupropion sustained release, venlafaxine extended release, mirtazapine, or psychotherapy is followed in incomplete or non-responders by combination therapy, electroconvulsive therapy, atypical antipsychotics, and novel treatments.

Concordance

Non-concordance (non-compliance or non-adherence in older literature) with antidepressant treatment has been recognized since the early days of these drugs' use (Blackwell, 1976; Johnson, 1986; Rashid, 1982) but is less well researched in psychiatry than similar problems in schizophrenia. The terminology varies with fashion in political correctness, some clinicians use the term adherence rather than concordance, others concordance (Myers and Midence, 1998).

Lingam and Scott (2002) performed a systematic review of the prevalence, predictors and methods for improving medication adherence in unipolar and bipolar affective disorders, between 1976 and 2001. They found estimates of medication non-adherence for unipolar and bipolar disorders which ranged from 10% to 60% (median 40%), and commented that this had not changed since the introduction of SSRIs and other new medications. They confirm that attitudes and beliefs are at least as important as side effects in predicting adherence. There are few empirical studies of how to improve medication adherence in affective disorders, compared with a much wider literature for schizophrenia, perhaps reflecting a paucity of data on factors contributing to the problem in depression. Non-adherent patients cost more to health care delivery organizations (Revicki et al., 1998). In general, patients who do not regularly swallow their medication can be assumed to have a worse prognosis, although this cannot be necessarily assumed in milder depressive conditions in general practice (Thompson et al., 2000). Demonstrating adherence rates with newly introduced treatments can be difficult, both technically and because discontinuation rates in randomised controlled trials (RCTs) do not reflect the rates observed in naturalistic studies.

Simon et al. (1995) criticized conventional RCTs as not being adequate to reflect effectiveness (as opposed to treatment efficacy) under 'real world' conditions, a problem was first noted by Schwartz and Lellouch in 1967 and expanded by others (Sackett and Gent, 1979; Feinstein, 1983; Diamond and Denton, 1993). Simon and colleagues suggested the use of 'quasi-experimental designs'.

Simon et al. (1996) reported the results of one such study in depressed patients. They studied a group of depressed patients from a HMO in Seattle. 65 000 patients, predominantly from low-income groups, from a catchment population of 400 000 were studied, generating 536 treated patients considered suitable for treatment with an antidepressant, who were willing to be randomized. This must now be seen as the definitive study of concordance and direct costs of antidepressant treatment. Prospectively identified primary care depressives registered with the HMO were randomized to treatment with either imipramine, desipramine or fluoxetine and then followed up naturalistically over a six-month period.

Non-concordance with desipramine and imipramine was significantly more likely than with fluoxetine. 61% of patients on fluoxetine received at least 90 days' treatment at an adequate dose, compared to 49% on desipramine and 48% on imipramine (both comparisons significant). An important finding, given the debate started by Song et al. (1993), is the rate of treatment discontinuation because of side effects. 9% discontinued on fluoxetine, 27% and 28% respectively on desipramine and imipramine, a highly significant difference. Clinical outcome was similar for all groups, although this must be understood in the context of the patients being able to switch treatment from that originally allocated – a significantly higher proportion of patients switched from a tricyclic to fluoxetine than vice versa.

The results of longer-term follow-up (at 9, 12, 18 and 24 months) were more difficult to interpret as patients intolerant of TCAs switched to the SSRI (Simon et al., 1999).

Choice of Antidepressant

Although in general, all antidepressants are considered equally effective as first-line treatment in major depression, individual differences in susceptibility to and ability to tolerate side effects are sometimes marked. Choice of antidepressant is an art guided by science. The BAP guidelines (Anderson et al., 2000) suggest matching the drug with individual patient's requirements, taking into account likely short-term and long-term effects. In the absence of special factors, antidepressants should be chosen that are better tolerated, safer in overdose and more likely to be prescribed at effective doses. It suggests consideration be given to a history of response to previously given drugs, both positive and adverse; the likely side-effect profiles (e.g. sedation, weight gain); choice of low lethality drugs if there is a history or likelihood of overdose; current physical illness, condition or medication that may interact with the antidepressant drug; associated psychiatric disorder that may specifically respond to a particular class of antidepressant (e.g. obsessive-compulsive disorder and SSRIs); and patient preference. It states that SSRIs, lofepramine, mirtazapine, nefazodone, reboxetine and venlafaxine are all relatively safe and well-tolerated and advises that in situations where maximizing efficacy is of overriding importance, an older TCA or venlafaxine at a dose of 150 mg or greater in preference to an SSRI or MAOI should be considered.

Relative Efficacy of Antidepressants

Some 60–70% of patients with major depressive disorder respond to any given anti-depressant, whether it be the older TCAs and MAOIs, or SSRIs or newer drugs (Healy, 1997). Progress since the 1950s has largely been in the domains of safety and tolerability, with no huge advances in efficacy, although the ability to safely prescribe effective doses with confidence and expect reasonable concordance have contributed to effectiveness. Although increased efficacy may be achieved with augmentation with agents such as lithium or thyroxine, a single effective agent is desirable. There are suggestions that, rather than improved efficacy, the SSRIs are less effective antidepressants in severe depression, compared to TCAs such as clomipramine. The goal of selectivity was to remove the undesirable effects, particularly of histaminic and muscarinic blockade. However, it was thought that mixed reuptake inhibition at 5-HT and noradrenergic sites might retain the benefits of the TCAs without the adverse effects. It was therefore hoped that drugs such as venlafaxine might show improvements in responder rates beyond the 60–70% barrier (Clerc et al., 1994).

Systematic reviews, using different methodologies, have examined differences in efficacy between antidepressants and have reached differing conclusions. Geddes et al. (2000) found statistical heterogeneity (systematic differences between studies) in treatment effects estimated in different studies, but not significant benefit for any one agent compared with others. Other systematic reviews have suggested that SSRIs may be less effective than TCAs, especially amitriptyline (Anderson, 1998, 2000), TCAs (in inpatients). Anderson suggests this may be related to the dual mechanism of action of the TCAs, a suggestion lent support by Thase et al. (2001a), who show superior efficacy of venlafaxine compared to SSRIs. Smith et al. (2002) performed a meta-analysis of 32 studies and showed a superior efficacy of venlafaxine over all other antidepressants as a group and against SSRIs, but no superiority over TCAs. NICE (2004) have examined differences between the commonly used SSRIs and TCAs, MAOIs and dual-acting drugs such as mirtazapine and venlafaxine (Table 10.1). They performed a meta-analysis of venlafaxine against SSRI studies and have stratified by dose (75 mg/day, <150 mg/day and ⩾150 mg/day of venlafaxine). Venlafaxine was not superior to the SSRIs at any of these doses for the three dose ranges, or overall, for mean endpoint score. Analysis of responders showed numerical inferiority for 75 mg and numerical superiority at <150 mg venlafaxine, compared to SSRIs. For doses ⩾150 mg/day of venlafaxine response was more likely with venlafaxine (0.82 CI 0.68–0.98). For studies reporting remission, venlafaxine was superior at doses of ⩾150 mg/day (0.92 CI 0.86–0.99) but not at lower doses. In inpatients, presumed more severely ill, venlafaxine was comparable in efficacy to TCAs (imipramine) with a trend towards better tolerability. Compared to SSRIs venlafaxine was marginally more effective in inpatients (−0.58 CI −1.07 to −0.09) but this is based on a single study against fluoxetine with 34 patients in each group. Venlafaxine was superior in efficacy to some TCAs (imipramine but not clomipramine) in outpatient care settings, where it was also superior to fluoxetine in five studies comparing a total of 617 patients on venlafaxine and 618 on fluoxetine (0.85 CI 0.72–1.00). In primary care studies venlafaxine did not differ on any measure of efficacy, but was more poorly tolerated, compared to SSRIs.

Parker et al. (1999) rated a range of antidepressant medication using a clinical panel judgement. ECT was judged as effective for both melancholic and non-melancholic depression. Antipsychotics were rated as effective, more so for non-melancholic depression. TCAs and irreversible MAOIs were rated as more effective than SSRIs, venlafaxine, mianserin or moclobemide. The superiority of TCAs over the SSRIs was specific to the melancholic patients. In a separate study, Parker et al. (2001)

TABLE 10.1   Meta-analysis results comparing SSRIs with other antidepressants in primary
care and secondary care (inpatient and outpatient) settings. Data taken from NICE (2004)

Comparison	Setting	Result	Odds ratio
SSRIs vs. TCAs	inpatients	No difference	0.12 CI − 0.01 to 0.24
SSRIs vs. TCAs	outpatients	No difference	0.02 CI − 0.07 to 0.10
SSRIs vs. TCAs	1° care	No difference	0.00 CI − 0.52 to 0.52
SSRIs vs. venlafaxine or mirtazapine	2° care	SSRI inferior	0.13 CI 0.06 to 0.19
SSRIs vs. venlafaxine or mirtazapine	1° care	No difference	0.08 CI − 0.05 to 0.22
SSRIs vs. MAOIs	inpatients	Favours SSRI	− 0.16 CI − 0.71 to 0.38

followed a naturalistic cohort of depressed patients for 12 months of treatment and
assessed patients' views of efficacy. In melancholic depression, ECT and irreversible
MAOIs were the most effective treatments, whilst the reversible inhibitor of MAOI
(RIMA) moclobemide was the least effective. TCAs were at the more effective end
of the spectrum, whilst SSRIs were towards the less effective end. In non-melancholic
depression, SSRIs were as effective as older antidepressants.

Onset of Action of Antidepressants

Traditional wisdom dictates that antidepressants produce a reduction in depressive
symptoms after two to three weeks. There is much evidence, going back to the first
antidepressant, imipramine, to suggest that this is an oversimplification, and that
some patients, and indeed some symptoms within individual patients, improve
more rapidly than others. There are several methodologies which have emerged to
establish speed of onset of action. Using pattern analysis, there is evidence for more
rapid onset with venlafaxine, fluoxetine, mirtazapine and nefazodone. Using
survival analysis, there is emerging evidence for several drugs including venlafaxine
and fluoxetine. In addition, adding other drugs to augment the spped of onset has
been studied. The best evidence is with the beta-blocker pindolol. Ballesteros and
Callado (2004) performed a meta-analysis of RCTs comparing pindolol plus
SSRIs with placebo plus SSRIs. In nine adequate trials, the pindolol augmentation
groups showed a better outcome after two weeks of treatment (OR 2.8; 95%
CI 1.4–5.7), but this benefit over SSRIs alone had disappeared by four to six weeks
(OR 1.4; 95% CI 0.8–2.7). This strongly supports the notion that pindolol speeds up
the onset of action of SSRIs.

Side Effects of Antidepressants

In general, the pharmacological profiles of antidepressants determine their adverse
effects and toxicity and hence their tolerability in clinical use. The side effects relate

to the affinity of these drugs at neurotransmitter receptors and transporters/reuptake sites in the brain and body.

The most obvious receptor affinity related effect is sedation, which may be either a wanted or unwanted effect in different circumstances: it is often a desirable effect during acute treatment, especially in agitated or anxious individuals, but is undesirable during continuation and maintenance treatment where it compromises a range of functions. Sedation is in general mediated by blockade of histaminic receptors, especially the H1 receptor, which is also involved in producing weight gain. Many of the more undesirable side effects of older tricyclic antidepressants are mediated by blockade of the muscarinic acetylcholine receptors, the predominant type of acetylcholine receptors in the brain which mediate many functions including memory and learning. The affinity of antidepressants for these receptors is shown in Figure 10.1. Muscarinic blockade is closely related to ongoing psychological deficits during treatment with tricyclic antidepressants and may relate to risk of accidents including road traffic accidents and falls in the elderly. Although H1 mediated sedation also contributes to the risk of accidents, muscarinic effects are more pernicious as patients are less aware of them. In general, the older tricyclics (especially amitriptyline and dothiepin) show high affinity), while the newer tricyclic lofepramine shows lower affinity. The SSRIs in general show very low affinity, except for paroxetine which has an affinity only marginally lower than that for the prototype tricyclic imipramine. The affinity of venlafaxine is similar to paroxetine, while the other SSRIs, mirtazapine, nefazodone and reboxetine show very low affinities. Blockade at the m1 muscarinic receptors produces blurred vision, dry mouth, sinus tachycardia, constipation, urinary retention and a range of psychological deficits especially in memory. Figure 10.2 shows the propensity of antidepressants, in recovered depressives on continuation treatment, to impair information processing as indicated by prolonged critical flicker fusion (CFF), while Figure 10.3 shows the relationship between muscarinic side effects with TCAs and impairment of CFF (Hale and Pinniniti, 1995).

Systematic reviews and meta-analyses have attempted to compare side-effect profiles of older and newer drugs, often with the intention of determining value-for-money of the newer drugs. One systematic review compared TCAs and SSRIs in people with all severities of depression (Trindade and Menon, 1998). Some studies have attempted to compare side effects and tolerability within drug groups, for example between different SSRIs. One large cohort study of people receiving four different SSRIs (fluvoxamine, fluoxetine, sertraline and paroxetine) in UK primary care found that reports of common adverse events (nausea/vomiting, malaise/lassitude, dizziness and headache/migraine) varied between SSRIs, with fluvoxamine coming out worst (relative risks verses fluvoxamine: fluoxetine RR 0.29 CI 0.27–0.32; paroxetine RR 0.35 CI 0.33–0.37; sertraline RR 0.26 CI 0.25–0.28), although this reflects commonly appreciated clinical knowledge (Mackay et al., 1997). A study of spontaneous reports to the UK Committee on Safety of Medicines found no difference in safety profiles between the same four SSRIs (Price et al., 1996).

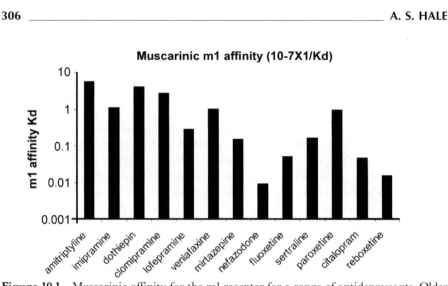

Figure 10.1 Muscarinic affinity for the m1 receptor for a range of antidepressants. Older tricyclics show high affinity. The affinity of venlafaxine and paroxetine are only marginally lower than that for the prototype tricyclic imipramine. The newer tricyclic lofepramine shows lower affinity, while the other SSRIs, mirtazapine, nefazodone and reboxetine show very low affinities. Blockade at the m1 muscarinic receptors produces blurred vision, dry mouth, sinus tachycardia, constipation, urinary retention and a range of psychological deficits especially in memory. Drawn from data in Leonard and Richelson (2000)

Antidepressant Tolerance

There is a considerable anecdotal literature on the loss of efficacy during continuation treatment with antidepressants (referred to as tolerance, tachyphylaxis, 'breakthrough depression'). It has been reported more frequently since the introduction of SSRIs and a notion has developed that there is a tendency for the effect of SSRIs to wane, so-called 'Prozac poop-out'. Byrne and Rothschild (1998) suggest that such tachyphylaxis is seen in 9–33% of patients on currently accepted maintenance and continuation doses of antidepressants, but may be more likely to occur with MAOIs and SSRIs. Quitkin et al. (1993) suggested that, for older TCAs and MAOIs, a considerable proportion of relapses in the first three months of treatment may be be due to loss of placebo effects. However, other explanations have been put forward, including unrecognized rapid cycling, pharmacological tolerance, pharmacokinetic changes, lack of prophylactic effect, an increase in underlying disease severity, and prior repeated drug trials (Sharma, 2001). Strategies for the management of tolerance include increasing the dose of antidepressant, reducing the dose, discontinuing treatment (for a drug holiday or indefinitely), augmentation or combination therapy, switching to an alternative antidepressant (including high-dose MAOI; Cohen and Baldessarini, 1985) and ECT. Of these, increasing the dose of the existing antidepressant is the commonest first-line

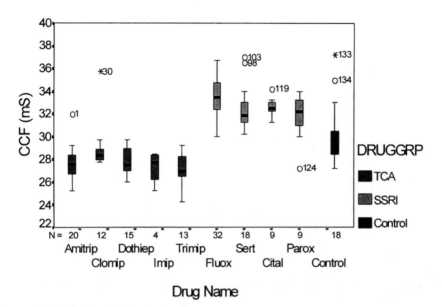

Figure 10.2 Critical flicker fusion frequency (cycles per second) in remitted depressed patients on maintenance antidepressant medication (older tricyclics and selective serotonin reuptake inhibitors) and drug-free controls. Graph shows box and whisker plot with outliers for each drug. Amitrip = amitriptyline; Clomip = clomipramine; Dothiep = dothiepin; Imip = imipramine; Trimip = trimipramine; Fluox = fluoxetine; Sert = sertraline; Cital = citalopram; Parox = paroxetine. Data from Hale and Pinniniti (1995)

strategy (Byrne and Rothschild, 1997). Sharma (2001) describes a series of 15 patients who showed loss of response to repeated trials of antidepressants and subsequent substitution, augmentation and ECT, who responded to discontinuation of antidepressants and substitution of a mood stabilizer, with a sustained response. Sharma argues that tolerance in such patients, at least in this open series, may represent unmasking of a bipolar diathesis by aggressive antidepressant treatment. Amsterdam and Hornig-Rohan (1996) suggest that unrecognized bipolarity is a common reason for treatment refractoriness.

Withdrawal

Withdrawal effects are well established for older antidepressants, described for TCAs very soon after their introduction (Kramer et al., 1961). Dilsaver et al. (1983) described gastrointestinal overactivity, insomnia, drowsiness or anxiety and agitation, irritability, apathy, headaches and moodiness. They attributed these symptoms to central cholinergic overactivity following withdrawal of

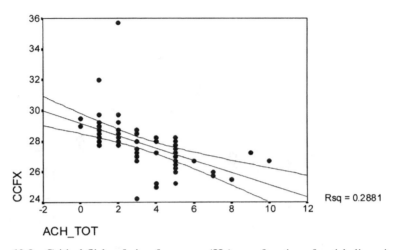

Figure 10.3 Critical flicker fusion frequency (Hz) as a function of anticholinergic side-effect score in remitted depressives on maintenance treatment with tricyclic antidepressants, demonstrating a close relationship between the two variables ($r = 0.537$, $p<0.001$). Data from Hale and Pinniniti (1995)

anticholinergic blockade with consequent up-regulation of central cholinergic function. They demonstrated how such effects could be treated with anticholinergic drugs. Hypomania was also described as an occasional consequence of TCA withdrawal (Mirin et al., 1981).

More recently, withdrawal symptoms have been described for SSRIs. Zajecka et al. (1998) examined discontinuation of fluoxetine ($n = 96$) versus continued treatment ($n = 299$) after 12 weeks' treatment. Sudden discontinuation was associated with increased dizziness (7% vs. 1%), dysmenorrhoea (3% vs. 0%), rhinitis (10% vs. 3%), and somnolence (4% vs. 0%), although high drop-out rates make these underestimates. Fluoxetine has a long half-life and so is the least likely of the SSRIs to show withdrawal effects. Stahl et al. (1997) reported the rate of spontaneous reports of suspected withdrawal worldwide for the first eight years after the introduction of fluoxetine, and showed higher rates for paroxetine than for sertraline or fluoxetine. The most common withdrawal effects reported for SSRIs were dizziness, nausea, paraesthesia, headache, and vertigo. Reporting rates are sensitive to the Weber effect, where spontaneous adverse events reports are highest shortly after the introduction of a new drug. As paroxetine and sertraline were launched after fluoxetine, this may bias the rates in favour of fluoxetine. Withdrawal does not seem to be any more frequent or severe in the elderly. Rosenbaum et al. (1998) conducted a double-blind placebo substitution study in remitted depressives on open label maintenance treatment with SSRIs. Patients were on placebo for five to eight days. Fewer fluoxetine patients experienced withdrawal than either paroxetine, and to a lesser extent sertraline, patients, both in terms of emergent somatic symptoms or symptoms of depression. Withdrawal reactions have also been described with other antidepressants such as venlafaxine (Parker and Blennerhassett, 1998). Slow taper of the shorter half-life drugs seems to reduce the risk of withdrawal. There is some evidence that pharmacodynamic differences among patients related to 5-HT$_{2A}$ receptor variants determine paroxetine intolerance rather than pharmacokinetics. Murphy et al. (2003a) showed that a susceptibility to paroxetine withdrawal seems to be strongly associated with the HTR2A C/C genotype.

Suicide

Early debates about increased suicidality and aggression have largely been resolved in favour of the SSRIs (Beasley et al., 1991; Heiligenstein et al., 1993), although disinhibition of underlying personality traits and recognition of a tendency to produce extrapyramidal side effects in a few patients (Hale, 1996) leaves open the question of self-harm precipitated by the dysthymia associated with akathisia (Wirshing et al., 1992). Jick et al. (1995) showed in general practice that the risk of suicide was higher in people who received fluoxetine (19/10 000 person years, CI 9–34) than those receiving dothiepin (RR of suicide vs. dothiepin 2.1, CI 1.1–4.1), but this was a historical cohort study and probably reflects the widespread knowledge that, unlike the TCAs, all SSRIs appear safe in overdose (Henry, 1994), and therefore patients at risk of suicide were preferentially given SSRIs. Concerns raised about abuse potential seem unfounded although there is some enhancement of psychometric performance not associated with activation or euphoria (Hale and Pinniniti, 1995).

Individual Antidepressants

Tricyclic Antidepressants (TCAs)

Tricyclic antidepressants (TCAs) are iminodibenzyl derivatives, first developed in the 1940s. Kuhn (1958) first noted the antidepressant properties of imipramine. Their antidepressant efficacy has been well established, with a response rate of up to 70%, although meta-analysis suggests a general response rate of closer to 60%, only 50% greater than placebo (Depression Guideline Panel, 1993). In the 18 years after imipramine was introduced, TCAs became available from two classes, tertiary amines (e.g. imipramine, amitriptyline, clomipramine) with two terminal methyl groups on the sidechain; and secondary amines (e.g. desipramine, nortriptyline), which are desmethylated derivatives of the tertiary amines. Tertiary amines are generally quite sedating while secondary amines are less so. TCAs also differ in the ratio of their inhibition of the uptake of noradrenaline to 5-HT. Nortriptyline, protriptyline, desipramine, maprotiline and lofepramine are predominantly noradrenaline reuptake inhibitors whilst clomipramine, imipramine, amitriptyline and dothiepin show a more equal ratio, although clomipramine's demethlyated metabolite is selective for 5-HT, giving clomipramine the most SSRI-like profile in clinical practice (Baldessarini, 1983). TCAs have five major pharmacological properties. They inhibit the reuptake of 5-HT and noradrenaline, are ml muscarinic antagonists, α-1 adrenoceptor antagonists and histamine H1 antagonists. Benefits and side effects are largely predictable from their binding and reuptake profiles.

Treatment with TCAs is initiated at low dose and titrated up slowly (every three or four days) to avoid side effects, especially postural hypotension (mediated by α-1 blockade) and the anticholinergic side effects of dry mouth, constipation, blurred vision and urinary retention. The dose–response curves for most TCAs are known and plasma level monitoring is useful to achieve the optimal balance between benefits and side effects (Perry et al., 1994). Lower doses are often required in elderly patients, but even in this group TCA doses below 75 mg daily are unlikely to be effective. Where response is seen at below the usual minimum effective dose in younger adults, increase up to this dose for maintenance is advocated (Anderson et al., 2000).

The utility of TCAs is limited by a high toxicity in overdose (Henry, 1994) mediated by arrhythmias caused by a quinidine-like effect on fast sodium channels in the heart. Pretreatment ECGs should be performed on at risk populations, which includes all children, adults over 40, and a history of heart problems. Paradoxically, the secondary TCA nortriptyline has been shown to be safer than the SSRI fluoxetine in elderly patients and those with heart disease (Roose, 1992).

This and the side-effect burden in general, have led to a general underdosing with tricyclics, especially in general practice (Bridges, 1983). Donoghue and Tylee (1996) showed a mean dose of 57 mg per day of tricyclics used in general practice in the UK despite recommendations that the minimum effective dose is 125–150 mg daily (1985). This leads to apparent treatment resistance, which may respond simply by increasing the dose of the TCA, achieving a more effective plasma level (Nelson et al., 1982).

A more recently developed TCA, available in some countries, is lofepramine, a selective noradrenaline reuptake inhibitor which has achieved some recent popularity as an alternative to the SSRIs. A tertiary amine, chemically related to imipramine, it is metabolized to the secondary amine desipramine, itself a selective noradrenaline reuptake inhibitor. Lofepramine has been available in many countries for longer than the SSRIs and is used because of a benign side-effect profile, related to a lack of free —NH_2 group in the sidechain which gives it minimal anticholinergic activity (Katona _et al._, 1993), and confers safety in overdose (Henry, 1994). These advantages are similar to those claimed for the SSRIs. The efficacy of lofepramine was reviewed by Lancaster and Gonzalez (1989) and an extensive and authoritative meta-analysis (and in some cases re-analysis) of clinical trial results was published by Kerihuel and Dreyfus (1991), who suggested that the risk/benefit ratio for lofepramine is superior to amitriptyline, imipramine, clomipramine, maprotiline and desipramine. Lofepramine is marketed as though 70 mg lofepramine is equivalent to 50 mg of imipramine, suggesting a minimum effective dose of 175–210 mg daily for lofepramine. Adequate dose-ranging data are not available due to the antiquity of many studies.

MAOIs

A second, older class of antidepressants is the monoamine oxidase inhibitors (MAOIs). These were introduced in the 1950s but concerns over both efficacy and safety have limited their popularity as a first-line treatment for major depression (Paykel and White, 1989). In major depression MAOIs are generally limited to third- or fourth-line treatments, essentially used for treatment-resistant depression (Nolen et al., 1988; Nolen, 1997). Three irreversible, non-selective (for MAO A and B) MAOIs are most commonly prescribed, phenelzine and isocarboxazid, which are derivatives of the hepatotoxic compound hydrazine, and tranylcypromine. MAOIs are in general activating, especially tranylcypromine, and traditionally given in divided doses early in the day. Phenelzine and tranylcypromine are structurally related to amphetamine, long thought responsible for their stimulant properties and causing concerns about their addiction potential. However, neither drug seems to possess addictive or euphoriant properties in normal clinical use (Mallinger and Smith, 1991; Thase et al., 1995). They are potentially metabolized to amphetamine, but current evidence suggests that the opening of the cyclopropyl ring structure of tranylcypromine, to form amphetamine, is not significant at usual doses (Sherry et al., 2000).

Prevailing clinical opinion of available controlled data suggests that all antidepressants have equal efficacy, approximately 60% to 70% in any given trial. However, it has also been believed for some time that MAOIs are less effective in major depression than TCAs, while MAOIs are superior in atypical depression. A systematic review of 55 randomized controlled trials comparing MAOIs with TCAs in several subgroups of people with depression (Thase et al., 1995) found that MAOIs were less effective in people with severe major depressive disorders but may be more effective in atypical depressive disorders (depressive disorders with reversed biological features, for example, increased appetite and weight, increased sleep, mood reactivity, and sensitivity to rejection). A six-month continuation therapy study with either phenelzine or imipramine in chronic atypical depressives initially stabilized on either drug for six months (Stewart et al., 1997) again shows benefit for phenelzine but not imipramine, again suggesting a special place for MAOIs with atypical depression. MAOIs may also be more effective than TCAs in very chronically depressed patients. Stewart et al. (1993) showed 70% of such patients to respond to phenelzine, 46% to imipramine and 17% to placebo. However, they also showed that a substantial proportion of these patients fitted the Columbia criteria for atypical depression.

A number of more selective MAOIs have been developed, but the only compound available in most countries is moclobemide. Two meta-analyses did not show any differences in efficacy between moclobemide and TCAs (Woggon, 1993; Angst et al., 1995). It has also been found equipotent to the SSRI fluoxetine in major depression, but superior to fluoxetine in atypical depression (Lonnqvist et al., 1994). One significant study found moclobemide inferior to TCAs in major depressive inpatients (DUAG, 1993). Moclobemide has developed a reputation for lack of efficacy in major depression and has been developed for a range of anxiety indications. Whether the reputation in depression is deserved or is a function of underdosing in clinical practice remains unclear.

SSRIs

The selective serotonin reuptake inhibitors (SSRIs) were the first of the newer 'designer' antidepressants, introduced throughout the world in the 1980s. The SSRIs differ in the potency of reuptake inhibition, but this shows no clear relationship to apparent effective clinical dose and so is of dubious relevance to efficacy. There is no convincing evidence that these compounds differ systematically in either efficacy (overall or for subpopulations of depressives) or in their side-effect profile, although one would expect minor differences from consideration of their receptor blocking and uptake inhibition profiles (Hyttel, 1994), which show minor effects on inhibition of dopamine reuptake with sertraline and noradrenaline reuptake with paroxetine. Clinical studies comparing the different SSRIs have rarely shown major differences. A recent study which compared the effectiveness of three SSRIs (paroxetine, fluoxetine, and sertraline) in depressed primary care patients, in an open-label, randomized, intention-to-treat trial (Kroenke et al., 2001) found responses to the three SSRIs comparable on all measures and at all time points, with similar incidences of adverse effects and discontinuation rates. Prospective head-to-head comparisons have produced similar results (Aguglia et al., 1993; Bennie et al., 1995; Newhouse and Richter, 1996; Tignol, 1992; Geretsegger et al., 1994; Patris et al., 1996). Escitalopram is a recently introduced SSRI. Escitalopram is the single isomer responsible for the serotonin reuptake inhibition produced by the racemic antidepressant citalopram. There is some data suggesting better efficacy than an equivalent dose of racemic citalopram (Gorman, 2002; Burke et al., 2002), perhaps suggesting the presence of the other isomer to be unhelpful in terms of efficacy.

A major benefit with several SSRIs is ease of dosing, as steep dose–response curves mean that a single or narrow range of doses can be advocated for most patients, usually in once-daily dose form. This ease of use has largely overcome the well-documented tendency in general practice to prescribe doses of a third to a half of effective therapeutic dose (Donoghue and Tylee, 1996), whilst still leaving some latitude for higher doses in secondary care (Hale and Stokes, 1991).

The SSRIs may be much less likely to trigger mania in bipolar patients than TCAs (Peet, 1994). Moclobemide seems also unlikely to trigger switches (Calabrese, Rapport et al., 1999). Boerlin et al. (1998) suggest that older MAOIs are more likely than SSRIs to trigger switch. Vieta et al. (2002) provide evidence that switch is much more likely with venlafaxine than with the SSRI paroxetine. The addition of lithium, but not anticonvulsant mood stabilizers, appears to further reduce the rate of switch in patients treated with an SSRI (Henry et al., 2001).

NARIs

Desipramine, lofepramine, and nortryptiline are examples of tricyclic antidepressant compounds from the first generation of antidepressants that exert their effects predominantly by blockade of noradrenaline reuptake, as does maprotiline, a nontricyclic compound. However, these antidepressants are also associated with interactions with muscarinic, histaminergic, and adrenergic receptors, leading to a range of undesirable side effects. Reboxetine is a selective noradrenaline reuptake inhibitor (NARI). It is a racemic mixture of two enantiomers, the (*S,S*)-enantiomer being the more potent inhibitor. It has little affinity for muscarinic acetylcholine receptors and does not block serotonin reuptake, α-1 or muscarinic receptors. Like most other antidepressants, it is a functional antagonist at the human $5\text{-}HT_{3A}$ receptor (Eisensamer et al., 2003). It does not inhibit monoamine oxidase activity, nor inhibit or induce hepatic cytochrome P450 enzymes and shows linear pharmacokinetics. Absorption is rapid and the terminal elimination half-life is about 13 hours. It seems safe in overdose. It has little sedative effect and minimal effect on sexual function (Clayton et al., 2003). It shows evidence of acute and long-term clinical efficacy and safety from double-blind, placebo-controlled, and active comparator studies, which show that it is significantly more effective than placebo and as effective as fluoxetine in reducing depressive symptoms (Schatzberg, 2000). Much has been made of its benefit for social adjustment, compared to that seen with SSRIs. This is in accord with its ability to bias in favour of positive rather than negative self-perception and to promote social bonding in normal volunteers (Harmer et al., 2003; Tse and Bond, 2003) and there is some evidence of its benefit in social phobics (Atmara et al., 2003). Montgomery et al. (2003) reviewed four placebo-controlled RCTs of reboxetine 8–10 mg/day for four to eight weeks in severe major depression (17 item HDRS $\geqslant$ 25). The responder rate was much higher than with placebo in these patients, 63% (56–74%) with reboxetine and 36% (20–52%) with placebo. One of these four trials, however, did not show superiority over placebo, and recent clinical studies conducted in the USA and Canada, prompted by the FDA, resulted in a letter of non-approval in the US. Overall, reboxetine was superior to placebo in only 5 of 12 placebo-controlled studies (Hajos et al., 2004). The current evidence for the NICE review on the treatment of depression (NICE, 2004) shows comparable efficacy when compared to fluoxetine and reboxetine (odds ratios -0.15 [CI -0.45 to 0.16] and -0.05 [CI -0.25 to 0.12]) respectively, in fact favouring reboxetine as a trend. Efficacy therefore remains under review for this compound.

Venlafaxine

Venlafaxine is a derivative of phenylethylamine and is a mixed serotonin and nor-adrenaline reuptake inhibitor (SNRI). Conceptually it offers the benefits of a TCA without the anticholinergic side effects. There is evidence for good efficacy, with two recent meta-analyses showing superior efficacy to all other antidepressants except for TCAs (Thase et al., 2001a; Smith et al., 2002). There is also some evidence for a more rapid onset of action than other commonly used antidepressants (Guelfi et al., 1995), and of efficacy in treatment resistant depression (Nierenberg et al., 1994). There is evidence for a dose–response effect, with the highest potency observed in doses $\geqslant 225$ mg/day of venlafaxine (Entsuah, 2003). Response rates in this meta-analysis were 61–66% for venlafaxine, 57% for SSRIs and 42% for placebo. Other dual action antidepressants have been developed, such as milnacipran, the efficacy of which was reviewed by Kasper et al. (1996) and Rouillon et al. (2000a); and duloxetine (Detke et al., 2002; Thase et al., 2003; Goldstein et al., 2002; Schatzberg, 2004). Duloxetine and milnacipran have a more balanced reuptake ratio than venlafaxine (5-HT/NE ratios 9, 2, and 30 respectively) (Wong and Bymaster, 2002), but the significance of this for clinical practice is unclear. Such ratios are similar to those seen with tricyclics such as amitriptyline and imipramine. All of these dual action antidepressants also appear to have beneficial effect in pain, both associated with depression and persistent pain syndromes (Iyengar et al., 2003; Davis and Smith, 1999).

Mirtazapine

Mirtazapine is a presynaptic α-2 antagonist with a dual action, increasing nor-adrenergic and serotonergic neurotransmission. Enhanced serotonergic neurotransmission is mediated via 5-HT_1 receptors, as mirtazapine antagonizes postsynaptic serotonergic 5-HT_2 and 5-HT_3 receptors. Mirtazapine has only a weak affinity for 5-HT_1 receptors and has very weak muscarinic anticholinergic and histamine (H_1) antagonist properties. These properties suggest efficacy and good potential tolerability. In systematic reviews, mirtazapine has proven to be superior to placebo, and equivalent in efficacy to the tricyclic antidepressants amitriptyline, doxepin and clomipramine, but with an improved tolerability profile (Fawcett and Barkin, 1998). There is some evidence for a rapid onset of antidepressant action, but equal efficacy, when compared to fluoxetine (Wheatley et al., 1998) and to paroxetine (Benkert et al., 2000). Guelfi et al. (2001) conducted a comparison of mirtazapine and venlafaxine, in high doses, in hospitalized melancholic depressives. There were no statistically significant differences but the results numerically favoured mirtazapine. Mirtazapine lacks the sexual and gastrointestinal side effects of the SSRIs and is often better tolerated, although it causes considerable weight gain and it is sedative, especially at lower doses, because of very potent antihistamine effects. Van der Flier and Schutte (2003) have performed a meta-analysis comparing the tolerability of mirtazapine with that for SSRIs and venlafaxine, showing better tolerability for mirtazapine. Thase (2003) showed in a meta-analysis significant remission rates with mirtazapine (38.8%) compared to SSRIs (34.7%), which was largely explained by a significantly faster onset of action for mirtazapine in the 12 double-blind RCTs reviewed. This faster onset of action has been confirmed in a further meta-analysis by Thompson et al. (2004). The meta-analysis by NICE (2004) showed mirtazapine to achieve better end point mean scores than SSRIs (-0.13 CI -0.27 to 0.00) but not to differ significantly in responder or remission rates.

Nefazodone

This phenylpiperazine drug has a mixed mechanism of action, showing both serotonin reuptake inhibition and $5\text{-}HT_{2a}$ receptor antagonism. It has been shown to be effective in placebo-controlled RCTs and compared to imipramine and fluoxetine, with a favourable profile compared to SSRIs in alleviating anxiety associated with depression (Zajecka, 1996). It is generally well tolerated, with favourable sexual and gastrointestinal profile compared to the SSRIs, but causing weight gain (Hale, 1997). However, there have been increasing concerns about hepatotoxicity (Stewart, 2002) and nefazodone has recently been withdrawn.

Bupropion

Bupropion is a weak inhibitor of biogenic amine reuptake. The mechanisms of action of bupropion as an antidepressant are not fully understood, but both dopaminergic and noradrenergic mechanisms are implicated. Bupropion inhibits dopamine reuptake and has a weaker effect on noradrenaline reuptake, but also has an effect on adrenergic neurotransmission in the locus coeruleus. There are minimal effects on serotonin reuptake, and no effect on serotonin, adrenergic, cholinergic or histaminic receptors (Sanchez and Hyttel, 1999). The hydroxybupropion metabolite has a half-life of 22 hours (compared to 10 hours for the parent compound) and this and the threoamino alcohol metabolite accumulates and contributes significantly to the antidepressant activity (Ascher et al., 1995). The efficacy of bupropion was established in six clinical trials in the 1970s and 1980s (Horst & Prescorn 1998), which showed benefit at doses of between 300 and 750 mg/day. Efficacy in maintenance treatment of depression has been demonstrated (Weihs et al., 2002). There is a relationship between response and plasma levels, with a therapeutic window between 50 and 100 ng/ml (Preskorn, 1983). There is a potential for inducing seizures, especially at high plasma levels (Pesola and Avasarala, 2002) and hence plasma level monitoring is advisable. A meta-analysis of studies against imipramine and placebo showed benefit over placebo and comparable efficacy to imipramine (Workman and Short, 1993). Bupropion has efficacy comparable to or superior to SSRIs (Coleman et al., 1999). Switching to bupropion has efficacy in patients resistant to treatment with other antidepressants including fluoxetine (Fava et al., 2003), while there is also evidence for augmentation of SSRIs or venlafaxine with bupropion (DeBattista et al., 2003). Adverse effects of bupropion include dry mouth, headache, insomnia and nausea but are mostly mild or moderate in intensity (Settle et al., 1999). Few patients discontinue treatment as a result. There is minimal effect on sexual function and some dose-related weight loss. The potentially life-threatening dermatological side effect, erythema multiforme, has been reported both with the standard and the sustained release preparations (Lineberry et al., 2001). There have been suggestions of drug-induced mania with bupropion but a comparison of switching in SSRIs versus bupropion (Joffe et al., 2002) failed to find any difference.

St John's Wort (Hypericum perforatum)

Hypericum perforatum (St John's wort) is a widely used over-the-counter herbal preparation taken as an alternative therapy for depression, sometimes in an attempt to avoid adverse effects associated with prescription antidepressants. There is some uncertainty about which of the many chemicals found in the parent plant are important and hence which preparations are optimal, with consequent uncertainty about dose.

Two meta-analyses have examined the efficacy and safety of St John's wort. Linde and Mulrow (2000) showed that in mild to moderately severe depressives, St John's wort was significantly superior to placebo (responder rates, 57% and 25% respectively), but no different to comparator antidepressants. A second analysis (Whiskey et al., 2001) extended this review by applying different inclusion and exclusion criteria but came to similar conclusions, showing response rates for St John's wort in comparison to antidepressants to be between 43.3% and 76.4%, and 40.1% and 72.2% respectively. When comparing St John's wort with placebo, response rates were 40.0–80% and 0–63% respectively. In general, most studies have found St John's wort to be comparable to active controls, such as amitriptyline (Wheatley, 1997), imipramine (Vorbach et al., 1997; Philipp et al., 1999; Woelk et al., 2000), and fluoxetine (Schrader et al., 2000), and superior to placebo. Whiskey et al. (2001) showed a relative risk of responding to treatment of 1.00 (CI 0.91–1.11) for St John's wort compared to standard antidepressants in nine adequate RCTs included, and of 1.59 (CI 1.40–1.80) compared to placebo in 14 studies included.

A recent adequately powered study ($n = 340$) comparing *H. perforatum* 900 to 1500 mg daily with sertraline 50–100 mg daily and placebo, during an eight-week acute study with an 18-week double-blind continuation phase in moderately severe depressives, with a minimum HDRS at baseline of 20, throws doubt on the efficacy of St John's wort (Davidson et al., 2002). This study finds St John's wort to be numerically inferior to placebo on the primary outcome measure. Sertraline also performs badly in a responder analysis (perhaps because of a low dose) but the effect size for sertraline on the HAM-D total score was consistent with reported effect sizes for standard antidepressants and for three other sertraline studies on the HAM-D change from baseline. Side effects of St John's wort were more frequent anorgasmia, swelling, and urination relative to placebo, although these were mild. However, a meta-anlysis by NICE (2004) which includes seven adequate studies, has shown St John's wort to be superior to placebo both in terms of mean end-point scores and responder status, for all levels of severity of depression including severe depression. Studies reviewed by NICE comparing St John's wort with other antidepressants found it inferior overall (1.20 CI 1.00–1.44) mainly due to the superiority of amitriptyline. Again, St John's wort had comparable efficacy to comparitors at all levels of severity.

Linde and Mulrow (2000) found that adverse events were poorly reported in the trials. They were reported by 26% of people on St John's wort compared with 45% of people on standard antidepressants and 15% on combinations of St John's wort and valerian, compared with 27% on amitriptyline or desipramine. Whiskey et al. (2001) noted headaches, restlessness, fatigue, and dizziness, as the most commonly reported side effects, which they comment seem to resemble SSRIs more than TCAs, except that St John's wort does not seem to prolong cardiac conduction (Czekella et al., 1997). There has been a report of three cases of possible mania induction associated with St John's wort (Moses and Mallinger, 2000). A review by Ernst et al. (1998) included RCTs and observational postmarketing surveillance studies of St John's wort. The most common adverse effects of St John's wort in the included trials were gastrointestinal symptoms, dizziness/confusion, tiredness/sedation, and dry mouth, although all occurred less frequently than on conventional drugs. Findings from observational studies were consistent with these findings.

Interactions with other drugs are possible and should be considered. These include HIV protease inhibitors, HIV non-nucleoside reverse transcriptase inhibitors, warfarin, cyclosporin, oral contraceptives, anticonvulsants, digoxin and theophylline, and perhaps also hormone-replacement therapies and several hormonal cancer therapeutics, including tamoxifen for breast cancer and medroxyprogesterone for lung cancer. These interactions are likely to be mediated via St John's wort's effect on cytochrome P450 enzymes where it acts as an enzyme inhibitor on certain subtypes and as an inducer on others (Whiskey et al., 2001).

Predictors of Antidepressant Treatment Response

Psychomotor retardation or agitation, pervasive anhedonia and non-reactive mood predict treatment response to TCAs (Fawcett et al., 1983; Hale and Stokes, 1991; Parker and Hadzi-Pavlovic, 1993). Interaction between endogenicity and severity produces a curvilinear relationship between endogenicity and acute TCA treatment response (Joyce and Paykel, 1989). The best treatment response to TCAs is shown by patients with endogenous symptoms but moderate severity. However, melancholic features may predict a poorer treatment response to SSRIs (Anderson and

Tomenson, 1994; Roose et al., 1994; Montes et al., 2004). Men may have better response to and tolerance of tricyclic antidepressants (Hamilton, 1995). Women may show better response and tolerance to SSRIs (Kornstein, 1997). There is a complex relationship between precipitating life events, coping styles and outcome of antidepressant treatment (Mazure et al., 2000). Adverse achievement events were predictors of poor outcome. While adverse interpersonal life events were associated with good outcome, this may reflect a large interpersonal network being more likely to provide a trigger event whilst at the same time also providing more opportunities for support.

A variety of biological markers have been thought to predict response to either antidepressants in general, or to particular groups of antidepressants, such as tricyclics (Hale et al., 1989), noradrenergic versus serotonergic antidepressants (Schatzberg, 1998) and MAOIs (Georgotas et al., 1987). The liability of patients with particular genotypes to respond selectively to particular drugs is under intensive investigation. For example, the presence of the APOE ε-4 allele predicts rapid response to mirtazapine but not to paroxetine in cognitively intact older patients with major depression (Murphy et al., 2003b).

ECT

Electroconvulsive therapy (ECT) remains a controversial treatment, at least as far as the public are concerned. It is an acute treatment, with time-limited benefit. Naturalistic studies show that the relapse rate during the 6 to 12 months following ECT exceeds 50% (Aronson et al., 1987; Sackeim et al., 1990). There are studies of 'maintenance treatment' using various top-up regimes, or on the use of drugs as maintenance therapy after ECT has produced remission. Sackeim et al. (2001) have pointed out that much of this work was done when ECT was considered a first-line treatment, and may not be applicable now that ECT is often reserved for a more treatment-resistant population. Several studies have shown that medication resistance is especially predictive of post-ECT relapse (Sackeim et al., 1990). Sackeim et al. (2001) show that continuation treatment in unipolar depressives with a combination of lithium and the noradrenergic TCA nortriptyline is clearly superior to nortriptyline alone or placebo, relapse rates being 39%, 60% and 84% respectively at six months, the latter two figures being substantially higher than with the earlier studies cited. However, they also pointed out that, in the post-SSRI era, patients are much less likely to have received an adequate trial of a TCA prior to ECT. The only placebo-controlled trial of lithium monotherapy continuation therapy after ECT in unipolar patients found no protective effects during the first six months (Coppen et al., 1981).

Janicak et al. (1985) performed a meta-analysis of the available 'simulated' ECT studies then available and found patients given real ECT more likely to respond to treatment (NNT 3, CI 2–5). Wijeratne et al. (1999) come to similar conclusions from 11 more recent studies. In general, ECT is reserved for patients with psychotic depression, patients with severe suicidal drive where a rapid response is required, or patients who cannot tolerate or have not responded to drug treatment.

Duration of Continuation Treatment

Traditional wisdom, reflected in most treatment guidelines, suggests continuation treatment for major depressives with an effective antidepressant for a period in the range of three to nine months after recovery. This is thought to reflect the natural history of depression, the patient remaining at risk of relapse if during the period of remission after responding to treatment, the antidepressant is discontinued before underlying recovery has occurred (Frank, 1991). Loonen et al. (1991) conducted a meta-analysis of six RCTs of continuation treatment, showing a reduction in the risk of relapse by nearly a half if antidepressants were continued for four to six months after acute treatment. Reimherr et al. (1998) examined whether this remained true for newer antidepressants, using a design with multiple, rather than a single, discontinuation point. They conducted a four-arm study in patients who had responded to 12–14 weeks of open label treatment with 20mg fluoxetine. They substituted placebo at either 0, 14, 38 or 50 weeks. Relapse rates were lower in the drug than the placebo groups after 24 total weeks of treatment (26.4% and 48.6% respectively), and after 38 total weeks of treatment (9.0% and 23.2%). After 62 total weeks of treatment, relapse rates were similar (10.7% and 16.2%). They therefore conclude that the traditional wisdom is correct, continuation treatment with fluoxetine being necessary for at least six months after remission is achieved with three months' acute treatment.

Whether this wisdom applies equally to all subtypes of depression is less clear. Stewart et al. (1997) conducted a placebo-controlled discontinuation study in atypical chronic depressives and showed that stopping phenelzine at six months after remission led to relapse.

Maintenance Treatment

It is apparent from a large body of work examining the relationship of life events to depression that the sensitivity to life events increases with each successive depressive episode (Brown et al., 1994). The impact of significant life events on the triggering of depressive illness is most apparent at the first episode. Thereafter, progressively smaller stresses, which may be indistinguishable from 'normal life', may trigger subsequent episodes, showing evidence of sensitization. The speed of sensitization increases with age. Maj et al. (1992) showed a pattern of increasing severity from index episode over three subsequent episodes followed prospectively. Shea et al. (1992) showed that 50% of patients relapsed within two years if imipramine was discontinued after achieving acute remission with 16 weeks' treatment. Half of all depressives only ever have one episode, although during the three years following an acute episode the suicide risk is increased. The risk of recurrence after an acute episode is 33% within the first year, 50% within the first five years and a 70% lifetime risk (Thase, 1992). For individuals who have already experienced a recurrence, there is a 40% risk of a further episode within two years of recovery rising to 60% after five years (Keller and Boland, 1998) with an 80% lifetime risk. Individuals who have experienced three previous episodes have a 90% lifetime risk (Thase, 2001). The risk of a subsequent episode thus increases with the number already experienced, in keeping with the life event and sensitization model cited above. There is some suggestion of a curvilinear relationship between risk of recurrence and age of onset, with a higher risk of recurrence for those experiencing their first episode before the age of 21 and after the age of 60. Greden (1993) has suggested that lifetime pharmacological maintenance may be indicated for patients 50 years or older at first episode, 40 years or older with two or more prior episodes, or for those with three or more prior episodes. This would suggest an algorithm such as shown in Table 10.2 (Hale, 1997a). Where recurrence is undesirable, prophylactic maintenance therapy should be considered. Evidence of efficacy with TCAs for up to five years exists, but few studies with newer drugs extend beyond one to two years.

A meta-analysis of maintenance treatment for two years in older depressives was conducted by the Old Age Depression Interest Group (1993), who found a 55% reduction in the risk of relapse over two years' treatment. There is no similar published meta-analysis in younger adults.

The definitive study of maintenance treatment with imipramine, the Pittsburg Maintenance Study, part of the NIMH Treatment of Depression Collaborative Research Programme, examined the benefits of three years' active antidepressant treatment versus placebo in a five-arm study which also included interpersonal psychotherapy (Frank et al., 1990). Patients were randomized after showing remission during 12 weeks of acute treatment with imipramine. Only 10% of patients who received neither antidepressant nor psychotherapy during the maintenance phase were free of recurrence during the three-year period, compared to just under 80% in the drug and combined drug and psychotherapy arms. The psychotherapy alone or with placebo arms showed three year survival around 30%. Of patients surviving at three-years in the imipramine arm, 20 were then re-randomized to either a further two-year continuation or placebo. 90% survived on imipramine compared to 10% on placebo (Kupfer et al., 1992). They concluded that, even after three years' remission on maintenance antidepressants, there was little or no protection against recurrence once treatment stops; and that patients with an episode frequency < 2 years should not be discontinued from active medication for at least five years.

More recent studies addressing maintenance treatment with modern antidepressants have been somewhat difficult to interpret due to high drop-out rates (e.g., Keller et al., 1998a). However, it is worth examining such studies as the burden of side effects with the older drugs is a major consideration in treatment choice with long-term treatment. Gilaberte et al. (2001) compared fluoxetine and placebo over 48 weeks of double-blind maintenance study in responders to 32 weeks of open label treatment with fluoxetine. 80% of the fluoxetine group survived compared to 60% of the placebo group, and the symptom-free period was significantly longer for patients treated with fluoxetine versus placebo (295 vs. 192 days). Hochstrasser et al. (2001) conducted a comparison of citalopram and placebo in a two-year maintenance study in younger recurrent depressive adults, with a 75% survival rate for citalopram versus 37% for placebo in those staying in the study for 500 days or longer. However, the dropout rate at this point was 91%, perhaps illustrating the difficulty of conducting such studies. Keller et al. (1998a) conducted a 76-week maintenance study comparing sertraline and placebo, showing 95% survival with sertraline compared with 70% on placebo, difficult to interpret because of the success of the placebo arm. Terra and Montgomery (1998) demonstrated the benefit of maintenance treatment with fluvoxamine for one year. Franchini et al. (1998) compared 20 and 40 mg daily doses of paroxetine in a two-year maintenance study of patients responding to acute treatment with the higher dose, finding that recurrences were significantly fewer with the higher dose (lending credence to the saying 'the dose that gets you well keeps you well'). In a one-year maintenance study Thase et al. (2001b) compared mirtazapine and placebo, with greater survival in the active drug arm (80%) than the placebo arm (56%). Rouillon et al. (2000b) showed statistical benefit for maintenance treatment over one year with the dual-action milnacipran. This study showed a very high placebo response rate, but the drug–placebo differences were more marked in comparison of various quality of life measures (Rouillon et al., 2000b). There is some evidence, from pooled data, for lower relapse rates with venlafaxine compared with placebo at one year (Entsuah et al., 1996) but dropout rates are very high in both groups.

A long-term maintenance study was also conducted in older patients (over 50 but mean age 67), who had recovered on a combination of nortriptyline and interpersonal psychotherapy (IPT). They were randomized to four treatment arms (drug+IPT; drug+clinic visit; IPT+ placebo; clinic visit+placebo) and followed up over three years (Reynolds et al., 1999). Time to recurrence of a major depressive episode for all three active treatments was significantly better than for placebo. Recurrence rates over three years were 20% for nortriptyline and IPT; 43% for nortriptyline+clinic visits; 64% for IPT+placebo; and 90% for placebo+clinic

TABLE 10.2   Duration of antidepressant treatment for major depression

	Age at first episode		
	≤39	40–49	≥50
First episode	6–9 months	6–9 months	Indefinitely
Second episode	6–9 months	4–5 years	Indefinitely
Second episode with complications	4–5 years	Indefinitely	Indefinitely
Third or subsequent episode	Indefinitely	Indefinitely	Indefinitely

visits. Combined treatment with nortriptyline+IPT was significantly more effective than IPT+placebo and showed a trend to superiority over nortriptyline alone. Older patients (>70years) relapsed more often and more quickly than those aged <70.

Psychological Treatments

The preference of patients for non-physical treatments, especially for milder forms of depression in primary care settings, together with a failure to demonstrate clear benefit of psychodynamically based psychotherapy and the limited availability of labour-intensive, long-term psychotherapy, have led to the development of a range of 'brief' psychotherapies, which have been evaluated for depressive disorders in recent years. Evidence from such studies of brief psychological treatments in depression have generally found that, for mild to moderately severe depression, psychological treatments are about as effective as drug treatment, but take a little longer to work. With more severe and/or melancholic depression, drug treatments are more effective (Thase and Friedman, 1999). There is strong evidence for this with cognitive-behaviour therapy, and similar evidence is emerging for several other therapies including interpersonal therapy, problem-solving therapy, and brief non-directive counselling. Similar evidence exists across the age range but is less robust with older people. The generalizability of the studies of psychological treatments is as uncertain as is sometimes the case with drug studies. In particular, drug doses in these comparative studies are often quite low, leading to criticisms that the drugs were handicapped by the drugs not reaching therapeutic concentrations. This is the case for most of the studies cited in a meta-analysis by Dobson (1989), where in addition many studies quoted were not blind and many were carried out in CBT centres, leading to potential bias.

Cognitive-Behaviour Therapy (CBT)

CBT, originally developed by Beck, aims to counter negative thoughts and cognitions, and may be seen as a form of re-educational therapy. By educating patients to challenge their negative thinking, and to consider rational, positive alternative interpretations, the cycle of repetitive negative thinking may be broken. Whether this leads to global improvement and recovery from depression clearly depends on the place of negative thinking in the aetiology and maintenance of a depressive episode. Gloaguen et al. (1998) performed a systematic review of 48 RCTs of psychological therapies (total $n = 2765$) mainly of outpatients in secondary care with mild to moderate depression, including dysthymia; people with psychotic or bipolar symptoms were excluded. Of these, 20 RCTs compared CBT with waiting list or placebo controls and 17 compared CBT with drug treatment. 79% of people receiving placebo were more symptomatic than the average person receiving CBT.

65% of people treated with CBT were less symptomatic than the average person treated with antidepressant drugs ($p < 0.0001$). They conclude that CBT is effective in mild to moderate depression, more so than waiting-list placebo or indeed antidepressants. No major adverse effects of CBT are reported. RCTs in primary care suggest limited acceptability to some patients. Recently it has been suggested that it may be possible to deliver CBT for depression in primary care or even home-based settings using computer programs as the delivery systems, e.g., 'Beating the Blues', which have more limited need for clinical supervision (Marks, 1999). If promising preliminary results are borne out in larger controlled trials, this could revolutionize the availability of psychological treatments for depression, which are at present severely limited by the need for intensive training and by the labour-intensive nature of the interventions. Some studies suggest that, although in milder cases CBT may be as effective as antidepressants, in more severe cases CBT may be scarcely more effective than placebo (Elkin et al., 1989). This is shown in Figure 10.4. The speed of recovery is usually slower with CBT than with an antidepressant, which may have significant health economic implications.

CBT has been studied in older adults with depression, systematically reviewed by McCusker et al. (1998). They described four RCTs in older adults that compared psychological treatments versus no treatment. None of the RCTs found a significant difference between treatment and no treatment, measured on the Hamilton Depression Rating Scale. It also found six RCTs comparing different psychological treatments. Five of six comparisons of 'rational' treatments (including cognitive-behaviour therapy) versus no treatment in older adults found significant benefit with treatment. Combined, the 'rational' treatments performed significantly better than no treatment, with a mean difference in the Hamilton Depression Rating Scale score of -7.25 (95% CI -10.1 to -4.4), but were not significantly different from the 'non-specific attention' control. None of the RCTs found significant differences in effectiveness between psychological treatments.

Interpersonal Psychotherapy (IPT)

IPT was developed in the USA by Weissman, Klerman and colleagues, as a pragmatic, effective, feasible and testable alternative to psychoanalysis and other psychodynamic psychotherapies. It was specifically designed to help patients with mild to moderate unipolar depression. It places emphasis on current interpersonal relationships and on strategies to improve them, helping the patient identify, understand and solve current problems and to develop constructive and positive ways of relating to others. Gloaguen et al. (1998) conducted a large RCT in patients with mild to moderate depression, a 16-week study comparing IPT versus drug treatment or placebo plus clinical management. Recovery rates were similar for IPT and imipramine (43% and 42% respectively), both significantly superior to the 'placebo' condition of clinical management. No adverse effects have been reported with IPT but its use is limited in comparison to medication by the need for extensive training. Maintenance treatment with IPT has been discussed above in the three and five-year comparison with imipramine (Frank et al., 1990; Kupfer et al., 1992). Agosti and Ocepek-Welikson (1997) examined the effectiveness of CBT, IPT, imipramine and clinical management in a re-analysis of those patients in the NIMH Treatment of Depression Collaborative Research programme who suffered from early-onset chronic depression. In this cohort of patients they found no evidence of differential response to the four treatment arms, in contrast to earlier results for major depressives as a whole. Elkin et al. (1989) showed that, as with CBT, IPT was significantly less effective than antidepressant treatment in more severe cases.

Problem-solving Therapy

A brief therapy involving cycles of problem identification, solution generation and testing. There are several small studies comparing problem-solving therapy with drug treatment of mildly depressed patients in primary care settings (Mynors-Wallis et al., 1995; Thase et al., 1997), finding the treatments equally effective. Problem-solving therapy shows little adverse effect and requires less training than CBT or IPT. Benefit in more severe depression or as a combined package with medication has yet to be systematically evaluated.

Non-directive Counselling/Supportive Psychotherapy

Where this differs from the brief therapies described above, which may be delivered under this label, it encompasses psychological treatments for patients with chronic and disabling conditions, for whom basic and fundamental change is not seen as a realistic goal, or attempts to ensure that reasonably healthy people stay healthy. As such, it could perhaps not be expected to effect remission or recovery from depression and might be reserved only for the most chronic and treatment-resistant of cases. It is, however, widely used, especially in primary care settings (King et al., 1994). Churchill et al. (1999) reviewed five RCTs comparing counselling with routine GP management of depression in UK primary care. No consistent advantage was seen for counselling in the main outcomes studied, although RCTs found greater satisfaction with counselling versus routine care. A recent Norwegian study compared adding either sertraline, mianserin or placebo to general practice based counselling in a double-blind RCT (Malt et al., 1999). They concluded that the combined drug and psychological treatment (counselling, emotional support, and close 24-week follow-up) was more effective than psychological treatment alone, in particular for those with recurrent depression, and more so in women than men. For cases of major depression in primary care, counselling is not an effective treatment, having been described as no more effective than a waiting list (Friedli et al., 1997; Harvey et al., 1998).

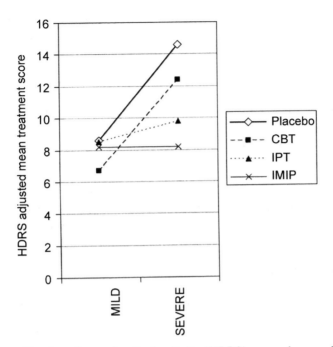

Figure 10.4 Hamilton Depression Rating Scale (HDRS) mean change with treatment with placebo, cognitive-behaviour therapy (CBT), interpersonal psychotherapy (IPT) or pharmacotherapy with imipramine (IMIP) as a function of initial severity of illness. Pharmacotherapy is clearly superior in more severe depression, with the two psychotherapies of intermediate benefit and placebo the least

Combined drugs and Talking Treatment

In more severe depression, where psychological treatments alone are not effective, there is strong evidence that combining antidepressant drug treatment with either interpersonal or cognitive therapy is more effective than either of the psychological therapies alone. Such an effect was absent in mild to moderate depression. Thase et al. (1997) conducted a meta-analysis of six RCTs totalling 595 patients. In mild to moderate depression there was no advantage in combining drug and specific psychological treatments, but in more severe depression, combined treatment was superior. A study with the modern drug nefazodone (Keller et al., 2000) compared it over three months treatment with cognitive-behaviour therapy or the combination and showed a clear and impressive superiority for the combined treatment (NNT 5, CI 3–6). In another comparison with modern antidepressants, Thase et al. (2000) randomized male patients to a 16-week, open label trial of CBT, fluoxetine or bupropion, with crossover for non-responders at eight weeks. The response rate was much higher in the drug-treated patients (87%) compared to the CBT group (54%), with the benefit from medication particularly apparent in chronic depressives.

The issue of maintenance treatment is perhaps even more crucial here than with monotherapies, but outcome data are patchy and it is unclear exactly what constitutes a 'maintenance' treatment with the various psychotherapies. Fava et al. (1998) examined the related issue of the efficacy of sequential use of CBT after successful treatment with antidepressants. They randomized recovered recurrent major depressives, tapering and discontinuing their antidepressants after randomizing to CBT or clinical management, with a 20-week intervention. Levels of residual symptoms were significantly lower in the CBT group than in the clinical management group after stopping medication. At two-year follow-up, the CBT group had a lower relapse rate (25%) than the clinical management group (80%) over the next two years, significant using survival analysis. This study thus suggests a protective effect of CBT which persists during a treatment-free follow-up period.

BIPOLAR DISORDERS

The treatment of bipolar disorders has seen major changes in recent years. In the not too distant past, lithium was the only licensed and evidence-based mood stabilizer, bipolar depression was not routinely recognized as requiring a different treatment approach to unipolar depression and mania was managed with typical antipsychotics. Now there are an ever-expanding number of mood stabilizers available, with a developing understanding of in which subtypes of bipolar illness to use each; there is much debate over when and which antidepressant to use in the acute depressed phase of bipolar illness; and atypical neuroleptics are not only replacing typical neuroleptics as anti-manic agents, but are seen as having putative mood stabilizing and antidepressant properties.

Nevertheless, for the acute depressive phase of bipolar illness, the evidence base remains somewhat thin, as there has been until recently little research, despite considerable evidence that the biology of bipolar and unipolar depression are very different. Bipolar depression is a very disabling condition, one recent study showing that patients with bipolar disorder spend about half of their lives with symptoms of illness, of which two-thirds of the time is spent depressed, a further 13% in mixed states (Judd et al., 2002).

Bipolar Depression

Bipolar depression is often misdiagnosed as unipolar depression, requiring more than 10 years of symptoms before correct diagnosis (American Psychiatric Association, 2002). Initial unipolar presentation in adolescent or young adult life shows a progressive rate of conversion to bipolar diagnosis with the appearance of hypomanic or manic symptoms, 25% and 16% of cases respectively converting over a

15-year period (Goldberg et al., 2001). Bipolar depression is difficult to treat effectively, with a lengthy period under treatment before treatment response is seen, often becoming treatment-resistant. Thase's group has shown that the median time to remission in outpatients with bipolar I depression treated with treatment guideline directed care was eight months (Hlastala et al., 1997). Ghaemi et al. (2001) showed that acute non-response to antidepressant treatment was commoner in bipolar than unipolar depression (RR 1.6, CI 0.8–3.4), irrespective of whether antidepressants were used alone or in combination with a mood stabilizer. There were non-significant differences in response rate between different classes of drug in bipolar patients, with the best response shown to SSRIs, then tricyclics and bupropion, and the worst response to 'miscellaneous' drugs. They also showed that the late development of tolerance was commoner (RR 3.4, CI 1.2–10.0), and relapse into depression on cessation of treatment was less frequent (RR 0.2, CI 0.1–0.5), in bipolar compared with unipolar depression. Rapid cycling and switch into mania occurred only in bipolar depressives.

The development of rapid cycling and manic switching seem to be common when treating depression in bipolar patients with an antidepressant alone, although they may be somewhat less likely with modern antidepressants or when used in conjunction with mood stabilizers (Bottlender et al., 2001; Ghaemi et al., 2001; Nemeroff et al., 2001; Altshuler et al., 1995), but controversy remains in this area (Henry et al., 2001; Preda et al., 2001; Post et al., 2001; Goldberg and Truman 2003). Traditional wisdom suggests that the risk of antidepressant-induced switch is one-third of that seen with TCAs (11.2%) and with SSRIs (3.7%) (Peet, 1994). However, recent data from the STEP-BD programme suggest that this may be an underestimate of the risk, especially in patients who have already shown at least one previous manic switch, in which the lowest switch rates were seen with MAOIs and mirtazapine (Truman et al., 2003) (Table 10.3). Risk factors of switch include multiple previous episodes of illness and being female (Boerlin et al., 1998); a history of previous drug induced switch (Fogelson et al., 1992); and multiple previous antidepressant trials or comorbid alcohol abuse (Goldberg and Whiteside, 2002). Some risks apply only to particular drugs: increased risk in early onset cases may apply only to TCAs, increased risk in those with a bipolar family history only with SSRIs (Howland, 1996); and the risk of switch with TCAs may be greater in bipolar II than bipolar I, with the reverse being the case with MAOIs (Boerlin et al., 1998; Himmelhoch et al., 1991). The genotype of the serotonin transporter protein gene may confer vulnerability to switch, the short form being associated with violent suicide, anxiety and SSRI response in addition to switching (Mundo et al., 2001).

Most treatment guidelines still advise against treatment of the acute depressive phase of bipolar illness with an antidepressant alone and advise that, in previously unmedicated non-psychotic individuals, treatment should commence with a mood stabilizer as monotherapy (Francis et al., 1998; American Psychiatric Association, 2002). Where this monotherapy is inadequate, Young et al. (2000) advocate the addition of a second mood stabilizer. The British Association of Psychopharmacology guidelines (Goodwin, 2003) advise initiation of an SSRI antidepressant combined with lithium, valproate or an antipsychotic. The rationale for this is the avoidance of manic switch or precipitation of rapid cycling which may be caused by an antidepressant used alone. Thase and Sachs (2000) suggest that the intrinsic antidepressant effect of some mood stabilizers used alone may be an adequate treatment, and where it is not, a mood stabilizer will be required anyway as prophylaxis against recurrence of either phase of illness. They also suggest that antidepressant monotherapy may be contraindicated only in bipolar I depressives, and safe in bipolar II individuals.

Where antidepressants are used in bipolar depression, second-generation drugs or MAOIs are usually favoured. Monotherapy with SSRIs has in general been found to produce response in 60–65% of bipolar cases although this is less consistant with paroxetine where Nemeroff (2001) showed a failure of both paroxetine and imipramine to differentiate from placebo when added to lithium (although paroxetine was more effective than placebo or lithium where lithium plasma levels were < 0.8 mmol/L), and Vieta (2002) showed low response rate for both paroxetine and venlafaxine (43% and 48% respectively). Himmelhoch et al. (1991) showed tranylcypromine to have a response rate of 81% compared to 48% with imipramine, in line with Thase et al. (1992a) who showed a tranylcypromine response rate of 75%.

Bupropion has found itself a niche for treating bipolar depression, based on scant evidence. A small double-blind study by Sachs et al. (1994) compared nine patients taking bupropion with 10 taking desipramine, with a 55% response rate with the former and 50% response rate with the latter drug, although the switch rate was low at 11% with bupropion compared to 50% with desipramine. An open label study of six bipolar II patients showed no switch and 100% efficacy (Haykel and Akiskal, 1990). Add-on studies supplementing existing antidepressant or mood stabilizer treatment with bupropion have also suggested efficacy (Erfurth et al., 2002).

Where an antidepressant is used in combination with a mood stabilizer, recent evidence suggests that the recurrence rate over one year increases very considerably if the antidepressant is discontinued (Altschuler et al., 2003), although preliminary one-year results for a five-year outcome study of discontinuation do not confirm this (Hsu et al., 2004).

Most North American treatment guidelines still caution against the use of antidepressants as first-line treatment. The American Psychiatric Association guidelines (Hirschfield et al., 2002), Francis et al. (1998) and Sachs et al. (2000) all advocate initial use of lithium or valproate preparations (divalproex in most US studies) as first-line treatment in acute bipolar depression. Lithium is generally favoured over divalproex as, although both treatments are effective in mania, only the former has unequivocally demonstrated efficacy in bipolar depression. However, a systematic review of nine early placebo-controlled crossover designed studies of lithium in acute bipolar depression (Zornberg and Pope, 1993) showed only a modest response rate of 36%. Divalproex monotherapy has not yet been extensively studied in controlled randomized studies, although in a review of four open label studies the response rate of 30% appears to be comparable to lithium treatment (McElroy and Keck, 1993).

Two key studies suggest that monotherapy with lamotrigine, at doses of between 50 and 300 mg daily, is an effective and generally well-tolerated treatment for an acute episode of bipolar depression. Calabrese et al. (1999) treated 195 patients with bipolar I depression in an RCT comparing three treatment arms, lamotrigine 50 mg/day or 200 mg/day, or placebo, over seven weeks. The two lamotrigine groups were well tolerated and both showed superior efficacy to placebo, with a trend in favour of the 200-mg/day group, but because of gradual titration the high dose group only had three weeks on the top dose, so a longer study may have shown a dose–response relationship. Switch rates were similar between groups (placebo 5%, lamotrigine 50 mg/day 3%, lamotrigine 200 mg/day 8%). Headache was the only notable side effect in the lamotrigine groups.

Frye et al. (2000) conducted an RCT in patients with treatment refractory bipolar disorder in various phases of illness. Patients were randomized in a series of cross-over trials to six weeks' treatment with lamotrigine (mean dose 274 mg/day), gabapentin (mean dose 3987 mg/day), or placebo. The lamotrigine group showed significant reductions in depressive symptoms compared to patients on placebo.

ECT has been extensively used in bipolar depression, with many studies performed from the mid-1960s to the late 1980s; the majority of these found ECT superior in efficacy to TCAs or MAOIs. It has not been systematically compared to newer antidepressants, antidepressant combinations with mood stabilizers or antipsychotics.

A recent development has been evidence for the mood stabilizing effects of atypical antipsychotics. At present, the only atypical antipsychotic studied in the depressive phase of bipolar illness is olanzapine. An RCT in bipolar depression compared olanzapine (5–20 mg/day, mean dose 9 mg/day), one of three fixed-dose combinations of olanzapine (mean dose 7 mg/day) and fluoxetine (mean dose 38 mg/day) (olanzapine/fluoxetine combination, OFC), and placebo in an eight-week trial among 833 patients with bipolar I depression with an initial MADRS score ≥ 20 (Tohen et al., 2003). This was the first RCT to show the efficacy of mono-therapy with an atypical antipsychotic in acute bipolar depression. Active treatment arms showed significantly bigger decrease in depressive symptoms than did the placebo group, beginning at week 1, with the OFC group showing significantly

TABLE 10.3   Rates of switch into mania after antidepressant treatment in patients with ≥ 1 previous manic switch studied in the STEP-BD programme (after Truman et al., 2003)

DRUG	n	Switch rate (%)
MAOIs	14	14
Mirtazapine	14	16.7
Nefazodone	29	17.2
Venlafaxine	38	26.3
ECT	14	28.6
Bupropion	67	34.3
Heterocyclics	34	38.2
SSRIs	67	58.2

larger decrease in MADRS total scores than the olanzapine only group at weeks 4, 6, and 8. Remission ($\geqslant 50\%$ decrease in MADRS score) was seen in 24.5% of patients on placebo, 32.8% of the olanzapine group, and 48.8% of the OFC group. There were no significant differences in switch rates. However, significantly more patients in the active treatment groups than in the placebo group had weight gain, appetite increase, dry mouth and asthenia.

Space does not permit a discussion of maintenance treatments for bipolar illness. An adequate mood stabilizer will prevent relapse into either depression, mania or hypomania, will not promote switching or rapid cycling and will treat both the manic/hypomanic and the depressive acute phases of illness (ECNP consensus 2000). Table 10.4 shows putative mood stabilizers and their efficacy in the different phases of bipolar illness and in preventing switching or rapid cycling. There is some evidence of yet more subtle distinctions, for example lithium may be less effective where depression is the first presentation in a new episode after a period of euthymia, rather than mania.

Psychological Treatments for Bipolar Disorder

Psychoeducation

Both brief and more extensive individual psychoeducational interventions have been shown to improve knowledge and attitudes to mood stabilizing medication (Soares et al., 1997; Colom et al., 1998) but there is little direct evidence of improved medication concordance.

Cognitive-Behaviour Therapy

Four RCTs have examined efficacy in bipolar patients. Perry et al. (1999) showed reduced relapse only for manic episodes at 12 and 18 months following 17–20 sessions, with improved social functioning and employment. Scott et al. (2001) showed stronger effects for preventing relapse for depression than mania, but the intervention was a mixture of up to 25 sessions of CBT with additional psychoeducation. Lam et al. (2000, 2003) showed reduction in episode number for depression, mania and hypomania with improvements in mood, social functioning and medication concordance at six months after 12–20 sessions of mixed CBT and psychoeducation. Zaretsky et al. (1999) compared CBT in bipolar and unipolar depressives after 20 sessions using the Basco and Rush (1996) therapy manual. There was improvement in mood in both groups. All these studies showed evidence of effectiveness but are small and do not adequately control for therapist time.

Two further studies have reported group CBT interventions (Palmer et al., 1995; Patelis-Siotis et al., 2001). Symptomatic improvement was reported in both but there was no follow-up data and so there is no evidence of benefit in preventing relapse.

Interpersonal and Social Rhythm Therapy

This technique is a modification of the IPT technique used with unipolar depression, with a focus on defining problems, emotional processing, and problem solving, over 12–20 sessions (Frank et al., 1994). In the first outcome study Frank et al., 1997 report that therapy stabilized social rhythms relative to 'normal clinical management' controls, but a later study by the same group failed to replicate this, but showed benefit for subsyndromal symptoms (Frank, 1999, 2001).

Family Therapy

Zaretsky (2004) has shown that focused family therapy is more effective than crisis management in the treatment of bipolar depressives. Benefits for family-focused treatment (FFT) have been shown to reduce relapse rates for bipolar depressives stable on medication, in two sub-analyses of a controlled study where two psycho-education sessions and as required crisis management were offered to the control families (Simoneau et al., 1999; Miklowitz et al., 2000). However, as the treatment group received 21 sessions of the full package, therapist exposure was not adequately matched. A two year follow-up (Miklowitz et al., 2003) showed that the FFT group had a lower relapse rate (35% vs. 54%) and better episode-free survival intervals (73.5±28.8 vs. 53.2±39.6 weeks) than controls (odds ratio, 0.38 CI 0.20–0.75). FFT also produced greater improvement in mood and better medication concordance.

VanGent and Zwart (1991) showed brief psychoeducational joint marital treatment to decrease relapse at follow-up in a small sample with nonspecific outcome assessment. Honig et al. (1997) showed that a eight-session family psychoeducational intervention was able to reduce expressed emotion (EE) in a small subgroup of relatives who had high EE at baseline in a moderately sized study, but they did not report symptomatic benefit for the patient.

Psychoanalytic Psychotherapy

Jones (2004) reviews the evidence for a psychoanalytic approach to bipolar disorder and finds it to be impressionistic and based on a few very small case series. Joffe (2002) comes to similar conclusions: 'the use of psychodynamically orientated psychotherapy was widely practiced with uncertain results'.

Group Therapy

Jones (2004) reviews four studies of group psychotherapy in bipolar patients, all of which were open trials and only one used blind assessment. Two of the studies

TABLE 10.4 Putative mood stabilizers showing efficacy against the different criteria for a full mood stabilizer

	Lithium	Divalproate	Carbamazepine	Lamotrigine	Topiramate	Olanzapine	Quetiapine	Risperidone
Acute mania	+	+	+	?+	?+	+	+	+
Bipolar depression	?++	?+	?+	++	?.	+	?.	?.
Prophylaxis mania	++	?++	?++	?+	?+?+	?+	?.	?+
Prophylaxis depression	+	?.	?.	+	?.	?+	?.	?.
Do not worsen mania/dep	+	+	+	+	+	+	+	+

reviewed, reporting on mixed bipolar and schizophrenic patient groups, showed reduced average rates of relapse at follow-up. The other two studies reported positive outcomes in terms of subjective benefit or group attendance and did not assess clinical outcome. These loose studies of generally open groups give mainly impressionistic support for the intervention and do not define clearly the necessary duration of treatment or elements of therapy. Four of the five studies reviewed by Joffe (2002) were not covered by Jones. Some showed reduced hospitalization rates as well as improved concordance. Joffe concludes 'nonetheless, group psychotherapy of various types appears to be useful as an adjunct to medication in the treatment of various phases of bipolar illness including depression'.

CONCLUSIONS

Advances in both pharmacological and psychotherapeutic treatment of depressive disorders have led to a clearer understanding of the benefits of selected treatments and combinations of treatments in different disorders and different phases of the disorders. For unipolar major depression, the initial treatment of choice remains antidepressants, and SSRIs and other newer compounds have rapidly replaced older drugs due to improved tolerability and safety in overdose. There are some doubts about the potency of SSRIs in the most severe cases, but venlafaxine and mirtazapine are proving useful alternatives to older tricyclic drugs in these cases. The need not only for adequate duration of continuation treatment, to prevent relapse within an episode, but also for maintenance treatment for many years in some recurrent depressives, is now understood and efficacy for both these purposes is now established for many antidepressants. However, it is also apparent that many patients still prefer talking therapy to drugs, and there is now a much clearer understanding of the place of brief psychotherapies in the management of milder depressive episodes, and as augmentation treatment with antidepressants. For bipolar disorder, the depressive phase of illness remains difficult to manage and there is ongoing debate about the place for antidepressants in the acute management of the disorder. A range of newer mood stabilizers now have evidence for efficacy and it has recently become apparent that atypical antipsychotics have considerable efficacy as mood stabilizers. The advent of the first depot preparation of an atypical antipsychotic may have important implications for maintenance treatment in poor compliers, but will not replace the need for psychological interventions including psychoeducational approaches.

REFERENCES

Agosti V, Ocepek-Welikson K (1997) The efficacy of imipramine and psychotherapy in early-onset chronic depression: a reanalysis of the National Institute of Mental Health Treatment of Depression Collaborative Research Program. *J Affect Disord* **43**: 181–186.

Aguglia E, Casacchia M, Cassano GB, et al. (1993) Double-blind study of the efficacy and safety of sertraline versus fluoxetine in major depression. *Int Clin Psychopharmacology* **8**: 197–202.

Altschuler LL, Post RM, Leverich GS, Mikalauskas K, Rosoff A, Ackerman L (1995) Anti-depressant-induced mania and cycle acceleration: a controversy revisited. *Am J Psychiatry* **152**: 1130–1138.

Altshuler L, Suppes T, Black D, Nolen WA, Keck PE Jr, Frye MA, McElroy S, Kupka R, Grunze H, Walden J, Leverich G, Denicoff K, Luckenbaugh D, Post R (2003) Impact of antidepressant discontinuation after acute bipolar depression remission on rates of depressive relapse at 1-year follow-up. *Am J Psychiatry* **160**(7): 1252–1262.

American Psychiatric Association (2000) *Practice Guideline for the Treatment of Patients with Major Depressive Disorder*. Second Edition. American Psychiatric Association, Arlington, VA.

American Psychiatric Association (2002) Practice guideline for the treatment of patients with bipolar disorder (revision). *Am J Psychiatry* **159** (4 Suppl): 1–50.

Amsterdam JD, Hornig-Rohan M (1996) In Amsterdam JD, Hornig-Rohan M (eds) *Psychiatric Clinics of North America* Vol 19: *Treatment Algorithms in Treatment Resistant Depression*. Philadelphia: WB Saunders, pp. 371–386.

Anderson IM (1998) RIS versus tricyclic antidepressants in depressed inpatients: a meta-analysis of efficacy and tolerability. *Depress Anx* **7**(Suppl 1): 11–17.

Anderson IM, Nutt DJ, Deakin JFW, on behalf of the Consensus Meeting and endorsed by the British Association for Psychopharmacology (2000) Evidence-based guidelines for treating depressive disorders with antidepressants: a revision of the 1993 British Association for Psychopharmacology guidelines. *J Psychopharmacol* **14**(1): 3–20.

Anderson IM, Tomenson BM (1994) The efficacy of selective serotonin re-uptake inhibitors in depression: a meta-analysis of studies against tricyclic antidepressants. *J Psychopharmacol* **8**: 238–249.

Angst J, Amrein R, Stabl M (1995) Moclobemide and tricyclic antidepressants in severe depression: meta-analysis and prospective studies. *J Clin Psychopharmacol* **15**(4 Suppl 2): 16S–23S.

Anton RF, Sexauer JD (1983) Efficacy of amoxapine in psychotic depression. *Am J Psychiatry* **140**: 1344–1347.

Aronson TA, Shukla S, Gujavarty K, et al. (1988) Relapse in delusional depression: a retrospective study of the course of treatment. *Comp Psychiatry* **29**: 12–21.

Aronson TA, Shukla S, Hoff A (1987) Continuation therapy after ECT for delusional depression: a naturalistic study of prophylactic treatments and relapse. *Convulsive Ther* **3**: 251–259.

Ascher JA, Cole JO, Colin J-N, Feighner JP, et al. (1995) Bupropion: a review of its mechanism of antidepressant activity. *J Clin Psychiatry* **56**(9): 395–401.

Atmaca M, Tezcan E, Kuloglu M (2003) An open clinical trial of reboxetine in the treatment of social phobia. *J Clin Psychopharmacol* **23**(4): 417–419.

Baldessarini RJ (1983) *Biomedical Aspects of Depression and its Treatment*. Washington, DC: American Psychiatric Press.

Ballesteros J, Callado LF (2004) Effectiveness of pindolol plus serotonin uptake inhibitors in depression: a meta-analysis of early and late outcomes from randomised controlled trials. *J Affective Dis* **79**: 137–147.

Basco MR, Rush AJ (1996) *Cognitive-Behavioral Therapy for Bipolar Disorder*. New York: Guilford.

Beasley CM Jr, Dornseif BE, Bosomworth JC, et al. (1991) Fluoxetine and suicide: a meta-analysis of controlled trials of treatment for depression. *BMJ* **303**: 685–692.

Benkert O, Grunder G, Wetzel H, Hackett D (1996) A randomized, double-blind comparison of a rapidly escalating dose of venlafaxine and imipramine in inpatients with major depression and melancholia. *J Psychiatr Res* **30**(6): 441–451.

Benkert O, Szegedi A, Kohnen R (2000) Mirtazapine compared with paroxetine in major depression. *J Clin Psychiatry* **61**(9): 656–663.

Bennie EH, Mullin JM, Martindale JJ (1995) A double-blind multicentre trial comparing sertraline and fluoxetine in outpatients with major depression. *J Clin Psychiatry* **56**: 229–237.

Blackwell B (1976) Treatment adherence. *Br J Psychiatry* **129**: 513–531.

Boerlin HL, Gitlin MJ, Zoellner LA, Hammen CL (1998) Bipolar depression and antidepressant-induced mania: a naturalistic study. *J Clin Psychiatry* **59**(7): 374–379.

Bottlender R, Rudolf D, Strauss A, Moller HJ (2001) Mood stabilizers reduce the risk of developing antidepressant induced maniform states in acute treatment of bipolar I depressed patients. *J Affect Disord* **63**: 79–83.

Breggin PR (1991) *Toxic Psychiatry: Why Therapy, Empathy, and Love Must Replace the Drugs, Electroshock, and Biochemical Theories of the New Psychiatry.* New York: St Martins Griffin. ISBN 0-312-11366-8.

Bridges PK (1983) '. . . and a small dose of an antidepressant might help'. *Br J Psychiatry* **142**: 626–628.

Brown GW, Harris TO, Hepworth C (1994) Life events and endogenous depression. A puzzle re-examined. *Arch Gen Psychiatry* **51**(7): 525–534.

Burke WJ, Gergel I, Bose A (2002) Fixed-dose trial of the single isomer SSRI escitalopram in depressed outpatients. *J Clin Psychiatry* **63**(4): 331–336.

Byrne S, Rothschild AJ (1997) Psychiatrists' responses to failure of maintenance therapy with antidepressants. *Psychiatr Serv* **48**: 835–837.

Byrne S, Rothschild AJ (1998) Loss of antidepressant efficacy during maintenance therapy: possible mechanisms and treatment. *J Clin Psychiatry* **59**: 279–288.

Calabrese JR, Bowden CL, Sachs GS, Ascher JA, Monaghan E, Rudd (1999) A double-blind placebo-controlled study of lamotrigine monotherapy in outpatients with bipolar I depression. Lamictal 602 Study Group. *J Clin Psychiatry* **60**: 79–88.

Calabrese JR, Rapport DJ, Kimmel SE, Shelton MD (1999) Controlled trials in bipolar I depression: focus on switch rates and efficacy. *Eur Neuropsychopharmacol* **9**(Suppl 4): S109–S112.

Chilvers C, Dewey M, Fielding K, Gretton V, Miller P, Palmer B, Weller D, Churchill R, Williams I, Bedi N, Duggan C, Lee A, Harrison G (2001) Antidepressant drugs and generic counselling for treatment of major depression in primary care: randomised trial with patient preference arms. *BMJ* **322**: 772–775.

Churchill R, Dewey M, Gretton V, et al. (1999) Should general practitioners refer people with major depression to counsellors? A review of current published evidence. *Br J Gen Pract* **49**: 738–743.

Clayton AH, Zajecka J, Ferguson JM, Filipiak-Reisner JK, Brown MT, Schwartz GE (2003) Lack of sexual dysfunction with the selective noradrenaline reuptake inhibitor reboxetine during treatment for major depressive disorder. *Int Clin Psychopharmacol* **18**(3): 151–156.

Clerc GE, Rujmy P, Verdeau-Paillès J, on behalf of the Venlafaxine French Inpatient Study Group (1994) A double-blind comparison of venlafaxine and fluoxetine in patients hospitalized for major depression and melancholia. *Int Clin Psychopharmacol* **9**: 139–143.

Cohen B, Baldessarini R (1985) Tolerance to therapeutic effects of antidepressants. *Am J Psychiatry* **142**: 489–490.

Coleman CA, Cunningham LA, Foster VJ, Batey SR, Donahue RMJ, Houser TL, Ascher JA (1999) Sexual dysfunction associated with the treatment of depression: a placebo-controlled comparison of bupropion sustained release and sertraline treatment. *Ann Clin Psychiatry* **11**: 205–215.

Colom E, Vieta E, Martinez A, et al. (1998) What is the role of psychotherapy in the treatment of bipolar disorder? *Psychother Psychosom* **67**: 3–9.

Coppen A, Abou-Saleh MT, Milln P, et al. (1981) Lithium continuation therapy following electroconvulsive therapy. *Br J Psychiatry* **139**: 284–287.

Corominas A, Bonet P, Nieto E (1998) Recurrent brief depression successfully treated with lithium. *Biol Psychiatry* **44**(9): 927–929.

Corya SA, Andersen SW, Detke HC, Kelly LS, Van Campen LE, Sanger TM, Williamson DJ, Dubé S (2003) Long-term antidepressant efficacy and safety of olanzapine/fluoxetine combination: a 76-week open-label study. *J Clin Psychiatry* **64**: 1349–1356.

Czekella J, Gastpar M, Hubner WD, Jager D (1997) The effect of hypericum extract on cardiac conduction as seen in the electrocardiogram compared to that of imipramine. *Pharmacopsychiatry* **30**(Suppl): 86–88.

Davidson JRT, Gadde KM, Fairbank JA, et al. (2002) Effect of *Hypericum perforatum* (St John's wort) in major depressive disorder: a randomized controlled trial. *JAMA* **287**(14): 1807–1814.

Davis JL, Smith RL (1999) Painful peripheral diabetic neuropathy treated with venlafaxine HCl extended release capsules. *Diabetes Care* **22**: 1909–1910.

DeBattista C, Solvason HB, Poirier J, Kendrick E, Schatzberg AF (2003) A prospective trial of bupropion SR augmentation of partial and non-responders to serotonergic antidepressants. *J Clin Psychopharmacol* **23**(1): 27–30.

Depression Guideline Panel (1993) *Depression in Primary Care* Vol 2: *Treatment of Major Depression* (AHCPR Publication No. 93-0551). Rockville, MD: US Department of Health and Human Services, Agency for Health Care Policy and Research.

Detke MJ, Lu Y, Goldstein DJ, Hayes JR, Demitrack MA (2002) Duloxetine 60mg once daily for major depressive disorder, a randomized, double-blind, placebo-controlled trial. *J Clin Psychiatry* **53**(4): 308–315.

Diamond G, Denton TA (1993) Alternative perspectives on the biased foundations of medical technology assessment. *Ann Intern Med* **118**: 455–464.

Dilsaver SC, Feinberg M, Greden J (1983) Antidepressant withdrawal symptoms treated with anticholinergic agents. *Am J Psychiatry* **140**: 249–251.

Dobson KS (1989) A meta-analysis of the efficacy of cognitive therapy for depression. *J Consult Clin Psychol* **57**(3): 414–419.

Donoghue JM, Tylee A (1996) The treatment of depression: prescribing patterns of antidepressants in primary care in the UK. *Br J Psychiatry* **168**: 164–168.

Doraiswamy PM, Khan ZM, Donahue RM, Richard NE (2001) Quality of life in geriatric depression: a comparison of remitters, partial responders and non-responders. *Am J Geriatr Psychiatry* **9**: 423–428.

DUAG (1993) Moclobemide: a reversible MAO-A-inhibitor showing weaker antidepressant effect than clomipramine in a controlled multicenter study. Danish University Antidepressant Group. *J Affect Disord* **28**(2): 105–116.

Dunlop SR, Dornseif BE, Wernick JF, Potvin JH (1990) Pattern analysis shows beneficial effect of fluoxetine treatment in mild depression. *Psychopharmacol Bull* **26**: 173–180.

Dunner DL, Schmaling KB, Hendrickson H, Becker J, Lehman A, Bea C (1996) Cognitive therapy versus fluoxetine in the treatment of dysthymic disorder. *Depression* **4**(1): 34–41.

Eastman CI, Young MA, Fogg LF, Liu L, Meaden PM (1998) Bright light treatment of winter depression: a placebo-controlled trial. *Arch Gen Psychiatry* **55**(10): 883–839.

ECNP (2000) ECNP consensus on the Optimal Definition of a Mood Stabilizer, Nice 2000. *Eur Neuropsychopharmacol* **11**: 79–88.

Eisensamer B, Rammes G, Gimpl G, Shapa M, Ferrari U, Hapfelmeier G, Bondy B, Parsons C, Gilling K, Zieglgansberger W, Holsboer F, Rupprecht R (2003) Antidepressants are functional antagonists at the serotonin type 3 (5-HT3) receptor. *Mol Psychiatry* **8**(12): 994–1007.

Elkin I, Shea MT, Watkins JT, et al. (1989) National Institute of Mental Health treatment of depression collaborative research program: general effectiveness of treatments. *Arch Gen Psychiatry* **46**: 971–982.

Entsuah AR (2003) Remission rates with various venlafaxine doses verses SSRIs in MDD. *American Psychiatric Association 156th Annual Meeting.* NR461.

Entsuah AR, Rudolph RL, Hackett D, Miska S (1996) Efficacy of venlafaxine and placebo during long-term treatment of depression: a pooled analysis of relapse rates. *Int Clin Psychopharmacol* **11**(2): 137–145.

Erfurth A, Michael N, Stadtland C, Arolt V (2002) Bupropion as add-on strategy in difficult-to-treat bipolar depressive patients. *Neuropsychobiology* **45**(Suppl 1): 33–36.

Ernst E, Rand JI, Barnes J, et al. (1998) Adverse effects profile of the herbal antidepressant St John Wort (*Hypericum perforatum* L). *Eur J Clin Pharmacol* **54**: 589–594.

Fava GA, Rafanelli C, Grandi S, Conti S, Belluardo P (1998) Prevention of recurrent depression with cognitive behavioral therapy: preliminary findings. *Arch Gen Psychiatry* **55**(9): 816–820.

Fava M, Papakostas GI, Petersen T, Mahal Y, Quitkin F, Stewart J, McGrath P (2003) Switching to bupropion in fluoxetine-resistant major depressive disorder. *Ann Clin Psychiatry* **15**(1): 17–22.

Fawcett J, Barkin RL (1997) Efficacy issues with antidepressants. *J Clin Psychiatry* **58**(Suppl 6): 32–39.

Fawcett J, Barkin RL (1998) Review of the results from clinical studies on the efficacy, safety and tolerability of mirtazapine for the treatment of patients with major depression. *J Affect Disord* **51**: 267–285.

Fawcett J, Clark DC, Scheftner WA, Hedeker D (1983) Differences between anhedonic and normally hedonic depressive states. *Am J Psychiatry* **140**(8): 1027–1030.

Feighner J, Targum SD, Bennett ME et al. (1998) A double-blind, placebo-controlled trial of nefazodone in the treatment of patients hospitalized for major depression. *J Clin Psychiatry* **59**: 246–253.

Feinstein A (1983) An additional basic science for clinical medicine II: The limitations of randomized trials. *Ann Intern Med* **99**: 544–550.

Fogelson DL, Bystritsky A, Pasnau R (1992) Bupropion in the treatment of bipolar disorders: the same old story? *J Clin Psychiatry* **53**(12): 443–446.

Frances AJ, Kahn DA, Carpenter D, Docherty JP, Donovan SL (1998) The Expert Consensus Guidelines for treating depression in bipolar disorder. *J Clin Psychiatry* **59** (Suppl 4): 73–79.

Franchini L, Gasperini M, Perez J, Smeraldi E, Zanardi R (1998) Dose–response efficacy of paroxetine in preventing depressive recurrences: a randomized, double-blind study. *J Clin Psychiatry* **59**(5): 229–232.

Frank E (1991) Response, remission, recovery, relapse, recurrence. *J Clin Psychiatry* **52**(suppl 2): 12–16.

Frank E (2001) Interpersonal and social rhythm therapy. In *Fourth International Conference on Bipolar Disorder*. Pittsburg, USA. http://www.hsls.pitt.edu/about/libraries/wpic/bipolar4.html

Frank E, Hlastala S, Ritenour A, Houck P, Tu XM, Monk TH, Mallinger AG, Kupfer DJ (1997) Inducing lifestyle regularity in recovering bipolar disorder patients: results from the maintenance therapies in bipolar disorder protocol. *Biol Psychiatry* **41**(12): 1165–1173.

Frank E, Kupfer DJ, Ehlers CL et al. (1994) Interpersonal and social rhythm therapy for bipolar disorder: integrating interpersonal and behavioural approaches. *Behav Ther* **17**: 143–149.

Frank E, Kupfer DJ, Perel JM, Cornes C, Jarrett DB, Mallinger AG, Thase ME, McEachran AB, Grochocinski VJ (1990) Three year outcomes for maintenance therapies in recurrent depression. *Arch Gen Psychiatry* **47**(12): 1093–1099.

Frank E, Swartz HA, Kupfer DJ (2000) Interpersonal and social rhythm therapy: managing the chaos of bipolar disorder. *Biol Psychiatry* **48**(6): 593–604.

Frank E, Swartz HA, Mallinger AG, Thase ME, Weaver EV, Kupfer DJ (1999) Adjunctive psychotherapy for bipolar disorder: effects of changing treatment modality. *J Abnorm Psychol* **108**(4): 579–587.

Freeman EW, Rickels K, Sondheimer SJ, Polanski M (1999) Differential response to anti-depressants in women with premenstrual syndrome/premenstrual dysphoric disorder: a randomized controlled trial. *Arch Gen Psychiatry* **56**: 932–939.

Freeman EW, Rickels K, Yonkers KA, Kunz NR, McPherson M, Upton GV (2001) Venlafaxine in the treatment of premenstrual dysphoric disorder. *Obstet Gynecol* **98** 5(1): 737–744.

Friedli K, King MB, Lloyd M, Horder J (1997) Randomised controlled assessment of non-directive psychotherapy versus routine general-practitioner care. *Lancet* **350**(9092): 1662–1665.

Frye MA, Ketter TA, Kimbrell TA, Dunn RT, Speer AM, Osuch EA, Luckenbaugh DA, Cora-Ocatelli G, Leverich GS, Post RM (2000) A placebo-controlled study of lamotrigine and gabapentin monotherapy in refractory mood disorders. *J Clin Psychopharmacol* **20**(6): 607–614.

Geddes JR, Freemantle N, Mason J, Eccles MP, Boynton J (2000) SSRIs versus other antidepressants for depressive disorder. *Cochrane Database Syst Rev 2000*. CD001851.

Georgotas A, McCue RE, Cooper TB, Nagachandran N, Friedhoff A (1989) Factors affecting the delay of antidepressant effect in responders to nortriptyline and phenelzine. *Psychiatry Res* **28**(1): 1–9.

Georgotas A, McCue RE, Friedman E, Cooper T (1987) Prediction of response to nortriptyline and phenelzine by platelet MAO activity. *Am J Psychiatry* **144**(3): 338–340.

Geretsegger C, Bohmer F, Ludwig M (1994) Paroxetine in the elderly depressed patient: randomised comparison with fluoxetine of efficacy, cognitive and behavioural effects. *Int Clin Psychopharmacol* **9**: 25–29.

Ghaemi SN, Lennox MS, Baldessarini RJ (2001) Effectiveness and safety of long-term antidepressant treatment in bipolar disorder. *J Clin Psychiatry* **62**: 565–569.

Gilaberte I, Montejo AL, de la Gandara J, Perez Sola V, et al. (2001) Fluoxetine in the prevention of depressive recurrences: a double-blind study. *J Clin Psychopharmacol* **21**: 417–424.

Gloaguen V, Cottraux J, Cucherat M, et al. (1998) A meta-analysis of the effects of cognitive therapy in depressed people . *J Affect Disord* **49**: 59–72.

Goldberg JF, Harrow M, Whiteside JE (2001) Risk for bipolar illness in patients initially hospitalized for unipolar depression. *Am J Psychiatry* **158**: 1265–1270.

Goldberg JF, Truman CJ (2003) Antidepressant-induced mania: an overview of current controversies. *Bipolar Disord* **5**(6): 407–420.

Goldberg JF, Whiteside JE (2002) The association between substance abuse and anti-depressant-induced mania in bipolar disorder: a preliminary study. *J Clinical Psychiatry* **63**(9): 791–795.

Goldstein DJ, Mallinckrodt C, Lu Y, Demitrack MA (2002) Duloxetine in the treatment of major depressive disorder: a double-blind clinical trial. *J Clin Psychiatry* **63**: 225–231.

Goodwin GM (2003) For the Consensus Group of the British Association for Psychopharmacology. Evidence-based guidelines for treating bipolar disorder: recommendations from the British Association for Psychopharmacology. *J Psychopharmacol* **17**(2): 149–173.

Gorman J (2002) Placebo-controlled efficacy comparison of escitalopram and citalopram. *Eur Psychiatry* **17**(Suppl 1): 97.

Greden JF (1993) Antidepressant maintenance medications: when to discontinue and how to stop. *J Clin Psychiatry* **54**(Suppl): 39–45.

Guelfi JD, Ansseau M, Timmerman L, Korsgaard S (2001) Mirtazapine versus venlafaxine in hospitalized severely depressed patients with melancholic features. *J Clin Psychopharmacol* **21**(4): 425–431.

Guelfi JD, White C, Hackett D, Guichoux JY, Magni G (1995) Effectiveness of venlafaxine in patients hospitalized for major depression and melancholia. *J Clin Psychiatry* **56**(10): 450–458.

Hajos M, Fleishaker JC, Filipiak-Reisner JK, Brown MT, Wong EH (2004) The selective norepinephrine reuptake inhibitor antidepressant reboxetine: pharmacological and clinical profile. *CNS Drug Rev* **10**(1): 23–44.

Halbreich U, Smoller JW (1997) Intermittent luteal phase sertraline treatment of dysphoric premenstrual syndrome. *J Clin Psychiatry* **58**: 399–402.

Hale AS (1996) Dopamine and the use of SSRIs for conditions other than depression. *Hum Psychopharmacol* **11**(Suppl 2): 103–108.

Hale AS (1997a) ABC of mental health: depression. *BMJ* **315**(7099): 43–46.

Hale AS (1997b) The treatment of depression: the reuptake inhibitors. In Honig A, van Praag HM (eds) *Depression: Neurobiological, Psychopathological and Therapeutic Advances*. Chichester, UK: John Wiley, pp. 365–383.

Hale AS, Hannah P, Sandler M, Bridges PK (1989) Tyramine conjugation test for prediction of treatment response in depressed patients. *Lancet* **8632**: 234–236.

Hale AS, Pinniniti NR (1995) Critical flicker fusion threshold and anticholinergic effects of chronic antidepressant treatment in remitted depressives. *J Psychopharmacol* **9**: 258–266.

Hale AS, Stokes P (1991) The utility of serotonin reuptake inhibitors in endogenous and severe depression. In Freeman HL (ed) *The Uses of Fluoxetine in Clinical Practice*. Royal Society of Medicine International Congress and Symposium Series Vol 189, pp. 15–25.

Hamilton JA (1995) Sex and gender as critical variables in psychotropic drug research. In Brown B, Rieker P, Willie C (eds) *Racism and Sexism and Mental Health*. Pittsburgh, PA: University of Pittsburgh Press, pp. 297–350.

Harmer CJ, Hill SA, Taylor MJ, Cowen PJ, Goodwin GM (2003) Toward a neuropsychological theory of antidepressant drug action: increase in positive emotional bias after potentiation of norepinephrine activity. *Am J Psychiatry* **160**(5): 990–992.

Harvey I, Nelson SJ, Lyons RA, Unwin C, Monaghan S, Peters TJ (1998) A randomized controlled trial and economic evaluation of counselling in primary care. *Br J Gen Prac* 1998 **48**(428): 1043–48.

Haykal RF, Akiskal HS (1990) Bupropion as a promising approach to rapid cycling bipolar II patients. *J Clin Psychiatry* **51**(11): 450–455.

Healy D (1997) *The Antidepressant Era*. London: Harvard University Press.

Heiligenstein JH, Beasley CM Jr, Potvin JH (1993) Fluoxetine not associated with increased aggression in controlled clinical trials. *International Clinical Psychopharmacology* **8**(4): 277–280.

Henry C, Sorbara F, Lacoste J, Gindre C, Leboyer M (2001) Antidepressant-induced mania in bipolar patients: identification of risk factors. *J Clin Psychiatry* **62**: 249–255.

Henry JA (1994) Antidepressants and overdose toxicity. *Hum Psychopharmacol* **9**(Suppl 1): 37–41.

Himmelhoch JM, Thase ME, Mallinger AG, Houck P (1991) Tranylcypromine versus imipramine in anergic bipolar depression. *Am J Psychiatry* **148**(7): 910–916.

Hlastala SA, Frank E, Mallinger AG, Thase ME, Ritenour AM, Kupfer DJ (1997) Bipolar depression: an underestimated treatment challenge. *Depress Anx* **5**: 73–83.

Hochstrasser B, Isaksen PM, Koponen H, Lauritzen L, et al. (2001) Prophylactic effect of citalopram in unipolar, recurrent depression: placebo-controlled study of maintenance therapy. *Br J Psychiatry* **178**: 304–310.

Honig A, Hofman A, Rozendaal N, Dingemans P (1997) Psycho-education in bipolar disorder: effect of expressed emotion. *Psychiatry Res* **72**: 17–22.

Horst WD, Preskorn SH (1998) Mechanisms of action and clinical characteristics of three atypical antidepressants: venlafaxine, nefazodone, bupropion. *J Affective Dis* **51**(3): 237–254.

Howland RH (1996) Induction of mania with serotonin reuptake inhibitors. *J Clin Psychopharmacol* **16**(6): 425–427.

Hsu DJ, Ghaemi N, El-Mallakh RS, et al. (2004) Antidepressant discontinuation and mood episode relapse in bipolar disorder. *American Psychiatric Association 157th Annual Meeting.* NR26.

Hyttel J (1994) Pharmacological characterization of selective serotonin reuptake inhibitors (SSRIs). *Int Clin Psychopharmacol* **9**(Suppl 1): 19–26.

Iyengar S, Bymaster FP, Webster AA, Simmons RMA, Hemrick-Luecke S (2003) Efficacy of duloxetine in models of persistent pain. *American Psychiatric Association 156th Annual Meeting.* N289.

Janicak PG, Davis JM, Gibbons RD, et al. (1985) Efficacy of ECT: a meta-analysis. *Am J Psychiatry* **142**: 297–302.

Jick SS, Dean AD, Jick H (1995) Antidepressants and suicide. *BMJ* **310**: 215–218.

Johnson DAW (1986) Non-compliance with antidepressant therapy – an underestimated problem. *Int Med Sup* **11**: 14–19.

Joffe RT (2002) Psychotherapeutic approaches to bipolar depression. *Clin Neuroscience Res* **2**: 252–255.

Joffe RT, MacQueen GM, Marriott M, Robb J, Begin H, Young LT (2002) Induction of mania and cycle acceleration in bipolar disorder: effect of different classes of antidepressant. *Acta Psychiatr Scand* **105**(6): 427–430.

Jones R, Yates WR, Williams S, Zhou M, Hardman L (1999) Outcome for adjustment disorder with depressed mood: comparison with other mood disorders. *J Affect Disord* **55**: 55–61.

Jones S (2004) Psychotherapy of bipolar disorder: a review. *J Affective Dis* **80**: 101–114.

Joyce PR, Paykel ES (1989) Predictors of drug response in depression. *Arch Gen Psychiatry* **46**(1): 89–99.

Judd LL, Akiskal HS, Schettler PJ, Endicott J, Maser J, Solomon DA, Leon AC, Rice JA, Keller MB (2002) The long-term natural history of the weekly symptomatic status of bipolar I disorder. *Arch Gen Psychiatry* **59**: 530–537.

Kasper S, Pletan Y, Solles A, Tournoux A (1996) Comparative studies with milnacipran and tricyclic antidepressants in the treatment of patients with major depression: a summary of clinical trial results. *Int Clin Psychopharmacol* **11**(Suppl 4): 35–39.

Katona CLE, Robertson MM, Abou-Saleh MT, Nairac BL, et al. (1993) Placebo-controlled trial of lithium augmentation of fluoxetine and lofepramine. *Int Clin Psychopharmacol* **8**: 323.

Keller MB, Boland RJ (1998) Implications of failing to achieve successful long-term maintenance treatment of recurrent unipolar major depression. *Biol Psychiatry* **44**: 348–360.

Keller MB, Gelenberg AJ, Hirschfeld RM, Rush AJ, Thase ME, Kocsis JH, Markowitz JC, Fawcett JA, Koran LM, Klein DN, Russell JM, Kornstein SG, McCullough JP, Davis SM, Harrison WM (1998a) The treatment of chronic depression, part 2: a double-blind, randomized trial of sertraline and imipramine. *J Clin Psychiatry* **59**(11): 598–607.

Keller MB, Kocsis JH, Thase ME, et al. (1998b) Maintenance phase efficacy of sertraline for chronic depression: a randomized controlled trial. *JAMA* **280**: 1665–1672.

Keller MB, McCullough JP, Klein DN, et al. (2000) A comparison of nefazodone, the cognitive behavioral-analysis system of psychotherapy, and their combination for the treatment of chronic depression. *N Engl J Med* **342**: 1462–1470.

Kennedy SH, Lam RW, Cohen NL, Ravindran AV, CANMAT Depression Work Group (2001) Clinical guidelines for the treatment of depressive disorders. IV. Medications and other biological treatments. *Can J Psychiatry* **46**(Suppl 1): 38S–58S.

Kerihuel JC, Dreyfus JF (1991) Meta-analysis of the efficacy and tolerability of the tricyclic antidepressant lofepramine. *J Int Med Research* **19**: 183–201.

King M, Broster G, Lloyd M, Horder J (1994) Controlled trials in the evaluation of counselling in general practice. *Br J Gen Pract* **44**: 382 229–382 232.

Kocsis JH, Frances AJ, Voss C, Mann JJ, Mason BJ, Sweeney J (1988) Imipramine treatment for chronic depression. *Arch Gen Psychiatry* **45**(3): 253–257.

Kocsis JH, Friedman RA, Markowitz JC, Leon AC, Miller NL, Gniwesch L, Parides M (1996) Maintenance therapy for chronic depression. A controlled clinical trial of desipramine. *Arch Gen Psychiatry* **53**(9): 769–774.

Kornstein SG (1997) Gender differences in depression: implications for treatment. *J Clin Psychiatry* **58**(Suppl 15): 12–18.

Kramer JC, Klein DF, Fink M (1961) Withdrawal symptoms following discontinuation of imipramine therapy. *Am J Psychiatry* **118**: 549–550.

Kramer PD (1993) *Listening to Prozac: A Psychiatrist Explores Antidepressant Drugs and the Remaking of the Self*. London: Penguin Psychology. ISBN 0-14-026671-2.

Kroenke K, West S, Swindle R, Gilsenan A, Eckert GJ, Dolor R, Stang P, Zhou X-H, Hays R, Weinberger M (2001) Similar effectiveness of paroxetine, fluoxetine, and sertraline in primary care: a randomized trial. *JAMA* **286**: 2947–2955.

Kuhn R (1958) The treatment of depressive states with G-22355 (imipramine hydrochloride). *Am J Psychiatry* **115**: 459–464.

Kupfer DJ, Frank E, Perel JM, Cornes C, Mallinger A, Thase M (1992) Five-year outcome for maintenance therapies in recurrent depression. *Arch Gen Psychiatry* **49**: 769–773.

Lam D, Bright J, Jones S, Hayward P, Schuck N, Chisholm D, Sham P (2000) Cognitive therapy for bipolar illness — a pilot study of relapse prevention. *Cogn Ther Res* **24**: 503–520.

Lam DH, Jones S, Hayward P, Bright J (1999) *Cognitive Therapy for Bipolar Disorders: A Therapist's Guide to Concepts, Methods and Practice*. Chichester, UK: John Wiley.

Lam DH, Watkins ER, Hayward P, Bright J, Wright K, Kerr N, Parr-Davis G, Sham P (2003) A randomized controlled study of cognitive therapy for relapse prevention for bipolar affective disorder: outcome of the first year. *Arch Gen Psychiatry* **60**(2): 145–152.

Lam RW, Gorman CP, Michalon M, Steiner M, Levitt AJ, Corral MR, Watson GD, Morehouse RL, Tam W, Joffe RT (1995) Multicenter, placebo-controlled study of fluoxetine in seasonal affective disorder. *Am J Psychiatry* **152**(12): 1765–1770.

Lancaster SG, Gonzalez JP (1989) Lofepramine: a review of its pharmacodynamic and pharmacokinetic properties, and therapeutic efficacy in depressive illness. *Drugs* **37**: 123–140.

Lapierre YD (1994) The pharmacological therapy of dysthymia. *Acta Psychiatrica Scand* **89**(Suppl 383): 42–48.

Lecrubier Y, Boyer P, Turjanski S, Rein W (1997) Amisulpride versus imipramine and placebo in dysthymia and major depression. Amisulpride Study Group. *J Affect Disord* **43**(2): 95–103.

Leonard B, Richelson E (2000) Synaptic effects of antidepressants: relationship to their therapeutic and adverse effects. In Buckley PF, Warrington JL (eds) *Schizophrenia and Mood Disorders: The New Drug Therapies in Clinical Practice*. Oxford: Butterworth-Heinemann.

Liebowitz MR, Quitkin FM, Stewart JW, McGrath PJ, Harrison WM, Markowitz JS, Rabkin JG, Tricamo E, Goetz DM, Klein DF (1988) Antidepressant specificity in atypical depression. *Arch Gen Psychiatry* **45**(2): 129–137.

Linde K, Mulrow CD (2000) St John's wort for depression. In *The Cochrane Library*, Issue 4. Oxford: Update Software. Search date 1998.

Linde K, Ramirez G, Mulrow CD, Pauls A, Weidenhammer W, Melchart D (1996) St. John's wort for depression. *BMJ* **313**: 253–258.

Lineberry TW, Peters GE Jr, Bostwick JM (2001) Bupropion-induced erythema multiforme. *Mayo Clin Proc* **76**(6): 664–666.

Lingam R, Scott J (2002) Treatment non-adherence in affective disorders. *Acta Psychiatrica Scandinavica* **105**(3): 164–172.

Lonnqvist J, Sihvo S, Syvalahti E, Kiviruusu O (1994) Moclobemide and fluoxetine in atypical depression: a double-blind trial. *J Affect Disord* **32**(3): 169–177.

Loonen AJ, Peer PG, Zwanikken GJ (1991) Continuation and maintenance therapy with antidepressive agents: meta-analysis of research. *Pharm Week Sci* **13**: 167–175.

Mackay FJ, Dunn NR, Wilton LV, et al. (1997) A comparison of fluvoxamine, fluoxetine, sertraline and paroxetine examined by observational cohort studies. *Pharmacoepidemiol Drug Safety* **6**: 235–246.

Maj M, Veltro F, Pirozzi R, Lobrace S, Magliano L (1992) Pattern of recurrence of illness after recovery from an episode of major depression: a prospective study. *Am J Psychiatry* **149**(6): 795–800.

Mallinger AG, Smith E (1991) Pharmacokinetics of monoamine oxidase inhibitors. *Psychopharmacol Bull* **27**: 493–502.

Malt UF, Robak OH, Madsbu H-P, Bakke O, Loeb M (1999) The Norwegian naturalistic treatment study of depression in general practice (NORDEP) – I: Randomised double blind study *BMJ* **318**: 1180–1184.

Marks IM (1999) Computer aids to mental health care. *Can J Psychiatry* **4**: 548–555.

Mason J, Freemantle N, Eccles M (2000) Fatal toxicity associated with antidepressant use in primary care. *Br J Gen Pract* **50**: 366–370.

Mazure CM, Bruce ML, Maciejewski PK, Jacobs SC (2000) Adverse life events and cognitive-personality characteristics in the prediction of major depression and antidepressant response. *Am J Psychiatry* **157**: 896–903.

McCusker J, Cole M, Keller E, et al. (1998) Effectiveness of treatments of depression in older ambulatory people. *Arch Intern Med* **158**: 705–712.

McElroy S, Keck PE (1993) Treatment guidelines for valproate in bipolar, schizoaffective disorders. *Can J Psychiatry* **38**: S62–S66.

Miklowitz DJ, George EL, Richards JA, Simoneau TL, Suddath RL (2003) A randomized study of family-focused psychoeducation and pharmacotherapy in the outpatient management of bipolar disorder. *Arch Gen Psychiatry* **60**(9): 904–912.

Miklowitz DJ, Simoneau TL, George EL, Richards JA, Kalbag A, Sachs-Ericsson N, Suddath R (2000) Family-focused treatment of bipolar disorder: 1-year effects of a psychoeducational program in conjunction with pharmacotherapy. *Biol Psychiatry* **48**(6): 582–592.

Miller IW, Keitner GI, Schatzberg AF, et al. (1998) The treatment of chronic depression, part 3: Psychosocial functioning before and after treatment with sertraline or imipramine. *J Clin Psychiatry* **59**: 608–619.

Miodownik C, Lerner V (2000) Risperidone in the treatment of psychotic depression. *Clin Neuropharmacol* **23**(6): 335–337.

Mirin SM, Schatzberg AF, Creasey DE (1981) Hypomania and mania after withdrawal of tricyclic antidepressants. *Am J Psychiatry* **138**: 87–89.

Montes JM, Ferrando L, Saiz-Ruiz J (2004) Remission in major depression with two antidepressant mechanisms: results from a naturalistic study. *J Affective Dis* **79**: 229–234.

Montgomery S, Ferguson JM, Schwartz GE (2003) The antidepressant efficacy of reboxetine in patients with severe depression. *J Clin Psychopharmacol.* **23**(1): 45–50.

Moses EL, Mallinger AG (2000) St John's wort: three cases of possible mania induction. *J Clin Psychopharmacol* **20**: 115–117.

Mulrow CD, Williams JW, Chiqueete E, et al. (2000) Efficacy of newer medications for treating depression in primary care people. *Am Med J* **108**: 54–64.

Mundo E, Walker M, Cate T, Macciardi F, Kennedy JL (2001) The role of serotonin transporter protein gene in antidepressant-induced mania in bipolar disorder: preliminary findings. *Arch Gen Psychiatry* **589**(6): 539–544.

Murphy GM Jr, Kremer C, Rodrigues HE, Schatzberg AF (2003a) Pharmacogenetics of antidepressant medication intolerance. *Am J Psychiatry* **160**(10): 1830–1835.

Murphy GM, Kremer C, Rodrigues H, Schatzberg AF (2003b) Mirtazapine versus Paroxetine Study Group. The apolipoprotein E epsilon-4 allele and antidepressant efficacy in cognitively intact elderly depressed patients. *Biol Psychiatry* **54**(7): 665–673.

Myers L, Midence K (1998) Methodological and conceptual issues in adherence. In Myers L, Midence K (ed.) *Adherence to Treatment in Medical Conditions.* Chichester, UK: John Wiley, pp. 1–24.

Mynors-Wallis LM, Gath DH, Lloyd-Thomas, AR, et al. (1995) Randomised controlled trial comparing problem solving treatment with amitriptyline and placebo for major depression in primary care. *BMJ* **310**: 441–445.

National Depressive and Manic-Depressive Association (1996) *Consensus Conference on the Undertreatment of Depression.* January.

Nelson JC (1997) Safety and tolerability of the new antidepressants. *J Clin Psychiatry* **58**(Suppl 6): 26–31.

Nelson JC, Jatlow P, Quinlan DM, et al. (1982) Desipramine plasma concentration and anti-depressant response. *Arch Gen Psychiatry* **39**: 1419–1422.

Nemeroff CB, Evans DL, Gyulai L, et al. (2001) Double-blind placebo-controlled comparison of imipramine and paroxetine in the treatment of bipolar depression. *Am J Psychiatry* **158**: 906–912.

Newhouse PA, Ko G, Richter EM (1996) Comparison of sertraline and fluoxetine in depressed geriatric outpatients: plasma levels and efficacy. *XXth CINP Congress, Melbourne, Australia.* Abstract P-1-4.

NICE (2004) *Depression, NICE Guideline, Second Consultation.* http://www.nice.org.uk/pdf/Depression_Appendix_19c_2ndconsultation.pdf.

Nierenberg AA, Feighner JP, Rudolph R, Cole JO, Sullivan J (1994) Venlafaxine for treatment-resistant unipolar depression. *J Clin Psychopharmacol* **14**(6): 419–423.

Nierenberg AA, Wright EC (1999) Evolution of remission as the new standard in the treatment of depression. *J Clin Psychiatry* **60**(Suppl 22): 7–11.

Nolen WA (1997) Classical and selective monoamine oxidase inhibitors in the treatment of depression. In Honig A, van Praag H (eds) *Depression, Neurobiological, Psychopathological and Therapeutic Advances.* Chichester, UK: John Wiley, pp. 385–395.

Nolen WA, Van de Putte JJ, Dijken WA, et al. (1988) Treatment strategy in depression II; MAO inhibitors in depression resistant to cyclic antidepressants: two controlled studies with tranylcypromine versus 1-5-hydroxytryptophan and nomifensine. *Acta Psychiatrica Scand* **78**: 676–683.

Ohayon MM, Schatzberg AF (2002) Prevalence of depressive episodes with psychotic features in the general population. *Am J Psychiatry* **159**(11): 1855–1861.

Old age depression interest group (1993) How long should the elderly take antidepressants? A double-blind placebo-controlled study of continuation/prophylaxis therapy with dothiepin. *Br J Psychiatry* **162**: 175–182.

O'Reardon JP, Amsterdam JD (1998) Treatment-resistant depression: progress and limitations. *Psychiatr Ann* **28**: 633–640.

Oxman TE, Barrett JE, Sengupta A, Katon W, Williams JW, Frank E, Hegel M (2001) Status of minor depression or dysthymia in primary care following a randomized controlled treatment. *Gen Hosp Psychiatry* **23**: 301–310.

Palmer AG, Williams H, Adams M (1995) CBT in a group format for bipolar affective disorder. *Behav Cogn Psychother* **23**: 153–168.

Pande AC, Birkett M, Fechner-Bates S, Haskett RF, Greden JF (1996) Fluoxetine versus phenelzine in atypical depression. *Biol Psychiatry* **40**(10): 1017–1020.

Pande AC, Sayler ME (1993) Severity of depression and response to fluoxetine. *Int Clin Psychopharmacol* **8**: 243–245.

Parker G, Blennerhassett J (1998) Withdrawal reactions associated with venlafaxine. *Aust NZ J Psychiatry* **32**: 291–294.

Parker G, Mitchell P, Wilhelm K, Menkes D, Snowdon J, Schweitzer I, Grounds D, Skerritt P, Roy K, Hadzi-Pavlovic D (1999) Are the newer antidepressant drugs as effective as established physical treatments? Results from an Australasian clinical panel review. *Aust NZJ Psychiatry* **33**: 874–881.

Parker G, Roy K, Hadzi-Pavlovic D, et al. (1992) Psychotic (delusional) depression: a meta-analysis of physical treatment. *J Affective Dis* **24**: 17–24.

Parker G, Roy K, Wilhelm K, Mitchell P (2001) Assessing the comparative effectiveness of antidepressant therapies: a prospective clinical practice study. *J Clin Psychiatry* **62**: 117–125.

Patelis-Siotis I, Young LT, Robb JC, Marriott M, Bieling PJ, Cox LC, Joffe RT (2001) Group cognitive behavioural therapy for bipolar disorder: a feasibility and effectiveness study. *J Affect Disord* **65**: 145–153.

Patris M, Bouchard J-M, Bougerol T, et al. (1996) Citalopram versus fluoxetine: a double-blind, controlled, multicentre Phase III trial in patients with unipolar major depression treated in general practice. *Int Clin Psychopharmacol* **11**: 129–136.

Paykel ES, Freeling P, Hollyman JA (1987) Predictors of therapeutic benefit from amitripty-line in mild depression: a general practice placebo controlled trial. *J Affect Disord* **14**: 83–95.

Paykel ES, Hart D, Priest R (1998) Changes in public attitudes to depression during the defeat depression campaign. *Br J Psychiatry* **173**: 519–522.

Paykel ES, Ramana R, Cooper Z, et al. (1995) Residual symptoms after partial remission: an important outcome in depression. *Psychol Med* **25**: 1171–1180.

Paykel ES, White JL (1989) A European study of views on the use of monoamine oxidase inhibitors. *Br J Psychiatry* **155**: 9–17.

Pearlstein T (2002) Selective serotonin reuptake inhibitors for premenstrual dysphoric disorder: the emerging gold standard? *Drugs* **62**(13): 1869–1885.

Peet M (1994) Induction of mania with selective serotonin re-uptake inhibitors and tricyclic antidepressants. *Br J Psychiatry* **164**: 549–550.

Perry A, Tarrier N, Morriss R, McCarthy E, Limb K (1999) Randomised controlled trial of efficacy of teaching patients with bipolar disorder to identify early symptoms of relapse and obtain treatment. *BMJ* **16**:318(7177): 149–153.

Perry PJ (1996) Pharmacotherapy for major depression with melancholic features: relative efficacy of tricyclic versus selective serotonin reuptake inhibitor antidepressants. *J Affect Disord* **39**(1): 1–6.

Perry PJ, Zeilmann C, Arndt S (1994) Tricyclic antidepressant concentrations in the plasma: an estimate of their sensitivity and specificity as a predictor of response. *J Clin Psychopharmacology* **14**: 230–240.

Perugi G, Frare F, Toni C, Ruffolo G, Torti C (2002) Open-label evaluation of venlafaxine sustained release in outpatients with generalized anxiety disorder with comorbid major depression or dysthymia: effectiveness, tolerability and predictors of response. *Neuropsychobiology* **46**(3): 145–149.

Peselow ED, Sanfilipo MP, Difiglia C, Fieve RR (1992) Melancholic/endogenous depression and response to somatic treatment and placebo. *Am J Psychiatry* **149**(10): 1324–1334.

Pesola GR, Avasarala J (2002) Bupropion seizure proportion among new-onset generalized seizures and drug related seizures presenting to an emergency department. *J Emerg Med* **22**(3): 235–239.

Philipp M, Kohner R, Hiller KO (1999) Hypericum extract versus imipramine or placebo in patients with moderate depression. *BMJ* **319**: 1534–1539.

Post RM, Altshuler LL, Frye MA, Suppes T, Rush AJ, Keck PE, et al. (2001) Rate of switch in bipolar patients prospectively treated with second-generation antidepressants as augmentation to mood stabilizers. *Bipolar Disord* **3**: 259–265.

Preda A, MacLean RW, Mazure CM, Bowers MB (2001) Antidepressant-associated mania and psychosis in psychiatric admissions. *J Clin Psychiatry* **62**: 30–33.

Preskorn SH (1983) Antidepressant response and plasma concentrations of bupropion. *J Clin Psychiatry* **44**(5 Pt 2): 137–139.

Preskorn SH, Fast GA (1993) Beyond signs and symptoms: the case against a mixed anxiety and depression category. *J Clin Psychiatry* **54**(Suppl): 24–32.

Price JS, Waller PC, Wood SM, et al. (1996) A comparison of the post marketing safety of four selective serotonin reuptake inhibitors including the investigation of symptoms occurring on withdrawal. *Br J Clin Pharmacol* **42**: 757–763.

Priest RG, Vize C, Roberts A, Roberts M, Tylee A (1996) Lay people's attitudes to treatment of depression: results of opinion poll for Defeat Depression Campaign just before its launch. *BMJ* **313**: 858–859.

Quitkin FM (1985) The importance of dosage in prescribing antidepressants. *Br J Psychiatry* **147**: 593–597.

Quitkin FM, Stewart JW, McGrath PJ, Nunes E, Ocepek-Welikson K, Tricamo E, Rabkin JG, Ross D, Klein DF (1993) Loss of drug effects during continuation therapy. *Am J Psychiatry* **150**: 562–565.

Ranjan R, Meltzer HY (1996) Acute and long-term effectiveness of clozapine in treatment-resistant psychotic depression. *Biol Psychiatry* **40**(4): 253–258.

Rashid A (1982) Do patients cash their prescriptions. *Br Med J* **284**: 24–26.

Rausch JL, Hobby HM, Shendarkar N, Johnson ME, Li J (2001) Fluvoxamine treatment of mixed anxiety and depression: evidence for serotonergically mediated anxiolysis. *J Clin Psychopharmacol* **21**(2): 139–142.

Ravindran AV, Anisman H, et al. (1999) Treatment of primary dysthymia with group cognitive therapy and pharmacotherapy: clinical symptoms and functional impairments. *Am J Psychiatry* **156**: 1608–1617.

Ravindran AV, Judge R, Hunter BN, Bray J, Morton NH (1997) A double-blind, multicenter study in primary care comparing paroxetine and clomipramine in patients with depression and associated anxiety. Paroxetine Study Group. *J Clin Psychiatry* **58**(3): 112–118.

Reimherr FW, Amsterdam JD, Quitkin FM, Rosenbaum JF, Fava M, Zajecka J, Beasley CM Jr, Michelson D, Roback P, Sundell K (1998) Optimal length of continuation therapy in depression: a prospective assessment during long-term fluoxetine treatment. *Am J Psychiatry* **155**: 1247–1253.

Revicki D, Simon G, Chan K, Katon W, Heiligenstein J (1998) Depression, health-related quality of life, and medical cost outcomes of receiving recommended levels of anti-depressant treatment. *J Fam Pract* **47**: 446–452.

Reynolds CF, Frank E, Perel JM, Imber SD, Cornes C, Miller MD, Mazumdar S, Houck PR, Dew MA, Stack JA, Pollock BG, Kupfer DJ (1999) Nortriptyline and interpersonal psychotherapy as maintenance therapies for recurrent major depression: a randomized controlled trial in patients older than 59 years. *JAMA* **281**: 39–45.

Roose SP (1992) Modern cardiovascular standards for psychotropic drugs. *Psychopharmacology Bull* **28**: 35–43.

Roose SP, Glassman AH, Attia E, Woodring S (1994) Comparative efficacy of selective serotonin reuptake inhibitors and tricyclics in the treatment of melancholia. *Am J Psychiatry* **51**: 1735–1739.

Rosenbaum JF, Fava M, Hoog SL, Ascroft RC, Krebs WB (1998) Selective serotonin reuptake inhibitor discontinuation syndrome: a randomized clinical trial. *Biol Psychiatry* **44**: 77–87.

Rosenzweig AS, Pasternak RE, Prigerson HG, Miller MD, Reynolds CF (1996) Bereavement-related depression in the elderly. Is drug treatment justified? *Drugs Aging* **8**(5): 323–328.

Rothschild AJ (1996) Management of psychotic, treatment-resistant depression. *Psychiatric Clin NA* **19**: 237–252.

Rothschild AJ (2003) Challenges in the treatment of depression with psychotic features. *Biological Psychiatry* **53**: 680–690.

Rothschild AJ, Bates KS, Boehringer KL, Syed A (1999) Olanzapine response in psychotic depression. *J Clin Psychiatry* **60**(2): 116–118.

Rothschild AJ, Duval SE (2003) How long should patients with psychotic depression stay on the antipsychotic medication? *J Clin Psychiatry* **64**(4): 390–396.

Rothschild AJ, Samson JA, Bessette B, et al. (1996) Efficacy of the combination of fluoxetine and perphenazine in the treatment of psychotic depression. *J Clin Psychiatry* **54**: 338–342.

Rouillon F, Berdeaux G, Bisserbe JC, Warner B, Mesbah M, Smadja C, Chwalow J (2000a) Prevention of recurrent depressive episodes with milnacipran: consequences on quality of life. *J Affect Disord* **58**(3): 171–180.

Rouillon F, Warner B, Pezous N, Bisserbe JC (2000b) Milnacipran efficacy in the prevention of recurrent depression: a 12-month placebo-controlled study. Milnacipran recurrence prevention study group. *Int Clin Psychopharmacol* **15**(3): 133–140.

Rush AJ, Trivedi MH (1995) Treating depression to remission. *Psychiatric Annals* **25**: 704–709.

Sackeim H, Haskett RF, Mulsant BH, Thase ME, Mann JJ, Pettinati HM, Greenberg RM, Crowe RR, Cooper TB, Prudic J (2001) Continuation pharmacotherapy in the prevention of relapse following electroconvulsive therapy: a randomized controlled trial. *JAMA* **285**(10): 1299–1307.

Sackeim HA, Prudic J, Devanand DP, et al. (1990) The impact of medication resistance and continuation pharmacotherapy on relapse following response to electroconvulsive therapy in major depression. *J Clin Psychopharmacol* **10**: 96–104.

Sackett D, Gent M (1979) Controversy in counting and attributing events in clinical trials. *N Engln J Med* **301**: 1410–1412.

Sachs GS, Lafer B, Stoll AL, et al. (1994) A double-blind trial of bupropion versus desipramine for bipolar depression. *J Clin Psychiatry* **55**(9): 391–393.

Sachs GS, Printz DJ, Kahn DA, Carpenter D, Docherty JP (2000) The expert consensus guidelines series: Medication Treatment of Bipolar Disorder 2000. *Postgrad Med Spec Rep* **April**: 1–104.

Sanchez C, Hyttel J (1999) Comparison of the effects of antidepressants and their metabolites on reuptake of biogenic amines and on receptor binding. *Cell Mol Neurobiol* **19**(4): 467–489.

Schatzberg AF (1998) Noradrenergic versus serotonergic antidepressants: predictors of treatment response. *J Clin Psychiatry* **59** (Suppl 14): 15–18.

Schatzberg AF (2000) Clinical efficacy of reboxetine in major depression. *J Clin Psychiatry* **61**(Suppl 10): 31–38.

Schatzberg AF (2003) Efficacy and tolerability of duloxetine, a novel dual reuptake inhibitor, in the treatment of major depressive disorder. *J Clin Psychiatry* **64**(Suppl 13): 30–37.

Schatzberg AF, Flores B, Solvason HB, et al. (2004) Mifeprostone in psychotic major depression. *APA 176th Annual Meeting.* NR 397.

Schrader E (2000) for the Study Group. Equivalence of St. John's wort extract (Ze 117) and fluoxetine. *Int Clin Psychopharmacol* **15**: 61–68.

Schwartz D, Lallouch J (1967) Explanatory and pragmatic attitudes to clinical trials. *J Chronic Dis* **20**: 637–648.

Scott J, Eccleston D, Boys R (1992) Can we predict the persistence of depression? *Br J Psychiatry* **161**: 633–637.

Scott J, Garland A, Moorhead S (2001) A pilot study of cognitive therapy in bipolar disorders. *Psychol Med* **31**(3): 459–467.

Settle EC, Stahl SM, Batey SR, Johnston JA, Ascher JA (1999) Safety profile of sustained-release bupropion in depression: results of three clinical trials. *Clin Ther* **21**(3): 454–463.

Sharma V (2001) Loss of response to antidepressants and subsequent refractoriness: diagnostic issues in a retrospective case series. *J Affective Disord* **64**: 99–106.

Shea MT, Elkin I, Imber SD, et al. (1992) Course of depressive symptoms over follow up. *Arch Gen Psychiatry* **49**: 782–787.

Shelton RC, Davidson J, Yonkers KA, Koran L, Thase ME, Pearlstein T, Halbreich U (1997) The undertreatment of dysthymia. *J Clin Psychiatry* **58**(2): 59–65.

Shelton RC, Tollefson GD, Tohen M, Stahl S, Gannon KS, Jacobs TG, et al. (2001) A novel augmentation strategy for treating resistant major depression. *Am J Psychiatry* **158**: 131–134.

Sherry RL, Rauw G, McKenna KF, Paetsch PR, Coutts RT, Baker GB (2000) Failure to detect amphetamine or 1-amino-3-phenylpropane in humans or rats receiving the MAO inhibitor tranylcypromine. *J Affect Disord* **61** (1–2): 23–29.

Simon GE, Heiligenstein J, Revicki D, VonKorff M, Katon WJ, Ludman E, Grothaus L, Wagner E (1999) Long-term outcomes of initial antidepressant drug choice in a 'real world' randomized trial. *Arch Fam Med* **8**: 319–325.

Simon GE, vonKorff M, Heiligenstein JH, Revicji DA, Grothaus L, Katon W, Wagner EH (1996) Initial antidepressant choice in primary care. Effectiveness and cost of fluoxetine vs tricyclic antidepressants. *JAMA* **275**: 1897–1902.

Simon GE, Wagner EH, vonKorff M (1995) Cost-effectiveness comparisons using 'real world' randomized trials: the case of new antidepressant drugs. *J Clin Epidemiol* **48**: 363–373.

Simoneau TL, Miklowitz DJ, Richards JA, Saleem R, George EL (1999) Bipolar disorder and family communication: effects of a psychoeducational treatment program. *J Abnorm Psychol* **108** (4): 588–597.

Smith D, Dempster C, Glanville J, Freemantle N, Anderson I (2002) Efficacy and tolerability of venlafaxine compared with selective serotonin reuptake inhibitors and other antidepressants: a meta-analysis. *Br J Psychiatry* **180**: 396–404.

Soares JJF, Stintzing CP, Jackson C, Skoldin B (1997) Psychoeducation for patients with bipolar disorder: an exploratory study. *Nordic J Psychiatry* **51**: 439–446.

Sogaard J, Lane R, Latimer P, et al. (1999) A 12 week study comparing moclobemide and sertraline in the treatment of outpatients with atypical depression. *J Psychopharmacol* **13**: 406–414.

Song F, Freemantle N, Sheldon TA et al. (1993) Selective serotonin reuptake inhibitors: meta-analysis of efficacy and acceptability. *BMJ* **306**: 683–687.

Spiker DG, Weiss JC, Dealy RS, et al. (1985) The pharmacological treatment of delusional depression. *Am J Psychiatry* **142**: 430–436.

Stahl MM, Lindquist M, Pettersson M, Edwards IR, Sanderson JH, Taylor NF, Fletcher AP, Schou JS (1997) Withdrawal reactions with selective serotonin reuptake inhibitors as reported to the WHO system. *Eur J Clin Pharmacol* **53**: 163–169.

Stahl SM (1993) Mixed anxiety and depression: clinical implications. *J Clin Psychiatry* **54** (Suppl): 33–38.

Stamenkovic M, Blasbichier T, Riederer F, Pezawas L, Brandstätter N, Aschauer HN, Kasper S (2001) Fluoxetine treatment in patients with recurrent brief depression. *Int Clin Psychopharmacol* **16**: 221–226.

Stamenkovic M, Pezawas L, de Zwaan M, Aschauer HN, Kasper S (1998) Mirtazapine in recurrent brief depression. *Int Clin Psychopharmacol* **13** (1): 39–40.

Stewart DE (2002) Hepatic adverse reactions associated with nefazodone. *Can J Psychiatry* **47**: 375–377.

Stewart JW, McGrath PJ, Quitkin FM (1992a) Can mildly depressed outpatients with atypical depression benefit from antidepressants? *Am J Psychiatry* **149** (5): 615–619.

Stewart JW, McGrath PJ, Quitkin FM, Rabkin JG, Harrison W, Wager S, Nunes E, Ocepek-Welikson K, Tricamo E (1993) Chronic depression: response to placebo, imipramine, and phenelzine. *J Clin Psychopharmacol* **13** (6): 391–396.

Stewart JW, Quitkin FM, Klein DF (1992b) The pharmacotherapy of minor depression. *Am J Psychother* **46** (1): 23–36.

Stewart JW, Tricamo E, McGrath PJ, Quitkin FM (1997) Prophylactic efficacy of phenelzine and imipramine in chronic atypical depression: likelihood of recurrence on discontinuation after 6 months' remission. *Am J Psychiatry* **154**: 31–36.

Stoll AL, Mayer PV, Kolbrener M, et al. (1994) Antidepressant associated mania: a controlled comparison with spontaneous mania. *Am J Psychiatry* **151**: 1642–1645.

Stratta P, Bolino F, Cupillari M, Casacchia M (1991) A double-blind parallel study comparing fluoxetine with imipramine in the treatment of atypical depression. *Int Clin Psychopharmacol* **6**(3): 193–196.

Terra JL, Montgomery SA (1998) Fluvoxamine prevents recurrence of depression: results of a long-term, double-blind, placebo-controlled study. *Int Clin Psychopharmacol* **13**(2): 55–62.

Thase ME (1992) Long-term treatments of recurrent depressive disorders. *J Clin Psychiatry* **53**(Suppl 9): 32–44.

Thase ME (2001) Preventing the long term complications of depression. In Montgomery SA (chair) *Understanding Depression: A Long-term, Recurring Disorder. J Clin Psychiatry* **62**: 379–392.

Thase ME (2003) Effectiveness of antidepressants: comparative remission rates. *J Clin Psychiatry* **64**(Suppl 2):3–7.

Thase ME, Entsuah AR, Rudolph RL (2001a) Remission rates during treatment with venlafaxine or selective serotonin reuptake inhibitors. *Br J Psychiatry* **178**: 234–241.

Thase ME, Fava M, Halbreich U, Kocsis JH, Koran L, Davidson J, Rosenbaum J, Harrison W (1996) A placebo-controlled, randomized clinical trial comparing sertraline and imipramine for the treatment of dysthymia. *Arch Gen Psychiatry* **53**(9): 777–784.

Thase ME, Friedman ES (1999) Is psychotherapy an effective treatment for melancholia and other severe depressive states? *J Affect Disord* **54**: 1–19.

Thase ME, Friedman ES, Fasiczka AL, Berman SR, Frank E, Nofzinger EA, Reynolds CF (2000) Treatment of men with major depression: a comparison of sequential cohorts treated with either cognitive-behavioral therapy or newer generation antidepressants. *J Clin Psychiatry* **61**: 466–472.

Thase ME, Greenhouse JB, Frank E, et al. (1997) Treatment of major depression with psychotherapy or psychotherapy – pharmacotherapy combinations. *Arch Gen Psychiatry* **54**: 1009–1015.

Thase ME, Lu Y, Joliat M, Detke MJ (2003) Remission in placebo-controlled trials of duloxetine with an SSRI comparitor. *American Psychiatric Association 156th Annual Meeting.* NR840.

Thase ME, Mallinger AG, McKnight D, Himmelhoch JM (1992a) Treatment of imipramine-resistant recurrent depression, IV: a double-blind crossover study of tranylcypromine for anergic bipolar depression. *Am J Psychiatry* **149**(2): 195–198.

Thase ME, Nierenberg AA, Keller MB, Panagides J, et al. (2001b) Efficacy of mirtazapine for prevention of depressive relapse: a placebo-controlled double-blind trial of recently remitted high-risk patients. *J Clin Psychiatry* **62**(10): 782–788.

Thase ME, Sachs GS (1992b) Bipolar depression: pharmacotherapy and related therapeutic strategies. *Biol Psychiatry* **48**: 558–572.

Thase ME, Simons AD, McGeary J, et al. (1992) Relapse after cognitive behaviour therapy of depression: potential implications for longer courses of treatment. *Am J Psychiatry* **149**: 1046–1052.

Thase ME, Sloan DM, Kornstein SG (2002) Remission as the critical outcome of depression treatment. *Psychopharmacology Bull* **6**(4 suppl 3): 12–25.

Thase ME, Trivedi MH, Rush AJ (1995) MAOIs in the contemporary treatment of depression. *Neuropsychopharmacology* **12**: 185–219.

Thompson C, Peveler RC, Stephenson D, McKendrick J (2000) Compliance with antidepressant medication in the treatment of major depressive disorder in primary care: a randomized comparison of fluoxetine and a tricyclic antidepressant. *Am J Psychiatry* **157**: 338–343.

Thompson C, van Willigenberg AP, Janssens CJ, et al. (2004) Mirtazepine versus SSRIs: a meta-analysis on onset of antidepressant activity. *American Psychiatric Association 157th Annual Meeting.* NR388.

Tignol J (1992) A double-blind, randomised multi-centre study comparing paroxetine 20 mg daily versus fluoxetine 20 mg daily in the treatment of adults with major depression. *Clin Neuropharmacol* **15**(Suppl B): 177.

Tiller J, Schweitzer I, Maguire K, Davies B (1989) A sequential double-blind controlled study of moclobemide and diazepam in patients with atypical depression. *J Affect Disord* **16**(2–3): 181–7.

Tohen M, Vieta E, Calabrese J, Ketter T, et al. (2003) Efficacy of olanzapine and olanzapine–fluoxetine combination in the treatment of bipolar I depression. *Arch Gen Psychiatry* **60**(11): 1079–1088.

Trindade E, Menon D (1998) Selective serotonin reuptake inhibitors differ from tricyclic antidepressants in adverse events. *Selective Serotonin Reuptake Inhibitors (SSRIs) for Major Depression. Part I. Evaluation of the Clinical Literature.* Ottawa: Canadian Coordinating Office for Health Technology Assessment, 1997 August Report 3E. *Evidence-Based Mental Health* **1**: 50.

Trivedi MH, Kleiber BA (2001) Algorithm for the treatment of chronic depression. *J Clin Psychiatry* **62**(Suppl 6): 22–29.

Truman CJ, Baldessano CF, Goldberg JF, et al. (2003) History of antidepressant-induced mania in the STEP 500. *American Psychiatric Association 156th Annual Meeting.*

Tse WS, Bond AJ (2003) Reboxetine promotes social bonding in healthy volunteers. *J Psychopharmacol* **17**(2): 189–195.

Tylee A, Gastpar M, Lepine JP, Mendlewicz J (1999) Identification of depressed patient types in the community and their treatment needs: findings from the DEPRES II (Depression Research in European Society II) survey. DEPRES Steering Committee. *Int Clin Psychopharmacol* **14**(3): 153–165.

Uhlenhuth EH, Balter MB, Ban TA, Yang K (1999) International study of expert judgment on therapeutic use of benzodiazepines and other psychotherapeutic medications: VI. Trends in recommendations for the pharmacotherapy of anxiety disorders, 1992–1997. *Depress Anxiety* **9**(3): 107–116.

Van der Flier S, Schutte AJ (2003) Tolerability of mirtazapine verses other antidepressants in patients with major depression. *American Psychiatric Association 156th Annual Meeting.* NR479.

Vanelle JM, Attar-Levy D, Poirier MF, Bouhassira M, Blin P, Olie JP (1997) Controlled efficacy study of fluoxetine in dysthymia. *Br J Psychiatry* **170**: 345–350.

VanGent EM, Zwart FM (1991) Psychoeducation of partners of bipolar manic patients. *J Affect Dis* **21**: 15–18.

Vieta E, Martinez-Aran A, Goikolea JM, Torrent C, Colom F, Benabarre A, Reinares M (2002) A randomized trial comparing paroxetine and venlafaxine in the treatment of bipolar depressed patients taking mood stabilizers. *J Clin Psychiatry* **63**(6): 508–512.

Vorbach EU, Arnoldt KH, Hubner WE (1997) Efficacy and tolerability of St. John's wort extract LI 160 versus imipramine in patients with severe depressive episodes according to ICD-10. *Pharmacopsychiatry* **30**(Suppl 2): 81–85.

Weihs KL, Houser TL, Batey SR, Ascher JA, Bolden-Watson C, Donahue RM, Metz A (2002) Continuation phase treatment with bupropion SR effectively decreases the risk for relapse of depression. *Biol Psychiatry* **51**(9): 753–761.

Wheatley D (1997) LI-160, an extract of St. John's wort, versus amitriptyline in mildly to moderately depressed outpatients: a controlled 6-week clinical trial. *Pharmacopsychiatry* 1997 **30**: 77–80.

Wheatley DP, van Moffaert M, Timmerman L, Kremer CM (1998) Mirtazapine: efficacy and tolerability in comparison with fluoxetine in patients with moderate to severe major depressive disorder. Mirtazapine–Fluoxetine Study Group. *J Clin Psychiatry* **59**(6): 306–312.

Wheeler Vega JA, Mortimer AM, Tyson PJ (2000) Somatic treatment of psychotic depression: review and recommendations for practice. *J Clin Psychopharmacol* **20**: 504–519.

Whiskey E, Werneke U, Taylor D (2001) A systematic review and meta-analysis of *Hypericum perforatum* in depression: a comprehensive clinical review. *Int Clin Psychopharmacol* **16**(5): 239–252.

Wijeratne C, Halliday GS, Lyndon RW (1999) The present status of electroconvulsive therapy: a systematic review. *Med J Austr* **171**: 250–254.

Wirshing WC, Van Putten T, Rosenberg J, Marder S, Ames D, Hicks-Gray T (1992) Fluoxetine, akathisia, and suicidality: is there a causal connection? *Archives of General Psychiatry* **49**(7): 580–581.

Woelk H (2000) for the Remotiv/Imipramine Study Group. Comparison of St. John's wort and imipramine for treating depression. *BMJ* **321**: 536–539.

Woggon B (1993) The role of moclobemide in endogenous depression: a survey of recent data. *Int Clin Psychopharmacol* **7**(3–4): 137–139.

Wong DT, Bymaster FP (2002) Dual serotonin and noradrenaline uptake inhibitor class of antidepressants potential for greater efficacy or just hype? *Prog Drug Res* **58**: 169–222.

Workman EA, Short DD (1993) Atypical antidepressants versus imipramine in the treatment of major depression: a meta-analysis. *J Clin Psychiatry* **54**(1): 5–12.

Yonkers KA (1997) Antidepressants in the treatment of premenstrual dysphoric disorder. *J Clin Psychiatry* **58**(Suppl 14): 4–10.

Young LT, Joffe RT, Robb JC, MacQueen GM, Marriott M, Patelis-Siotis I (2000) Double-blind comparison of addition of a second mood stabilizer versus an antidepressant to an initial mood stabilizer for treatment of patients with bipolar depression. *Am J Psychiatry* **157**: 124–126.

Zajecka JM (1996) The effect of nefazodone on comorbid anxiety symptoms associated with depression: experience in family practice and psychiatric outpatient settings. *J Clin Psychiatry* **57** (Suppl 2): 10–14.

Zajecka J, Fawcett J, Amsterdam J, et al. (1998) Safety of abrupt discontinuation of fluoxetine: a randomised, placebo controlled study. *J Clin Psychopharmacol* **18**: 193–197.

Zaretsky AE (2004) Family focused therapy is more effective than crisis management for preventing relapse after a bipolar episode. *Evid Based Ment Health* **7**: 49.

Zaretsky AE, Segal ZV, Gemar M (1999) Cognitive therapy for bipolar depression: a pilot study. *Can J Psychiatry* **44**(5): 491–494.

Zisook S, Shuchter SR (1993) Uncomplicated bereavement. *J Clin Psychiatry* **54**(10): 365–372.

Zornberg GL, Pope HG (1993) Treatment of depression in bipolar disorder: new directions for research. *J Clin Psychopharmacol* **13**: 397–408.

11

Psychological Treatments of Depression

Jeffrey Roelofs and Peter Muris

University of Maastricht, Maastricht, The Netherlands

INTRODUCTION

In Freud's classic paper 'Mourning and Melancholia' (Freud, 1917), melancholic depression was conceptualized as internalized anger about the emotional loss of the mother during childhood. In 1923, Freud revised his theory of depression in his publication *The Ego and the Id* (Freud, 1923), in which he postulated that melancholic patients have a stringent superego, which would install strong feelings of guilt about aggressive thoughts and behaviours towards loved ones (see Gabbard, 2000). Lloyd Silverman (1976, 1985) attempted to empirically test Freud's theoretical notions of depression. Silverman reasoned that when depression is the result of anger towards loved ones, confrontation with this repressed material would lead to an increase of depressive symptoms. In one of his experiments, female depressed patients were confronted with neutral (e.g., 'people walking') and aggressive statements (e.g., 'destroy mother'). These statements were presented subliminally, which means that patients were not consciously aware of the content of the statements due to a very brief exposure time. A measure of depression was completed before and after the presentation of the statements. In line with Silverman's expectations, subliminally presented aggressive statements, but not neutral statements, enhanced patients' depression scores. Although these findings at first sight seem to be in line with the psychoanalytic theory of depression, it is important to note that there are alternative and more plausible explanations for these results. More precisely, Silverman's findings can be well explained in terms of an emotional priming effect. That is, presenting negative stimuli may prime individuals towards a negative mood, which is reflected in elevated depression scores. As an aside, it should be mentioned that attempts to replicate Silverman's findings have been largely unsuccessful (e.g., Oliver and Burkham, 1982). Thus, altogether, there is little evidence for the empirical basis of the psychoanalytic theory of depression. This does not mean,

Mood Disorders: Clinical Management and Research Issues. Edited by E. J. L. Griez, C. Faravelli, D. J. Nutt and J. Zohar.
©2005 John Wiley & Sons Ltd. ISBN 0 470 09426 5.

however, that the discipline of psychology can be discarded in the case of depressive psychopathology.

The learning theoretical perspective and the cognitive-behavioural perspective of depression have a clearly formulated theoretical foundation, which has formed the basis for experimental research and contributed to our knowledge of the treatment of depressed patients. Although psychological interventions for depression have traditionally been regarded as difficult and unrewarding due to the relentless negativism, lack of energy, and low motivation of the depressed patient (Hammen, 1997), several effective psychotherapeutic treatments for depression have been developed in the past decades. In this chapter, we explore three of the most widely used psychological treatment interventions for depression, namely behavioural therapy, cognitive therapy, and interpersonal psychotherapy. The term 'depression' refers in this chapter to major depressive disorder and dysthymic disorder. For each intervention, the theoretical background is briefly described and the content of treatment and its goals are discussed. We conclude this chapter with a comprehensive overview of research on the effectiveness of these types of psychological treatment. The fact that we focus on these three psychological treatments does not imply that other methods (e.g., psychoanalytic psychotherapy) are inferior, only that they have not been as widely studied and evaluated.

BEHAVIOURAL TREATMENT

Theoretical Foundation

Lewinsohn's Reinforcement Theory

From a learning theoretical perspective, depression should be viewed as the result of a specific learning history. In particular, operant learning processes are assumed to play a key role in the pathogenesis of depression. Skinner (1953) was probably the first who launched the idea that depression can best be regarded as a diminution of the frequency of normal behaviour. In terms of his operant theory of learning, this diminution is caused by a decrease in positive reinforcement of that behaviour. In terms of the 'law of effect', normal behaviour simply extinguishes because it is not followed by positive consequences.

This point of view was elaborated most extensively by Lewinsohn (1975) in his learning theory of depression. According to this theory (which is comprehensively discussed by van Son and Hoevenaars, 1998), there are two types of stimuli that are associated with the emergence of feelings of dysphoria, fatigue, and other somatic complaints. The first type of stimulus involves a deficit of positive reinforcement and the second type is concerned with the administration of punishment. In terms of learning theory, both types of stimulus are regarded as unconditioned stimuli that irrevocably elicit the unconditioned response of depression.

The lack of positive reinforcement may be caused by a number of factors. First, it may well be the case that, for some reason, there are no positive reinforcers available in the depressed patient's environment. Otherwise, the deficit in reinforcement may be due to the fact that the person has not learned the behaviour to acquire positive reinforcement. In this context, one should especially think about persons who have not learned adequate social skills and as a result elicit few positive reinforcers in interaction with other people (i.e., social reinforcers). A final possibility is that the person has not learned to actually view positive consequences as reinforcers. In a similar vein, the increase of punishment may be provoked by a triad of factors. First, the person may live in an environment that is characterized by high levels of aversiveness and punishment. Second, the person displays behaviour that elicits aversive reactions in the environment. Third and finally, the person has learned to interpret a lot of events as aversive or as punishment (see Figure 11.1).

Taken together, low levels of reinforcement and high levels of punishment may be the result of a constellation of environmental and personal features as can be illustrated in the following example of a depressed adolescent.

> Jim is seventeen years old as he is diagnosed with a severe major depressive disorder. The boy is shy, has no friends, and has always found it difficult to make contact with peers. At home, he lives with his depressed mother, an irritable woman who has always

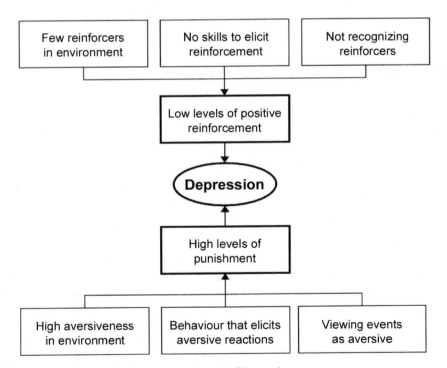

Figure 11.1 Lewinsohn's behavioural model of depression

criticized and punished Jim for almost everything he does. His father was quite different. He was Jim's buddy and used to do all kinds of pleasurable activities with him. Unfortunately, father died in a car accident, about one year ago. Although Jim has coped adequately with this loss, he misses father almost every day. At school, his performance is deteriorating. One of his teachers has tried to approach him, but Jim refused his help: 'Why do you pick on me? There are other students who do worse!'

Lewinsohn's (1975) theory does not only account for the emergence of the depression, but also for the continuation of the disorder. That is, the first sign of a depression frequently involves a dejected or dysphoric mood and the environment usually reacts with sympathy and concern, thereby unintentionally reinforcing the depressive behaviour and thus enhancing its frequency. As time goes by, the depressive behaviour will increasingly elicit aversion in the environment and people will start to avoid the depressed patient. This further decreases the level of reinforcement and aggravates the depression.

Others have formulated variations of Lewinsohn's learning theory of depression. For example, Costello (1972) has suggested that it is not a decrease in the amount of reinforcement that gives cause to a depression, but rather a decline of the value or attractiveness of reinforcers, which has been labelled as 'loss of reinforcer-effectiveness'. In a similar vein, Rehm (1977) argues that depressed patients have a negative view of themselves and as a consequence frequently evaluate their behaviour in a negative way. In terms of learning theory, depressed patients can be characterized by low levels of self-reinforcement and high levels of self-punishment.

Seligman's Learned Helplessness Model

A final theory that should be mentioned when discussing learning theory models of depression, is Seligman's (1974, 1975) initial formulation of the learned helplessness theory. This view was based on observational experiments of animals who received electric shocks in two different situations. In the first part of the experiment, some dogs were put in a box with electric grids in the flooring and subjected to numerous painful electric shocks from which they could not escape. In the second part, these animals as well as dogs who did not have this prior experience with inescapable shock, were placed in a similar box. However, there was one important difference: that is, painful shock could be avoided by jumping over to another compartment of the box as soon as the dogs heard a warning signal (e.g., a buzzer). Seligman observed that the behaviour of the dogs was markedly affected by whether they were previously exposed to inevitable shock. Animals who did not have the earlier experience became quite upset when they received the first electric shocks, but soon learned to jump to the other compartment when they heard the warning signal (i.e., conditioned stimulus), thereby avoiding further painful shocks. In contrast, the animals that had prior experience with inescapable shock behaved quite differently. Soon after receiving the first shocks, they stopped running around in a distressed way. Instead they seemed to give up and passively accepted the painful stimulation.

Not surprisingly, they did not acquire the avoidance response adequately: in fact, they lay down in a corner and whined. Apparently, these animals seemed to have acquired a 'sense of helplessness' when confronted with uncontrollable stressful stimulation. This helplessness later seriously affected their performance in stressful situations that could be controlled. They appeared to lose their ability and motivation to learn to respond in an effective way to painful stimulation.

Seligman (1974, 1975) noted clear similarities between the learned helplessness of animals and human depression. He proposed that the disconnection of behaviour, on the one hand, and the receipt of reinforcement and punishment, on the other hand, plays a key role in the pathogenesis of depression. Like the helpless animals, depressed patients appear passive in the face of stress and fail to initiate action that may allow them to deal with the aversive situation.

Although the learning theoretical formulations as put forward by Lewinsohn and Seligman seem to cover some important aspects of depression, it is also clear that both models have significant shortcomings in explaining the full depressive syndrome. As a result, both theories have been revised repeatedly, mostly by incorporating elements of the cognitive theory. An example can be found in the next section, in which we will briefly address the cognitive-learning formulation of Seligman's learned helplessness theory of depression.

Content of Treatment

Given the focus of learning theories of depression on reinforcement and punishment, the major goal of behaviourally oriented treatments involves increasing the positive reinforcement and decreasing punishment received by the depressed patient. In this context, a number of different treatment approaches have been described, all of which share this common goal. Furthermore, behavioural approaches to the treatment of depression share a number of other commonalities (Hoberman and Lewinsohn, 1985). For example, depressed patients are required to monitor activities, mood, and thoughts. They are encouraged to set achievable goals in order to ensure successful early experiences, and to give themselves rewards for attaining these goals. Finally, most behavioural approaches involve training designed to correct various performance and skill deficits of depressed patients.

Increasing Pleasant Activities

This behavioural approach consists of four steps. First, the depressed patient receives a clear account of the rationale of this treatment approach. Mood is directly associated with behaviour. For example, when you do something pleasurable, you feel good. But when you do something unpleasurable, you feel bad. People can influence their mood by changing their behaviours. As a depressed person, your activity level is probably rather low. As a result, you also engage in few positive activities and as a consequence your mood deteriorates. The purpose of this treatment is to increase the frequency of your positive activities, thereby eventually improving your mood.

The second step in this treatment involves self-observation. The depressed patient is instructed to find out which activities have either a positive or a negative effect on mood. This is done by means of a diary in which the patient rates the pleasurableness and mood associated with various activities. The purpose of this step is to demonstrate the patient that there is a clear link between behaviour and mood.

The third step is concerned with the identification of activities, events and persons that are potentially reinforcing for the patient. The Pleasant Events Schedule (PES; MacPhillamy and Lewinsohn, 1971) may be a useful tool for this purpose. The PES is a questionnaire consisting of 320 items describing interactions with the environment that many people find to be pleasant (e.g., being with friends, being told that you are loved, going to a restaurant, having sex). The patient first indicates the frequency of each event's occurrence during the past month and then rates the subjective enjoyability of the event. In this way, the individual's rate of engagement in person–environment interactions, his/her potential for positive reinforcement, as well as the total amount of experienced positive reinforcement can be assessed. Most importantly, scores on the PES can be used to provide an individualized list of 'target' pleasant events.

The fourth and final step is concerned with the actual increase of pleasant activities. The therapist selects activities that according to the PES do occur and provide a high level of reinforcement, and then stimulates the patients to engage in these activities by giving him/her homework assignments.

Social Skills Training

Based on the assumption that depressed patients display deficits in their social skills and as a consequence elicit low levels of positive reinforcement and high levels of punishment (see supra), it has been suggested that social skills training can be useful in the treatment of these patients. A good example of such a training is the programme developed by Becker et al. (1987). This programme focuses primarily on three specific behavioural repertoires that appear to be particularly relevant to depressed patients: negative assertion, positive assertion, and conversational skills. Negative assertion involves behaviours that allow persons to stand up for their rights. Thus, training in negative assertion concerns learning how to refuse unreasonable demands, how to request others to change their inconvenient behaviour, and how to compromise and negotiate solutions. Positive assertion refers to the expression of positive feelings about others, as well as offering appropriate apologies. Conversational skills involve initiating conversations, asking questions, making appropriate self-disclosures, and ending conversations gracefully. In all of these areas, depressed patients are given direct behaviour training as well as training in social perception. Next, patients are encouraged to practise the skills and behaviours across different situations, interacting with various persons (strangers, family members, friends, people at work/school). Finally, depressed patients are trained to evaluate their behaviour more objectively and to administer appropriate self-reinforcement.

This section has described a number of frequently employed behavioural treatment approaches for depression. All these treatments focus on changing the patient's interaction with the social environment in order to increase the amount of received positive reinforcement. Available evidence indeed suggests that there is little doubt about the effectiveness of these interventions (Gotlib and Hammen, 1992): increasing pleasant activities and social skills training both typically lead to a significant reduction of depressive symptomatology. In clinical practice, pure behaviour treatment of depression is not frequently provided. In most cases, this treatment is combined with cognitive elements, which will be the focus of the next section.

COGNITIVE THERAPY

Theoretical Foundation

In the past decades, psychopathology researchers have increasingly advocated the use of diathesis–stress models for understanding the development of depression. The basic idea of this model is that individuals, who eventually develop depression, differ in some underlying way from those who do not become depressed. This underlying difference is referred to as their diathesis (or predisposition). Among those with the diathesis, only those who experience stress will actually develop the disorder. Originally it was assumed that the diathesis was constitutional or biological in origin (e.g., Meehl, 1962; Rosenthal, 1963), but depression researchers have also proposed diatheses that are cognitive in nature (e.g., Metalsky et al., 1982). Two diathesis–stress models in which cognitive diatheses are conceived as important vulnerability factors for depression (i.e., the cognitive model as proposed by Beck (1967) and the reformulated helplessness model of depression) are discussed here.

The Cognitive Theory of Beck

The first cognitive diathesis discussed here was provided by Aaron T. Beck, a psychiatrist who became disenchanted with psychodynamic theories of depression early in his career and later developed his own cognitive theory of depression. A central tenet of this theory is the presence of depressogenic schemas. A schema is an organized representation of knowledge about a concept or about some stimulus, which is helpful in guiding the processing of current information. At the basis of depressogenic schemas, individuals have negative dysfunctional beliefs or depressogenic assumptions that are rigid, extreme, and counterproductive. An example of a dysfunctional belief is 'To be happy, I must be accepted by

all people at all times' (Beck, 1976). A psychosocial stressor merely serves to activate these depressogenic schemas with dysfunctional beliefs that have previously
been dormant. Thus, the schemas and beliefs are thought to serve as the underlying diathesis or vulnerability to develop depression, although they may lie
dormant for years in the absence of significant stressors. When current stressors
activate depressogenic schemas, the negative cognitive triad becomes apparent
and is experienced by the depressed individual in the form of negative automatic
thoughts. These thoughts involve unpleasant pessimistic predictions centred on
the three themes of the negative triad: (a) negative thoughts about the self
(e.g., 'I'm nothing'); (b) negative thoughts about one's experiences and the
surrounding world (e.g., 'People don't like me'); and (c) negative thoughts
about one's future (e.g., 'It's hopeless because things will always be this way').
As a consequence of the negative cognitive triad, a depressed individual may
experience affective (e.g., depressed mood), behavioural and motivational (e.g.,
withdrawal from social activities), cognitive (e.g., worrying), and physical symptoms (e.g., change in appetite and sleep). Figure 11.2 illustrates Beck's cognitive
theory of depression: activation of dysfunctional beliefs may lead to negative
automatic thoughts (cognitive triad), which may in turn induce affective, behavioural and motivational, cognitive, and physical symptoms. These symptoms
serve to maintain the negative automatic thoughts.

Recent extensions of the cognitive theory elaborate on the notion of specific
vulnerability. Two types of schemas (belief systems) have been proposed that may
interact with two classes of stressors to provoke a depressive reaction (Beck, 1983,
1991; Sacco and Beck, 1995). 'Sociotropy' refers to the tendency to value closeness,
acceptance, dependency, and sharing. Individuals whose cognitive schemas are
highly developed around sociotropic themes should be more likely to become
depressed when confronted with sociotropic trauma, such as social deprivation or
rejection. 'Autonomy' refers to the tendency to value independent functioning,
mobility, choice, and achievement. Individuals whose cognitive schemas are highly
developed around autonomous themes are expected to be vulnerable to depression
when exposed to stressors such as failure or immobilization.

Along with dysfunctional beliefs that fuel the cognitive triad once they are
activated, Beck also postulates that the negative cognitive triad tends to be
maintained by a variety of cognitive biases or distortions. The cognitive biases
are listed below:

(1) Dichotomous thinking (i.e., a tendency to think in black-or-white or all-or-
    nothing).
(2) Selective abstraction (i.e., a tendency to focus on a negative detail in a situation
    and to conceptualize the entire experience on the basis of this negative fragment).
(3) Arbitrary inference (i.e., jumping to a conclusion based on minimal or no
    evidence).
(4) Overgeneralization (i.e., a tendency to draw a conclusion from a single perhaps
    rather unimportant event).

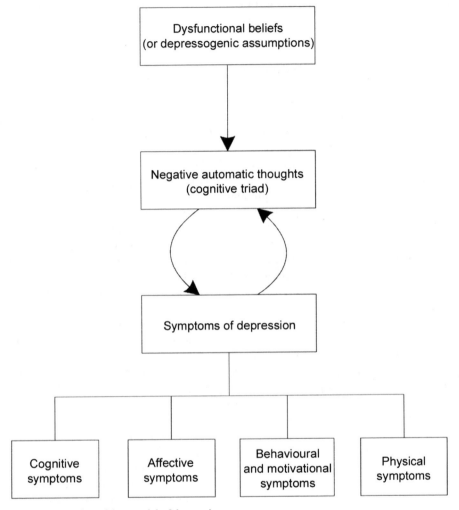

Figure 11.2 Cognitive model of depression

(5) Magnification and minimization (i.e., a tendency to overestimate the significance or magnitude of undesirable events, and to underestimate the significance or magnitude of desirable events).

(6) Personalization (i.e., a tendency to relate external events to oneself without evidence).

Although the cognitive theory of depression is focused on an intrapsychic mechanism to describe the development and maintenance of depression, the role of interpersonal factors in depressive disorders is also acknowledged (Beck et al., 1979;

Beck, 1988, 1991; Sacco and Beck, 1995). The role of interpersonal factors will be discussed in the next section on interpersonal psychotherapy.

The Reformulated Helplessness Model of Depression

Beck's theory originated from his clinical observations of the pervasive patterns of negative thinking in depressed patients. The reformulated learned helplessness model of depression, the second cognitive diathesis discussed here, was based on observations in an animal research laboratory (see supra). The central tenet of this model is a depressogenic attributional style. Seligman (1974, 1975) first proposed that learned helplessness might provide a useful model for depression. Abramson and colleagues proposed a reformulated helplessness theory (Abramson et al., 1978). They theorized that people with a depressive or pessimistic attributional style, which involves a tendency to make internal, stable, and global attributions for negative (uncontrollable) events, are prone to experience depression following a negative life event. A pessimistic or depressive attribution for receiving a low grade on an exam, for example, would be 'I'm stupid'. The cause is internal ('I'), stable (intelligence is not likely to change much) and global (stupidity is likely to affect a wide range of issues in one's life). A more optimistic attribution for the same event would be 'The teacher made up the test in a bad mood and made it especially difficult'. The cause is external (the teacher), unstable (the teacher hopefully is not always in a bad mood), and specific (only the teacher on this course) (Carson et al., 1996). Thus, individuals who have a pessimistic or depressive attributional style (diathesis) are at risk for depression when faced with uncontrollable negative events. In 1989, a further revision of this theory was presented, known as the hopelessness theory (Abramson et al., 1989). The revised theory implies that a pessimistic or depressive attributional style in conjunction with one or more negative uncontrollable events may not be sufficient to produce depression unless one has first experienced a state of hopelessness. Thus, depressed individuals may have no control over what is going to happen and have the absolute certainty that an important bad outcome is going to occur or that a highly desired good outcome is not going to occur.

Cognitive Therapy

Based on the cognitive approach of Beck and colleagues (Beck et al., 1979), a depression-specific psychotherapy has been developed (see for a detailed overview Sacco and Beck, 1995). This form of psychotherapy also accounts for the attributional style that depressed individuals have. Three assumptions underlie cognitive therapy interventions. First, a depressed individual's affect and behaviour are largely determined by the way in which he or she views the world. Second, cognitions can be self-monitored and communicated. Third, modification of cognitions should lead to changes in affect and behaviour (Sacco and Beck, 1995). Cognitive therapy is a short-term treatment (15 to 25 sessions of about 50 minutes at weekly intervals) that focuses on here-and-now problems.

The first step in a cognitive therapy is to provide a rationale for the treatment. A therapist can do this by providing the following hypothetical situation. Suppose someone is lying in bed at night and suddenly, there is a noise. This person who is lying in bed may think: 'There is a burglar in the house'. Then the therapist may ask the depressed patient: 'What would this person feel and what would he or she do?' After the patient has provided an answer to this question, the therapist may continue: 'Suppose the person in bed thought that the cat threw the vase. What would this person feel and do?' By means of this example, the relations between thoughts, feelings and behaviour are explained.

The second step in cognitive therapy for depression has to do with the identification of automatic negative thoughts. Depressed individuals are often unaware of these thoughts and once they are brought to their attention, they consider them as accurate representations of reality, even though they are often unreasonably negative. Diaries can be used for self-monitoring automatic thoughts and the associated feelings and behaviours. In the process of identification of automatic thoughts, collaborative empiricism can be applied, in which unrealistic thoughts are raised as tentative hypotheses, to be tested by data-gathering techniques, such as homework assignments. The therapist encourages the depressed patient to identify automatic thoughts but does not argue the reasonableness of these thoughts.

The third step involves challenging the reasonableness of the automatic thoughts. On this step, the depressed patient is taught to think as a scientist who tests the hypothesis that the automatic thoughts are illogical and inaccurate. The cognitive biases or distortions that lie at the basis of the negative automatic thoughts are identified and corrected. The therapist may use Socratic dialogue to examine the logic or the premises on which conclusions are based. Behavioural experiments are designed to gather data bearing on the validity of the automatic thought. The credibility of each of the thoughts can be measured (from 0 to 100%) before and after such an experiment, so that depressed individuals learn to distance themselves from their thoughts. Alternative interpretations are obtained by means of a 'brainstorm'. Depressed patients also learn to recognize their tendency to attribute the cause of negative events erroneously to internal, stable, and global factors. Next, depressed patients are taught to ask themselves what would happen if their worst fear would come true. This confrontation with the worst case scenario, makes depressed patients realize that they can cope with negative events and that these events occur to all people. Often depressed individuals gain a more realistic perspective. Finally, depressed patients learn to substitute more reasonable interpretations for the irrational negative automatic thoughts. They are encouraged to write down their dysfunctional thoughts and to formulate rational counter-responses, rather than simply processing them in their minds.

The fourth step consists of the identification of the dysfunctional beliefs (or depressogenic assumptions) that make up the core of a schema. Dysfunctional beliefs are also termed 'silent assumptions', as depressed individuals are often unaware of the existence of these beliefs. Identification of dysfunctional beliefs usually occurs as a product of the examination of automatic thoughts. Modification of these beliefs involves the same process as modification of negative automatic thoughts. Dysfunctional beliefs are less accessible when the depressed individual is no longer experiencing the depressive disorder. Thus, it is important to begin the process of identifying these underlying beliefs while symptoms are still present (Sacco and Beck, 1995).

In sum, cognitive therapy consists of highly structured systematic attempts to teach individuals with depression to evaluate their beliefs and negative automatic thoughts. Patients are also taught to identify and correct biases or distortions of information processing, and to uncover and correct their underlying depressogenic assumptions. Cognitive therapy heavily relies on an empirical approach, in that patients are taught to treat their beliefs as hypotheses that can be tested through the use of behavioural experiments.

INTERPERSONAL THERAPY

Theoretical Foundation

Interpersonal therapy (IPT) is a symptom-directed, time-limited, individual psychotherapy method that has been developed by Klerman et al. (1984). IPT is an intervention with an eclectic character, which means that this method borrows theoretical notions and treatment principles from various other psychotherapeutic schools. The basic assumption of IPT is that the interpersonal context plays a crucial role in the pathogenesis of depression. Although not supported by an idiosyncratic theory about the origins of depression, there are several empirical findings showing that difficulties in the social and interpersonal context are associated with depression.

Attachment Theory

Early in life, children develop an attachment relationship to the caregiver. More specifically, through interactions with primary caregivers, children develop expectations about their caregivers' availability, which serve as the basis for internal working models of the self and the other. When experiences lead to the expectation that caregivers will be loving and responsive, children develop a model of the self as loved and valued, and a model of the other as warm and loving (Bretherton, 1985). This confidence allows children to develop secure strategies for seeking out their caregivers when distressed or in need, with the expectation that their needs will be met. In contrast, when children have experiences that lead them to expect caregivers to be rejecting or unreliable, they develop a model of the self as unloved and rejected, and a model of the other as unloving and rejecting. These children do not expect that caregivers will be available when needed, and they develop alternative, insecure strategies for coping with their distress.

Bowlby (1969) assumes that attachment status (i.e., secure vs. insecure) and associated working models provide the foundation for all later social relationships. Indeed, research has shown that insecurely attached individuals are more likely to have interpersonal problems than their securely attached counterparts (see Cassidy and Shaver, 1999). Moreover, there is abundant evidence showing that insecure attachment is associated with high levels of depression symptoms or even depressive disorders (e.g., Bifulco et al., 2002). Altogether these findings seem to indicate that interpersonal problems mediate the link between insecure attachment and depression, a conclusion that is in keeping with the basic assumptions of IPT.

Social Origins Theory

Brown and Harris (1978) carried out a large-scale study of depressed women in England. Great care was taken as to the methods of this study. That is, the researchers used a detailed interview and carefully trained interviewers to question the subjects about any recent adversities that had distressed them. The truthfulness of the women's reports was checked by interviewing relatives. Furthermore, trained members of the research staff rated the stressfulness of the events, rather than relying on the respondents' estimations. Using these methods, Brown and Harris found that 61% of depressive women but only 25% of the control subjects had experienced a severely disturbing life event in the nine months prior to the interview. Most pertinent to the present discussion, many of these events had an interpersonal character, for example separation from a key person (i.e., the husband) and serious illness or death of someone close. Moreover, social support appeared to be crucial. When the women were divided into those who had an intimate friend in whom they confided and those who did not have a close friend, the impact of the stressful life events were quite different. Only 10% of the women with an intimate relationship got depressed after the life event, whereas this figure was 37% for the women without a confidant. These results seem to suggest that interpersonal difficulties put people at risk for developing depression, whereas interpersonal resilience may buffer against such disorder.

Contents of Treatment

Stages of Treatment

The Dutch psychiatrist Peeters (1999) has provided a comprehensive description of IPT. Briefly, he describes IPT as a relatively short-lasting intervention method consisting of 15 to 20 sessions that can be allocated to three stages. During the first stage, which usually takes up to three sessions, the therapist devotes a lot of attention to the diagnostics of the depression and the provision of psycho-education about this mental disorder. The diagnosis is discussed within a medical context in which depression is conceived as a disease from which the patient suffers. A significant amount of time is spent on what is called the 'interpersonal anamnesis', during which the therapist checks whether the patient's personal environment has changed prior to the development of the depression. Of particular importance are the relationships of the patient with significant others, both in the present and in the past. The therapist will try to link the patient's interpersonal problems to the current depression.

IPT distinguishes four areas in which interpersonal problems can be classified: (1) grief, (2) interpersonal conflict, (3) role change, and (4) interpersonal deficit. These areas can serve as focuses (i.e., targets) of the therapy.

(1) Grief can be a focus of IPT when the beginning of the depression is related to the decease of a significant other. In most cases, the problem involves pathological grief in which ambivalent feelings for the deceased person play a key role. The therapist primes the process of mourning by encouraging the patient to address positive as well as negative feelings in relation to the deceased person. When these feelings are sufficiently expressed, it is important that the patient invests in relationships with familiar and unfamiliar people.

(2) Interpersonal conflict concerns a conflict between the patient and a significant other, and can be a focus of IPT when it is associated with the origins or maintenance of the depressive disorder. The purpose of IPT is to clear out the conflict and to examine whether there are possibilities of coming to a more positive relationship with the other. In most cases, the patient is taught to deal in a different way with the conflict or to redefine the relationship, thereby changing his expectations in relation to the other.

(3) Role change might be a focus of IPT when the depression is linked to important changes in the patient's social life. This has frequently to do with major transitions in the life cycle such as moving into rooms, having children, children leaving the parental home, or going into retirement. The patient has to give up his old role and should learn to play a new one. It may well be the case that the patient has to acquire certain skills so that he can play his new role adequately.

(4) Interpersonal deficits refer to a lack of skills in relationships with others, which lead to strong feelings of insufficiency and social isolation. When chosen as a target for treatment, the main purpose of IPT is to reduce the social deprivation. To accomplish this goal, the therapist carefully analyses the patient's relationships in the past: What went wrong? Why were relationships broken off? Following this, the therapist tries to stimulate the patient to enter into new relationships, thereby giving directions in order to counteract interpersonal deficits.

Because IPT is intended as a brief intervention, the therapist and the patient agree on the fact that during therapy only one or two of these focuses will be addressed. The therapist will first choose a focus that has a direct and evident link to the actual problems of the patient and which can be changed in the short term.

The purpose of the second stage, which has a duration of about 10 sessions, is to solve the interpersonal problems that are chosen as focuses. First, the patient's problems and associated feelings and thoughts are explored. Then, the therapist and the patient will think up new ways of dealing with these problems, and, finally, the patient will implement these solutions in his daily functioning.

The third and final stage of IPT is concerned with finishing treatment and consists of only a couple of sessions. During these sessions, the patient has to give up his relationship with the therapist and increasingly relies on his own strengths and competences for dealing with interpersonal challenges. Therapist and patient also discuss potential future problems and ways in which these can be resolved.

Techniques

As mentioned earlier, IPT employs various techniques that are also used in other psychological interventions. The following techniques are of particular importance to IPT as they fit rather well in the short-lasting and focal nature of this intervention (Klerman et al., 1984): (a) exploration, which primarily refers to an analysis of the patient's interpersonal relationships; (b) encouragement of the expression of affect may help to reduce the emotional flatness of the depressed patient, which frequently hinders relationships with others; (c) clarification; by means of summaries and the discussion of inconsistencies, the patient may gain new insights; (d) communication analysis may help the patient to understand why interpersonal problems arise or continue; (e) role play can also be used to reconstruct interpersonal events in order to get better insight into problems and difficulties and to practise new behaviours; (f) use of the therapeutic relationship; although the relationship between the patient and his social environment is the main target of an IPT treatment, it is possible that a patient's social contacts are so poor that it may be necessary to take behaviours and interactions during the therapy sessions into consideration; and (g) giving advice and directives may be useful especially in the beginning of treatment, when indecisiveness may be a prominent feature of the depression. In the further course of the treatment, the therapist will become more supportive and stimulating in order to prompt new activities for the depressed patient.

IPT is a less well-known treatment method for depression than behavioural and cognitive therapy. Nevertheless, as we will see in the next section, therapy outcome studies demonstrate that IPT should be considered as an effective psychological intervention for depression.

DISCUSSION

From a biomedical point of view, depression is conceptualized as a 'medical illness'. In the United States but also in many other countries, medication is the most commonly delivered treatment for depression (Narrow et al., 1993). In contrast to the illness model, several psychological models have been proposed, resulting in interventions such as behaviour therapy, cognitive therapy, and IPT, which have been evaluated as being effective in reducing depressive symptoms. Yet, these effective non-drug strategies are often ignored by medical practitioners (Altrocchi et al., 1986).

Most research on the effectiveness of psychotherapy has relied on cognitive therapy in which principles of behaviour therapy such as behavioural experiments are incorporated. Several studies have shown that in the acute phase of depression, cognitive therapy is more effective than antidepressant medication (e.g., Blackburn et al., 1981; Rush et al., 1977, 1982). Other studies have shown that cognitive therapy is equally effective as antidepressant medication (e.g., Hollon et al., 1992) or combined cognitive–drug treatment (e.g., Beck et al., 1985; Blackburn et al., 1981; Covi and Lipman, 1987; Evans et al., 1992; Hollon et al., 1992). A number of other studies suggest that cognitive therapy adds to the efficacy of standard anti-depressants drug treatment (e.g., Bowers, 1990; Dunn, 1979; Miller et al., 1989; Teasdale et al., 1984).

Several meta-analyses (e.g., Steinbrueck et al., 1983; Dobson, 1989; Conte et al., 1986; Nietzel et al., 1987; Robinson et al., 1990; Hollon et al., 1991) reported in the psychiatric and psychological literature, which cover multiple studies with thousands of patients, have consistently supported the perspective that psychotherapy is at least as effective as medication in the treatment of depression (see for a critical discussion, Antonuccio et al., 1995). Although these meta-analyses were conducted independently, there was some overlap of included studies. Except for the meta-analyses conducted by Dobson (1989) and Hollon et al. (1991) who specifically focused on the effectiveness of cognitive-behavioural interventions, the meta-analyses combined all brands of psychotherapy for depression.

With respect to effectiveness in the long-term (e.g., relapse), several studies have shown that psychotherapy is at least as effective as medication treatments (e.g., Blackburn et al., 1981, 1986; Evans et al., 1992; Greenberg et al., 1992; Hersen et al., 1984; Hollon et al., 1991, 1992; McLean and Hakstian, 1990; McLean and Taylor, 1992; Rush et al., 1977, 1978; Shea et al., 1992a; Simons et al, 1986; Weissman et al., 1981). However, the effectiveness of all treatments on the long-term are some-what disappointing given that a substantial part of the patients show a return of the depression. With respect to IPT, Weissman and Markowitz (1994) indicated that IPT can be used in dysthymic disorder, geriatric depressed patients, and depressed primary care patients. Although IPT is not as well studied as cognitive therapy, research has supported its effectiveness in the acute phase of depression as well as during follow-up (e.g., DiMascio et al., 1979; Weissman et al., 1979; Elkin et al., 1989; Weissman et al., 1981; Shea et al., 1992b; Frank et al., 1989).

The effectiveness of medication treatment in combination with psychotherapy has not yet been convincingly demonstrated (AHCPR, 1993; Manning and Frances, 1990). However, patients suffering from severe recurrent depression may benefit from a combined treatment (Thase et al., 1997). To prevent relapse in these patients, effective maintenance interventions of cognitive therapy and IPT have been developed (e.g., Fava et al., 1996; Frank et al., 1993) as well as prolonged treatments with depressive medication (e.g., Janicak et al., 1997). However, more research regarding the effectiveness of psychotherapy in the long run, and particularly in combination with medication treatment, is warranted.

Three individual studies are particularly noteworthy so that they will be discussed in more detail here. In the first study, conducted by the Treatment of Depression Collaborative Research Program (Elkin et al., 1989), 239 depressed individuals were randomly assigned to receive either cognitive therapy, IPT, imipramine, or placebo in combination with clinical management. Cognitive therapy, IPT, and imipramine significantly reduced depression symptoms. However, re-analyses of the results from this study by means of a random regression model showed that cognitive therapy was less effective than IPT and imipramine in severely depressed individuals (Elkin et al., 1995). A second important study analysed data on 595 individuals with major depressive disorder derived from six independent studies (Thase et al., 1997). Of the total sample, 243 individuals received psychotherapy (cognitive therapy or IPT) and 352 received a combination of IPT and pharmacotherapy. Results from this study indicated that recovery rates for psychotherapy versus combined treatment did not differ for less severe cases. In more severe cases, combined treatment showed significantly higher recovery rates than psychotherapy (rates were 43% and 25% respectively). A third important study has been conducted by the United States Department of Health and Human Services (AHCPR, 1993), which investigated the effectiveness of different types of antidepressants, placebo, behavioural therapy, cognitive therapy, IPT, and another psychological intervention, namely brief dynamic therapy. The results showed that except for placebo and brief dynamic therapy (which were least effective), all treatments were equally effective in reducing depressive symptoms. Figure 11.3 shows a visual representation of the effectiveness of the various interventions in this study.

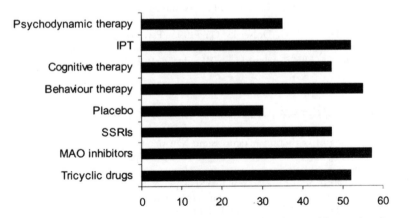

Figure 11.3 The AHCPR (1993) study: percentages of patients with a major depressive disorder recovering after various treatments. *Note.* SSRI = selective serotonin reuptake inhibitor, MAO = monoamine oxidase

In summary, this chapter has focused on psychological treatments for depression (i.e., behavioural treatment, cognitive treatment, IPT). Behaviour treatment aims to increase positive reinforcement and decrease punishment thereby reducing levels of depression and improving dysfunctional skills and problem-solving. Behaviour treatment is often incorporated in cognitive treatment, commonly known as 'cognitive-behavioural treatment'. This type of treatment stresses changing negative automatic thoughts and the underlying depressogenic assumptions. IPT focuses on interpersonal problems as the cause of depression. Research on the effectiveness of these interventions indicates that particularly cognitive-behavioural interventions and IPT are at least as effective as medication in the treatment of unipolar depression. Future research should address some issues that have not been resolved. For example, it remains to be established whether a combined intervention of medication and psychotherapy is superior to an intervention that only relies on one of these approaches, whether psychological treatments such as cognitive therapy and IPT are equally effective as medication in the treatment of severely depressed patients, and what individual characteristics predict good treatment response to psychological interventions.

REFERENCES

Abramson LY, Metalsky GI, Alloy LB (1989) Hopelessness depression: a theory-based subtype of depression. *Psych Rev* **96**: 358–372.

Abramson LY, Seligman MEP, Teasdale JD (1978) Learned helplessness in humans: critique and reformulation. *J Abnorm Psychol* **87**: 49–74.

AHCPR (1993) *Depression Guideline Panel. Depression in Primary Care.* Vol 2. Treatment of Major Depression. Clinical practice guidelines 5 (AHCPR Publication 93-0551). Rockville, MD: Department of Health and Human Services.

Altrocchi J, Antonuccio DO, Miller G (1986) Nondrug prescriptions for adult outpatient depression. *Postgraduate Med* **79**: 164–181.

Antonuccio DO, Danton WG, DeNelsky GY (1995) Psychotherapy versus medication for depression: challenging the conventional wisdom with data. *Professional Psychology: Research and Practice* **26**: 574–585. Retrieved from World Wide Web: http://www.apa.org/journals/anton.html.

Beck AT (1967) *Depression: Clinical, Experimental and Theoretical Aspects.* New York: Harper & Row.

Beck AT (1976) *Cognitive Theory and the Emotional Disorders.* New York: International Universities Press.

Beck AT (1983) Cognitive therapy of depression: New perspectives. In Clayton PJ, Barrett JE (Eds) *Treatment of Depression: Old Controversies and New Approaches.* New York: Raven Press, pp. 265–284.

Beck AT (1988) *Love is Never Enough.* New York: Harper & Row.

Beck AT (1991) Cognitive therapy: a 30-year retrospective. *Am Psychologist* **46**: 368–375.

Beck AT, Hollon SD, Young JE, Bedrosian RC, Budenz D (1985) Treatment of depression with cognitive therapy and amitriptyline. *Arch Gen Psychiatry* **42**: 142–148.

Beck AT, Rush AJ, Shaw BF, Emery G (1979) *Cognitive Therapy of Depression.* New York: Guilford Press.

Becker RE, Heimberg RG, Bellack AS (1987) *Social Skills Training Treatment for Depression*. New York: Pergamon Press.

Bifulco A, Moran PM, Ball C, Bernazzani O (2002) Adult attachment style. I: Its relationship to clinical depression. *Soc Psychiatry Psychiatr Epidem* **37**: 50–59.

Blackburn IM, Bishop S, Glen AIM, Whalley LJ, Christie JE (1981) The efficacy of cognitive therapy in depression: a treatment trial using cognitive therapy and pharmacotherapy, each alone and in combination. *Br J Psychiatry* **139**: 181–189.

Blackburn IM, Eunson KM, Bishop S (1986) A two-year naturalistic follow-up of depressed patients treated with cognitive therapy, pharmacotherapy, and a combination of both. *J Affect Dis* **10**: 67–75.

Bowers WA (1990) Treatment of depressed in-patients: cognitive therapy plus medication, relaxation plus medication, and medication alone. *Br J Psychiatry* **156**: 73–78.

Bowlby J (1969) *Attachment and Loss, I: Attachment*. New York: Basic Books.

Bretherton I (1985) Attachment theory. Retrospect and prospect. In Bretherton I, Waters E (eds) *Growing Points of Attachment Theory and Research*. Monographs of the Society for Research into Child Development, Vol 50, pp. 3–35.

Brown GW, Harris T (1978) *Social Origins of Depression*. London: Free Press.

Carson RC, Butcher JN, Mineka S (1996) *Abnormal Psychology and Normal Life*. New York: HarperCollins.

Cassidy J, Shaver PR (1999) *Handbook of Attachment. Theory, Research, and Clinical Applications*. New York: Guilford Press.

Conte HR, Plutchik R, Wild KV, Karasu TB (1986) Combined psychotherapy and pharmacotherapy for depression: a systematic analysis of the evidence. *Arch Gen Psychiatry* **43**: 471–479.

Costello CG (1972) Depression: loss of reinforcer effectiveness? *Behav Ther* **3**: 240–247.

Covi L, Lipman RS (1987) Cognitive behavioral group psychotherapy combined with imipramine in major depression. *Psychopharmacol Bull* **23**: 173–176.

DiMascio A, Weissman MM, Prusoff BA, Neu C, Zwilling M, Klerman GL (1979) Differential symptom reduction by drugs and psychotherapy in acute depression. *Arch Gen Psychiatry* **36**: 1450–1456.

Dobson KS (1989) A meta-analysis of the efficacy of cognitive therapy for depression. *J Consult Clin Psychol* **57**: 414–419.

Dunn RJ (1979) Cognitive modification with depression-prone psychiatric patients. *Cogn Ther Res* **3**: 307–317.

Elkin I, Gibbons RD, Shea MT, Sotsky SM, Watkins JT, Pilkonis PA, Hedeker D (1995) Initial severity and differential treatment outcome in the National Institute of Mental Health Treatment of Depression Collaborative Research Program. *J Consult Clin Psychol* **63**: 841–847.

Elkin I, Shea T, Watkins JT, Imber SD, Sotsky SM, Collins JF, Glass DR, Pilkonis PA, Leber WR, Docherty JP, Fiester SJ, Parloff MB (1989) National Institute of Mental Health Treatment of Depression Collaborative Research Program: general effectiveness of treatments. *Arch Gen Psychiatry* **46**: 971–982.

Evans MD, Hollon SD, DeRubeis RJ, Piasecki JM, Grove WM, Garvey MJ, Tuason VB (1992) Differential relapse following cognitive therapy and pharmacotherapy for depression. *Arch Gen Psychiatry* **49**: 802–808.

Fava G, Grandi S, Zielezny M, Rafanelli C, Canestrari R (1996) Four-year outcome for cognitive behavioral treatment of residual symptoms in major depression. *Am J Psychiatry* **42**: 945–947.

Frank E, Kupfer DJ, Cornes C, Morris S (1993) Maintenance interpersonal psychotherapy for recurrent depression. In Klerman G, Weissman M (eds) *New Applications of Interpersonal Psychotherapy*. Washington, DC: American Psychiatric Press, pp. 75–102.

Frank E, Kupfer DJ, Perel JM (1989) Early recurrence in unipolar depression. *Arch Gen Psychiatry* **46**: 397–400.

Freud S (1917) *Mourning and Melancholia.* In The standard edition of the complete psychological works of Sigmund Freud, Vol 14. Translated and edited by J. Strachey. London: Hogarth Press, 1963, pp. 237–260.

Freud S (1923) *The Ego and the Id.* In The standard edition of the complete psychological works of Sigmund Freud, Vol. 19. Translated and edited by J. Strachey. London: Hogarth Press, 1963, pp. 1–66.

Gabbard GO (2000) *Psychodynamic Psychiatry in Clinical Practice.* Washington, DC: American Psychiatric Press.

Gotlib IH, Hammen CL (1992) *Psychological Aspects of Depression: Toward a Cognitive–Interpersonal Ontegration.* Chichester, UK: John Wiley.

Greenberg RP, Bornstein RF, Greenberg MD, Fisher S (1992) As for the kings: a reply with regard to depression subtypes and antidepressant response. *J Consult Clin Psychol* **60**: 675–677.

Hammen CL (1997) Depression. In Brewin CR (ed) *Clinical Psychology: A Modular Course.* Hove: Psychology Press.

Hersen M, Bellack AS, Himmelhoch JM, Thase ME (1984) Effects of social skills training, amitriptyline, and psychotherapy in unipolar depressed women. *Beh Ther* **15**: 21–40.

Hoberman HM, Lewinsohn PM (1985) The behavioral treatment of depression. In Beckham EE, Leber WR (eds) *Handbook of Depression: Treatment, Assessment, and Research.* Homewood, IL: Dorsey Press.

Hollon SD, DeRubeis RJ, Evans MD, Wiemer MD, Garvey MJ, Grove WM, Tuason VB (1992) Cognitive therapy and pharmacotherapy for depression: single and in combination. *Arch Gen Psychiatry* **49**: 774–781.

Hollon SD, Shelton RC, Loosen PT (1991) Cognitive therapy and pharmacotherapy for depression. *J Consult Clin Psychol* **59**: 88–99.

Janicak P, Davis J, Preskorn S, Ayd F (1997) *Principles and Practice of Psychopharmacotherapy* (2nd edn). Baltimore, MD: Williams & Wilkins.

Klerman GL, Weissman MM, Rounsaville BJ, Chevron ES (1984). *Interpersonal Psychotherapy for Depression.* New York: Basic Books.

Lewinsohn PM (1975) The behavioral study and treatment of depression. In Hersen M, Eisler RM, Miller PM (eds) *Progress in Behavior Modification.* New York: Academic Press.

MacPhillamy DJ, Lewinsohn PM (1971) The pleasant events schedule. Unpublished manuscript, University of Oregon, Eugene.

Manning D, Frances A (eds) (1990) *Combined Pharmacotherapy and Psychotherapy for Depression* (Vol 26). Washington, DC: American Psychiatric Association.

McLean PD, Hakstian AR (1990) Relative endurance of unipolar depression treatment effects: longitudinal follow-up. *J Consult Clin Psychol* **58**: 482–488.

McLean PD, Taylor S (1992) Severity of unipolar depression and choice of treatment. *Beh Res Ther* **30**: 443–451.

Meehl PE (1962) Schizotaxia, schizotypy, schizophrenia. *Am Psychologist* **17**: 827–838.

Metalsky GI, Abramson LY, Seligman MEP, Semmel A, Peterson CR (1982) Attributional styles and life events in the classroom: vulnerability and invulnerability to depressive mood reactions. *J Pers Soc Psychol* **43**: 612–617.

Miller IW, Norman WH, Keitner GI, Bishop SB, Dow MG (1989) Cognitive-behavioral treatment of depressed inpatients. *Beh Ther* **20**: 25–47.

Narrow WE, Regier DA, Rae DS, Manderscheid RW, Locke BZ (1993) Use of services by persons with mental and addictive disorders: findings from the National Institute of Mental Health Epidemiological Catchment Area Program. *Arch Gen Psychiatry* **50**: 95–107.

Nietzel MT, Russell R, Hemmings K, Gretter M (1987) Clinical significance of psychotherapy for unipolar depression. A meta-analytic approach to social comparison. *J Consult Clin Psychol* **55**: 151–161.

Oliver JM, Burkham R (1982) Subliminal psychodynamic activation in depression: a failure to replicate. *J Abnorm Psychol* **92**: 337–342.

Peeters F (1999) Stemmingsstoornissen. In Smeets G, Bögels SM, van der Molen HT, Arntz A (eds) *Klinische psychologie. Diagnostiek en therapie*. Groningen: Wolters-Noordhoff.

Rehm LP (1977) A self-control therapy program for treatment of depression. In Clarkin JF, Glazer HJ (eds) *Depression. Behavioral and Directive Intervention Strategies*. New York: Garland.

Robinson LA, Berman JS, Neimeyer RA (1990) Psychotherapy for the treatment of depression: a comprehensive review of controlled outcome research. *Psych Bull* **108**, 30–49.

Rosenthal D (1963) *The Genain Quadruplets*. New York: Basic Books.

Rush AJ, Beck AT, Kovacs M, Hollon SD (1977) Comparative efficacy of cognitive therapy and pharmacotherapy in the treatment of depressed outpatients. *Cogn Ther Res* **1**: 17–37.

Rush AJ, Beck AT, Kovacs M, Weissenburger J, Hollon SD (1982) Comparison of the effects of cognitive therapy and pharmacotherapy on hopelessness and self-concept. *Am J Psychiatry* **139**: 862–866.

Rush AJ, Hollon SD, Beck AT, Kovacs M (1978) Depression: must psychotherapy fail for cognitive therapy to succeed? *Cogn Ther Res* **2**: 199–206.

Sacco WP, Beck AT (1995) Cognitive theory and therapy. In Beckham EE, Leber WL (eds) *Handbook of Depression*. New York: Guilford Press, pp. 329–351.

Seligman MEP (1974) Depression and learned helplessness. In Friedman RJ, Katz MM (eds) *The Psychology of Depression: Contemporary Theory and Research*. Washington, DC: Hemisphere.

Seligman MEP (1975) *Helplessness: On Depression, Development, and Death*. San Francisco: Freeman.

Shea MT, Elkin I, Imber SD, Sotsky SM, Watkins JT, Collins JF, Pilkonis PA, Beckham E, Glass DR, Dolan RT, Parloff MB (1992a) Course of depressive symptoms over follow-up: findings from the National Institute of Mental Health treatment of depression collaborative research program. *Arch Gen Psychiatry* **49**: 782–787.

Shea MT, Widiger TA, Klein MH (1992b) Comorbidity of personality disorders and depression: implications for treatment. *J Consult Clin Psychol* **60**: 857–868.

Silverman LH (1976) Psychoanalytic theory. The reports of my death are greatly exaggerated. *American Psychol* **31**: 621–637.

Silverman LH (1985) Comments on three recent subliminal psychodynamic activation investigations. *J Abnorm Psychol* **94**: 640–643.

Simons AD, Murphy GE, Levine JL, Wetzel RD (1986) Cognitive therapy and pharmaco-therapy for depression: sustained improvement over one year. *Arch Gen Psychiatry* **43**: 43–48.

Skinner BF (1953) *Science and Human Behavior*. New York: Macmillan.

Steinbrueck SM, Maxwell SE, Howard GS (1983) A meta-analysis of psychotherapy and drug therapy in the treatment of unipolar depression with adults. *J Consult Clin Psychol* **51**: 856–863.

Teasdale JD, Fennell MJV, Hibbert GA, Amies PL (1984) Cognitive therapy for major depressive disorder in primary care. *Br J Psychiatry* **144**: 400–406.

Thase ME, Greenhouse JB, Frank E, Reynolds CF, Pilkonis PA, Hurley K, Grochocinski V, Kupfer DJ (1997) Treatment of major depression with psychotherapy or psychotherapy–pharmacotherapy combinations. *Arch Gen Psychiatry* **54**: 1009–1015.

Van Son M, Hoevenaars J (1998) Het operante model. In Albersnagel FA, Emmelkamp PMG, van den Hoofdakker RH (eds) *Depressie. Theorie, Diagnostiek & Behandeling*. Houten: Bohn Stafleu Van Loghum.

Weissman MM, Klerman GL, Prusoff BA, Sholomskas D, Padian N (1981) Depressed outpatients. Results one year after treatment with drugs and/or interpersonal psychotherapy. *Arch Gen Psychiatry* **38**: 51–55.

Weissman MM, Markowitz JC (1994) Interpersonal psychotherapy. *Arch Gen Psychiatry* **51**: 599–606.

Weissman MM, Prusoff BA, DiMascio A, Neu C, Goklaney M, Klerman GL (1979) The efficacy of drugs and psychotherapy in the treatment of acute depressive epidodes. *Am J Psychiatry* **136**: 555–558.

12

Treatment-resistant Mood Disorders: from Diagnosis to Treatment

Daniel Souery[1], Pierre Oswald[2] and Joseph Zohar[3]

[1]University Clinics of Brussels, Brussels, Belgium
[2]Erasmus Hospital, Free University of Brussels, Brussels, Belgium
[3]Tel Aviv University, Sackler School of Medicine, Tel Aviv, Israel

INTRODUCTION

Depression remains a highly prevalent disorder, with significant personal and socioeconomic implications. Moreover, depression is still under-diagnosed and consequently undertreated. When adequately treated, up to half of all patients do not respond adequately to first-line monotherapy and 60–70% of depressed patients fail to reach complete remission, despite rapid development in the therapeutic armamentarium of mood disorders since the late 1980s. Selective serotonin reuptake inhibitors (SSRIs), reboxetine, a selective norepinephrine reuptake inhibitor (SNRI), and newer antidepressants with dual actions, both on serotonergic and noradrenergic systems, such as venlafaxine, mirtazapine and milnacipran have been proposed as a replacement to the older tricyclic antidepressants (TCAs), and although they are safer and better tolerated, they have not significantly altered the rate of improvement in depressive symptoms.

Considered in a broad sense, treatment-resistant depression (TRD) incorporates well over a third of depressed patients. However, the poor level of attention previously paid to any conceptual examination of TRD has resulted in unsystematic research and uncontrolled clinical trials, which in turn have led to a degree of confusion. An analysis of the existing publications on TRD highlights the absence of a standardized definition and operational criteria (Schatzberg et al., 1983, 1986; Ayd, 1983; Fawcett and Kravitz, 1985; Feighner, 1985; Roose et al., 1986; Links and Akiskal, 1987; McGrath et al., 1987; Fink, 1991; Montgomery, 1991; Nelson and Dunner, 1993; Thase and Rush 1995; Souery et al., 1999; Sackeim, 2001). Thus, a substantial number of definitions have been employed in clinical trials and have

Mood Disorders: Clinical Management and Research Issues. Edited by E. J. L. Griez, C. Faravelli, D. J. Nutt and J. Zohar.
©2005 John Wiley & Sons Ltd. ISBN 0 470 09426 5.

given rise to various treatment guidelines. This may explain why it remains difficult in clinical practice to treat resistant patients using any systematic algorithms.

Recently, research in this field has focused on the more fundamental aspects of TRD. These aspects include methodological considerations, predictive factors, neurochemistry, and biological markers. Methodological advances have contributed to the achievement of a reasonable level of consensus on the general concept of resistance and they allow an improved understanding of the issues of characterization and definition.

However, methodological advances have not been considered extensively in other resistant mood disorders, namely resistant bipolar disorders and 'resistant' dysthymia, where many of the conceptual definitions are currently derived from the approach used in unipolar major depression. Hence, treatment-resistant bipolar depression is largely unstudied and many of the treatment strategies for bipolar depression are based on guidelines derived from studies on unipolar TRD, which are not necessarily applicable to resistant bipolar. In various treatment phases, some patients will have a different level of resistance to a given therapeutic strategy or agent, reflecting their response or resistance to acute treatment and their post-recovery maintenance or relapse. This observation, if taken into consideration, may assist in the differentiation of acute and long-term resistance.

We will review here methodological issues in TRD and extend it to treatment-resistance on two specific psychiatric disorders, dysthymia and bipolar disorder. Current knowledge on biological factors implicated in TRD will be described as well. Finally the therapeutic aspect will be covered with a special attention to clinical management of TRD.

METHODOLOGICAL CONSIDERATIONS IN TREATMENT-RESISTANT DEPRESSION (TRD)

Before any assumption about treatment-resistance is made, different factors must be considered which may give rise to 'pseudo-resistant' depression.

Misdiagnosis of Depression and Subtypes of Depression

Misdiagnosis leads to treatment of patients considered as resistant when, in fact, they are suffering from a primary psychiatric disorder other than depression.

The major subtypes of affective disorder respond in different ways to the available therapies and the failure to recognize these subtypes is one of the most common factors contributing to non-response. Important differential diagnoses that may influence the treatment response in TRD are the primary–secondary classifications, melancholic depression, psychotic depression, atypical depression, and bipolar depression. Guscott and Grof (1991) conducted a comprehensive review of the over-diagnosis of primary affective disorders in patients who were defined as having resistant depression. Evidence exists that the misdiagnosis of primary non-affective disorders accounts for a substantial proportion of patients classified as having resistant depressive disorders (Levine, 1986; MacEwan and Remick, 1988; Nelsen and Dunner, 1995). Careful attention should be paid both to the identification and appropriate treatment of primary non-affective disorders. In these conditions, the pharmacological treatment of secondary depression can differ from that of primary depression in terms of dosage, duration, and onset of response. Melancholic depression, characterized by an absence of mood reactivity, severe neurovegetative symptoms and psychomotor retardation, appears to show a greater degree of response to tricyclic antidepressants (TCAs) and electroconvulsive therapy (ECT) (Nelson et al., 1990) than to other antidepressant therapies. In atypical depression, which is characterized by mood reactivity, hypersomnia, hyperphagia, and increased sensitivity to environmental events and rejection, evidence supports the use of specific treatment choices. Adequate treatment of atypical depression should include a trial of a monoamine oxidase inhibitor (MAOI) (Liebowitz et al., 1988; Zisook et al., 1985; Quitkin et al., 1991; Benazzi, 2002). In bipolar depression, the treatment of choice depends on whether psychotic symptoms are present and on the severity of depression. The first line of treatment in cases of severe psychotic bipolar depression remains ECT or a mood stabilizer, combined with an antidepressant and an antipsychotic. The use of antidepressants alone in less severe bipolar depressive episodes is not recommended (Thase and Kupfer, 1996). Specific forms of treatment that relate to affective disorder subtypes are reviewed elsewhere in more detail (Amsterdam and Hornig-Rohan, 1996).

Psychiatric Comorbidity

Comorbid psychiatric disorders that are often seen with mood disorders include substance abuse or dependence, personality disorders, eating disorders, obsessive–compulsive disorders, and panic or generalized anxiety disorders (Hirschfeld et al., 1988; Maser and Cloninger, 1990; Corruble et al., 1996). In treatment failure, a thorough evaluation of these conditions should always be considered. Comorbidity entails the treatment of complex syndromes of which depression forms only a part. It has been observed that in depression, concomitant personality disorders, widely ranging from 20% to 80% among depressed patients, reduce the efficacy of antidepressant treatments and may contribute towards treatment-resistance (Pfohl et al., 1984; Black et al., 1988; Shea et al., 1990, 1992; Nelson et al., 1994). It is not clear, therefore, whether the observed 'treatment-resistance' relates to the depressive state or to the comorbid personality disorder (Thase, 1996). The complexity of the subject is illustrated by the extremely heterogeneous nature of the diagnosis in some published reports, involving patients whose diagnostic characteristics include a wide range of personality disorders. Moreover, the relationship between personality disorder and depression is likely to be complex. So far, hypotheses have implicated a direct predisposition to depression in patients with pathological personality, a modification of depressive symptoms when suffering from personality disorder or, on the other hand, the fact that a long-term unremitted depression may have an enduring impact on personality. Some authors have also put forward that personality disorder could constitute an attenuated form of depression (Shea and Hirschfeld, 1996; Thase, 1996). In patients with comorbid psychiatric condition, some psychotherapeutic interventions may be beneficial. For example, a combination of psychotherapy and somatic treatment should be considered in resistant patients with concomitant personality disorders.

Concurrent Medical Condition

A variety of concurrent medical conditions may also contribute to TRD. Depressed patients with comorbid medical disorders tend to have worse depression outcomes than depressed patients without comorbid medical illness (Koike et al., 2002). Among them, thyroid dysfunction seem to be the most supported in the literature (Gold et al., 1981; Hatterer and Gorman, 1990; Howland, 1993). After the classic paper by Asher (1949) on 'myxedematous madness', hypothyroidism has been clearly described to be associated with depression. Overall, 7% to 10% of depressed patients appear to have subclinical hypothyroidism as defined by an elevated basal TSH or an augmented TSH response to TRH (Reus, 1993). The association between depression and hyperthyroidism is less clear. Kathol et al. (1986) rather describe features of generalized anxiety disorder in these patients.

Other medical conditions have been implicated as organic causes of depression and require documentation and exclusion in TRD (Levine, 1986; Gruber et al., 1996). These conditions should be labelled as mood disorder due to a general medical condition according to the DSM-IV (APA, 1994). Examples of such conditions are Cushing's syndrome, Parkinson's disease, neurological neoplasms, pancreatic carcinoma, connective-tissue disorders, vitamin deficiencies and certain viral infections. Several types of medication also, such as immunosuppressants, steroids and sedatives, may precipitate or contribute to chronic depression and adversely affect remission and response. Hence it is essential to elicit a thorough medical history when evaluating treatment-resistance. Although some patients with major depression induced by a medical condition may respond to antidepressant treatment (Primeau, 1988), diagnosis of secondary depression is associated with a major factor of chronicity despite adequate treatments (Keller, 1984; Dinan and Mobayed, 1992).

Poor Compliance

Between 30% and 60% of patients do not take their medication as prescribed (Cramer, 1995; Demyttenaere, 1997). Reasons for this include the occurrence of adverse effects, guilt feeling about taking medication, treatment discontinuation once symptoms begin to improve, fear of drug dependency or loss in effectiveness and social stigma (Mendlewicz, 2001).

Treatment Inadequacy

Treatment adequacy in terms of dose, duration and compliance remains one of the key issues in dealing with resistant patients. In terms of criteria for adequate dose and duration of treatment, only about 25% of patients in clinical practice are adequately treated when they are prescribed antidepressants (Katon et al., 1992; Lepine et al., 1997), even with SSRIs (Dunn et al., 1998). Furthermore, a significant proportion of cases referred to university settings for 'refractory depression' have not received even a single adequate antidepressant trial (Bridges, 1983). A systematic review of the adequacy of previous courses of treatment is required prior to any decision on the management of resistant cases. Clinical trials on antidepressant efficacy in major depression suggest response rates reaching 80% (Anderson and Tomenson, 1994) but this promise is largely not realized in clinical practice, owing to the complex interaction between patients and health care provider resulting in inadequate treatment of depression (Mendlewicz, 2001).

For major depressive disorders, specific recommendations on antidepressant dosage and the duration of treatment should be based on literature data and practice guidelines (Phillips and Nierenberg, 1994; Amsterdam and Hornig-Rohan, 1996). In the course of time, the recommendation of adequate dosage has increased from 150 mg/ day to 250–300 mg/day of imipramine or its equivalent (Ayd, 1983; Nierenberg et al., 1991). Imipramine, desipramine, and nortriptyline should be monitored using plasma levels, which have been demonstrated to relate accurately to clinical outcome (Roose and Glassman, 1994). Moreover, blood levels should be measured because a significant proportion of the general population are slow metabolizers of nortryptiline. For other antidepressants, plasma levels can be used to assess a patient's compliance with treatment. When appropriate, plasma levels should also be used for patients who do not respond to adequate doses of antidepressants, so that possible individual variations in pharmacokinetic characteristics can be documented. In such patients, dosage adjustments, based on blood levels, may produce a treatment-response (Amsterdam et al., 1980; Glassman, 1994).

The maximum tolerated dose should be used, according to dosage recommendations. Before treatment-resistance is considered, the recommended daily doses of standard treatment that should be attained are 300 mg of imipramine, 90 mg of phenelzine or the equivalent therapeutic regimens with at least four weeks of treatment at the optimal dose (verified by blood level where appropriate). For some antidepressants, the need to reach maximal doses to consider non-response is less clear. For instance, no greater subsequent response was observed when increasing dose from 20 mg to 60 mg of fluoxetine after non-response to three weeks of treatment as compared to maintenance on the original 20 mg (Schweiser et al., 1990). On the other hand, patients who had failed to respond to eight weeks of treatment with 20 mg of fluoxetine were analysed in a double-blind randomized study (Fava et al., 1994). Patients treated with high doses of fluoxetine (40–60 mg) responded significantly better than patients treated with fluoxetine plus lithium and those treated with fluoxetine plus desipramine.

The adequate duration of an antidepressant trial has also evolved over the years from three to six weeks (Quitkin, 1984). Some studies have suggested that prolonged trials of treatment, lasting more than 10 or 12 weeks (Greenhouse et al., 1987; Georgotas et al., 1989), can lead to a therapeutic response in certain resistant patients. However, there is a lack of evidence to support the advantage of prolonged trials over eight weeks as compared to switching strategies. In current reports on TRD, the absence of a standardized pattern for dosage and duration of treatment is more a question of the study design and selection criteria than a conceptual inconsistency. More detailed analyses of this issue have been published showing that the point at which treatment alteration should be considered in light of the degree of improvement in previous weeks (Quitkin et al., 1996).

The efficacy of pharmacotherapy in mood disorders may vary according to the treatment phase (see Figure 12.1). Treatment is generally divided into acute, continuation and maintenance phases (Thase and Kupfer, 1996).

Not only should resistance to the acute treatment phase be examined, but also to the continuation and maintenance phases of therapy. Some patients, who respond to the acute phase of pharmacotherapy, may be resistant to long-term treatment with high rates of recurrence, exhibiting 'continuation' or 'maintenance resistance'. As in the acute treatment phase, treatment adequacy should also be considered in the long-term treatment of depression. Recommendations on dosages and the duration of treatment are essential for a successful outcome in the continuation and maintenance phases. In particular, compliance should be assessed in maintenance resistance, since many patients reduce or end their treatment following remission of their symptoms.

The criteria most widely applied for defining 'responders' and 'non-responders' are based on standardized rating scales, which are used to assess the severity of depression. In clinical trials, the criteria classically used to indicate response to treatment are the following: a minimum rating of 'much improved' on the Clinical Global Impression (CGI) scale; a minimum reduction of 50% on the Hamilton Depression Rating Scale (HAM-D); a score of 9 or less on the Beck Depression Inventory scale and a score of 15 on the Montgomery–Asberg Depression Rating Scale (MADRS). Remission is also frequently defined as a score of 7 or less on the HAM-D. The process of defining these criteria in TRD is a complex one, due to the marked variability in the severity and morbidity of resistant depression as well as to

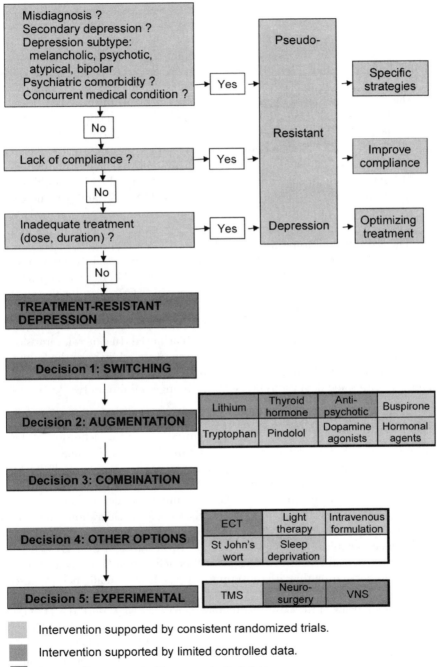

Figure 12.1 Decision tree.

variations in the therapeutic objectives. It is more likely that resistance to treatment will occur along a continuum, which could complicate the use of pre-specified thresholds, particularly in very severe pretreatment major depression. In such cases, even with a 50% reduction in symptoms, significant residual symptoms may remain. It is important also to define therapeutic objectives according to the patient's quality of life and in the context of subjective evaluation by the patient and other family members. A moderate improvement, as measured on a given rating scale for depressive symptoms, can be sufficient to give a noticeable improvement in the quality of life of some depressive patients. A moderate improvement in long-term and chronic resistant depression, as recorded on scales such as the CGI, HAM-D or MADRS, should be associated with an improved quality of life evaluation. The general rule in epidemiological studies and clinical trials, should be the joint use of thresholds (e.g. a score of 6 or less on the HAM-D) and percentages of improvement (e.g. a minimum 50% reduction in the baseline scores on the HAM-D). In addition to this, improvement should be assessed on more than one rating scale. The advantage of using the HAM-D is that it covers the whole spectrum of depressive symptoms, while the MADRS and CGI are more sensitive to improvement, measuring change (Galinowski and Lehert, 1995). No appropriate instrument exists to examine specific symptoms in relation to the therapeutic response or to non-response. Discovering a solution to this last issue should be a major objective in TRD research. Finally, the minimum length of response required before remission can be considered to have been achieved. In general, remission is defined as a response of at least two weeks' duration. In addition to the failure to respond to treatment, the duration of the episode without response has also been examined, with some definitions of TRD specifying a minimum two-year period for this (Feighner et al., 1985).

In the literature on TRD, a controversial subject is the number and type of adequate antidepressant treatment trials required before the definition of TRD can be considered. The classification of resistant depression in stages has been proposed, based on the previous treatment response (Schatzberg et al., 1986; Nierenberg et al., 1991; Thase and Rush, 1995), where increasing resistance is equated with an increased failure to respond to the less common antidepressant treatments, such as augmentation strategies or ECT. For theoretical considerations, all of these definitions may be acceptable but do not provide an operational tool that can be easily applied to clinical practice and research. For instance, if ECT is essential to be eligible for resistance status, clinicians will be left with a large segment of the affectively ill population that are resistant to several drugs and augmentation strategies yet cannot be characterized. Another controversial issue is the requirement for consecutive trials of the same or different classes of drugs. With the TCAs, the benefits of switching treatment from one of the group members to another has not been supported by the available data (Charney et al., 1986; Reimherr et al., 1984). Conversely, there is emerging evidence that some patients, who do not respond to a selective serotonin reuptake inhibitor (SSRI) may respond to a second trial with a different SSRI or to a trial with a TCA (Brown and Harrison, 1992; Zarate et al.,

1996; Joffe et al., 1996; Thase and Rush, 1997). Although more controlled data are needed to document the effectiveness of TCAs in SSRI resistance, some studies suggest that this strategy is effective (Peselow et al., 1989). SSRI response in TCA resistant outpatients has been documented in several studies with response rates of between 30% and 70% (Delgado et al., 1988; Faravelli et al., 1988; Nolen et al., 1998; White et al., 1990; Gagiano et al., 1993).

TREATMENT RESISTANCE IN DYSTHYMIC DISORDER

Previously known as 'depressive neurosis', dysthymic disorder affects 3% to 6% (Kessler et al., 1994) of the general population. One-quarter of patients with depression are thought to have dysthymia, a condition called 'double depression' in which dysthymia is considered as a comorbid disorder upon which depression is surimposed (Sanderson et al., 1990). Moreover 40% of dysthymic patients have been found to have a double depression (Keller and Shapiro, 1985; Weissman et al., 1988). Patients with double depression pursue a highly recurrent course (Akiskal, 1994). Being viewed as a chronic and characterologic form of mood disorder, dysthymia is still a condition undertreated (Keller, 1993; Shelton et al., 1997). On the other hand, there are several double-blind, placebo-controlled randomized studies showing the efficacy of antidepressants in dysthymic and 'neurotic' depression (Alpert and Lagomisano, 2001, for review). Even in double depression, most antidepressants have shown a good response. Interestingly, Kocsis et al. (1996) have demonstrated a similar response to an initial open-label treatment with desipramine during a randomized, double-blind maintenance phase of up to two years in three groups of dysthymics, double depressives and chronic major depressives. Thus, if naturalistic studies tent to suggest that dysthymia implies a poorer diagnosis, clinical trials show evidence for similar response between dysthymia, double depression and depression alone.

If dysthymia is 'treatable' in a significant proportion of patients, the issue of therapy-resistance should also be considered in this disorder. For example, most recent studies have identified risk factors to develop a poorer response to antidepressant treatment in dysthymia: lower-levels of education, high neuroticism, more severe medical illness and being an older female (Katon et al., 2002).

However, several methodological problems are encountered when studying this condition. First, until now no clear definition of remission in dysthymia has been stated. Indeed, using criteria of 50% reduction in total HAM-D score or a HAM-D score of less than 8, patients are still dysthymic (Thase et al., 1996). Some studies suggest that minor depressive symptoms tend to remain in dysthymia when compared to major depression (Keller et al., 1983). Dysthymia is a chronic disorder, often present for many years. It is thus possible that the delay of onset of action of antidepressant is longer than for treating unipolar affective disorder. As prospective data on the evolution of response of patients during the course of antidepressant treatment are lacking, it is not possible to speculate on the 'adequate duration' of an antidepressant treatment in this condition. There are also little data on long-term treatment and on response to switching and augmentation strategies on dysthymic disorder. Harrison et al. (1986) observed in a randomized, placebo-controlled, continuation study that antidepressant treatment should be maintained for at least six months.

TREATMENT-RESISTANCE IN BIPOLAR DISORDER

The concept of resistance to the treatment is particularly complex in bipolar disorders, this by reason of the many clinical situations that are to be managed in the short and long term.

The natural course of bipolar disorder is characterized by marked severity of acute affective episodes, followed by high rates of relapse and recurrence. Thus, the primary goals of treatment in bipolar disorder are to treat both acute phases of the illness as well as to prevent recurrence. Treatment may be required for acute mania, for acute depression, or to prevent recurrence of such states. Treatment phases remain a function of the subtype of bipolar disorder considered, such as rapid cycling or mixed states. In order to prevent recurrence, long-term or lifetime prophylactic strategies may be necessary. Lithium has been considered to be the effective reference prophylactic treatment, but newer medications offer promising advantages in the acute and long-term management of this disorder.

While consensus definitions have been well established for treatment phases in unipolar recurrent depression (Frank et al., 1991), such advances are still lacking for bipolar disorder. This is mainly due to the polarity of the disorder, and the diversity of clinical presentations in either depressed or manic states. However, extrapolation of unipolar treatment phase criteria can be made, yet adjustment is required to take into account the particular aspects of bipolar disorder. A breakdown of different phases of treatment can be made accordingly: acute, continuation and maintenance (Thase and Kupfer, 1996). The acute phase of bipolar disorder consists of the treatment duration of classic euphoric mania, mixed episodes, hypomania, rapid cycling, and depression. The duration of acute treatment may vary between two and six weeks. The continuation phase consists of the initial period lasting approximately two to six months after the acute symptoms have remitted, the goal being relapse prevention. During the maintenance phase that follows continuation, the aim is to prevent the occurrence of any new episodes by prophylactic treatment with a mood stabilizer. Thus lifelong, long-term treatment may be necessary for a significant proportion of patients.

The clinical heterogeneity of bipolar disorder makes it difficult to generalize about treatment strategies. The bipolar disorder spectrum includes bipolar I and bipolar II disorders, and cyclothymic disorder, as enumerated by DSM-IV. A patient with bipolar I may present with only a single manic episode, or a combination of manic and depressive episodes where the most recent episode is either manic, hypomanic, mixed, or depressed. Patients with bipolar II may present with either hypomanic or depressive episodes. The clinician is faced with a heterogeneous group of patients who represent the spectrum of bipolar disorder, yet exhibit different features and degrees of severity of the illness. Moreover, these patients may be seen at different moments in their illness, presenting with different acute episodes that require different treatment strategies. Even among a group of patients receiving the diagnosis of bipolar I, there are a variety of clinically relevant features that may predict treatment choice, its outcome and the overall course of the illness. Such clinical features include psychosis, catatonia, a seasonal pattern, or rapid cycling, for example. Other episode specifiers include melancholic features, atypical features, post-partum onset and length on episode. These clinical manifestations may imply different treatment modalities.

Working clinical definitions for treatment refractory bipolar illness have been suggested (Sachs, 1996). These definitions are proposed as a starting point and need validation through controlled studies, as well as for TRD criteria. Treatment-refractory bipolar depression is defined by the lack of remission of a depressive state despite two adequate trials of standard antidepressant agents (six weeks each), with or without augmentation strategies. This last definition suffers the same limitations as the definition proposed for TRD. Moreover, adequate antidepressant trial for bipolar depression is not well defined, in particular for the use of mood stabilizers.

Treatment-refractory mania is defined as a manic episode without remission despite six weeks of adequate therapy with at least two antimanic agents (lithium, neuroleptic, anticonvulsant) in the absence of antidepressant or other mood-elevating agents. The Young Mania Rating Scale (YMRS) is widely used in clinical trials to evaluate treatment response. A total score of 12.5 on the YMRS has been described as reflecting the median euthymic rating, 15 as the lower limits of mania, 20 as mania of moderate severity and 25 as the lower limit of mania of sufficient severity to require hospitalization. Treatment-refractory mood cycling may be defined as continued cycling despite maximal tolerated lithium in combination with valproate or carbamazepine for a period of three times the average cycle length, or six months, whichever is longer, in the absence of antidepressants or other cycle-promoting agents. The definitions of treatment-refractory mania and mood cycling should also be examined regarding all methodological considerations discussed above for TRD. Lastly, resistance to long-term treatment or 'maintenance resistance' can be of particular relevance in bipolar affective disorder.

The growing number of therapeutic strategies available in bipolar disorders results in an increase in the chances of response to the treatment in the various phases of the disease. Beyond the traditional treatments like lithium, the antiepileptics and the typical neuroleptics, the new antiepileptics and atypical antipsychotics must be considered in particular clinical situation.

The treatment of choice for classic, euphoric mania is lithium, while valproate is preferred for a mixed episode, mania with dysphoric mood or for mania in rapid cycling bipolar disorder. For rapid stabilization of severe mania, valproate is recommended because therapeutic blood levels can be attained quickly through a loading dose strategy of 20 mg/kg per day. Valproate may also be used to treat classic mania if it is preferred because of its side-effect profile or a previous non-response to lithium. Similarly, carbamazepine may be effective for mixed episodes or for rapid cycling as opposed to valproate if it is preferred due to its side-effect profile or the patient's previous treatment history. Combinations of antimanic agents may also be necessary, particularly in treatment-resistant manic, mixed and hypomanic episodes.

New molecules, and in particular lamotrigine, have been tested in bipolar disorder. The effectiveness of lamotrigine is now established in the depressive phases and in maintenance and this in placebo-controlled studies among bipolar patients I and II, with or without fast cycles. Calabrese et al. showed an antidepressant effectiveness compared with placebo among depressive bipolar patients. This molecule is particularly tempting because of its good long-term tolerance. Nevertheless, one described cutaneous rashes at the beginning of treatment, with increased risk of Stevens–Johnson syndrome. To avoid this adverse effect, a diagram of progressive administration is recommended, to be adapted according to the pre-existing treatment. Indeed, valproate inhibits the metabolism of lamotrigine, while carbamazepine accelerates it. Moreover, lamotrigine does not seem to induce manic or hypomanic states nor to increase the frequency of the cycles. On the other hand, studies in bipolar disorders could not confirm antimanic effectiveness. The recent data obtained with lamotrigine suggest that this is a treatment of choice in bipolar patients for whom the burden of the disease is mainly explained by their depressive episodes or symptomatology. It may also become a first-line treatment for acute bipolar depression. Lamotrigine was superior to placebo in a seven-week blinded, randomized trial on most analyses, although the Hamilton Rating Scale for Depression, which was the primary rating instrument, did not indicate a significant difference from placebo (Calabrese et al., 1999). Lamotrigine has been studied in three placebo-controlled maintenance trials in bipolar disorder. In rapid cycling patients, among bipolar II patients, lamotrigine was significantly superior to placebo in delaying time to intervention, with most benefit seen for delay in intervention for emerging depression. Lamotrigine was not significantly different from placebo among bipolar I patients (Calabrese et al., 2000). The study suggests that the prophylactic effect of lamotrigine is seen when depression, not mania, is the primary illness characteristic. Lamotrigine was studied in two 18-month trials, one of which enrolled currently or recently manic patients, the other, recently depressed patients. In both studies, lamotrigine as monotherapy, but not lithium, delayed time to intervention for depression. Lamotrigine also reduced average depressive symptomatology in comparison with placebo (Bowden et al., 2000; Calabrese et al., 2003). Among over 1000 patients studied in blinded, randomized, placebo-controlled trials, there was no evidence that lamotrigine destabilized mood, or precipitated mania or hypomania. If confirmed, those data may offer new therapeutic strategies in resistant bipolar disorders. In the acute phase in treating depressive episodes and in 'maintenance resistance', preventing depressive phases when the burden of the disease is explained by the high rate of depressive recurrences.

Just like the traditional neuroleptics, the atypical antipsychotics (AAP) are effective in the control of agitation and the psychotic symptoms associated with the manic state. More recent studies highlighted the fact that the AAP would have a specific antimanic effect independent of the antipsychotic action. This observation explains why the main target of clinical trials with atypical antipsychotics used to be pure mania. Data are available in this direction for olanzapine, risperidone, ziprasidone, quetiapine and clozapine. Olanzapine has been recognized by the Food and Drug Administration (FDA) for the indication 'acute mania' on the basis of a randomized, placebo-controlled study which shows an acute effectiveness within three to four weeks among manic or mixed bipolar patients. Other studies show the effectiveness of olanzapine in combination with lithium or valproate among patients not responding to these treatments. A controlled study shows the comparable effectiveness of risperidone (6 mg) compared to haloperidol (10 mg) and lithium (900–1200 mg) in mania. For risperidone, the majority of the studies relates to the effectiveness in combination with conventional mood stabilizers (add one therapy). Although it may be less relevant for registration purposes, as far as clinical needs are concerned it is of importance that most atypical antipsychotics have also been tested in combination treatments. Finally, first data are now available on the long-term prophylactic efficacy of atypical antipsychotics. These combined efficacy data definitely support the use of atypical antipsychotics in bipolar disorder, and offer new possibilities in bipolar resistant patients.

BIOLOGICAL FACTORS OF TRD

During the last decades, a large amount of data have permitted substantial advances in the understanding of psychiatric disorders and specifically in the field of affective disorders. Unfortunately, substantial studies are lacking in TRD. But emerging methods, such as pharmacogenomics and brain imaging, will help to improve knowledge and management of TRD. We will include in this section well-studied data in neuroendocrinology and psychoimmunology and will review studies implicating serotonin in TRD. Finally, an update in the field of pharmacogenetics will be presented.

Endocrine Aspects in Resistant Depression

Hypothalamic–Pituitary–Adrenal (HPA) Axis

The HPA axis seems to be the most common biological abnormality in major depression (Amsterdam et al., 1989). The HPA axis was also suggested to be involved in the maintenance of depression, in a longer duration of the actual depressive episode and in the pathogenesis of TRD. Amsterdam et al. (1994) have demonstrated that patients who have failed several treatment trials are more likely to demonstrate enhanced HPA axis activity compared with patients with non-resistant depression. Nevertheless, the pathophysiologic significance remains unclear. For example, hypercortisolaemia, assessed basally or after dexamethasone suppression test, has not been found to be associated with acute antidepressant response (APA Task Force on Laboratory Tests in Psychiatry, 1987). More largely, corticosteroids affect brain and have influence on mood and behaviour (Wolkowitz, 1992). Moreover, corticosteroids could affect several brain systems such as the serotonin pathway, even though the interactions are complex (Van Praag, 1996), and could also work as regulators of transcription of specific genes (Holsboer, 1989). Regarding treatment, it has been hypothesized that medication that decreases the HPA axis system activity could act as an antidepressant. Cushing's syndrome, a condition associated with a high incidence of fatigue, irritability and decreased cognitive ability and libido, showed a improvement in depression scales, even complete remission, when treated with medication aiming at lower cortisol levels (Reus et al., 1997; Kiraly et al., 1997). In major depression, results are promising but only on small sample sizes (Reus and Wolkowitz, 2001). Ketoconazole, which is the most studied antiglucocorticoid, has shown moderate to high response rates (Wolkowitz et al., 1993; Amsterdam et al., 1994; Thakore and Dinan, 1995; Wolkowitz et al., 1999a).

Dehydroepiandrosterone (DHEA) is the most important adrenal corticosteroid and has focused attention since a synthesis *de novo* has been demonstrated in the brain, since DHEA has been shown to have intrinsic activity at brain $GABA_A$ and other receptors (Wolkowitz et al., 2000) and since elevation of the cortisol-DHEA ratio in drug-free depressed patients has been recently shown (Young et al., 2002). Recent double-blind, placebo-controlled trials of DHEA in major depression and dysthymia showed an improvement of depressive symptoms (Wolkowitz et al., 1999b; Bloch et al., 1999) but further, larger studies are needed to clearly demonstrate an positive effect of DHEA in depression and TRD. DHEA could probably also be effective in the management of depressive and anxiety symptoms in other disorders, such as schizophrenia (Strous et al., 2003).

Thyroid

Even hypothyroidism seems to be more frequent in depressed patients than in the non-affected (see above); only a few case series have suggested that thyroid dysfunction could be a predictor of treatment-response (Joffe, 1999). Gewirtz et al. (1988) found a comorbid thyroid disorder in approximately 40% of TRD patients studied. Joffe and Levitt (1992) showed a response rate of 16% in patients with subclinical hypothyroidism as opposed to 54% in the sample of patients with normal basal TSH level. In clinical practice, thyroid hormones have been widely used as a potentiator of antidepressant treatment in TRD. Several studies have proved the efficacy of triiodothyronine (T_3) 25 to 50 µg a day in such a cases (review in Wolkowitz and Reus, 2001). At a molecular level, links between thyroid function and neurotransmitters implicated in antidepressant response remains unclear. Further studies are thus needed to explore these interactions.

Oestrogen

Several authors have suggested an implication of oestrogen in TRD since extracts of animal ovarian tissue were administered to oophorectomized women at the end of the nineteenth century to alleviate psychological symptoms thought to be related to the removal of the ovaries (Stoppe and Doren, 2002). Several arguments tend to show an interaction between oestrogen and several neurotransmitters. McEwen et al. (1995) suggested that serotonergic, cholinergic, dopaminergic, GABAergic, adrenergic and opioid systems could respond to oestrogen. Gonzales and Carrillo (1993) showed a positive correlation between estradiol levels and whole blood serotonin levels. Oestrogen is also thought to influence the production of tryptophan hydroxylase, the rate-limiting enzyme in the synthesis of serotonin, in female rhesus monkeys (Pecins-Thomson et al., 1996). Finally, several studies have demonstrated the involvement of oestrogen on serotonin receptors in rat brain (for review see Sherwin, 2001).

Most clinical trials showed a modest effect on symptoms of depression. A 'tonic' effect on well-being in non-depressed or mildly depressed women should not be regarded as true antidepressant effect (Stoppe and Doren, 2002). So far, oestrogen could thus be regarded as a potentiator of the effects of an antidepressant drug (Sherwin, 2001). Concerning TRD, large studies investigating the efficacy of oestrogen as an adjunct to antidepressant treatment are lacking. Prange et al. (1976) showed a faster response (although non-significant) of the combination of 150 mg imipramine and 50 µg ethinyl estradiol when compared to a combination of 150 mg imipramine and placebo. Zohar et al. (1985) failed to demonstrate a beneficial effect of oestrogen in combination with imipramine in female TRD patients when compared to the combination of imipramine and placebo, although a few patients had a remarkable response.

Inflammatory Response System and TRD

The status of the immune system in depression has been studied since the 1980s. Results suggest that antidepressants of several classes decrease the production of pro-inflammatory cytokines such as interferon-gamma and tumour necrosis factor-alpha, and increase that of interleukin-10, an anti-inflammatory cytokine. Studies with animal models and cytokine immune therapy in humans suggest that pro-inflammatory cytokines induce depressive symptomatology. Moreover, these depressive symptoms can be effectively reversed by antidepressant treatment (Kenis and Maes, 2002). Sluzewska et al. (1996a) studied acute phase proteins (APP) in depressive patients. They showed that 75% of patients within this sample showed elevated levels of APPs. Moreover, patients considered as stage 2 or 3 resistant (see above) showed a specific glycosylation pattern of α-1-acid glycoprotein (AGP) and α-1-chimotrypsine (ACT), linked to the longest illness and episode duration. The same group also found a positive correlation between morning cortisol levels and concentration of interleukin-6, AGP and ACT in TRD patients (Sluzewska, 1996b). On a clinical aspect, lithium augmentation in TRD patients has been found to modulate and to 'normalize' APP levels, according to response/non-response in TRD (Sluzewska, 1994). This phenomenon might be related to elevation of glucocorticoids in TRD, suggesting that some TRD patients with an immune disturbance could take advantage of a treatment that modulates glucocorticoid levels (Amsterdam et al., 1994; Sluzewska et al., 2001).

Serotonin and TRD

Serotonin (5-HT) has been studied for decades in depression. Several lines of evidence have established that 5-HT plays a key role in the occurrence and the management of depression (Maes and Meltzer, 1995). In TRD, possible causes have been identified that could explain the lack of response when prescribing a anti-depressant (for review see Meltzer et al., 1994). Tryptophan (TRP), the precursor of 5-HT, determines in part the synthesis of central 5-HT (Fernstrom et al., 1973). Even TRP alone is not sufficient in depression and TRD, studies have reported TRP to augment the antidepressant effect of MAOIs (Pare, 1963). A limited availability or an excessive clearance of plasma TRP could therefore explain a insufficient response to antidepressants. On the other side, different attempts to study the serotonergic system in patients, e.g. platelet measures such as 5-HT uptake and uptake sites, hormone or temperature responses to TRP or cerebrospinal fluid (CSF) 5-hydroxyindolacetic acid (5-HIAA) level, the major serotonin metabolite, have been proposed in order to examine possible serotonergic predictors of response or non-response but no consistent pattern has emerged (Meltzer et al., 1994). For example, a classic work from Van Praag et al. (1978) demonstrated that depressed patients with low CSF 5-HIAA respond better than patients with normal CSF 5-HIAA to treatment to 5-hydroxytryptophan. We can therefore conclude that, even

though the serotonergic system plays a major role in depression, no clear serotonergic exist so far that could predict response to treatment.

Pharmacogenetics

Besides environmental factors, family, twin, adoption and segregation studies have
evidenced the genetic implication in mood disorders and major depression
(Mendlewicz, 1994). Nevertheless, it becomes more and more obvious that the
pattern of inheritance is complex, involving genetic and environmental interactions. Hundreds of linkage and case–control association studies have been
conducted since the late 1970s in the field of genetics of affective disorders (Souery
et al., 2001). Pharmacogenetics is the study of genetically determined, interindividual differences in therapeutic response to drugs and susceptibility to adverse
effects (Lerer, 2002). For a few years, pharmacogenetics has focused interest since it
has been substantially supported in the literature that genetic factors play a role in
response to antidepressants (Lerer and Macciardi, 2002).

Most recent studies studied mainly genes implicated in serotonergic pathway (for
exhaustive review see Lerer and Macciardi, 2002). From the initial observation of
Smeraldi et al. (1998) who determined that the serotonin transporter (5-HTT)
linked polymorphic region (5-HTTLPR) was associated with response to fluvoxamine, several studies have confirmed the implication of 5-HTTLPR in
treatment-response. Other genes related to the serotonergic pathway, such as the
tryptophan hydroxylase (rate-limiting enzyme in the 5-HT biosynthesis) gene and
the 5-HT$_{2A}$ receptor gene, have been studied in case–control association studies but
replication studies are needed to confirm their implication in treatment response
(Serretti et al., 2001a, 2001b; Cusin et al., 2002).

A insertion-deletion (I/D) polymorphism has been identified within the angiotensin converting enzyme (ACE) gene. At a central level, the primary function of
ACE is the degradation of neuropeptides including substance P (SP), thought to be
associated with depression since an SP antagonist (MK-869) has been shown to
have a similar antidepressant profile to that of paroxetine in unipolar depressed
patients (Kramer et al., 1998). Baghai et al. (2001) have shown that the D-allele
carriers had better response to treatment and shorter duration of hospitalization.

Pharmacogenetics is currently a growing field. Despite methodological and
statistical issues (not discussed here), new tools and technologies in pharmacogenetics will help us in the search for genetic predictive factors in antidepressant
response.

TREATMENT STRATEGIES IN TRD

Treatment of resistant depression should entail a comprehensive treatment algorithm whereby treatment is optimized and comorbid conditions are identified

(O'Reardon and Amsterdam, 2001). In this context, TRD can be defined as failure to respond to two adequate trials of different classes of antidepressants (i.e. consecutive treatments with two different antidepressants, each given separately in an adequate dosage for a period of at least six to eight weeks). Evidence is available for TRD management in augmentation, switching and combination strategies. Other options are also considered.

Augmentation Strategies

In the augmentation strategy, the clinician seeks a synergistic interaction between different therapeutic agents. The most used augmentation agent is lithium since several studies have shown that the addition of 600 mg/day or more leads to better chances of response in TRD patients, with response rates of up to 50% (de Montigny et al., 1983; Heninger et al., 1983; Schopf et al., 1989; Stein and Bernadt, 1993). A lithium level of at least 0.6 mmol/l should be reached (O'Reardon and Amsterdam, 2001). However, side effects may limit its use in clinical practice. Another augmentation strategy that has focused attention is addition of thyroid hormones with a response range of 25% to 60% when associated with TCA in several randomized, double-blind, placebo-controlled studies (Goodwin et al., 1982; Joffe et al., 1993). Buspirone, dopaminergic drugs, psychostimulants, modafinil, atypical antipsychotics such as risperidone and olanzapine, anticonvulsants, inositol, opiates, oestrogen and DHEA have been proposed in augmentation management of TRD, but no definitive data are available on their efficacy. Finally, two open studies have suggested a possible use for pindolol augmentation in TRD (Artigas et al., 1994; Blier and Bergeron, 1995) but controlled studies have failed to confirm an advantage over placebo in this group of patients with pindolol augmentation (Moreno et al., 1997; Perez et al., 1999).

Switching Strategies

Switching between drugs is often simpler with less risk of drug–drug interaction. The question remains if one should switch within a class (i.e. from a failed SSRI treatment to a second SSRI) or out of the class to another antidepressant (i.e. from SSRIs to MAOIs, or from SSRIs to SNRIs). A number of studies support the value of switching from one SSRI to a different SSRI. Other strategies, for example, switching from a serotonergic to a noradrenergic agent, seem reasonable as they are related to the concepts of 'serotonergic' versus 'adrenergic' depression – that is to say, should some depressed patients who are not responding to serotonergic medication be switched to adrenergic medications and vice versa. As this hypothesis is not yet resolved, it deserves further research (Marengell, 2001).

Combination Strategies

Combination strategies are those involving the concomitant use of two agents with well-established antidepressant efficacy. The typical rationale is that of broadening the action on the central nervous system by combining agents affecting different neurotransmitter systems. For example, the combination of mirtazapine and SSRIs has been reported effective in a double-blind study of TRD patients (Carpenter et al., 2002). The combination of TCA and SSRIs may be effective in resistant patients (Kraus et al., 1996) but lower doses of TCAs are required, due to the competition at the cytochrome P450 2D6. Nevertheless, there is limited evidence, mostly in uncontrolled studies, supporting the efficacy of combination antidepressant treatment. Further randomized controlled trials with larger sample sizes are required to demonstrate the efficacy of a combination antidepressant strategy for patients with treatment-resistant depression (Lam et al., 2002).

Alternative Treatments

For delusional depression and treatment-refractory depression, electroconvulsive therapy (ECT) may be highly effective (Abrams, 1992). ECT is also helpful in moderate-to-severe depression.

Light therapy (e.g. 10 000 lux for 0.5–1 h/day or 2500 lux for 2–4 h/day) is the treatment of choice for seasonal affective disorder and, in combination with pharmacotherapy, a possible additive treatment strategy for non-seasonal depression (Kasper and Neumeister, 1998).

A few preparations of St John's wort in high concentration (e.g. Jarsin or Neuroplant 900 mg/day) have been demonstrated in controlled trials to be effective in mild-to-moderate depression (LaFrance et al., 2000). However, evidence of significant adverse drug interactions with St John's wort should not be overlooked (Boehnlein and Oakley, 2002).

Sleep deprivation (SD) has been studied in controlled trials in research settings, and appears to be effective in the treatment of some depressed patients, although the effects are short-lived (Giedke and Schwarzler, 2002).

When considering experimental approaches, transcranial magnetic stimulation (TMS) has been studied for its possible clinical applicability. Although statistically significant treatment effects have been found in open and controlled trials, a clinically meaningful response has not yet been demonstrated (McNamara et al., 2001; Schlaepfer et al, 2002). Technically, repeated rhythmic TMS (repetitive TMS or rTMS) seems to be the most effective technique. Further studies are necessary to clarify the relevant methodology and the regions of the brain that should be stimulated.

Some authors believe that vagus nerve stimulation (VNS) may ultimately prove useful, but this has to be proved in positive randomized controlled trials (Sackeim et al., 2001), but severe side effects including apathy may limit their future use (Matthews, 2003).

Finally, specific stereotactic techniques might prove to be helpful in the neurosurgical treatment of severe forms of TRD (Malhi and Bartlett, 2000).

CLINICAL DECISION TREE

Kasper, Zohar and Stein propose a possible way to deal with the treatment complexity of TRD via a 'decision tree', i.e. to provide a scheme of possibilities for the different stages of treatment, leaving the treating psychiatrist the flexibility to 'match' the best option according to the specific profile of the relevant patient (Kasper et al., 2002). See Figure 12.1. As there are different levels of evidence backing each intervention, each was coded by a colour signifying its confidence level (represented by different tints in Figure 12.1).

CONCLUSIONS

Treatment-resistant depression occupies more and more of psychiatrists' time, especially nowadays, when many depressed patients are being treated by GPs with SSRIs and are sent to psychiatrists only if they do not respond. These resistant patients also present a significant therapeutic challenge for the treating psychiatrists.

After careful review of issues such as diagnosis, dose, and treatment duration, and ruling out a possible medical condition, the diagnosis of resistant depression is warranted. Although the current knowledge about the biology of TRD is lacking, it is becoming increasingly clear that when the diagnosis is made, it does not mean that there is a 'bad' patient (who does not want to improve) or a 'bad' physician (a psychiatrist who does not know how to treat the patient). It actually means that the relevant patient belongs to a substantial group of patients (20–30%) who are truly treatment-resistant, and probably reflect one of several subtypes of depression which are yet to be identified. However, as neither the patient nor the psychiatrist can sit and wait for the full mystery of depression to be unfolded, clinical steps need to be taken. In this chapter, in Figure 12.1, we have given the different decisions that could be taken different weights of tint based on their 'confidence level' and placed them in a 'decision tree'. This might help the psychiatrist to build a 'road map' for future treatment. This plan, which should be carefully played out while taking into account the past history of the patient, the past response to treatment and the current medical condition (if there is a hepatic problem, to give medication that excretes by the kidney, if heart problem to choose antidepressants that do not affect the heart, if a female of child-bearing age, to try to take into account antidepressants which are not teratogenic etc.). Only then, and based on all the available data (i.e. 'confidence level'), appropriate steps should be initiated.

Although the data of what one should do beyond the second step is quite limited, there are some data that might help to decide what to do and what not to do, and in which order, taking into consideration the relative efficacy on one hand and the specific profile of the patient on the other.

The treatment should then be delivered, preferably after consultation with a trusted colleague, while making sure that each step that is taken is actually being tested thoroughly and adequately. At these stages, taking short cuts and jumping from one strategy to another not only deprives the psychiatrists of adequate information for future intervention, but also might hurt the therapeutic relationships – the confidence of the patient that he will be led along the rough road ahead by a competent guide.

It is clear that an additional effort should be put into research both of the biological basis as well as the therapeutic steps that need to be taken once a truly resistant patient is identified. This kind of research needs to be built on better and clearer concept and definition acknowledging the polymorphism of this difficult yet quite common phenomenon. Until then the therapeutic intervention should include, on top of a well-thought-out and carefully built plan of treatment, a fundamental value including empathy, comforting and support, along with a confidence, which might only derive from in-depth knowledge of the current state of the art in treating those difficult-to-treat patients.

This chapter has been aimed at pointing out the state of the art (including some of the current conceptual dilemmas) in this challenging area of psychiatry.

ACKNOWLEDGEMENT

The chapter is written on behalf of the treatment-resistant consortium and has been partially supported by an unrestricted educational grant from Lundbeck.

REFERENCES

Abrams R (1992) *Electroconvulsive Therapy* (2nd edition). New York: Oxford University Press.

Akiskal HS (1994) Dysthymic and cyclothymic depression: therapeutic considerations. *J Clin Psychiatry* 555 (4 (Suppl)): 46–52.

Alpert JE, Lagomisano IT (2001) Psychiatric comorbidity in treatment-resistant depression. In Amsterdam JD, Hornig M, Nierenberg AA (eds) *Treatment-resistant mood disorders*.

Amsterdam JD, Brunswick DJ, Mendels J (1980) The clinical application of tricyclic antidepressant pharmacokinetics and plasma levels. *Am J Psychiatry* 137: 653–662.

Amsterdam JD, Hornig-Rohan M (1996) Treatment algorithms in treatment-resistant depression. *Psychiatr Clin North Am* 19(2): 371–385.

Amsterdam JD, Maislin G, Gold P, Winokur A (1989) The assessment of abnormalities in hormonal responsiveness at multiple levels of the hypothalamic–pituitary–adrenocortical axis in depressive illness. *Psychoneuroendocrinology* 14: 43–62.

Amsterdam JD, Rosenzweig M, Mozley PD (1994) Assessment of adrenocortical activity in refractory depression: steroid suppression with ketoconazole. In Nolen WA, Zohar J, Roose SP, Amsterdam JD (eds) *Refractory Depression: Current Strategies and Future Directions.*

Anderson IM, Tomenson BM (1994) The efficacy of selective serotonin reuptake inhibitors in depression: a meta-analysis of studies against tricyclic antidepressants. *J Psychopharmacol* **8**: 238–249.

APA (1994) *Diagnostic and Statistical Manual of Mental Disorders* (DSM-IV) (4th edition). Washington, DC: American Psychiatric Association.

APA Task Force on Laboratory Tests in Psychiatry (1987) The dexamethasone suppression test: an overview of its current status in psychiatry. *Am J Psychiatry* **144**: 1253–1262.

Artigas F, Perez V, Alvarez E (1994) Pindolol induces a rapid improvement of depressed patients treated with serotonin reuptake inhibitors. *Arch Gen Psychiatry* **51**: 248–251.

Asher R (1949) Myxoedematous Madness. *Br Med J* **2**: 555–562.

Ayd FJ (1983) Treatment resistant depression. *Int Drug Ther Newsletter* **18**: 25–27.

Baghai TC, Schule C, Zwanzger, P, et al. (2001) Possible influence of the insertion/deletion polymorphism in the angiotensin I-converting enzyme gene on therapeutic outcome in affective disorders. *Mol Psychiatry* **6**: 258–259.

Benazzi F (2002) Can only reversed vegetative symptoms define atypical depression? *Eur Arch Psychiatry Clin Neurosci* **252**: 288–293.

Black DW, Bell S, Hubert J, et al. (1988) The importance of axis II in patients with major depression. *J Affect Disord* **14**: 115–122.

Blier P, Bergeron R (1995) Effectiveness of pindolol with selected antidepressant drugs in the treatment of major depression. *J Clin Psychopharmacol* **15**: 217–222.

Bloch M, Schmidt PJ, Danaceau MA, et al. (1999) Dehydroepiandrosterone treatment of midlife dysthymia. *Biol Psychiatry* **45**: 1533–1541.

Boehnlein B, Oakley LD (2002) Implications of self-administered St. John's wort for depression symptom management. *J Am Acad Nurse Pract* **14**: 443–448.

Bowden CL, Calabrese JR, McElroy SL, et al. (2000) A randomized, placebo-controlled 12-month trial of divalproex and lithium in treatment of outpatients with bipolar I disorder. *Arch Gen Psychiatry* **57**: 481–489.

Bridges PK (1983) '. . . and a small dose of an antidepressant might help.' *Br J Psychiatry* **142**: 626–628.

Brown WA, Harrison W (1992) Are patients who are intolerant to one SSRI intolerant to another. *Psychopharm Bull* **28**: 253–256.

Burrows GD, Norman TR, Judd FK (1994) Definition and differential diagnosis of treatment-resistant depression. *Intern Clin Psychopharm* **9**(2): 5–10.

Calabrese JR, Bowden CL, Sachs GS, et al. (1999) A double-blind placebo-controlled study of lamotrigine monotherapy in outpatients with bipolar I depression. *J Clin Psychiatry* **60**: 79–88.

Calabrese JR, Bowden CL, Sachs G, Yatham LN, Asghar SA, Hompland M, Montgomery P, Earl N, Smoot TM, DeVeaugh-Geiss J (2003) A placebo-controlled 18-month trial of lamotrigine and lithium maintenance treatment in recently manic or hypomanic patients with bipolar I disorder. *Arch Gen Psychiatry* **60**(4): 392–400.

Calabrese JR, Suppes T, Bowden CL, et al. (2000) A double-blind placebo-controlled prophylaxis study of lamotrigine in rapid cycling bipolar disorder. *J Clin Psychiatry* **61**: 841–850.

Carpenter LL, Yasmin S, Price LH (2002) A double-blind, placebo-controlled study of antidepressant augmentation with mirtazapine. *Biol Psychiatry* **51**: 183–188.

Charney DS, Price LH, Heninger GR (1986) Desipramine-yohimbine combination treatment of refractory depression: implications for the beta-adrenergic receptor hypothesis of antidepressant action. *Arch Gen Psychiatry* **43**: 1155–1161.

Corruble E, Ginestet D, Guelfi JD (1996) Comorbidity of personality disorders and unipolar major depression: a review. *J Affect Disord* **12**: 157–170.

Cramer JA (1995) Relationship between medication compliance and medical outcomes. *Am J Health Syst Pharm* **52**(14 Suppl 3): S27–S29.

Cusin C, Serretti A, Zanardi R, et al. (2002) Influence of monoamine oxidase A and serotonin receptor 2A polymorphisms in SSRI antidepressant activity. *Int J Neuropsychopharmacol* **5**: 27–35.

Delgado PL, Price LH, Charney DS, et al. (1988) Efficacy of fluvoxamine in treatment-refractory depression. *J Affect Disord* **15**: 55–60.

de Montigny C, Cournoyer G, Morissette R, et al. (1983) Lithium carbonate addition in tricyclic antidepressant-resistant unipolar depression. Correlations with the neurobiologic actions of tricyclic antidepressant drugs and lithium ion on the serotonin system. *Arch Gen Psychiatry* **40**: 1327–1334.

Demyttenaere K (1997) Compliance during treatment with antidepressants. *J Affect Disord* **43**: 27–39.

Dinan TG, Mobayed M (1992) Treatment resistance after head injury: a preliminary study of amitryptiline response. *Acta Psych Scand* **85**: 292–294.

Dunn RL, Donoghue JM, Ozminkowski RJ, et al. (1998) Selective serotonin reuptake inhibitor antidepressant prescribing in primary care in the United Kingdom. *Primary Care Psychiatry* **4**: 141–148.

Faravelli C, Albanesi G, Sessarego A (1988) Viqualine in resistant depression: A double-blind, placebo-controlled trial. *Neuropsychobiology* **20**: 78–81.

Fava M, Rosenbaum JF, McGrath PJ, et al. (1994) Lithium and tricyclic augmentation of fluoxetine treatment for major depression: a double-blind, contolled study. *Am J Psychiatry* **151**: 1372–1374.

Fawcett J, Kravitz HM (1985) Treatment refractory depression. In Schatzberg AF (ed) *Common Treatment Problems in Depression*. Washington, DC: American Psychiatric Press.

Feighner JP, Herbstein J, Damlouji N (1985) Combined MAOI, TCA, and direct stimulant therapy of treatment-resistant depression. *J Clin Psychiatry* **46**: 206–209.

Fernstrom JD, Larin R, Wurtman J (1973) Correlations between brain tryptophan and plasma neutral amino acid levels following food consumption in rats. *Life Sci* **13**: 517–524.

Fink M (1991) A trial of ECT is essential before a diagnosis of refractory depression is made. In Amsterdam JD (ed) *Advances in Neuropsychiatry and Psychopharmacology* Vol 2. *Refractory Depression*. New York: Raven Press, pp. 87–92.

Frank E, Prien RF, Jarrett R, et al. (1991) Conceptualization and rationale for consensus definitions of terms in major depressive disorder. *Arch Gen Psychiatry* **48**: 851–855.

Gagiano CA, Muller PGM, Gourie J, LeRoux JF (1993) The therapeutic efficacy of paroxetine: (a) an open study in patients with major depression not responding to antidepressants; (b) a double blind comparison with amitriptyline in depressed outpatients. *Acta Psychiatr Scand* **80**: 130–131.

Galinowski A, Lehert P (1995) Structural validity of MADRS during antidepressant treatment. *Intern Clin Psychopharmacol* **10**: 157–161.

Georgotas A, McCue RE, Cooper GL, et al. (1989) Factors affecting the delay of antidepressant effect in responders to nortryptiline and phenelzine. *Psychiatric Res* **28**: 1–9.

Gewirtz GR, Malaspina D, Hatterer JA, et al. (1988) Occult thyroid dysfunction in patients with refractory depression. *Am J Psychiatry* **145**: 1012–1014.

Giedke H, Schwarzler F (2002) Therapeutic use of sleep deprivation in depression. *Sleep Med Rev* **6**: 361–377.

Glassman AH (1994) Antidepressant plasma levels revisited. *Int Clin Psychopharmacology* **9**(Suppl 2): 25–30.

Gold MS, Pottash ALC, Extein I (1981) Hypothyroidism and depression. *JAMA* **245**: 1919–1922.

Gonzales GF, Carrillo C (1993) Blood serotonin levels in postmenopausal women: effects of age and serum oestradiol levels. *Maturitas* **17**: 23–29.

Goodwin FK, Prange AJ Jr, Post RM, et al. (1982) Potentiation of antidepressant effects by L-triiodothyronine in tricyclic nonresponders. *Am J Psychiatry* **139**: 34–38.

Greenhouse JB, Kupfer DJ, Franck E, et al. (1987) Analysis of time to stabilization in the treatment of depression: biological and clinical correlates. *J Affect Disord* **13**: 259–266.

Gruber AJ, Hudson JI, Pope HG (1996) The management of treatment-resistant depression in disorders on the interface of psychiatry and medicine. *Psychiatr Clin North Am* **19**(2): 351–361.

Guscott R, Grof P (1991) The clinical meaning of refractory depression: a review for the clinician. *Am J Psychiatry* **148**: 695–704.

Harrison W, Rabkin J, Stewart JW, et al. (1986) Phenelzine for chronic depression: a study of continuation treatment. *J Clin Psych* **47**: 346–349.

Hatterer JA, Gorman JM (1990) Thyroid function in refractory depression. In Roose SP, Glassman AH (eds) *Treatment Strategies for Refractory Depression*. Washington, DC: American Psychiatric Press, pp. 171–191.

Heninger GR, Charney DS, Sternberg DE (1983) Lithium carbonate augmentation of antidepressant treatment. An effective prescription for treatment-refractory depression. *Arch Gen Psychiatry* **40**: 1335–1342.

Hirschfeld RMA, Kosier T, Keller MB, et al. (1988) The influence of alcoholism on the course of depression. *J Affect Disord* **16**: 151–158.

Holsboer F (1989) Psychiatric implications of altered limbic–hypothalamic–pituitary–adrenocortical activity. *Eur Arch Psychiatry Neurol Sci* **238**: 302–322.

Howland RH (1993) Thyroid dysfunction in refractory depression: implications for pathophysiology and treatment. *J Clin Psychiatry* **54**: 47–54.

Joffe RT (1999) Peripheral thyroid hormone levels in treatment-resistant depression. *Biol Psychiatry* **45**: 1053–1055.

Joffe RT, Levitt AJ (1992) Major depression and subclinical (grade 2) hypothyroidism. *Psychoneuroendocrinology* **17**: 215–221.

Joffe RT, Levitt AJ, Bagby RM, et al. (1993) Predictors of response to lithium and triiodothyronine augmentation of antidepressants in tricyclic non-responders. *Br J Psychiatry* **163**: 574–578.

Joffe RT, Levitt AJ, Sokolov ST (1996) Response to an open trial of a second SSRI in major depression. *J Clin Psychiatry* **57**: 114–115.

Kasper S, Neumeister A (1998) Non-pharmacological treatments for depression: focus on sleep deprivation and light therapy. In Briley M, Montgomery S (eds) *Antidepressants Therapy: At the Dawn of the Third Millennium*. London: Martin Dunitz.

Kasper S, Zohar J, Stein DJ (2002) Pharmacotherapy of unipolar depression. In *Decision Making in Psychopharmacology*. London: Martin Dunitz, pp. 1–12.

Kathol RG, Delahunt JW (1986) The relationship of anxiety and depression to symptoms of hyperthyroidism using operational criteria. *Gen Hosp Psychiatry*. Jan; **8**(1): 23–28.

Katon W, Russo J, Frank E, et al. (2002) Predictors of nonresponse to treatment in primary care patients with dysthymia. *Gen Hosp Psychiatry* **24**: 20–27.

Katon W, von Korff M, Lin E (1992) Adequacy and duration of antidepressant treatment in primary care. *Med Care* **30**: 67–76.

Keller MB (1993) The difficult depressed patient in perspective. *J Clin Psychiatry* **54**(Suppl): S4–S8.

Keller MB, Lavori PW (1984) Double depression, major depression, and dysthymia: distinct entities or different phases of a single disorder? *Psychopharmacol Bull*. Summer, **20**(3): 399–402.

Keller MB, Lavori PW, Endicott J, et al. (1983) 'Double depression': two-year follow-up. *Am J Psychiatry* **140**: 689–694.

Keller MB, Shapiro RW (1985) Double depression: surimposition of acute depressive episodes on chronic depressive disorders. *Am J Psych* **139**: 794–800.

Kenis G, Maes M (2002) Effects of antidepressants on the production of cytokines. *Int J Neuropsychopharmacol* **5**: 401–412.

Kessler RC, McGonagle KA, Zhao S (1994) Lifetime and 12-month prevalence off DSM-III-R psychiatric disorderss in the United States: results from the National Comorbidity Survey. *Arch Gen Psychiatry* **51**: 8–19.

Kiraly SJ, Ancil RJ, Dimitrova G (1997) The relationship of endogenous cortisol to psychiatric disorder: a review. *Canad J Psychiatry* **42**: 415–420.

Kocsis JH, Friedman RA, Markowitz JC, et al. (1996) Maintenance therapy for chronic depression. A controlled clinical trial of desipramine. *Arch Gen Psychiatry* **53**: 769–774.

Koike AK, Unutzer J, Wells KB (2002) Improving the care for depression in patients with comorbid medical illness. *Am J Psychiatry* **159**: 1738–1745.

Kramer MS, Cutler N, Feighner J, et al. (1998) Distinct mechanism for antidepressant activity by blockade of central substance P receptors. *Science* **281**: 1640–1645.

Kraus RP, Diaz P, McEachran A (1996) Managing rapid metabolizers of antidepressants. *Depress Anxiety* **4**(6): 320–327.

LaFrance WC Jr, Lauterbach EC, Coffey CE, et al. (2000) The use of herbal alternative medicines in neuropsychiatry. A report of the ANPA Committee on Research. *J Neuropsychiatry Clin Neurosci* **12**: 177–192.

Lam RW, Wan DD, Cohen NL, Kennedy SH (2002) Combining antidepressants for treatment-resistant depression: a review. *J Clin Psychiatry* **63**: 685–693.

Lepine JP, Gastpar M, Mendlewicz J (1997) Depression in the community: the first pan-European study DEPRES (Depression Research in European Society). *Int Clin Psychopharmacol* **12**: 19–29.

Lerer B (2002) Genes and psychopharmacology: exploring the interface. In Lerer B (ed) *Pharmacogenetics of Psychotropic Drugs*.

Lerer B, Macciardi F (2002) Pharmacogenetics of antidepressant and mood-stabilizing drugs: a review of candidate-gene studies and future research directions. *Int J Neuropsychopharmacol* **5**: 255–275.

Levine S (1986) The management of resistant depression. *Acta. Psych Belgica* **86**: 141–151.

Liebowitz MR, Quitkin FM, Stewari JW, et al. (1988) Antidepressant specificity in atypical depression. *Arch Gen Psychiatry* **45**: 129–137.

Links PS, Akiskal HS (1987) Chronic and intractable depressions: terminology. classification and description of subtypes. In Zohar J, Belmaker RH (eds) *Treating Resistant Depression*. New York: PMA Publishing, pp. 1–22.

Maes M, Meltzer HY (1995) The Serotonin Hypothesis of depression. In: Bloom FE, Kupfer DJ. Psychopharmacology. The Fourth Generation of Progress. New York: Raven Press, pp. 933–944.

Marangell LB (2001) Switching antidepressants for treatment-resistant major depression. *J Clin Psychiatry* **62**(suppl 18): 12–17.

Maser JD, Cloninger RC (1990) *Comorbidity of Mood and Anxiety Disorders*. Washington, DC: American Psychiatric Press.

Matthews K, Eljamel MS (2003) Vagus nerve stimulation and refractory depression: please can you switch me on doctor? *Br J Psychiatry*, Sep; **183**: 181–183.

McEwan WG, Remick RA (1988) Treatment resistant depression: a clinical perspective. *Canad J Psychiatry* **33**: 788–792.

McEwen BS, Gould E, Orchinik M, et al. (1995) Oestrogens and the structural and functional plasticity of neurons: implications for memory, ageing and neurodegenerative processes. *Ciba Found Symp* **191**: 52–66; discussion 66–73.

McGrath PJ, Stewart JW, Harrison W, et al. (1987) Treatment of refractory depression with a monoamine oxidase inhibitor anti-depressant. *Psychopharmacol Bull* **23**: 169–173.

McNamara B, Ray JL, Arthurs OJ, Boniface S (2001) Transcranial magnetic stimulation for depression and other psychiatric disorders. *Psychol Med* **31**: 1141–1146.

Meltzer HY, Maes M, Elkis H (1994) The biological basis of refractory depression. In Nolen WA, Zohar J, Roose SP, Amsterdam JD (eds) *Refractory Depression: Current Strategies and Future Directions.*

Mendlewicz J (1994) The search for a manic depressive gene: from classical to molecular genetics. *Progr Brain Res* **100**: 255–259.

Mendlewicz J (2001) Optimising antidepressant use in clinical practice: towards criteria for antidepressant selection. *Br J Psychiatry* Sep; 42–51 (Suppl 42): S1–S3.

Montgomery SA (1991) Selectivity of antidepressants and resistant depression. In Amsterdam JD (ed) *Advances in Neuropsychiatry and Psychopharmacology*: Vol 2. *Refractory Depression.* New York: Raven Press, pp. 93–104.

Moreno FA, Gelenberg AJ, Bachar K, Delgado PL (1997) Pindolol augmentation of treatment-resistant depressed patients. *J Clin Psychiatry* **58**: 437–439.

Nelsen MR, Dunner DL (1993) Treatment resistance in unipolar depression and other disorders. *Psychiatr Clin North Am* **16**(3): 541–566.

Nelsen MR, Dunner DL (1995) Clinical and differential diagnostic aspects of treatment-resistant depression. *J Psychiatr Res* **29**(1):43–50.

Nelson JC, Mazure CM, Jatlow PI (1990) Does melancholia predict response in major depression? *J Affect Disord* **18**: 157–165.

Nelson JC, Mazure CM, Jatlow PI (1994) Characteristics of desipramine-refractory depression. *J Clin Psychiatry* **55**: 12–19.

Nierenberg AA, Keck PE, Samson J, et al. (1991) Methodological considerations for the study of treatment-resistant depression. In Amsterdam JD (ed) *Advances in Neuropsychiatry and Psychopharmacology*: Vol 2. *Refractory Depression.* New York: Raven Press, pp. 1–12.

Nolen WA, Van De Putte JJ, Dijken WA, et al. (1998) Treatment strategy in depression, I: tricyclic and selective reuptake inhibitors in resistant depression: a double-blind partial crossover study on the effects of oxaprotiline and fluvoxamine. *Acta Psychiatr Scand* **78**: 668–675.

O'Reardon JP, Amsterdam JD (2001) Overview of treatment-resistant depression and its management. In Amsterdam JD, Hornig M, Nierenberg AA (eds) *Treatment-resistant Mood Disorders.*

Pare CMB (1963) Potentiation of monoamine oxidase inhibitors by tryptophan. *Lancet* **ii**: 527–528.

Pecins-Thompson M, Brown NA, Kohama SG, Bethea CL (1996) Ovarian steroid regulation of tryptophan hydroxylase mRNA expression in rhesus macaques. *J Neurosci* **16**: 7021–7029.

Perez V, Soler J, Puigdemont D, et al. (1999) A double-blind, randomized, placebo-controlled trial of pindolol augmentation in depressive patients resistant to serotonin reuptake inhibitors. Grup de Recerca en Trastorns Afectius. *Arch Gen Psychiatry* **56**: 375–379.

Peselow ED, Filippi AM, Goodnick P, et al. (1989) The short- and long-term efficacy of paroxetine HCL, B: Data from a double-blind crossover study and from a year-long trial vs. imipramine and placebo. *Psychopharmacol Bull* **25**: 272–276.

Pfohl B, Stangl D, Zimmerman M (1984) The implications of DSM-III personality disorders for patients with major depression. *J Affect Disord* **7**: 309–318.

Phillips KA, Nierenberg AA (1994) The assessment and treatment of refractory depression. *J Clin Psychiatry* **55**(Suppl 2): S20–S26.

Prange AJ Jr, Wilson IC, Breese GR, Lipton MA (1976) Hormonal alteration of imipramine response: a review. In Sachar EJ (ed) *Hormones, Behavior and Psychopathology.*

Primeau F (1988) Post-stroke depression: a critical review of the literature. *Canad J Psychiatry* **8**(33): 757–765.

Quitkin FM, HarrisonW, StewartJW, et al. (1991) Response to phenelzine and imipramine in placebo non-responders with atypical depression. *Arch Gen Pychiatry* **48**: 319–323.

Quitkin FM, McGrath PJ, StewartJW, et al. (1996) Chronological milestones to guide drug change. When should clinicians switch antidepressants? *Arch Gen Psychiatry* **53**: 785–792.

Quitkin FM, Rabkin GJ, Ross D, et al. (1984) Duration of antidepressant treatment:What is an adequate treatment. *Arch Gen Psychiatry* **41**(3): 238–245.

Reimherr FW,Woods DR, Byerley B, et al. (1984) Characteristics of responders to fluoxetine. *Psychopharmacol Bull* **20**: 70–72.

ReusVI (1993) Psychiatric aspects of thyroid disease. InJoffe RT, Levitt AJ (eds) *The Thyroid Axis and Psychiatric Illness.*

Reus VI, Wolkowitz OM (2001) Antiglucocorticoid drugs in the treatment of depression. *Expert Opin Investig Drugs.* Oct: **10**(10): 1789–1796.

Reus VI, Wolkowitz OM, Frederick S (1997) Antiglucocorticoid treatments in psychiatry. *Psychoneuroendocrinology* **22**(Suppl 1): S121–124.

Roose SP, Glassman AH (1994) Treatment with tricyclic antidepressants: defining the refractory patient. In NolenWA, ZoharJ, Roose SP, AmsterdamJD (eds) *Refractory Depression: Current Strategies and Future Directions.*

Roose SP, Glasman AH, Walsh BT, et al. (1986) Tricyclic responders: phenomenology and treatment. *AmJ Psychiatry* **143**: 345–348.

Sachs GS (1996) Treatment-resistant bipolar depression. *Psychiatr Clin North Am* **19**(2): 215–236.

Sackeim HA (2001) The definition and meaning of treatment-resistant depression. *J Clin Psychiatry* **62**(Suppl 16): 10–17.

Sackeim HA, Rush AJ, George MS, et al. (2001) Vagus nerve stimulation (VNS) for treatment-resistant depression: efficacy, side effects, and predictors of outcome. *Neuropsychopharmacology* **25**: 713–728.

SandersonWC, Beck AT, BeckJ (1990) Syndrome comorbidity in patients with major depression or dysthymia: prevalence and temporal relationships. *AmJ Psychiatry* **147**: 1025–1028.

Schatzberg AF, ColeJO, Cohen BM, et al. (1983) Survey of depressed patients who have failed to respond to treatment. In DavisJM, MaasJW (eds) *The Affective Disorders.* Washington, DC: American Psychiatric Press, pp. 73–85.

Schatzberg AF, ColeJO, Elliott GR (1986) Recent views on treatment resistant depression. In Halbreich U, Feinberg SS (eds) *Psychosocial Aspects of Non-response to Antidepressant Drugs.* Washington, DC: American Psychiatric Press, pp. 95–109.

Schlaepfer TE, Kosel M, Nemeroff CB (2003) Efficacy of repetitive transcranial magnetic stimulation (rTMS) in the treatment of affective disorders. *Neuropsychopharmacology.* Feb; **28**(2): 201–205.

SchopfJ, Baumann P, Lemarchand T, Rey M (1989) Treatment of endogenous depressions resistant to tricyclic antidepressants or related drugs by lithium addition. Results of a placebo-controlled double-blind study. *Pharmacopsychiatry* **22**: 183–187.

Schweiser E, Rickels K, AmsterdamJD (1990) What constitutes an adequate treatment trial for fluoxetine? *J Clin Psychiatry* **51**: 8–11.

Serretti A, Zanardi R, Cusin C, et al. (2001b) Tryptophan hydroxylase gene associated with paroxetine antidepressant activity. *Eur Neuropsychopharmacol* **11**: 375–380.

Serretti A, Zanardi R, Rossini D, et al. (2001a) Influence of tryptophan hydroxylase and serotonin transporter genes on fluvoxamine antidepressant activity. *Mol Psychiatry* **6**: 586–592.

Shea MT, Hirschfeld RM (1996) Chronic mood disorder and depressive personality. *Psychiatr Clin North Am.* Mar; **19**(1): 103–120.

Shea MT, Pilkonis PA, Beckham E, et al. (1990) Personality disorder and treatment outcome in the NIMH treatment of depression collaborative research program. *AmJ Psychiatry* **147**: 711–718.

Shea MT, Wuidiger TA, Klein MH (1992) Comorbidity of personality disorders and depression: implications for treatment. *J Cons Clin Psychol* **60**: 857–868.

Shelton RC, Davidson J, Yonkers KA, et al. (1997) The undertreatment of dysthymia. *J Clin Psychiatry* **58**: 59–65.

Sherwin BB (2001) Estrogen and depressive illness in women. In Amsterdam JD, Hornig M, Nierenberg AA (eds) *Treatment-resistant Mood Disorders.*

Sluzewska A, et al. (2001) Immunologic factors. In Amsterdam JD, Hornig M, Nierenberg AA (eds) *Treatment-resistant Mood Disorders.*

Sluzewska A, Rybakowski J, Bosmans E, et al. (1996b) Indicators of immune activation in major depression. *Psychiatry Res* **64**: 161–167.

Sluzewska A, Rybakowski JK, Sobieska M, Amsterdam JD (1996a) Changes in concentration and microheterogeneity of two acute phase proteins in major depression. *Behav Pharmacol* **7**: 105–106.

Sluzewska A, Rybakowski JK, Sobieska M, Wiktorowicz K (1994) The effect of lithium, carbamazepine and fluoxetine on alpha-1-acid glycoprotein and alpha-1-chymotrypsin in depressed patients. *Neuropsychopharmacology* **10**: 202.

Smeraldi E, Zanardi R, Benedetti F, et al. (1998) Polymorphism within the promoter of the serotonin transporter gene and antidepressant efficacy of fluvoxamine. *Mol Psychiatry* **3**: 508–511.

Souery D, Amsterdam J, de Montigny C, et al. (1999) Treatment resistant depression: methodological overview and operational criteria. *Eur Neuropsychopharmacol* **9**: 83–91.

Souery D, Rivelli SK, Mendlewicz J (2001) Molecular genetic and family studies in affective disorders: state of the art. *J Affect Disord* **62**: 45–55.

Stein G, Bernadt M (1993) Lithium augmentation therapy in tricyclic-resistant depression. A controlled trial using lithium in low and normal doses. *Br J Psychiatry* **162**: 634–640.

Stoppe G, Doren M (2002) Critical appraisal of effects of estrogen replacement therapy on symptoms of depressed mood. *Arch Women Ment Health* **5**: 39–47.

Strous RD, Maayan R, Lapidus R, et al. (2003) Dehydroepiandrosterone augmentation in the management of negative, depressive, and anxiety symptoms in schizophrenia. *Arch Gen Psychiatry* **60**: 133–141.

Thakore JH, Dinan TG (1995) Cortisol synthesis inhibition: a new treatment strategy for the clinical and endocrine manifestations of depression. *Biol Psychiatry* **37**: 364–368.

Thase ME (1996) The role of axis II comorbidity in the management of patients with treatment resistant depression. *Psychiatr Clin North Am* **19**(2): 287–292.

Thase ME, Fava M, Halbreich U, et al. (1996) A placebo-controlled, randomized clinical trial comparing sertraline and imipramine for the treatment of dysthymia. *Arch Gen Psychiatry* **53**: 777–784.

Thase ME, Kupfer DJ (1996) Recent developments in the pharmacotherapy of mood disorders. *J Consult Clin Psychol* **64**(4): 646–659.

Thase ME, Rush AJ (1995) Treatment-resistant depression. In Bloom FE, Kupfer DJ (eds) *Psychopharmacology: The Fourth Generation of Progress.* New York: Raven Press.

Thase ME, Rush AJ (1997) When at first you don't succeed: sequential strategies for antidepressant nonresponders. *J Clin Psychiatry* **58**(Suppl 13): 23–29.

Tohen M, Waternaux CM, Tsuang MT (1990) Outcome in mania: a four year prospective follow-up of 75 patients utilizing survival analysis. *Arch Gen Psychiatry* **47**: 1106–1111.

Van Praag HM (1996) Faulty cortisol/serotonin interplay. Psychopathological and biological characterisation of a new, hypothetical depression subtype (SeCA depression). *Psychiatry Res* **65**: 143–157.

van Praag HM (1978) Neuroendrocrine disorders in depressions and their significance for the monoamine hypothesis of depression. *Acta Psychiatr Scand.* May; **57**(5): 389–404.

Weissman MM, Leaf PJ, Bruce ML, et al. (1988) The epidemiology of dysthymia in five communities: rates, risks, comorbidity and treatment. *Am J Psychiatry* **145**: 815–819.

White K, Wykoff W, Tynes LL, Schneider L, Zemansky M (1990) Fluvoxamine in the treatment of tricyclic-resistant depression. *Psychiatr J Univ Ottawa* **15**: 156–158.

Wolkowitz OM (1992) Prospective controlled studies of the behavioral and biological effects of exogenous corticosteroids. *Psychoneuroendocrinology* **19**: 233–255.

Wolkowitz OM, Brizendine L, Reus VI (2000) The role of dehydroepiandrosterone (DHEA) in psychiatry. *Psychiatric Annals* **30**: 123–128.

Wolkowitz OM, Reus VI (2001) Psychoneuroendocrine aspects. In Amsterdam JD, Hornig M, Nierenberg AA (eds) *Treatment-resistant Mood Disorders*.

Wolkowitz OM, Reus VI, Chan T, et al. (1999a) Antiglucocorticoid treatment of depression: double-blind ketoconazole. *Biol Psychiatry* **45**: 1070–1074.

Wolkowitz OM, Reus VI, Keebler A, et al. (1999b) Double-blind treatment of major depression with dehydroepiandrosterone. *Am J Psychiatry* **156**: 646–649.

Wolkowitz OM, Reus VI, Manfredi F, et al. (1993) Ketoconazole administration in hypercortisolemic depression. *Am J Psychiatry* **150**: 810–812.

Young AH, Gallagher P, Porter RJ (2002) Elevation of the cortisol-dehydroepiandrosterone ratio in drug-free depressed patients. *Am J Psychiatry* **159**: 1237–1239.

Zarate CA, Kando JC, Tohen M, Weiss MK, Cole JO (1996) Does intolerance or lack of response with fluoxetine predict the same will happen with sertraline? *J Clin Psychiatry* **57**(2): 67–71.

Zisook B, Braff DL, Click MA (1985) Monoamine oxidase inhibitors in the treatment of atypical depression. *J Clin Psychopharmacol* **5**: 131–137.

Zohar J, Shapria B, Oppenheim G, Ayd FJ, Belmaker RH (1985) Addition of estrogen to imipramine in female-resistant depressives. *Psychopharmacol Bull* **21**(3): 705–706.

Brain Stimulation in Depression

Thomas E. Schlaepfer[1,2] and Markus Kosel[1]

[1]University Hospital Bern, Bern, Switzerland
[2]The Johns Hopkins University School of Medicine, Baltimore, MD, USA

INTRODUCTION

It should be clear that pharmacologic treatments and special forms of psychotherapy have an important role to play in patients suffering from mood disorders. However, a large proportion of patients with depression do not improve substantially even after two treatment trials using antidepressant drugs of different classes for at least six weeks at a standard dose agreed on as being generally effective. Methods of direct or indirect stimulation of the brain have been evaluated and used for the treatment of these treatment-refractory forms of depression for about a century now. But only relatively recently, due to technical advances and better knowledge about the neurobiology of the stimulation effects, broad interest in these methods has emerged.

Currently one method is clinically used for the treatment of affective disorders (electroconvulsive therapy (ECT) and four more methodologies under investigation (repetitive transcranial magnetic stimulation (rTMS), magnetic seizure therapy (MST), vagus nerve stimulation (VNS) and deep brain stimulation (DBS)). Reflecting the current state of research we will focus on TMS and VNS because these methods have received most interest.

ECT has been in continuous use in psychiatry for almost 70 years, and remains the most effective and most rapidly acting treatment for severe depression with a very benign side-effect profile (Fink, 1985). In 1938, chemical induction methods were replaced by electrical induction. In the 1950s, the introduction of general anaesthesia greatly reduced morbidity from the treatment. The move from sine wave ECT to brief pulse stimulation during the 1980s significantly reduced the severity of cognitive side effects of the treatment, and provided the first clear demonstration that the type of electrical current applied to the scalp was a major determinant of side effects (Weiner et al., 1986). Recent research has extended that

Mood Disorders: Clinical Management and Research Issues. Edited by E. J. L. Griez, C. Faravelli, D. J. Nutt and J. Zohar.
©2005 John Wiley & Sons Ltd. ISBN 0 470 09426 5.

finding by showing that electrode placement interacts with electrical dosage in determining efficacy as well as side effects (Sackeim et al., 2000). Challenges facing the field of convulsive therapy today include maintaining response following an effective course of ECT and minimizing cognitive side effects. It is important to note, however, that these side effects are of minor importance when treating a life-threatening illness (Cuijpers and Smit, 2002) with a mortality rate of up to 20% (Wulsin et al., 1999). Still, it is of obvious importance to investigate the underlying mechanisms of the treatment in order to understand effect and side effects better and thus to improve acceptance of the therapy for patients and the public at large. One important avenue of research is the recent work on magnetic seizure therapy (MST), which is discussed in this chapter. This brain stimulation therapy has apparently a much more benign side-effect profile with hopefully the same efficacy as ECT.

One very recent development is the adoption of the method of deep brain stimulation (DBS) as a putative treatment for affective disorders. DBS is an important FDA-approved treatment of Parkinson's disease and other movement disorders (Mogilner et al., 2002). Development of this technique has opened a new avenue for research and treatment in neuropsychiatric disorders. The technical refinement, over the past 15 years, of DBS for the treatment of movement disorders has resulted in a renaissance in the field of functional neurosurgery. As with other brain stimulation techniques, the exact mechanism of action of brain stimulation remains unknown. Most likely, brain stimulation exerts its effects via a number of differing but interrelated mechanisms that come into play depending on the site of stimulation, the disease entity being treated, and the stimulation parameters used. DBS, at high frequencies (approximately 100 Hz or greater, as typically used clinically for movement disorders), has been proposed to inhibit transmission via one or more of the following actions: (1) depolarization blockade, (2) synaptic fatigue, or (3) 'neural jamming' (imposing a physiologically meaningless pattern of activity within the affected circuits). Any of these phenomena would in effect produce a 'functional lesion', mimicking the effect of an actual therapeutic lesion procedure via a nondestructive mechanism.

In the realm of neuropsychiatry, DBS has first been adopted for the treatment of refractory obsessive-compulsive disorders (Greenberg et al., 2000; Hollander et al., 2002). Interestingly, there are a few reports that DBS produced marked affective changes in movement disorder patients (Bejjani et al., 1999; Berney et al., 2002). This suggests that DBS can modulate activity in neural circuits important in psychopathological states or, potentially, in the response to treatment. As the intricate interplay of brain systems involved in the modulation of mood and affect becomes more clear (Keightley et al., 2003; Mayberg, 1997, 2002) it is obvious that DBS – which affords stimulation at subcortical localizations – will be used as a putative treatment for particularly refractory patients. It may well be, that DBS turns out to be the most efficacious brain stimulation technique in the treatment of affective disorders due to its focality. Studies researching this method are in an early planning stage in the USA and Europe.

TRANSCRANIAL MAGNETIC STIMULATION (TMS)

Principle of the Method

With the observation of Faraday in 1831, that a time-varying magnetic field can induce a current in a nearby conductor, the theoretical basis of inducing depolarizing currents by electromagnetic coils was established. The French scientist d'Arsonval reported on the first human application of transcranial magnetic stimulation (TMS) already in 1896. He was able to induce phosphenes (flickering-light sensation, not elicited by visual perception), vertigo and syncope in subjects whose head was placed in a large electromagnetic coil. In 1959, Kolin demonstrated for the first time that an alternating magnetic field is able to stimulate a sciatic frog nerve and could induce contractions of the gastrocnemic muscle. In 1965, Bickford was able to induce muscle twitching in humans by applying a pulsed magnetic field with a maximum field-strength of 20 000 to 30 000 gauss to ulnar, peroneal and sciatic nerves (Geddes, 1991).

Barker first demonstrated the induction of muscle potentials by magnetic stimulation of the central nervous system in 1985 (Barker et al., 1985). He induced muscle twitching with a coil of 10 cm diameter placed on the scalp over the motor cortex. A brief pulse of 110 μs with a peak current of 4000 amperes was applied and pulses at a maximal rate of 0.33 Hz were delivered.

With the possibility of stimulating the motor cortex non-invasively (Figures 13.1 and 13.2), TMS replaced high-voltage transcutaneous electrical stimulation used in clinical studies mainly to measure central motor conduction time. This variable may be altered by a variety of neurological disorders such as multiple sclerosis, amyotrophic lateral sclerosis, cervical myelopathy and degenerative ataxic disorders. It seems that TMS has great potential in the intraoperative monitoring of the integrity of motor tracts during surgery of the brain and spinal tract (Murray, 1991). TMS has subsequently found diagnostic use in neurology for disorders such as demyelinating diseases involving the excitability and the connections of the motor cortex with other parts of the nervous system involved in motor pathways (Ziemann and Hallett, 2000).

With recent technology, single- or paired-pulse techniques that are used to assess brain physiology and pathophysiology as well as repetitive TMS (rTMS, high-frequency rTMS: stimulation faster than 1 Hz, low-frequency rTMS: stimulation at 1 or less Hz) up to 80 Hz can be delivered.

Delivery of Repetitive Transcranial Magnetic Stimulation (rTMS)

The equipment necessary for delivering TMS consists basically of two parts: the stimulator, which generates brief pulses of strong electrical currents – frequency

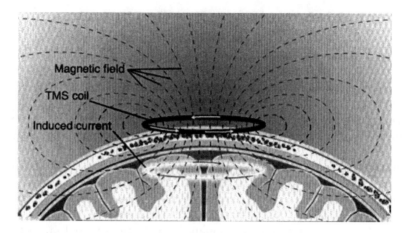

Figure 13.1 Transcranial magnetic stimulation (TMS): principle of action. A transient current in a magnetic stimulating coil over the scalp induces a small current in the brain, which is able to activate neural elements in the motor cortex

and intensity of the current pulses, as well as train duration and intertrain interval can be varied – and a stimulation coil connected to the stimulator.

The TMS stimulus interfering with the brain consists of very strong pulsating magnetic fields changing amplitude from 0 to 1.5 tesla in a few milliseconds. The shape of the magnetic field depends on the design of the coil. There are circular coils with a cylinder-shaped field, figure-8 coils with a more focal field (maximum strength at the intersection of the two circles) and iron core coils that also generate focal fields with a maximum strength in the centre of the coil. Older coil models using water or air-cooling have to be connected to water circulation or a ventilating system. The magnetic field generated by the coil is perpendicular to its surface and passes unimpeded through the skin and the skull. Since the strength of magnetic fields declines exponentially with distance from the inducing conductor, depolarizing of neurons occurs only to a distance of 2–3 centimetres from the surface of the coil. This is why only superficial structures of the brain can be directly interfered with. However, distant effects of the application of TMS, for example on regional cerebral blood flow, can be measured and might be important for biological effects. The cost of a device capable of delivering fast rTMS amounts to about $10 000– 40 000.

Side Effects of rTMS and Safety Considerations

Compared to ECT, MST, DBS and VNS, rTMS can be considered as relatively safe since it is non-invasive and the induction of convulsions are not required for a treatment. Therefore, side effects linked to anaesthesia and convulsion do not occur.

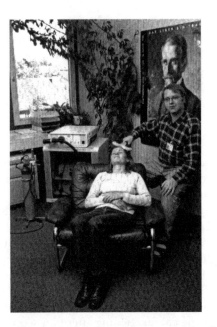

Figure 13.2 Practical use of repetitive transcranial magnetic stimulation (rTMS). This is a common setting for nonconvulsive rTMS studies in neuropsychiatry. Patients are awake, sitting relaxed in a chair while stimulation (here to the left dorsolateral prefrontal cortex) is applied. A typical stimulator, here with four booster modules, affording high-frequency stimulation is used. Note the oxygen tank nearby, which would be used as most important therapy in the event of a seizure developing. Having a Freud-like picture in the room as depicted here is not germane to maximizing treatment efficacy but is certainly helpful. (Photograph reproduced with permission)

There are, however, side effects directly linked to the application of rTMS or occurring up to a few hours later. Of major concern are involuntarily induced epileptic seizure, local pain during application, changes in auditory performance due to the noise generated in the coil and headache, as well as the concern of alterations of cognitive functions. Until now, in research applications, mainly short-term problems (application of TMS, follow-up of a few weeks) were addressed. But also long-term concerns have to be addressed. These might include long-lasting cognitive impairment which is the most frequent unwanted long-term side effect of ECT, sleep problems or potentially problems linked to effects of the influence of the strong magnetic fields on the brain.

Seizures

The risk of causing a seizure is the primary safety concern with TMS. Even though this risk is primarily associated with rTMS, single pulse stimulation has also been reported to produce seizures in patients with large cerebral infarcts, contusions or other structural brain lesions. According to Wassermann (Wassermann, 2000), in patients with completely subcortical lesions, no seizures are reported. According to the same author, there are a few articles reporting the induction of seizures in epilepsy patients without gross lesions.

Cognitive impairment

Mainly short-term observations concerning cognitive function after TMS administration are available. rTMS can produce transient disruption of various cerebral functions, depending on the site of stimulation. Observations reported include a significant decrease in a memory subtest within an hour after stimulation with 150 trains of rTMS at 15 Hz and 120% motor threshold delivered at four different positions (Flitman et al., 1998). Commenting on these results, Lorberbaum concludes, that these cognitive effects were due to subconvulsive epileptic activity or that the threshold for adverse effects on memory might be near that of seizure (Lorberbaum and Wassermann, 2000). Loo reported results from a study where 12 subjects suffering from major depression received rTMS during four weeks. No significant changes in neuropsychological functioning after four weeks were observed (Loo et al., 2001).

Hearing

No significant changes in auditory threshold were observed in a study involving 12 depressed subjects undergoing rTMS during four weeks when assessed for four weeks after the end of the study (Loo et al., 2001).

Headache

The application of TMS may cause local pain resulting from direct stimulation of muscles underlying the coil and from stimulation of facial and scalp nerves. It is generally more painful at higher intensities and frequencies. About 5–20% of subjects experience tension headache subsequently (George et al., 1999).

Potential Long-term Effects

There is of course legitimate concern whether the application of rTMS might cause brain damage in the widest sense. Mechanisms discussed are heating of neuronal tissue, exocitotoxicity and any influences of magnetic fields. As with other side effects, besides the occurrence of seizure, there are very few data and no thorough investigations available which would address these questions. There are, however, after the administration of TMS and rTMS to many thousand subjects, no indications that their application might cause brain damage.

Basic Effects Induced by TMS

Ji demonstrated that one single train of rTMS applied to rats *in vivo* induced c-fos and c-jun expression in different brain regions and among them in key regions controlling circadian biological rhythms (Ji et al., 1998). Similar stimulation parameters have earlier been shown to have efficacy in an animal model of depression (Fleischmann et al., 1995). These findings might point to a possible antidepressant mode of action of TMS effects via circadian rhythms. The finding that immediate–early gene expression is modified by TMS has been replicated and further examined recently by other authors, both *in vivo* and *in vitro* (Doi et al., 2001; Hausmann et al., 2001).

Keck measured modulatory effects of frontal rTMS in rat brain *in vivo* using intracerebral microdialysis (Keck et al., 2000). There was a continuous reduction in arginine vasopressin release of up to 50% within the hypothalamic paraventricular nucleus in response to rTMS. In contrast, the release of taurine, aspartate and serine was selectively stimulated within this nucleus by rTMS. Furthermore, in the dorsal hippocampus the extracellular concentration of dopamine was elevated in response to rTMS.

By using positron emission tomography (PET), a diminished ^{11}C raclopride binding to dopamine receptors in the left dorsal caudate nucleus could be measured in eight volunteers after left dorsolateral prefrontal cortex rTMS. This implies, that rTMS can trigger the dopamine release in these brain structures (Strafellea et al., 2001). Several studies documented the effect of rTMS on human blood hormone levels. They include effects on cortisol, prolactin and thyroid stimulating hormone (TSH). Actual results cannot be considered as conclusive. They indicate, however, that TMS might significantly influence endocrine functions of the brain (Cohrs et al., 1998; George et al., 1996; Szuba et al., 2001). TMS can transiently disrupt or induce activity in focal brain regions, depending on the region stimulated. Applied to the visual cortex for example, strong TMS can produce phosphenes and a stimulus of lower intensity may induce transient scotomas (Hallett, 2000). Also other functions, such as linguistic processing, can be investigated with rTMS (Flitman et al., 1998). Peinemann reported a neuromodulatory effect of subthreshold high-frequency rTMS in 10 subjects. After 1250 stimulations at 90% motor threshold, an intracortical inhibition could be measured which lasted at least 10 minutes after the rTMS stimulation (Peinemann et al., 2000).

The combination of non-invasive stimulation of the brain coupled with functional neuroimaging techniques offers new opportunities to investigate functions of the human brain. It also makes it possible to visualize effects of TMS which are documented to occur at distant sites from the stimulation (Paus et al., 1997). In another study, 10 medication-free subjects suffering from major depression (eight unipolar, two bipolar), received in a crossover, randomized study rTMS at the left prefrontal cortex, at 100% motor threshold, at 20 Hz or 1 Hz. With 20 Hz, an increase in rCBF in the prefrontal cortex left > right, cingulate gyrus left >> right, left amygdala, bilateral insula, basal ganglia, uncus hippocampus, para-hippocampus, thalamus, cerebellum was observed; with 1 Hz only decreases in rCBF: right prefrontal cortex, left medial cortex, left basal ganglia, left amygdala. Individuals that improved with one frequency concerning their depressive symptoms worsened with the other (Speer et al., 2000).

All these approaches from different areas of neuroscience convergingly show that TMS has prominent and reproducible effects on the brain, which is certainly encouraging and sets TMS apart from some other putative approaches to treating neuropsychiatric disorders (Hallett, 2000). The problem is, that the connection from cellular levels to complex behavioural changes – such as those observed in depression – is difficult to make. The field has suffered somewhat from a 'top down' approach in which early promising results in depression have led to an enthusiasm for clinical studies without sufficient neuroscientific foundations. Approaches integrating findings from all levels of biological systems are extremely important and should be undertaken in order to support the ongoing clinical research.

rTMS as a Putative Treatment for Mood Disorders

In 1987 Bickford made an observation which changed the whole field of neuropsychiatric TMS research. He described transient mood elevation in several normal volunteers receiving single pulse stimulations to the motor cortex (Bickford et al., 1987). This was the starting point of the scientific investigation of effects of depolarizing magnetic fields on a variety of neuropsychiatric disorders. Subsequently, unblinded pilot studies of TMS with depressed patients were done using single pulse stimulations at frequencies less than 0.3 Hz (Grisaru et al., 1994; Höflich et al., 1993; Kolbinger et al., 1995). In these studies relatively large areas under the vertex were stimulated bilaterally and all involved only a few subjects. More recent work has suggested that rTMS at 1 Hz with a round coil may have some value in depression (Klein et al., 1999).

After studies on mood alteration in healthy volunteers and open studies involving only very few subjects, the first subject-blinded, rTMS study involving 17 patients suffering from treatment-resistant major depression, psychotic subtype, was published by Pascual-Leone (Pascual-Leone et al., 1996). More recently, larger studies have been conducted and researchers have attempted to establish meaningful sham conditions. These include

(a) stimulations at different cortical sites (e.g. right prefrontal vs. left prefrontal cortex in depression),
(b) placement of the stimulation coil not tangentially to the head but tilted at 45° or
(c) 90°.

Therapeutic effects were not only investigates in mood disorders but also in other psychiatric disorders, such as anxiety, schizophrenia and tic disorders. Other studies investigated the basic neurobiology of TMS effects at different levels. TMS techniques also allowed investigations of neuronal connectivity and functionality of neural circuits (George et al., 2000b; Ziemann and Hallett, 2000). An important recent development is the combination of TMS with functional imaging; this approach affords testing of important novel hypotheses on TMS effects.

It is crucial to note that today rTMS is not indicated as a clinical treatment approach in any neuropsychiatric condition. The only disorder where a substantial body of information about clinical efficacy is available is major depression. For other disorders, only preliminary results are available or only small, non-conclusive studies have been conducted. rTMS has mainly been delivered to adult subjects, older than 20 and younger than 60 years old.

The dorsolateral prefrontal cortex (DLPFC) has been the most important target for stimulation in depression. Converging evidence from different areas of research support the hypothesis that mood is regulated by an interconnected network of brain regions encompassing prefrontal, cingulate, parietal, and temporal cortical regions as well as parts of the striatum, thalamus and hypothalamus. Lesions of this network from tumour, infarction or transient disruption may result in mood changes. In addition, alterations of cerebral blood flow and metabolism in the dorsolateral, ventrolateral, orbitofrontal, and medial frontal regions, as well as the subgenual prefrontal and anterior cingulate cortex have been demonstrated in patients suffering from major depression (Mayberg, 1997; Soares and Mann, 1997). Studies of rTMS in mood in healthy subjects (Mosimann et al., 2000) and treatment-refractory major depression selected the DLPFC as a region which is both a key part of the network discussed above and at the same time accessible to focally limited effects of TMS.

George reported the first open study of the antidepressant effects of rTMS in six treatment-resistant depressed patients treated with five daily rTMS sessions to the left DLPFC (George et al., 1995). He demonstrated that two patients in this study experienced substantial improvement as assessed by a drop of 26% in Hamilton Rating Scale for Depression (HRSD) scores. Open and blinded studies of rTMS to the left DLPFC followed with varying results. Figiel showed in a comparatively large open study that 42% of 56 patients responded to five daily rTMS sessions with a considerably lower response rate in the elderly (Figiel et al., 1998). Triggs demonstrated in a study of two weeks' treatment a 41% drop in HRSD in another open trial (Triggs et al., 1999). It is important to note that there are open studies which have failed to find any antidepressant activity of rTMS (Schouten et al., 1999).

Effect sizes have varied considerably in controlled, single-blinded studies of rTMS in treatment-resistant depression. George found only modest antidepressant efficacy of rTMS in a within-subject crossover sham-controlled study of 12 depressed patients who were treated for two weeks with stimulation to the left DLPFC (George et al., 1997). Berman found an antidepressant response in 20 subjects that was statistically different from sham stimulation using similar stimulation parameters in a parallel design, but still only of modest clinical impact (Berman et al., 2000). Both George and Berman used a low stimulation intensity of 80% of motor threshold. Generally, it seems that the higher intensity may have been more effective; however, Loo found no differences between active and sham rTMS using 110% of motor threshold (Loo et al., 1999). In a study looking at low frequency rTMS Klein demonstrated in a sham-controlled trial of 71 patients that 1 Hz stimulation to the _right_ DLPFC was significantly more effective than sham (Klein et al., 1999). It is unclear whether stimulation of the _left_ hemisphere at these parameters would have had the same effect. More recent work on rTMS treatment of acute mania suggests that right hemisphere treatment may be more effective in that condition (Grisaru et al., 1998). In a study looking at the effect of frequency, Padberg randomized 18 patients to single pulse TMS, 10 Hz rTMS and sham rTMS delivered to the left DLPFC and demonstrated a mild antidepressant effect with single pulse TMS (Padberg et al., 1999). George recently reported a sham-controlled trial in which 20 patients were randomly assigned to receive an equivalent number of pulses at 5 Hz or 20 Hz over two weeks. Both active groups had a 45% response and no patients responded to sham stimulation (George et al., 2000a). This suggests that lower frequencies may have therapeutic efficacy as well, which is important because slow rTMS is associated with a lower risk of seizure. An analysis of treatment response and cerebral metabolism suggests that patients with hypometabolism at baseline may respond better to high-frequency stimulation (20 Hz), whereas those with baseline hypermetabolism respond better to 1 Hz stimulation (Kimbrell et al., 1999); however, the effects of rTMS on mood examined in this study were not statistically significant.

In conclusion, the key findings in depression have not been systematically replicated. Effect sizes have often been small and variable. A recent systematic review of published and unpublished studies on the effectiveness of rTMS in the treatment of refractory major depression demonstrated both a relative lack in the overall quality of studies (compared to drug registration trials) and the lack of a main effect (Martin et al., 2003). Sources of variability across studies include differences in stimulation parameter settings, concomitant medications, and patient sample characteristics. In addition, simple and economical methods for precise and reliable coil placement are needed, as this factor is probably important for effectiveness (Kozel et al., 2000). In much of this work, the magnitude of antidepressant effects, while often statistically significant, has been below the threshold of clinical usefulness (Berman et al., 2000) and has not lived up to expectations raised by encouraging results in animal studies. The disparity between the human and animal studies on depression may relate to the differences in amount and site of stimulation between humans and rodents (see the section on animal studies above). Furthermore, the persistence of antidepressant effects beyond the one-to-two-week treatment period has rarely been examined. Initial evidence suggests that the beneficial effects may be transitory, making the development of maintenance strategies important if rTMS is to move to the clinic. Establishing whether nonconvulsive rTMS has antidepressant properties aside from their clinical usefulness is of theoretical importance, since positive data support the notion that focally targeted manipulations of cortical function can result in mood improvement. Nonetheless, as a clinical antidepressant intervention, the future of rTMS is far from certain.

Large multicentre studies assessing the therapeutic efficacy of TMS, for instance in major depression disorder, are urgently needed. To date, effects on mood improvement of TMS has not been compared in blinded studies against established treatments, such as pharmacotherapy and ECT.

Summary

rTMS is a relatively affordable and safe method of applying magnetic fields non-invasively to the human brain.

From the viewpoint of the *clinician*, the following comments can be made:

(a) Today data on clinical efficacy of rTMS in mood disorders are not unequivocal and results on other psychiatric disorders, such as schizophrenia and anxiety disorders have to be considered as very preliminary but nevertheless interesting and encouraging.

(b) For the therapeutic application in mood disorders, rigorously controlled and double-blinded multicentre trials are needed in order to address the question of the clinical efficacy of TMS. But before that can be done, technical problems in the application of TMS have to be solved, e.g. more satisfactory sham conditions have to be developed. Today, using analogies to pharmacological drug development, valid phase II trials have still to be conducted. Crucial open questions remain about medium- and long-term efficacy of TMS, prevention of relapse and medium- and long-term side effects. There is virtually no data on these issues since most trials have only assessed treatment response after two weeks. rTMS has not been demonstrated to be clinically equal or even superior to pharmacological treatment or to ECT. Double-blinded phase III trials, comparing established drug treatments and ECT with TMS, have still to be conducted.

(c) There is no consensus at all about possible mechanisms of action of antidepressant effects of TMS. However, this is also the case for many other treatments in psychiatry. rTMS research is basically empirical. Many variables play a role in rTMS and a large parameter space has therefore to be carefully explored in order to find the most efficacious treatment. It is likely that this complicated process will be very slow, since there is not a large amount of funding for such studies. Nevertheless, rTMS clearly has effects on the brain – which is certainly remarkable – and it might be that rTMS is a treatment modality in search of a suitable application in psychiatry. Therefore it is of utmost importance to continue on the long and difficult path of research on clinical rTMS applications.

(d) Today, different TMS methodologies have a place as diagnostic tools in neurological disorders, where neural conductivity is assessed in different, mainly demyelinating, disorders.

From the viewpoint of the *neuroscientist*, TMS is a methodology with great potential as a research tool (Hallett, 2000; Lisanby et al., 2000). This technique, by itself and combined with other methods such as EEG and neuroimaging, may be useful to test functional connectivity, neuroplasticity, information processing (for example in the visual system), indirect and direct motor control, and aspects of mood control. It affords testing of either general hypotheses of the function of the brain at different levels and hypotheses of the underlying pathology of neuropsychiatric disorders. Even if the early enthusiasm, which prevailed after early studies of clinical effects in the treatment of mood disorders settled down somewhat, rTMS will be even more useful as an investigational tool of basic and clinical research.

MAGNETIC SEIZURE THERAPY (MST)

Magnetic seizure therapy (MST) refers to the intentional induction of a seizure for therapeutic purposes using repetitive transcranial magnetic stimulation (rTMS). Like rTMS, DBS and VNS, MST is not at present FDA-approved for therapeutic application, but it is under investigation as a more focal form of convulsive therapy that has been hypothesized to carry fewer side effects than ECT.

Two observations led to the start of research about MST as a more targeted form of ECT: (a) there were some indications that rTMS stimulation at higher amplitudes might be more efficacious in the treatment of depressive disorder; (b) the established fact that therapeutic seizures have a strong and reliable effect in depression. Efficacy and side effects of ECT seem to be dependent upon the path of the current passed through the brain (Sackeim et al., 2000). Therefore, targeting seizures to focal cortical areas, such as regions of the prefrontal cortex, may reduce some side effects of convulsive treatment. The electrical field induced by magnetic stimulation is more focal than the one induced by ECT and only penetrates about 2 cm below the scalp, so its direct effects are confined to superficial cortex (Epstein, 1990). Thus, MST offers more precise control over current paths in the cortex than the transcranial application of electricity. MST has now been tested in proof of concept studies both in nonhuman primates and patients (Lisanby et al., 2001a, 2001b) and preliminary results on cognitive side effects of the treatment compared to those of ECT have been obtained (Lisanby et al., 2003). Much additional research is needed to evaluate the putative clinical efficacy of this approach and to determine whether it has significant advantages over ECT.

Preliminary studies in nonhuman primates carried out at Columbia University indicated that commercially available magnetic stimulators were not powerful enough to reliably induce seizures in an anaesthetized animal (Lisanby et al., 2001a). In order to overcome the anticonvulsant effects of anaesthesia, it was necessary to increase the maximal device output (60 Hz, 100% maximal intensity, 6.6 seconds). The first MST-induced seizure in an anaesthetized animal was performed in 1998 (Lisanby et al., 2001a). The first patient to receive MST was treated in 2000 in Bern, Switzerland, in the context of an IRB approved case study (Lisanby et al., 2001b). She was a 20-year-old inpatient with a severe major depressive episode referred for convulsive therapy due to failure to respond to adequate psychopharmacology. MST was administered in an ECT suite, under the same general anaesthetic regimen as used for ECT. The MST procedure was performed three times per week and was similar to clinical ECT procedures. Earplugs were inserted to protect hearing and EEG electrodes were modified to prevent heating that can be caused by MST. Following the induction of anaesthesia and muscular relaxation, the TMS coil was placed on the scalp and a single high-intensity train of magnetic stimulation was administered.

With high-intensity stimulation, MST induced generalized tonic-clonic seizures resembling ECT in their motor manifestations, but differing markedly from ECT in the speed of postictal recovery of orientation and in the lack of significant side effects. As this was the first human use of MST and its clinical efficacy was unknown, we only administered four MST treatments at the onset of her treatment course. Following these four treatments, the patient experienced a 50% drop in her depression scores. The treatments were well-tolerated and the only reported side effect was a mild headache after one of the treatments. There were no subjective complaints of memory problems. Mini Mental State Examination (MMSE) score remained unchanged throughout the treatment course, but more extensive neuropsychological testing was not performed. After completing her four MST sessions, the patient went on to receive ECT treatments to further reduce her symptoms and prevent relapse. Following this initial proof of concept case study, approval was obtained from the FDA and local IRB to conduct a feasibility trial of MST in the USA and another trial assessing efficacy of MST is under way in Switzerland. To date (2003) about two dozen patients suffering from refractory major depression have received MST in this trial.

MST is at present at a very early stage of development, and its ultimate clinical value in the treatment of major depression or other neuropsychiatric diseases is not yet known. Preliminary work in nonhuman primates and in patients with major depression demonstrates the feasibility of MST. Results to date suggest that seizures induced with MST differ from those induced with ECT in their length, degree of ictal expression, and degree of postictal suppression. While the number of patients receiving the treatment to date is small, there are preliminary suggestions that MST may have benefits over ECT in some measures of acute cognitive side effects, especially attention and orientation recovery (Lisanby et al., 2003). Clinical trials of the efficacy and side effects of a complete course of MST are under way, and will be important to determine whether MST has clinical value in the treatment of depression.

VAGUS NERVE STIMULATION (VNS)

Principle of VNS

Vagus nerve stimulation (VNS) in humans refers generally to stimulation of the left vagus nerve at the cervical level using the NeuroCybernetic Prosthesis (NCP, Cyberonics Inc., Houston, TX, USA) system. The first clinical investigations of VNS in humans with this system were carried out in 1988 for the treatment of intractable partial seizures (Penry and Dean, 1990). The development of the NCP was initiated on the basis of animal model experiments showing that stimulation of the vagus nerve aborted or reduced seizures (Terry et al., 1990). Since 1988, more than 16 000 NCP-systems have been implanted in patients suffering from epilepsy (Schachter, 2002). The FDA approved the NCP system in 1997 as an adjunctive therapy in reducing the frequency of seizures in adults and adolescents over 12 years of age with partial onset seizures that are refractory to antiepileptic medications. In 2001, VNS was approved for a CE mark (indicating compliance with safety and environmental regulations) in the member countries of the European Union for treatment of adults with treatment-resistant or treatment-intolerant chronic or recurrent depression, including unipolar and bipolar depression. Today VNS is an established and safe treatment of drug-resistant partial-onset seizures. In a recent *Cochrane Review* two randomized double-blind trials (both sponsored by Cyberonics Inc., results published by the VNS study group 1995 (E03-study) and by Handforth et al. (1998) (E05-study)) were analysed with regard to reduction in seizure frequency and side effects in patients suffering from drug-resistant partial epilepsy (Privitera et al., 2002).

The NCP system consists of three parts: (1) the implantable, multi-programmable bipolar NCP pulse generator which is similar to a cardiac pacemaker in size and shape. The pulse generator is housed in a hermetically sealed titanium case and is powered by a single battery (estimated life varying according to models and stimulation parameters between 0.49 and 16.4 years, at usual stimulation parameters about 5–10 years); (2) two helical electrodes which are wrapped around the left vagus nerve and are linked to the pulse generator by a bipolar lead; and (3) a programming wand linked to a computer running programming software which allows non-invasive programming, functional assessment (device diagnostics) and data retrieval. The pulse generator is implanted in a subcutaneous chest pocket just below the clavicle whereas the electrodes are attached to the vagus nerve made accessible by an incision at the level of the neck. Through a subcutaneous tunnel the electrodes are linked to the pulse generator. The implantation procedure has to be performed by a properly trained physician experienced in operating in the carotid sheath. The surgical procedure, including functional tests of the system is generally performed in about two hours in an outpatient setting. The system is able to deliver electrical impulses at frequencies between 1 and 145 Hz, at 0 to 12 mA with a pulse width varying from 130 to 1000 μs at on-times ranging from 7 to 270 s and off-times ranging from 0.2 to 180 min. A magnet allows the patient to induce VNS during an aura or at the beginning of a seizure by applying or passing the magnet over the pulse generator (Cyberonics Inc., 2001).

The left vagus nerve is the anatomical structure immediately influenced by the NCP system. In the neck, each vagus nerve lies within the carotid sheat, between the carotid artery and the jugular vein. The vagus nerves leave the skull through the jugular foramina and are attached by multiple rootlets to the medulla. They are mixed nerves, carrying about 80% afferent nerve fibres. In its cervical portion, the vagus nerves contain narrow-calibre, unmyelinated C-fibres, myelinated inter-mediate-calibre B-fibres and thicker A-fibres. Most of the cell bodies of the afferent cells are located in the vagal jugular and the nodose ganglia and project primarily to the nucleus tractus solitarius (NTS) but also to the area postrema, the spinal trigeminal nucleus, the medullary reticular formation, the dorsal nucleus of the vagus and the nucleus ambiguous (Henry, 2002). Neurons of the NTS nucleus project to numerous areas in the forebrain and the brainstem including indirect projections into the locus coeruleus and diffuse connections to the cortex. Important structures thought to mediate antiepileptic effects receiving projections from the NTS include the amygdala and the thalamus. The cell bodies of the efferent fibres are located in the nucleus ambiguous and the dorsal motor nucleus of the vagus nerve. They provide innervations of the heart, aorta, lungs, the gastrointestinal tract and also the voluntary striated muscles of the larynx and pharynx (George et al., 2000c; Vonck et al., 2001). The right vagal nerve mainly influences heart rate (Sitdikov et al., 2000). The build-up of the different parts of the vagal system – afferent and efferent parts, with their respective brainstem nuclei (NTS and nucleus ambiguous as well as the dorsal nucleus of the vagus nerve) and the asymmetric distribution of function with the right vagal nerve preferentially involved in the chronotropic regulation of the heart – has been conceptualized in an evolution-based concept, the polyvagal theory (Porges, 1995).

Mechanism of Action

The precise mechanisms by which VNS exerts its effects are not known. However, VNS influences the neuronal activities of different parts of the brain as investigated by animal and human studies during the last several years. It is probably along the anatomic distributions of vagal projections that the effects of VNS are exerted. In animal models of epilepsy, experiments suggest that the stimulation of efferent fibres does not mediate antiepileptic effects (Krahl et al., 2001). *In vivo* single cell record-ings of pyramidal neurons in the parietal association cortex of rats revealed that predominantly low-intensity trains of VNS activating predominantly myelinated fibres elicited a slow hyperpolarization, whereas the stimulation at higher intensities recruiting also unmyelinated fibres yielded a more pronounced response in some neurons but none in others (Zagon and Kemeny, 2000). Studies also performed in rats suggest that the locus coeruleus and the NTS are essentially involved in the regulation of epileptic excitability (Henry, 2002).

Studies in humans are performed by EEG methods, the measurement of evoked potentials, neuroimaging and investigations of the concentration of amino acid and phospholipid content of the cerebrospinal liquid (Henry, 2002). In 21 patients assessed with serial EEG at baseline, 3, 6 and 12 months after implantation of a VNS-system, serial electroencephalic (EEG) studies showed a progressive decrease in the number of spikes on EEG with time. In five patients who showed active spike and wave activity on baseline EEGs, a progressive increase in the duration of spike-free intervals and progressive decrease in duration and frequency of spikes and wave activity was found over time (Koo, 2001).

Investigations of possible effects of VNS in humans with brain-imaging methods yield contradictory results. Acute effects on brain activity were assessed in a blood oxygenation level dependent (BOLD) functional magnetic imaging (BOLD fMRI) study conducted in six adults with recurrent drug-resistant major depression. VNS applied for 7 seconds at 20 Hz resulted in a bilateral activation in the frontal cortex, the hypothalamus and the left globus pallidus. However, at stimulation of 5 Hz, the level of activation did not reach statistical significance compared to baseline recordings without stimulation. Brain regions activated by hearing a tone were also greater when VNS was applied at 20 Hz than at 5 Hz. These findings suggest a frequency-dependent activity of VNS (Lomarev et al., 2002). In a study investigating regional blood flow changes induced by VNS in 11 partial epilepsy patients using a positron emission tomography (PET) technique, only increase in left and right thalamic regional cerebral blood flow was correlated with seizure reduction (Henry et al., 1999). Recent similar results support this finding. In a single positron emission computed tomography/SPECT study involving 23 epilepsy patients in an acute effect setting, the left thalamus, right parahippocampal gyrus and right hippocampus were deactivated by VNS. In chronic conditions, acute stimulation resulted in a significant left thalamic activation (Van Laere et al., 2002).

The integration of the results of animal and human studies performed at different anatomical and functional levels using different methods in a unitary, straightforward model is not yet possible, either with respect to the antiepileptic activity of VNS or for its putative antidepressant effect. Putative mechanisms of antiepileptic activity in humans may be mediated through:

(a) increased synaptic activities in the thalamus and thalamocortical projection pathways, leading to increased arousal and possibly decreased synchrony of synaptic activities between and within cortical regions,

(b) through intermittently increased synaptic activity in the insula, hypothalamus and other components of the central autonomic system,

(c) through transiently decreased synaptic activities in the hypothalamus and other components of the limbic system or

(d) through intermittently increased release of norepinephrine over widespread cerebral regions (Henry, 2002).

Side Effects of VNS

Postoperative infection is estimated to occur in approximately 3% to 6% of patients (Ben-Menachem, 2001). Intraoperative ventricular asystole during the initial testing of the NCP device has been reported in nine patients. These episodes all resolved without further negative consequences for the patients (Schachter, 2002). The occurrence of such phenomena in patients with epilepsy was estimated to be 0.1% (Tatum et al., 1999). Peripheral nerves are vulnerable to injury, both from mechanical factors and electrical stimulation. Mechanical damage can be minimized by using snug-fitting, self-sizing electrodes with flexible cables and with provision for slack in the distal segment to avoid tension on the electrode array and nerve (Agnew and McCreery, 2000). Histological analysis of chronically stimulated human vagus nerves is lacking in the literature. In a case report, severe myelin loss, inflammation and fibrosis were described in a 5-year-old boy without clinical signs of vagus nerve dysfunction (stimulation at $0.25-1.5\,mA$ current, $20\,Hz$, $250\,ms$ pulse width, on-time $30\,s$ during the first three months of stimulation, off-times $15-30$ seconds, stimulation for eight months). It was not clear whether these results were a consequence of surgical manipulation or repeated stimulation (Tubbs et al., 2001).

The following side effects (percentage of a population of 95 patients) were reported in the E05-study (only side effects occurring in at least 10% of patients): voice alteration (66%), cough (45%), pharyngitis (35%), pain (28%), dyspnoea (25%), headache (24%), dyspepsia (18%), vomiting (18%), paraesthesia (18%), nausea (15%), accidental injury (13%), fever (12%), infection (12%). Voice alteration and dyspnoea were significantly higher in this stimulation group compared with the 103 patients in the low-stimulation group. One implanted patient of the high-stimulation group had postictal Cheyne–Stokes respiration that recurred also after device deactivation (Handforth et al., 1998).

One of the most frequent side effects is voice alteration. In a survey implicating 20 patients, 95% stated that they experienced vocal side effects. However, 100% of these patients would have the stimulator implanted again knowing the extent of the side effects (Charous et al., 2001). Hoarseness, cough and throat discomfort increase as output current and duty cycle increase (DeGiorgio et al., 2001).

Results available from measurements of cardiac rhythm with Holter monitoring, of respiratory function with respiratory function tests and of gastrointestinal effects with serum gastrin levels do not indicate significant effects of VNS during therapeutic stimulation (Handforth et al., 1998). Microwave transmission, cellular phones and airport systems to not affect the NCP system. However, the manufacturer advises reasonable caution in avoiding devices that generate strong electric or magnetic fields. He indicates that therapeutic radiation, external defibrillation, extracorporal shockwave lithotripsy and electrocautery surgery may damage the pulse generator's circuitry. Magnetic resonance imaging should not be performed with a magnetic resonance body coil in the transmit mode. According to the manufacturer's guidelines, an MRI should be done only using a transmit-and-receive type head of coil and specific precautions have to be observed (Cyberonics Inc., 2001).

VNS as a Putative Treatment for Affective Disorders

The first NCP system for treatment-resistant depression was implanted in 1998 at the Brain Stimulation Laboratory of the Medical University of South Carolina.

Several observations led to the systematic investigation of a possible therapeutic efficacy of VNS in depressive disorders:

(1) Improved mood and cognition were observed in epilepsy patients treated with VNS.
(2) Drugs used to treat epilepsy including carbamazepine, gabapentin, lamotrigine and valproate are also effectively used to treat mood disorders. VNS is an effective treatment of epilepsy.
(3) Positron emission tomography studies show that VNS affects the metabolism and thus the function of limbic structures in a way compatible with antidepressant function.
(4) Neurochemical studies in animals and humans reveal that VNS alters concentrations of monoamines within the central nervous system.
(5) The vagus nerve is anatomically linked to brain structures related to mood disorders (George et al., 2000b, 2000c).

To date (2003), published data of VNS in depressed patients include one open label, multicentre pilot study conducted in the USA. In this study, 30 patients were included and 30 patients were later added, of whom one patient had to be excluded from the study (Sackeim et al., 2001). Patients with a DSM-IV diagnosis of major depressive disorder or bipolar I or II disorder were included who suffered currently from a major depressive episode (MDE). The MDE had to be longer than two years in duration or the patient had to have at least four MDEs (the first 30 patients) in his or her lifetime. Patients had to score at least 3 on the Antidepressant Treatment History Form, indicating that they had failed in at least two medication trials during the current MDE using different medication classes. It was required that no substantial clinical improvement was detected in a psychotherapy trial of at least six weeks. The score on the Hamilton 28-item scale had to be at least 20 and scores on the Global Assessment of Function scale had to be 50 at maximum. Those with bipolar disorder had to have resistance, intolerance or a medical contraindication to lithium. Exclusion criteria included atypical or psychotic features in the current MDE; a history of schizophrenia, schizoaffective disorder or other non-mood-disorder psychosis; current rapid-cycling bipolar disorder; a current secondary diagnosis or signs of delirium, dementia, amnesia or other cognitive disorder; and clinically significant current suicidal intent. During the acute study (baseline period before VNS and 12-week period after the implantation) medication regimens were kept stable, except that that medication dosage could be decreased, but not increased (Sackeim et al., 2001).

In a follow-up study, the first 30 patients included were assessed until nine months after the three-month acute study. During this period, changes in psychotropic medication and VNS parameters were allowed. The response rate (defined as at least 50% reduction in baseline Hamilton rating) was 40% (12/30) and the remission rate (Hamilton rating score less than 10) increased from 17% (5/30) after the acute phase study to 29% (8/28) (Marangell et al., 2002).

Summary

In conclusion, preliminary available data suggest a sustained antidepressant effect in moderately medically resistant major depression. If these findings can be confirmed, VNS could become a key treatment in depression. Several applications in the field of neuropsychiatry are under research. Effects of VNS on memory appear to be complex. VNS could be implicated in the modulation of memory storage and enhance recognition memory in humans (Clark et al., 1999). There are indications that VNS might reversibly deteriorate figural but not verbal memory (Helmstaedter et al., 2001). Results of a pilot study suggest a positive effect of VNS on cognition in patients suffering from Alzheimer's disease (Sjogren et al., 2002). As a research tool, VNS suffers from its invasiveness. Implantation of an NCP system needs a clear indication. However, further insight into the mechanism of its action in depression, epilepsy and other neuropsychiatric disorder are expected.

REFERENCES

Agnew WF, McCreery DB (2000) Considerations for safety with chronically implanted nerve electrodes. *Epilepsia* **31**: S27–S32.

Barker AT, Jalinous R, Freeston IL (1985) Noninvasive magnetic stimulation of human motor cortex. *Lancet* **2**: 1106–1107.

Bejjani BP, Damier P, Arnulf I, et al. (1999) Transient acute depression induced by high-frequency deep-brain stimulation. *N Engl J Med* **340**: 1476–1480.

Ben-Menachem E (2001) Vagus nerve stimulation, side effects, and long-term safety. *J Clin Neurophysiol* **18**: 415–418.

Berman RM, Narasimhan M, Sanacora G, et al. (2000) A randomized clinical trial of repetitive transcranial magnetic stimulation in the treatment of major depression. *Biol Psychiatry* **47**: 332–337.

Berney A, Vingerhoets F, Perrin A, et al. (2002) Effect on mood of subthalamic DBS for Parkinson's disease: a consecutive series of 24 patients. *Neurology* **59**: 1427–1429.

Bickford RG, Guidi M, Fortesque P, Swenson M (1987) Magnetic stimulation of human peripheral nerve and brain: response enhancement by combined magnetoelectrical technique. *Neurosurgery* **20**: 110–116.

Charous SJ, Kempster G, Manders E, Ristanovic R (2001) The effect of vagal nerve stimulation on voice. *The Laryngoscope* **111**: 2028–2031.

Clark KB, Naritoku DK, Smith DC, Browning RA, Jensen RA (1999) Enhanced recognition memory following vagus nerve stimulation in human subjects. *Nature Neurosci* **2**: 94–98.

Cohrs S, Tergau F, Riech S, et al. (1998) High-frequency repetitive transcranial magnetic stimulation delays rapid eye movement sleep. *Neuroreport* **9**: 3439–3443.

Cuijpers P, Smit F (2002) Excess mortality in depression: a meta-analysis of community studies. *J Affect Disord* **72**: 227–236.

Cyberonics Inc. (2001) *Physician's Manual: NeuroCybernetic Prothesis System NCP Pulse Generator Models 100 and 101*, (May edition). Houston, TX: Cyberonics.

DeGiorgio CM, Thompson J, Lewis P, et al. (2001) Vagus nerve stimulation: analysis of device parameters in 154 patients during the long-term XE5 Study. *Epilepsia* **42**: 1017–1020.

Doi W, Sato D, Fukuzako H, Takigawa M (2001) c-Fos expression in rat brain after repetitive transcranial magnetic stimulation. *Neuroreport* **12**: 1307–1310.

Epstein C (1990) Localizing the site of magnetic brain stimulation in humans. *Neurology* **40**: 666–670.

Figiel GS, Epstein C, McDonald WM, et al. (1998): The use of rapid-rate transcranial magnetic stimulation (rTMS) in refractory depressed patients. *J Neuropsychiatry Clin Neurosci* **10**: 20–25.

Fink M (1985) *Convulsive Therapy.* New York: Raven Press.

Fleischmann A, Prolov K, Abarbanel J, Belmaker RH (1995) The effect of transcranial magnetic stimulation of rat brain on behavioral models of depression. *Brain Res* **699**: 130–132.

Flitman S, Grafman J, Wassermann E, et al. (1998) Linguistic processing during repetitive transcranial magnetic stimulation. *Neurology* **50**: 175–181.

Geddes LA (1991) History of magnetic stimulation of the nervous system. *J Clin Neurophysiol* **8**: 3–9.

George M, Nahas Z, Molloy M, et al. (2000a) A controlled trial of daily left prefrontal cortex TMS for treating depression. *Biol Psychiatry* **48**: 962–970.

George M, Sackeim H, Marangell L, et al. (2000b) Vagus nerve stimulation. A potential therapy for resistant depression? *Psychiatr Clin North Am* **23**: 757–783.

George M, Sackeim H, Rush A, et al. (2000c) Vagus nerve stimulation: a new tool for brain research and therapy. *Biol Psychiatry* **47**: 287–295.

George MS, Lisanby SH, Sackeim HA (1999) Transcranial magnetic stimulation: applications in neuropsychiatry. *Arch Gen Psychiatry* **56**: 300–311.

George MS, Wassermann EM, Williams WA, et al. (1995) Daily repetitive transcranial magnetic stimulation (rTMS) improves mood in depression. *Neuroreport* **6**: 1853–1856.

George MS, Wassermann EM, Kimbrell TA, et al. (1997) Mood improvement following daily left prefrontal repetitive transcranial magnetic stimulation in patients with depression: a placebo-controlled crossover trial. *Am J Psychiatry* **154**: 1752–1756.

George MS, Wassermann EM, Williams WA, et al. (1996) Changes in mood and hormone levels after rapid-rate transcranial magnetic stimulation (rTMS) of the prefrontal cortex. *J Neuropsychiatry Clin Neurosci* **8**: 172–180.

Greenberg BD, Murphy DL, Rasmussen SA (2000) Neuroanatomically based approaches to obsessive-compulsive disorder. Neurosurgery and transcranial magnetic stimulation. *Psychiatr Clin North Am* **23**: 671–686, xii.

Grisaru N, Amir M, Cohen H, Kaplan Z (1998) Effect of transcranial magnetic stimulation in posttraumatic stress disorder: a preliminary study. *Biol Psychiatry* **44**: 52–55.

Grisaru N, Yaroslavsky Y, Abarbanel JM, Lamberg T, Belmaker R (1994) Transcranial magnetic stimultation in depression and schizophrenia. *Eur Neuropsychopharmacol* **4**: 287–288.

Hallett M (2000) Transcranial magnetic stimulation and the brain. *Nature* **406**: 147–150.

Handforth A, DeGiorgio C, Schachter S, Uthman B, Naritoku D, Tecoma E (1998) Vagus nerve stimulation therapy for partial-onset seizures: a randomized active control trial. *Neurology* **51**: 48–55.

Hausmann A, Marksteiner J, Hinterhuber H, Humpel C (2001) Magnetic stimulation induces neuronal c-fos via tetrodotoxin-sensitive sodium channels in organotypic cortex brain slices in rat. *Neurosci Lett* **310**: 105–108.

Helmstaedter C, Hoppe C, Elger CE (2001) Memory alterations during acute high-intensity vagus nerve stimulation. *Epilepsy Res* **47**: 37–42.

Henry TR (2002) Therapeutic mechanisms of vagus nerve stimulation. *Neurology* **59**: S3–S14.

Henry TR, Votaw JR, Pennell PB, et al. (1999) Acute blood flow changes and efficacy of vagus nerve stimulation in partial epilepsy. *Neurology* **52**: 1166–1173.

Höflich G, Kasper S, Hufnagel A, Ruhrmann S, Möller HJ (1993) Application of transcranial magnetic stimulation in the treatment of drug-resistant major depression: a report of two cases. *Human Psychopharmacol* **8**: 361–365.

Hollander E, Bienstock CA, Koran LM, et al. (2002) Refractory obsessive-compulsive disorder: state-of-the-art treatment. *J Clin Psychiatry* **63**(Suppl 6): 20–29.

Ji RR, Schlaepfer TE, Aizenman CD, et al. (1998) Repetitive transcranial magnetic stimulation activates specific regions in rat brain. *Proc Natl Acad Sci USA* **95**: 15635–15640.

Keck ME, Sillaber I, Ebner K, et al. (2000) Acute transcranial magnetic stimulation of frontal brain regions selectively modulates the release of vasopressin, biogenic amines and amino acids in the rat brain. *Eur J Neurosci* **12**: 3713–3720.

Keightley ML, Winokur G, Graham SJ, Mayberg HS, Hevenor SJ, Grady CL (2003) An fMRI study investigating cognitive modulation of brain regions associated with emotional processing of visual stimuli. *Neuropsychologia* **41**: 585–596.

Kimbrell TA, Little JT, Dunn RT, et al. (1999) Frequency dependence of antidepressant response to left prefrontal repetitive transcranial magnetic stimulation (rTMS) as a function of baseline cerebral glucose metabolism. *Biol Psychiatry* **46**: 1603–1613.

Klein E, Kreinin I, Chistyakov A, et al. (1999) Therapeutic efficacy of right prefrontal slow repetitive transcranial magnetic stimulation in major depression: a double-blind controlled study. *Arch Gen Psychiatry* **56**: 315–320.

Kolbinger HM, Höflich G, Hufnagel A, Möller HJ, Kasper S (1995) Transcranial magnetic stimulation (TMS) in the treatment of major depression. *Human Psychopharmacol* **10**: 305–310.

Koo B (2001) EEG changes with vagus nerve stimulation. *J Clin Neurophysiol* **18**: 434–441.

Kozel FA, Nahas Z, de Brux C, et al (2000) How coil–cortex distance relates to age, motor threshold, and antidepressant response to repetitive transcranial magnetic stimulation. *J Neuropsychiatry Clin Neurosci* **12**: 376–384.

Krahl SE, Senanayake SS, Handforth A (2001) Destruction of peripheral C-fibers does not alter subsequent vagus nerve stimulation-induced seizure suppression on rats. *Epilepsia* **42**: 586–589.

Lisanby HS, Luber B, Schlaepfer TE, Sackeim HA (2003) Safety and feasibility of magnetic seizure therapy (MST) in major depression: randomized within-subject comparison with electroconvulsive therapy. *Neuropsychopharmacology* in press.

Lisanby SH, Luber B, Finck AD, Schroeder C, Sackeim HA (2001a) Deliberate seizure induction with repetitive transcranial magnetic stimulation in nonhuman primates. *Arch Gen Psychiatry* **58**: 199–200.

Lisanby SH, Luber B, Sackeim HA (2000) Transcranial magnetic stimulation: application in basic neuroscience and neuropsychopharmacology. *Int J Neuropsychopharmacol* **3**: 259–273.

Lisanby SH, Schlaepfer TE, Fisch HU, Sackeim HA (2001b) Magnetic seizure therapy of major depression. *Arch Gen Psychiatry* **58**: 303–305.

Lomarev MP, Denslow S, Nahas Z, Chae JH, George MS, Bohning DE (2002) Vagus nerve stimulation (VNS) synchronized BOLD fMRI suggests that VNS in depressed adults has frequency/dose dependent effects. *J Psychiat Res* **36**: 219–227.

Loo C, Mitchell P, Sachdev P, McDarmont B, Parker G, Gandevia S (1999) Double-blind controlled investigation of transcranial magnetic stimulation for the treatment of resistant major depression. *Am J Psychiatry* **156**: 946–948.

Loo C, Sachdev P, Elsayed H, et al. (2001) Effects of a 2- to 4-week course of repetitive transcranial magnetic stimulation (rTMS) on neuropsychologic functioning, electro-encephalogram, and auditory threshold in depressed patients. *Biol Psychiatry* **49**: 615–623.

Lorberbaum JP, Wassermann EM (2000) Safety concerns of TMS. In George MS, Belmaker R (eds) *Transcranial Magnetic Stimulation in Neuropsychiatry*. Washington, DC: American Psychiatric Press, pp. 141–161.

Marangell LB, Rush AJ, George MS, et al. (2002) Vagus nerve stimulation (VNS) for major depressive episodes: one year outcomes. *Biol Psychiatry* **51**: 280–287.

Martin JL, Barbanoj MJ, Schlaepfer TE, Thompson E, Perez V, Kulisevsky J (2003) Effectiveness of repetitive transcranial magnetic stimulation for the treatment of depression: systematic review and meta-analysis. *Br J Psychiatry* in press.

Mayberg HS (1997) Limbic-cortical dysregulation: a proposed model of depression. *J Neuropsychiatry Clin Neurosci* **9**: 471–481.

Mayberg HS (2002) Modulating limbic-cortical circuits in depression: targets of antidepressant treatments. *Semin Clin Neuropsychiatry* **7**: 255–268.

Mogilner A, Sterio D, Rezai A, Zonenshayn M, Kelly P, Beric A (2002) Subthalamic nucleus stimulation in patients with a prior pallidotomy. *J Neurosurgery* **96**: 660–665.

Mosimann UP, Rihs TA, Engeler J, Fisch HU, Schlaepfer TE (2000) Mood effects of repetitive transcranial stimulation (rTMS) of left prefrontal cortex in healthy volunteers. *Psychiatry Res* **94**: 251–256.

Murray NMF (1991) Magnetic stimulation of cortex: clinical applications. *J Clin Neurophysiol* **8**: 66–76.

Padberg F, Zwanzger P, Thoma H, et al. (1999) Repetitive transcranial magnetic stimulation (rTMS) in pharmacotherapy-refractory major depression: comparative study of fast, slow and sham rTMS. *Psychiatry Res* **88**: 163–171.

Pascual-Leone A, Rubio B, Pallardo F, Catala MD (1996) Rapid-rate transcranial magnetic stimulation of left dorsolateral prefrontal cortex in drug-resistant depression. *Lancet* **348**: 233–237.

Paus T, Jech R, Thompson CJ, Comeau R, Peters T, Evans AC (1997) Transcranial magnetic stimulation during positron emission tomography: a new method for studying connectivity of the human cerebral cortex. *J Neurosci* **17**: 3178–3184.

Peinemann A, Lehner C, Mentschel C, Münchau A, Conrad B, Siebner HR (2000) Subthreshold 5-Hz repetitive transcranial magnetic stimulation of the human primary motor cortex reduces intracortical paired-pulse inhibition. *Neurosci Lett* **296**: 21–24.

Penry JK, Dean JC (1990) Prevention of intractable partial seizures by intermittent vagal stimulation in humans: preliminary results. *Epilepsia* **31**: S40–S43.

Porges SW (1995) Orienting in a defensive world: mammalian modifications of our evolutionary heritage. A polyvagal theory. *Psychophysiology* **32**: 301–318.

Privitera MD, Welty TE, Ficker DM, Welge J (2002) Vagus nerve stimulation for partial seizures (*Cochrane Review*), Vol. issue 3. Oxford.

Sackeim HA, Prudic J, Devanand DP, et al. (2000) A prospective, randomized, double-blind comparison of bilateral and right unilateral electroconvulsive therapy at different stimulus intensities. *Arch Gen Psychiatry* **57**: 425–434.

Sackeim HA, Rush AJ, George MS, et al. (2001): Vagus nerve stimulation (VNS) for treatment-resistant depression: efficacy, side effects, and predictors of outcome. *Neuropsychopharmacology* **25**: 713–728.

Schachter SC (2002) Vagus nerve stimulation therapy summary – five years after FDA approval. *Neurology* **59**: S15–S20.

Schouten EA, D'Alfonso AA, Nolen WA, De Haan EH, Wijkstra J, Kahn RS (1999) Mood improvement from transcranial magnetic stimulation. *Am J Psychiatry* **156**: 669–670.

Sitdikov FG, Gil'mutdinova RI, Minnakhmetov RR, Zefirov TL (2000) Asymmetrical effects of vagus nerves on functional parameters of rat heart in postnatal ontogeny. *Bull Exp Biol Med* **130**: 620–623.

Sjogren MJ, Hellstrom PT, Jonsson MA, Runnerstam M, Silander HC, Ben-Menachem E (2002) Cognition-enhancing effect of vagus nerve stimulation in patients with Alzheimer's disease: a pilot study. *J Clin Psychiatry* **63**: 972–980.

Soares JC, Mann JJ (1997) The anatomy of mood disorders – review of structural neuroimaging studies. *Biol Psychiatry* **41**: 86–106.

Speer AM, Kimbrell TA, Wasserman EM, et al. (2000) Opposite effects of high and low frequency rTMS on regional brain activity in depressed patients. *Biol Psychiatry* **48**: 1133–1141.

Strafellea AP, Paus T, Barrett J, Dagher A (2001) Repetitive transcranial magnetic stimulation of the human prefrontal cortex induces dopamine release in the caudate nucleus. *J Neurosci* **21**(RC157): 1–4.

Szuba MP, O'Reordon JP, Rai AS, et al. (2001) Acute mood and thyroid stimulating hormone effects of transcranial magnetic stimulation in major depression. *Biol Psychiatry* **50**: 22–27.

Tatum WO, Moore DB, Stecker MM, et al. (1999) Ventricular asystole during vagus nerve stimulation for humans. *Neurology* **52**: 1267–1269.

Terry R, Tarver WB, Zabara J (1990) An implantable neurocybernetic prosthesis system. *Epilepsia* **31**: S33–S37.

Triggs WJ, McCoy KJM, Greer R, et al. (1999) Effects of left frontal transcranial magnetic simulation on depressed mood, cognition, and corticomotor threshold. *Biol Psychiatry* **45**: 1440–1445.

Tubbs RS, Patwardhan R, Palmer CA, et al. (2001) Histological appearance of a chronically stimulated vagus nerve in a pediatric patient. *Pediatr Neurosurg* **35**: 99–102.

Van Laere K, Vonck K, Boon P, Versijpt J, Dierckx R (2002) Perfusion SPECT changes after acute and chronic vagus nerve stimulation in relation to prestimulus condition and long-term clinical efficacy. *J Nucl Med* **43**: 733–744.

Vonck K, Van Laere K, Dedeurwaerdere S, Caemaert J, De Reuck J, Boon P (2001) The mechanism of action of vagus nerve stimulation for refractory epilesy: the current status. *J Clin Neurophysiol* **18**: 394–401.

Wassermann EM (2000) Side effects of repetitive transcranial magnetic stimulation. *Depress Anxiety* **12**: 124–129.

Weiner R, Rogers H, Davidson J, Squire L (1986) Effects of stimulus parameters on cognitive side effects. *Ann NY Acad Sci* **462**: 315–325.

Wulsin LR, Vaillant GE, Wells VE (1999) A systematic review of the mortality of depression. *Psychosom Med* **61**: 6–17.

Zagon A, Kemeny AA (2000) Slow hyperpolarization in cortical neurons: a possible mechanism behind vagus nerve stimulation therapy for refractory epilepsy. *Epilepsia* **41**: 1382–1389.

Ziemann U, Hallett M (2000) Basic neurophysiological studies with TMS. In George MS, Belmaker RH (eds) *Transcranial Magnetic Stimulation in Neuropsychiatry*. Washington, DC: American Psychiatric Press.

PART V
Research Issues
and Debates

Potential Targets for the Treatment of Depressive Disorders

Hans M. Rollema and Jeffrey Sprouse

Pfizer Global Research and Development, Groton, CT, USA

Despite increased knowledge of the factors that are implicated in the aetiology of mood disorders, the precise pathophysiology and cause of depression are still unknown. Since the mid-1960s, hypotheses of the pathophysiology of depression have been focused on the serotonergic and noradrenergic neurotransmitter systems, largely based on the fact that all current antidepressant drugs act via monoamine transmitter function, either by blockade of presynaptic transporters, by inhibition of monoamine oxidase, or by inhibition of receptors that regulate monoamine transmitter release. The monoamine hypothesis of depression still has a prominent place in theories on the aetiology of depression and has been further developed to include effects on autoreceptors and to explain the delayed onset of antidepressant effects. This hypothesis has guided antidepressant drug design and development for more than 40 years and led to the current first-line treatment of depression, the selective serotonin reuptake inhibitors (SSRIs). While the SSRIs have proven to be safe and effective, it is recognized that significant improvements can be made in drugs targeting monoamine transmitters and efforts to find novel antidepressants that are superior in terms of efficacy and devoid of serious side effects continue to focus on monoaminergic systems. Recent introductions or clinical studies of dual 5-HT/NE reuptake inhibitors, selective NE reuptake inhibitors, 5-HT reuptake inhibitors that incorporate affinities for other receptors and 5-HT autoreceptor antagonists are all examples of attempts to improve on the success of the SSRIs. Although restoring the balance in serotonergic and noradrenergic systems is clearly critical for a clinical response, it has been thought for a long time that alterations in monoamine levels can cause crucial post-receptor downstream changes. Recent hypotheses suggest that stress-induced disturbances in neurotrophic factors could play an important role in the aetiology of depression and that long-term effects of antidepressants are possibly mediated by changes in the post-receptor intracellular machinery. Studying the adaptive changes induced by antidepressants might therefore provide a better understanding of the neurobiological basis of depression. Results of several

Mood Disorders: Clinical Management and Research Issues. Edited by E. J. L. Griez, C. Faravelli, D. J. Nutt and J. Zohar.
©2005 John Wiley & Sons Ltd. ISBN 0 470 09426 5.

recent studies have supported this idea and suggested that abnormalities in cortico-tropin releasing factor, in cell transduction factors and neurotrophic factors may be underlying the pathophysiology of mood disorders, and accordingly represent potential novel drug targets.

This chapter discusses several novel approaches that target serotonergic, non-serotonergic and downstream systems, with an emphasis on the pharmacology of autoreceptor antagonists.

INTRODUCTION

Major depressive disorder is the most common mood disorder and a highly preva-lent brain disease. In the USA, about 19 million patients were diagnosed with depression during the year ending September 2002. Of these, 94% received drug treatment mainly with selective serotonin reuptake inhibitors (SSRIs), while more recently dual serotonin and norepinephrine reuptake inhibitors (SRI/NRIs) have been introduced, as well as a selective norepinephrine inhibitor (NRI). It is expected that because of increased recognition of the disease, the number of diag-nosed patients will continue to grow. Depression is often a chronic illness and because of the high comorbidity with other psychiatric disorders, such as general-ized anxiety disorder, panic disorders, social phobia, obsessive compulsive disorder, post-traumatic stress syndrome, it is one of the leading causes of disability. Adding to this burden is the high incidence of vegetative, somatic and cognitive symptoms, which are often associated with the core symptoms.

Given the limited access to psychotherapy and electroconvulsive therapy (ECT), pharmacotherapy with antidepressants is often the only practical treatment option. Although current first-line treatment with SSRIs has significantly improved the side-effect profile of the tricyclics (TCAs) and monoamine-oxidase inhibitors (MAOIs) and are considered to be safe, effective, and easily dosed, there are limita-tions to their utility, including delayed onset of action (four to six weeks) and the failure of approximately 30% of patients to respond to the first antidepressant treat-ment. In addition, SSRIs are associated with side effects that may limit their use, such as sexual dysfunction, gastrointestinal discomfort, somnolence and weight gain (Gummick and Nemeroff, 2000). There is thus room for improvements, but the design and development of novel antidepressants is hampered by the fact that the precise aetiology, pathophysiology and neurobiology of depression are not known. Therefore significant challenges exist to improve our understanding of depression and consequently its treatment. Multiple approaches are being pursued to address those challenges, several of which are discussed in more detail below.

Pathophysiology and Neurobiology of Depression

The precise pathophysiology and cause of depression are still obscure and a greater understanding is impeded in part by the different subtypes of depression. In fact, not much is known about the neurobiology of normal mood regulation. Studies on the genetic, neuroanatomical and biochemical correlates of the disease, often in heterogeneous and small patient populations, using different methodologies, are not easily replicated and have so far not resulted in any consistent findings.

Results of genetic linkage and chromosomal association studies have been equivocal and no abnormal genes have been found for this complex disease, possibly because the respective genes work in combination with others and the individual effects are relatively small.

The results of neuroanatomical studies are also difficult to replicate and have not shown a clear pattern of changes that might underlie mood disorders, with the possible exception of abnormalities in the volumes of subcortical white matter, which could be related to stress-induced neuronal loss (see under 'Novel Intracellular Targets'). In the future, it is likely that the technique of functional brain imaging will provide more insight into neuroanatomical abnormalities.

Likewise, there is no convincing evidence of a primary dysfunction of a specific monoaminergic system in depressed patients. The presumed perturbation of the serotonergic and noradrenergic systems could mediate the depressive symptoms, since restoring the balance in these systems seems to be critical for a clinical response. However, our understanding is limited to empirical findings with little to implicate causality. The hypothesis that an imbalance in neurotransmitter systems is responsible for depression was based on biochemical findings in patients (e.g. CSF levels of the serotonin metabolite 5-HIAA are reduced, patients relapse when tryptophan availability is limited) and on the pharmacological effects of drugs (e.g. LSD, reserpine, MAOIs, TCAs), which all increase synaptic concentrations of monoamine transmitters. One other consistent biochemical finding in depressed patients is increased cortisol release, likely to be the consequence of hyperactivity of the hypothalamus-pituitary-adrenal (HPA) axis.

Development of SSRIs and Related Antidepressants

After the serendipitous findings in the 1950s that a derivative of a phenothiazine antihistaminic drug, the TCA imipramine, and a tuberculostatic MAOI, iproniazid, had antidepressant effects, it was soon discovered that these drugs all block the reuptake or degradation of monoamines in the brain, thereby increasing the availability of neurotransmitter in the synaptic cleft to interact with postsynaptic receptors. This represented a breakthrough in the thinking about mood disorders, since it clearly indicated that a chemical could restore what was probably an imbalance in neurotransmitters in the brain of depressed patients. These findings led to the formulation of the 'monoamine hypothesis of depression', i.e. that the biological basis for depression is a deficiency of the monoamine neurotransmitters in the brain (Schildkraut, 1965; Bunney and Davis, 1965). Obviously, this led to a search for more selective inhibitors of monoamine transporters, especially for inhibitors of the serotonin transporter. Serotonin was singled out, because it was thought that the side effects of TCAs could be due to the inhibition of norepinephrine reuptake (NRI). The SSRIs that were subsequently developed also lacked affinity for adrenergic, cholinergic and histaminergic receptors which, as it turns out, were causing many of the side effects of TCAs. Maintaining antidepressant activity and being much safer, SSRIs have become the first-line antidepressant treatment (see Figure 14.1). Currently about 30 antidepressant drugs are available on the market: the SSRIs (fluvoxamine, fluoxetine, sertraline, paroxetine, citalopram), the dual SRI/NRIs (venlafaxine, milnacipran), a NRI/DRI (bupropion) and an $\alpha_2/5\text{-HT}_{2A}$ antagonist (mirtazapine). Second-line therapies include several generic TCAs (amitryptiline, clomipramine, desipramine, imipramine, etc.) and MAOIs (phenelzine, tranylcypromine, moclobemide).

IMPROVING SEROTONERGIC ANTIDEPRESSANTS

Efforts to improve antidepressant therapy are focused on designing new drugs that will have better efficacy (i.e. improved response rates or remission rates), faster onset of action and reduced side effects.

Improving Efficacy

Dual Reuptake Inhibitors

Results of comparative studies suggest that TCAs might be more efficacious antidepressants than SSRIs, possibly because TCAs increase the synaptic availability of both 5-HT and NE. When it was recognized that the poor side-effect profile of the TCAs was related to their histaminergic, adrenergic and cholinergic properties, rather than to inhibition of norepinephrine reuptake, it was concluded that combining norepinephrine and serotonin reuptake inhibition (SRI/NRI) might lead to compounds with the efficacy of TCAs, but without their side effects. Combined SRI/NRIs (milnacipran, venlafaxine) are now available, and although some trials seem to indicate that SRI/NRIs may have improved efficacy, more comparative studies are required to definitively establish whether these agents have indeed better efficacy. Since it is conceivable that the antidepressive effect of the TCAs stems more from blocking NE than 5-HT reuptake, selective NRIs are also being developed as antidepressants, such as reboxetine.

Finally, based on the well-established role of dopamine in reward mechanisms and the fact that anhedonia is a hallmark of depression, some investigators believe that blocking the reuptake of dopamine in addition to that of serotonin and norepinephrine, might lead to more efficacious antidepressants. Such compounds are not available yet and further studies will indicate if this is a good approach or if additional side effects are being introduced when all three monoamine transporters are blocked simultaneously.

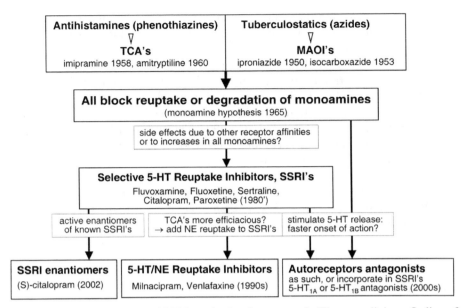

Figure 14.1 Development of SSRIs and related compounds. The serendipitous finding of antidepressant activity of tricyclics and monoamine oxidase inhibitors in the 1950s and the discovery that these compounds increase serotonergic neurotransmission, led to the formulation of the monoamine hypothesis of depression around 1965 and to the development of selective serotonin reuptake inhibitors in the 1980s. Since then, less selective reuptake inhibitors are being purposefully designed by incorporating additonal reuptake or autoreceptor antagonist properties in an SSRI. Recently, enantiomers of racemic SSRIs (sertraline and paroxetine were originally launched as the active enantiomer) have been developed

Recently the active enantiomers of the SSRIs that have been marketed so far as the racemates have been developed. This is not a novel pharmacological approach, but makes the SSRI 'cleaner' by removing the inactive or less active component from the racemic mixture. Obviously this was already the case for the two SSRIs that were originally launched as the active enantiomers, sertraline and paroxetine.

Augmentation Strategies

Another approach aimed at increasing the efficacy of SSRIs is the augmentation therapy, i.e. combining an SSRI with an antidepressant that has a different mechanism of action (e.g. co-administering an SSRI with the α_2 antagonist mirtazapine or with the 5-HT$_{1A}$ agonist buspirone). Although the combination of antidepressants with different biochemical mechanisms could theoretically result in a synergistic effect and thus increased efficacy, so far only results of small, open studies have been published and there is as yet little evidence for increased efficacy by such combinations.

Addition of a non-antidepressant drug (e.g. lithium, triodothyronine, antipsychotics) to SSRI treatment is also being investigated and recent clinical data suggest that the combined administration of atypical antipsychotics and SSRIs might be more efficacious than an SSRI alone, especially in treatment-resistant major depression (Ostroff and Nelson, 1999). The mechanism of this putative increase in efficacy of such drug combinations is not known and several preclinical studies are in progress to address this question.

Finally, several studies have been published on augmenting the SSRI response by potentiating the effect of the SSRI on extracellular 5-HT levels with 5-HT$_{1A}$ or 5-HT$_{1B}$ autoreceptor antagonists. The rationale for this approach is discussed in more detail below, under '5-HT antagonists'.

Faster Onset of Action

Despite the fact that SSRIs, like TCAs and MAOIs, interact with their targets almost immediately and produce a biochemical effect shortly after administration, it takes still four to six weeks until the effect of the treatment is apparent. There is a consensus that after the initial monoamine increase, secondary processes have to take place to produce the clinical effect. At present there are two hypotheses that account for the delayed onset of antidepressant action. One is that serotonergic autoreceptors, which are initially activated by elevated 5-HT levels, have to desensitize to eliminate the opposing effect they have on the SSRI-induced extracellular 5-HT levels. This hypothesis is discussed in detail below under '5-HT antagonists'. The other hypothesis is that the elevated monoamine levels trigger downstream signalling pathways that induce longer-term changes in transcription and gene expression that is responsible for the slow onset of the clinical effect. This hypothesis is briefly discussed below under 'Novel Intracellular Targets'.

The fact that the effect of SSRIs is mediated by 5-HT activation of postsynaptic 5-HT receptors, most of which may be of the 5-HT$_{1A}$ subtype, raises the interesting possibility that 5-HT$_{1A}$ agonists per se could be fast-acting antidepressants, since these compounds should immediately activate postsynaptic 5-HT$_{1A}$ receptors and produce an effect. However, clinically tested 5-HT$_{1A}$ receptor agonists (flesinoxan, buspirone) have only moderate antidepressant efficacy and do not have a faster onset of action. Possible explanations for this are *inter alia* that the compounds have insufficient receptor occupancy, that other than 5-HT$_{1A}$ receptors need to be activated, or that poor pharmacokinetic properties partially prevent their full potential clinical efficacy (Blier and Ward, 2003).

Reducing Side Effects

Sexual dysfunction is one of the side effects frequently associated with the use of serotonergic antidepressants and it is generally believed that the high incidence of sexual dysfunction results from activation of postsynaptic serotonergic receptors that might be involved in sexual behaviour. The antidepressant-induced sexual dysfunction can sometimes be managed by dose reduction, drug holidays, switching antidepressant drugs and by appropriate co-medication. Adding an α_2 antagonist, a 5-HT_2 antagonist or a dopamine agonist has in some cases yielded beneficial effects, probably because blockade or activation of these receptors can counteract sexual dysfunction, regardless of the cause. This concept is consistent with some reports that the antidepressant mirtazapine, which is an $\alpha_2/5\text{-HT}_{2A}$ antagonist, may produce less sexual dysfunction (Montejo et al., 2001). However, there is still a great need for effective antidepressants that do not produce sexual side effects. One of the possible strategies is the incorporation of additional receptor affinities in an SSRI, either antagonist affinities to block unwanted interactions of 5-HT with specific serotonin receptor types that are thought to mediate the sexual side effects, or agonist activities that will enhance sexual behaviour to counteract the side effects. As of yet there are no examples of such 'mixed' 5-HT reuptake inhibitors that have been shown to be effective antidepressants and to produce significantly less side effects.

INCORPORATING SEROTONIN AUTORECEPTOR ANTAGONISM

5-HT_{1A} Antagonists

Although acute SSRIs increase extracellular *5-HT levels* by blocking the 5-HT transporter, the extent of 5-HT release is hampered by the rising 5-HT levels in the cell body area, which activate somatodendritic 5-HT_{1A} autoreceptors resulting in reduced neuronal cell firing and release (see Figures 14.2 to 14.4). The net result of acute SSRIs is thus initially a diminished terminal 5-HT release, but during chronic SSRI treatment and hence continuous exposure to high 5-HT levels, the somatodendritic 5-HT_{1A} receptors are thought to desensitize over time. Since these autoreceptors are now activated to a smaller degree, they do not attenuate the effects of the SSRI on terminal 5-HT levels. If a 5-HT_{1A} antagonist were present in the brain, 5-HT_{1A} autoreceptors would be blocked (i.e. immediately 'desensitized'), so that the SSRI would produce a faster and more pronounced increase in terminal 5-HT release, allowing activation of the postsynaptic 5-HT receptors that mediate the clinical effects. This biochemical model for the delayed onset of activity was confirmed in several in vivo animal studies, measuring actual extracellular 5-HT levels in the brains of awake animals by microdialysis. In these experiments, 5-HT_{1A} antagonists were indeed found to potentiate the effect of a low dose of SSRI on extracellular 5-HT levels. These results prompted clinical studies on the effect of combining SSRIs with a 5-HT_{1A} antagonist, since a 5-HT_{1A} antagonist was already available in the clinic, the mixed 5-HT_{1A}, 5-HT_{1B} and β_2 antagonist, pindolol (Artigas, 1993; Blier and de Montigny, 1994; Perez et al., 1999).

Although the initial open label, as well as some double-blind studies reported very positive results, several later studies were equivocal or negative (for a review see Nelson, 2000). Taken together, the clinical data seem to suggest that pindolol may have some augmentation effects, but it is actually not certain whether those effects are indeed due to its 5-HT_{1A} blocking properties. In the first place, several in vitro and in vivo studies have shown that pindolol can act as a partial 5-HT_{1A} agonist rather than as a full antagonist. For instance, pindolol decreases cell firing of serotonergic neurons in the cell bodies in guinea pig, an effect that was completely blocked by the full 5-HT_{1A} antagonist, WAY 100635, suggesting 5-HT_{1A} partial agonist effects of pindolol in this in vivo model (Sprouse et al., 2000). Secondly, recent studies have provided evidence that the brain levels of pindolol after doses that are used in the augmentation studies (2.5 mg t.i.d.) are insufficient to effectively block 5-HT_{1A} receptors (Rabiner, 2001; Cremers, 2001). In the case of pindolol then, the 5-HT_{1A} hypothesis has not really been tested yet and is awaiting trials with a potent and more selective 5-HT_{1A} antagonist. That compound would need the additional selectivity of acting on pre- vs. postsynaptic 5-HT_{1A} receptors, if activation of postsynaptic 5-HT_{1A} sites is mediating the serotonergic effect, and in turn, the clinical benefits.

5-HT_{1B} antagonists

In addition to 5-HT_{1A} autoreceptors on the cell bodies that control cell firing, the serotonergic neurons also contain 5-HT_{1B} autoreceptors on the nerve terminals that regulate 5-HT release. Activation of the terminal autoreceptors by elevated 5-HT will reduce terminal 5-HT release and thus also oppose the acute effects of an SSRI. Following the same reasoning as above for 5-HT_{1A} antagonists, blocking terminal autoreceptors with a 5-HT_{1B} antagonist represents an alternative SSRI augmentation strategy. By immediately blocking the 5-HT_{1B} receptor, the SSRI-induced elevated 5-HT levels can no longer activate the release-regulating autoreceptors, so that when co-administered with an SSRI, the increase in 5-HT would be faster and more pronounced. That concept has also been confirmed in microdialysis animal studies in vivo (e.g. Rollema et al., 1996; Figure 14.3).

However, there is an important distinction between the 5-HT_{1B} and the 5-HT_{1A} antagonist approaches: 5-HT_{1A} antagonists have no effects on 5-HT release (i.e. they do not *increase* cell firing rates by themselves), while 5-HT_{1B} antagonists have been shown to increase terminal 5-HT release in guinea pig brain when given alone

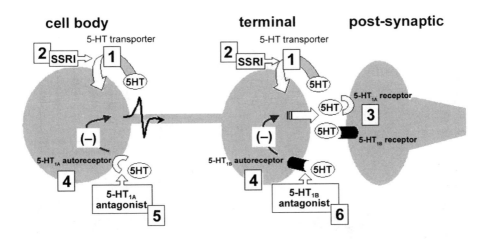

Figure 14.2 Effects of SSRIs and autoreceptor antagonists on the serotonergic system. The numbers in the schematic refer to sites where serotonergic drugs can affect 5-HT cell firing, extracellular 5-HT levels and 5-HT release. 1: 5-HT transporters in cell bodies and in nerve terminals remove 5-HT after it is released. 2: SSRIs block the 5-HT transporter and thereby increase extracellular 5-HT levels. 3: 5-HT can interact with different postsynaptic receptors (e.g. 5-HT_{1A}, 5-HT_{1B}, 5-HT_{2A}, etc.) mediating the serotonergic effects and in turn the clinical benefits. 4: At the same time the elevated 5-HT also activates autoreceptors, which will decrease cell firing (in cell bodies, 5-HT_{1A}) and 5-HT release (in terminals, 5-HT_{1B}), attenuating the SSRI effect on extracellular 5-HT levels. 5: 5-HT_{1A} antagonists block cell body autoreceptors and potentiate the SSRI effect. 6: 5-HT_{1B} antagonists block the terminal autoreceptor and potentiate the SSRI effect or produce an increase in terminal 5-HT release by themselves

(Rollema et al., 1996). Recently several studies have shown that compounds that act as *inverse agonists* at the 5-HT_{1B} (which have the opposite effect of agonists and also stimulate 5-HT release like antagonists) may be more efficacious under conditions of low serotonergic tone, as may be the case in depression (Middlemiss et al., 1999). It is thus conceivable that 5-HT_{1B} antagonists or 5-HT_{1B} inverse agonists will act as antidepressants on their own, with the advantage that in the absence of an SSRI there is no need for desensitization (or pharmacological blockade) of cell body 5-HT_{1A} autoreceptors, since there is in vivo electrophysiological evidence that 5-HT_{1B} antagonists do not affect cell firing (Sprouse et al., 1997; see Figure 14.4).

There could be additional advantages related to the presence of 5-HT_{1B} heteroreceptors, which are thought to regulate the release of other transmitters that may be involved in depression, such as DA, NE, ACh and GABA. The presence of postsynaptic 5-HT_{1B} receptors, which are thought to play a role in sexual behaviour, are another important consideration in the sense that blockade of these receptors by a 5-HT_{1B} antagonist may reduce certain sexual side effects. Finally, since

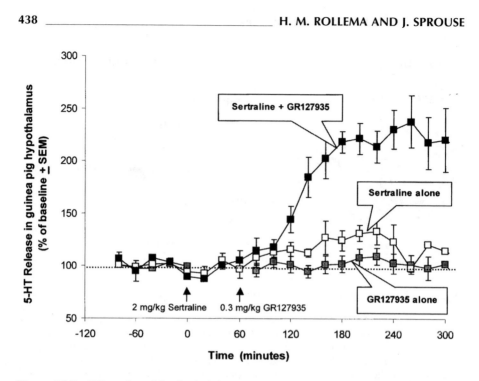

Figure 14.3 Effect of combined administration of an SSRI and a 5-HT$_{1B}$ antagonist on in vivo 5-HT release. Extracellular 5-HT levels were measured by in vivo microdialysis in the hypothalamus of awake guinea pigs and drug effects are expressed as percentages of the average pre-drug baseline levels (=100%). The SSRI sertraline and the 5-HT$_{1B}$ antagonist GR127935 are given s.c. (at arrows) at low doses, which when given alone have no or only a small effect on 5-HT release, but when given together produce a robust 5-HT increase. This synergistic effect demonstrates augmentation of the neurochemical SSRI response by 5-HT$_{1B}$ autoreceptor blockade in vivo (Rollema et al., 1996)

5-HT$_{1B}$ receptors have been postulated to play an important role in obsessive-compulsive disorder (El Mansari and Blier, 1996; Mundo et al., 2002), 5-HT$_{1B}$ antagonists might have additional therapeutic applications, similar to the SSRIs in this respect, but again with a more rapid course of action.

In summary, both 5-HT$_{1B}$ antagonist and SSRI treatment will produce the increases in serotonergic neurotransmission that are thought to be necessary for the alleviation of depressive symptoms. In the case of an SSRI, this is accomplished by blockade of the reuptake carrier followed by a gradual desensitization of the cell body and nerve terminal autoreceptors that inhibit 5-HT release. In the case of a 5-HT$_{1B}$ antagonist, blockade of the 5-HT$_{1B}$ autoreceptors occurs acutely and will increase 5-HT release, potentially leading to a more rapid clinical response.

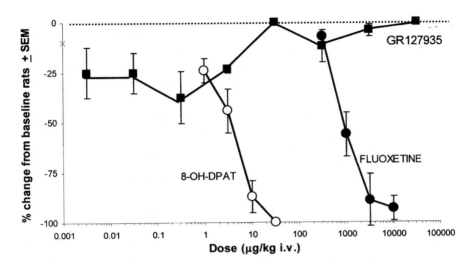

Figure 14.4   Effect of a 5-HT$_{1A}$ agonist, an SSRI and a 5-HT$_{1B}$ antagonist on in vivo 5-HT cell firing in the cell body area. Cell firing is measured in the cell body area (dorsal raphe) in anaesthetized guinea pigs and the effects of the drugs, measured after i.v. administration, are expressed as the percentage change from pre-drug baseline cell firing. Low doses of a full 5-HT$_{1A}$ agonist (8-OH-DPAT) completely shut down cell firing by direct activation of 5-HT$_{1A}$ autoreceptors, an SSRI (fluoxetine) decreases cell firing by indirect activation of 5-HT$_{1A}$ autoreceptors via elevated 5-HT levels, while the 5-HT$_{1B}$ antagonist (GR127935) has no effect on in vivo cell firing at any of the doses tested (Sprouse et al., 1997)

NOVEL NON-SEROTONERGIC ANTIDEPRESSANT TARGETS

Corticotropin-releasing Factor 1 (CRF$_1$) Antagonists

As mentioned before, there is general agreement that while all current antidepressant drugs target monoaminergic systems, it is likely that other neurobiological systems are involved in mediating the antidepressant effect. In view of the fact that many depressed patients hypersecrete cortisol, reflecting hyperactivity of the hypothalamus–pituitary–adrenal (HPA) axis, it has been suggested that drugs that can regulate HPA axis activity could be possible treatments for mood disorders. The activity of the HPA axis is determined by genetic and environmental factors and is under continuous feedback control of corticotropin-releasing factor (CRF), a 41 amino-acid neuropeptide that is released from the hypothalamus and stimulates the secretion of corticotropin (ACTH) from the anterior pituitary into the bloodstream. CRF plays thus a central role in the coordination of neuroendocrine, autonomic and behavioural responses to stress by regulating adrenal glucocorticoid activity and activating CRF receptors in various brain areas, such as hippocampus and amygdala (Figure 14.6). High CRF levels increase the activity of the HPA axis and so stimulate cortisol secretion, which may lead to detrimental effects, but in addition CRF can also produce several negative, depression-like behavioural responses (e.g. fear, decreased appetite, decreased sexual behaviour, increased blood pressure) by excessive stimulation of CRF_1 receptors (Arborelius et al., 1999; Holsboer, 1999). If the negative feedback control on hypothalamic CRF release is indeed decreased in depression, resulting in continuous hyperactivity of CRF neural circuits, then offsetting the negative effects of extreme CRF_1 receptor activation by blocking CRF_1 receptors with a selective, centrally acting CRF_1 antagonist could have an antidepressant effect (Figure 14.5).

Since potent competitive CRF antagonists have been available for some time, the rationale for CRF antagonists as novel antidepressants has been confirmed in a great number of behavioural and biochemical animal studies. However, the CRF antagonists that were used in these experiments were peptides (α-helical CRF_{9-41}, D-Phe-CRF_{2-41}), which are unsuitable as drug molecules because they lack selectivity and are limited by poor bioavailablity, requiring intracerebral administration to enter the CNS. It was thus necessary to design small, non-peptide molecules, which are orally bioavailable, long-acting and highly selective for the target receptor subtype (in this case CRF_1, the subtype that mediates CRF-induced psychopathology). Researchers at Pfizer were the first to synthesize and characterize such a small molecule, CP-154,526, a potent and selective CRF_1 antagonist (Schulz et al., 1996). Animal studies showed that CP-154,526 blocked the CRF-induced increases in ACTH release and in locus coeruleus cell firing. In behavioural models, CP-154,526 attenuated fear-potentiated startle responses and reduced escape deficits in the learned helplessness model, the latter supporting the utility of CRF antagonists in depression. Since then several CRF_1 antagonists have been synthesized and investigated, but only a few have entered clinical trials. So far only one small, open label study on the safety, toleration and neuroendocrine effects of a CRF_1 antagonist, R121919, in 20 patients with major depression has been published (Zobel, 2000). The results (Table 14.1) suggest an antidepressant effect of the CRF antagonist, showing a 12–16 points drop in the HAM-D and HAM-A scales after four weeks of treatment, which persuaded the authors to conclude that 'these findings, along with the observed worsening of affective symptomatology after drug discontinuation, suggests that the pharmacological principle of CRF_1 receptor antagonism has considerable therapeutic potential in the treatment and the prevention of diseases where exaggerated central CRF activity is present at baseline or following stress exposure' (Zobel et al., 2000).

The development of R121919 unfortunately had to be halted because of hepatotoxicity and future studies with other compounds are needed to determine whether the blockade of central CRF_1 receptors is a viable and safe approach for treatment of mood disorders.

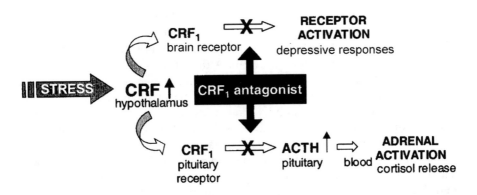

Figure 14.5. Schematic illustration of the potential antidepressant mechanism of CRF_1 receptor antagonists. CRF stimulates the secretion of ACTH that activates the adrenal cortex to release cortisol. Cortisol secretion is under tight negative feedback control, since hypersecretion may lead to neuronal damage. Blockade of pituitary CRF_1 receptors by antagonists attenuates cortisol secretion by preventing the effect of increased CRF release. In addition, too much stimulation of CRF_1 receptors in various brain areas can produce depression-like behavioural responses. By blocking brain CRF_1 receptors the detrimental effects of excessive CRF_1 release are prevented. The potential antidepressant effect of centrally acting CRF_1 antagonists is thought to be mediated via these mechanisms

TABLE 14.1   Results of an open label trial with the CRF_1 antagonist, R121919 (data taken from Zobel et al., 2000). Numbers represent the HAM-D and HAM-A scores at the start of the trial and after four weeks dosing patients with 5–40 mg/day or with 40–80 mg/day R121919

	R121919 5–20–40 mg/day	R121919 40–60–80mg/day
Antidepressant effect		
HAM-D score at start (Day 0)	26	28
HAM-D score at four weeks (Day 30)	15	11
Antianxiety effect		
HAM-A score at start (Day 0)	23	27
HAM-A score at four weeks (Day 30)	14	10

Neurokinin₁ (NK₁) Antagonists

The NK_1 receptor is one of the tachykinin receptors for substance P, a peptide neuro-transmitter that is involved in neuronal processing of various noxious and stressful stimuli, in modulating emesis and in the inflammation process. Naturally, there has been interest in designing substance P antagonists as potential therapeutics, but as in the case of the CRF antagonists, antagonists based on neuropeptides backbones lack good drug properties. More than 10 years ago, Pfizer scientists described the first non-peptide small molecule NK_1 antagonists, CP-96,345 and CP-99,994 (Snider et al., 1991; McLean et al., 1991). Although these and many other NK_1 antagonists were also screened in the standard antidepressant animal models at that time, no antidepressant effects were detected. Surprisingly, several years later, scientists at Merck reported that NK_1 antagonists might have antidepressant properties, an opportunistic finding made possible by noting a reduction in stress-induced vocalization in guinea pig pups (Kramer et al., 1998). These interesting findings prompted Phase II studies on the lead compound, MK869, which showed that this NK1 antagonist had antidepressant effects, comparable to the positive control paroxetine and significantly better than placebo (Kramer et al., 1998). A comparison of the side-effect profiles in the three patient groups shows a clearly reduced incidence of sexual side effects in MK869-treated patients compared with patients on paroxetine (Table 14.2).

If NK_1 antagonists indeed turn out to have antidepressant activity, the lack of sexual side effects could be one of the major advantages over SSRIs. Further studies with other NK_1 antagonists will show whether or not blockade of NK_1 receptors represents a useful alternative to SSRI treatment (Stout et al., 2001).

The exact antidepressant mechanism of NK_1 antagonists is not yet known, although recent evidence suggests that it is either related to inducing alterations in substance P release or to changes in serotonergic transmission. The substance P system may play a role in depression, since substance P-containing pathways (e.g. from amygdala to hypothalamus and periaqueductal grey) are important in the response to stressors and substance P is released in amygdala after stress. The notion

TABLE 14.2   Summary of results of a trial with the NK_1 antagonist, MK869 (data taken from Kramer et al., 1998). Numbers represent decreases in HAM-D scores (antidepressant effect) and percentage of patients with sexual side effects (adverse events) in patients treated with the NK_1 antagonist MK869, with the SSRI paroxetine, or with placebo

	MK-869 ($n=71$)	Paroxetine ($n=72$)	Placebo ($n=70$)
Antidepressant effect			
HAM-D-D21 decrease at 2 weeks	−9	−10	−5
HAM-D-D21 decrease at 6 weeks	−13	−12	−9
Sexual adverse events			
Libido decreased	0	6	0
General sexual dysfunction	0	8	0
Ejaculation disorder (% males)	3	20	7
Impotence (% males)	3	10	4
Sexual dysfunction (combined)	3	26	4

that the serotonergic system might be involved in the therapeutic effect of NK_1 receptor blockade, comes from the finding that dorsal raphe cell firing is increased when animals are treated with NK_1 antagonists and in NK_1 knock-out mice. An increase in neuronal activity is consistent with desensitization of $5\text{-}HT_{1A}$ autoreceptors in the cell body region, an effect that chronic SSRIs show as well (Santarelli et al., 2001). These data suggests that the substance P and 5-HT transmitter systems can interact with each other and that NK_1 antagonists have a similar acute effect on cell firing as chronic SSRIs. This would imply that NK_1 antagonists could have a faster onset of action, although it is clear that the initial clinical data from the MK869 study do not support a faster onset of antidepressant effect, as HAM-D scores follow similar time courses in the MK869 and paroxetine treated groups. Since this was only the first trial with an NK_1 antagonist, it is of course possible that further studies and more clinical trials may tell a different story.

NOVEL INTRACELLULAR TARGETS

Signal Transduction Pathways and Neurotrophic Factors

While all current antidepressant treatments modulate monoaminergic neurotransmission, this effect per se may not actually produce the antidepressant activity. Therefore, it has been hypothesized that instead, the increased monoamine levels could trigger changes in other pathways that ultimately mediate the antidepressant effect. Several studies are now focused on identifying secondary processes and pathways that may be linked to the mechanism of action of antidepressants and could represent some of the underlying factors in the pathophysiology of mood disorders. A current hypothesis (for reviews see Duman et al., 1997, 2000; Manji et al., 2001) is based on the notion that stress-induced neuronal damage in vulnerable brain areas early in life, may lead to depressive symptoms and that antidepressants can reverse that process by activating intracellular pathways that stimulate repair mechanisms.

This scenario implies a crucial role for intracellular transduction pathways and neurotrophic factors, which are potent regulators of neural plasticity and support the survival of adult neuronal and glia cells.

The transduction pathways form complex signalling networks that facilitate the system to respond to signals that are generated by receptor activation, e.g. resulting from elevated neurotransmitter levels after antidepressants. The sequence of events that is involved in such pathways can be briefly exemplified as follows (see Figure 14.6): when a receptor is activated by a neurotransmitter, the cyclic adenosine-3′,5′-monophosphate (cAMP) system (or another second messengers system, such as cGMP, inositol triphosphate, Ca^{++}) is activated, resulting in increased levels of cAMP and protein kinases (PKA), which in turn will stimulate the expression of the transcription factor CREB (cAMP-response-element-binding protein). Increased CREB expression will subsequently lead to up-regulation of specific target genes, such as BDNF (brain-derived neurotrophic factor) and its receptor, tyrosine kinase BDNF (trkB) in the hippocampus and cortex. Stress is believed to reduce the expression of neurotrophic factors and therefore to cause atrophy or cell death of vulnerable neurons in the hippocampus, resulting in depressive symptoms. When it was found that chronic treatment with different types of antidepressants actually increases expression of the proteins and factors that are involved in this intracellular signalling pathway, it was proposed that this effect could be a final common mechanism of action of antidepressants (Duman et al., 1997). Such a hypothesis would account for the delayed onset of antidepressants, since the up-regulation of transcription factors and target genes will take much longer than it takes to increase monoamine levels. This model is also consistent with recent neuroimaging observations of reduced volumes of certain brain areas in depressed patients, supporting the neurodegenerative aspect of the pathophysiology of depression (Bremner et al., 2000). Since it is quite possible that the neuronal damage caused by stress is mediated via increases in stress hormones, in particular by hypersecretion of corticosteroids, the neurotrophic mechanism could also readily be linked to the theory of hyperactivity of the HPA axis in depression.

This unifying hypothesis about depression accounts for the actions of serotonergic as well as novel non-serotonergic antidepressants and may thus provide a

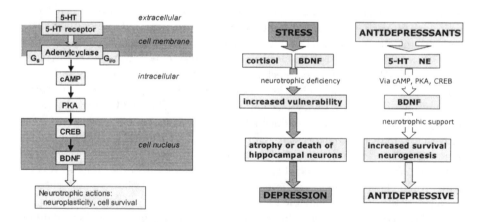

Figure 14.6 Schematic of the proposed role of transduction pathways and neurotrophic factors in the aetiology and treatment of depression. The left diagram illustrates how 5-HT receptor activation triggers a chain of events, starting with stimulation of second messengers (e.g. cAMP) via GPCRs ($G_{i/o}$ or G_s). This causes an increase in phosphokinase (PKA) activity, which in turn stimulates the expression of transcription factors (CREB) and ultimately of BDNF, which supports cell repair and survival. The diagram on the right shows how stress causes high cortisol secretion that can lead to neuronal atrophy or death in susceptible areas (e.g. hippocampus), especially if the protection by neurotrophic factors is insufficient. The neuronal damage that leads to depressive symptoms is thought to be reversed by enhancing neurotrophic support via stimulating BDNF formation, following increases in the signal transduction pathways after antidepressant treatment (Duman et al., 1997, 2000)

basis for new therapies. The numerous components of the signal transduction pathway, including the cAMP system, protein kinases, the transcription and neurotrophic factors and many others, provide a multitude of opportunities to intervene with drugs. These could be drugs that directly stimulate BDNF release or drugs that target upstream components that play a role in the regulation of BDNF expression. The rapidly increasing knowledge in this area could lead to the identification and validation of small molecules that target these sites, although it may take several years before such compounds will be available.

SUMMARY AND CONCLUSIONS

The precise pathophysiology and neurobiology of depression are still unknown and until recently hypotheses on depression focused on the serotonergic and noradrenergic neurotransmitter systems exclusively. Such a limited scope was fuelled by the knowledge that all currently used antidepressant drugs affect monoaminergic systems. At the same time, it is also recognized that the current antidepressant drugs, while being effective and safe, can be improved regarding their efficacy, onset of action and side-effect profile. Such improvements may be possible by incorporating certain desirable properties in SSRIs, essentially generating less selective uptake inhibitors with improved antidepressant profiles. Examples of such approaches are the dual reuptake inhibitors that block both the 5-HT and NE transporter, SSRIs with 5-HT$_{1A}$ or 5-HT$_{1B}$ receptor antagonist affinity and 5-HT$_{1B}$ antagonists or inverse agonists per se. Attempts to discover non-serotonergic antidepressants that will affect other than the monoaminergic systems, have been mainly focused on the development of selective, small molecule antagonists of the neuropeptides, CRF$_1$ and NK$_1$. Preliminary findings suggest that both CRF$_1$ and NK$_1$ antagonists might have antidepressant activities, but more studies are needed to confirm this and to show whether these compounds have distinct advantages over currently used SSRIs and SRI/NRIs. It is also now recognized that the initial effect of antidepressant drugs on the monoamines could be the starting point for further, later-occurring changes in downstream systems, such as the signalling transduction cascade and neurotrophic factors. Future developments will therefore target components of the intracellular signalling systems and the regulation of neurotrophic factors, but it will still take several years before novel compounds will be developed that can demonstrate the utility of this approach in the clinic. Increasing our knowledge and insights in the neurobiology of depression will help to guide the search for novel agents, but at the same time the reciprocal is also true, namely that the outcome of clinical studies with novel agents are in turn likely to improve our understanding of the pathophysiology and aetiology of depression.

A final comment about developing new antidepressant drugs from the point of view of the drug discovery and development process. Identifying new potential targets for antidepressant drugs is not the same as finding new antidepressant drugs, since it takes now on average 10–15 years and US$500–700 million from the identification of a target to marketing a new medication. This lengthy and costly process includes among others, the task of expressing the target for screening assays, synthesizing and identifying lead compounds, optimizing compounds to generate a suitable drug molecule, long-term toxicological studies, safety studies in healthy volunteers in Phase I, and finally several clinical trials in a great number of patients. Research on dual reuptake inhibitors, on $5\text{-}HT_{1A}$ and $5\text{-}HT_{1B}$ receptor antagonists and on CRF_1 and NK_1 receptors antagonists has already been going on for some time, so it is possible that novel antidepressants will initially come from these classes in the near future. However, targeting the intracellular pathways is a relatively new area and will take much longer before any compound of such a new class will be available.

REFERENCES

Arborelius L, Owens MJ, Plotsky PM, Nemeroff CB (1999) The role of corticotropin-releasing factor in depression and anxiety disorders. *J Endocrinol* **160**: 1–12.

Artigas F (1993) 5-HT and antidepressants: new views from microdialysis studies. *Trends Pharmacol Sci* **14**: 262.

Blier P (2001) Pharmacology of rapid-onset antidepressant treatment strategies. *J Clin Psychiatry* **62**(S15): 12–17.

Blier P, de Montigny C (1994) Current advances and trends in the treatment of depression. *Trends Pharmacol Sci* **15**: 220–226.

Blier P, Ward NM (2003) Is there a role for $5\text{-}HT_{1A}$ agonists in the treatment of depression? *Biol Psychiatry* **53**: 193–203.

Bremner JD, Narayan M, Anderson ER, Staib LH, Miller HL, Charney DS (2000) Hippo-campal volume reduction in major depression. *Am J Psychiatry* **157**: 115–118.

Bunney WE, Davis JM (1965) Noreprinephrine in depressive reactions. *Arch Gen Psychiatry* **13**: 483–494.

Cremers TIFH, Wiersma LJ, Bosker FJ, Den Boer JA, Westerink BHC, Wikstrom HK (2001) Is the beneficial antidepressant effect of co-administration of pindolol really due to somato-dendritic autoreceptor antagonism? *Biol Psychiatry* **50**: 13–21.

Duman RS, Heninger GR, Nestler EJ (1997) A molecular and cellular theory of depression. *Arch Gen Psychiatry* **54**: 597–606.

Duman RS, Malberg J, Nakagawa S, D'Sa C (2000) Neuronal plasticity and survival in mood disorders. *Biol Psychiatry* **48**: 732–739.

El Mansari M, Blier P (1996) Functional characterization of $5\text{-}HT_{1D}$ autoreceptors on the modulation of 5-HT release in guinea pig mesencephalic raphe, hippocampus and frontal cortex. *Br J Pharmacol* **118**: 681–689.

Farvolden P, Kennedy SH, Lam RW (2003) Recent developments in the psychobiology and pharmacotherapy of depression: optimizing existing treatments and novel approaches. *Expert Opin Investig Drugs* **12**: 65–86.

Gummick JS, Nemeroff CB (2000) Problems with currently available antidepressants. *J Clin Psychiatry* **61**: 5–15.

Holsboer F (1999) The rationale for corticotropin-releasing hormone receptor (CRH-R) antagonists to treat depression and anxiety. *J Psychiatr Res* **33**: 181–214.

Kramer MS, Cutler N, Feighner J, Shrivastava R, Carman J, Sramek JJ, Reines SA, et al. (1998) Distinct mechanism for antidepressant activity by blockade of central substance P receptors. *Science* **281**: 1640–1645.

Manji HK, Drevets WC, Charney DS (2001) The cellular neurobiology of depression. *Nature Med* **7**: 541–547.

McAskill R, Mir S, Taylor D (1998) Pindolol augmentation of antidepressant therapy. *Br J Psychiatry* **173**: 203–208.

McLean S, Ganong AH, Seeger TF, Bryce DK, Pratt KG, Reynolds LS, Siok CJ, Lowe JA III, Heym J (1991) Activity and distribution of binding sites in brain of a non-peptide substance P (NK1) receptor antagonist. *Science* **251**: 437–439.

Middlemiss DN, Göthert M, Schlicker E, Scott CM, Selkirk JV, Watson JM, Gaster LM, Wyman P, Riley G, Price GW (1999) SB-236057, a selective 5-HT$_{1B}$ receptor inverse agonist, blocks the human terminal 5-HT autoreceptor. *Eur J Pharmacol* **375**: 359–365.

Montejo AL, Llorca G, Izquierdo JA, Rico-Villademoros F (2001) Incidence of sexual dysfunction associated with antidepressant agents: a prospective multicenter study of 1022 outpatients. *J Clin Psychiatry* **62**(Suppl 3): 10–21.

Mundo E, Richter MA, Zai G, Sam F, McBride J, Macciardi F, Kennedy JL (2002) 5HT$_{1D}$-receptor gene implicated in the pathogenesis of obsessive-compulsive disorder: further evidence from a family-based association study. *Mol Psychiatry* **7**: 805–809.

Nelson JC (2000) Augmentation strategies in depression. *J Clin Psychiatry* **61**(Suppl 2): 13–19.

Nestler EJ, Barrot M, DiLeone RJ, Eisch AJ, Gold SJ, Moteggia LM (2002) Neurobioloy of depression. *Neuron* **34**: 13–25.

Ostroff RB, Nelson JC (1999) Risperidone augmentation for selective serotonin reuptake inhibitors in major depression. *J Clin Psychiatry* **60**: 256–259.

Perez V, Soler J, Puigdemont D, Alvarez E, Artigas F (1999) A double-blind, randomized, placebo-controlled trial of pindolol augmentation in depressive patients resistant to serotonin reuptake inhibitors. *Arch Gen Psychiatry* **56**: 375–379.

Rabiner EA, Bhagwaga Z, Gunn RN, Sargent PA, Bench CJ, Cowen PJ, Grasby PM (2001) Pindolol augmentation of selective serotonin reuptake inhibitors: PET evidence that the dose used in clinical trials is too low. *Am J Psychiatry* **158**: 2080–2082.

Rollema H, Clarke T, Sprouse JS, Schulz DW (1996) Combined administration of a 5-hydroxytryptamine (5-HT)$_{1D}$ antagonist and a 5-HT reuptake inhibitor synergistically increases 5-HT release in guinea pig hypothalamus in vivo. *J Neurochem* **67**: 2204–2207.

Santarelli L, Gobbi G, Debs PC, Sibille EL, Blier P, Hen R, Heath MJS (2001) Genetic and pharmacological disruption of neurokinin 1 receptor function decreases anxiety-related behaviors and increases serotonergic function. *Proc Nat Acad Sci USA* **98**: 1912–1917.

Schulz DW, Mansbach RS, Sprouse JS, Braselton JP, Collins J, Corman M, Dunaiskis A, Faraci S, Schmidt AW, Seeger T, Seymour P, Tingley FD, Winston EN, Chen YL, Heym J (1996) CP-154,526 a potent and selective non-peptide antagonist of corticotropin releasing factor receptors. *Proc Nat Acad Sci USA* **93**: 10477–10482.

Schildkraut JJ (1965) The catecholamine hypothesis of affective disorders: a review of the supporting evidence. *J Am Psychiatry* **122**: 509–521.

Snider RM, Constantine JW, Lowe JA III, Longo KP, Lebel WS, Woody HA, Drozda SE, Desai MC, Vinick FJ, Spencer RW, Hess H-J (1991) A potent non-peptide antagonist of the substance P (NK1) receptor. *Science* **251**: 435–437.

Sprouse JS, Braselton J, Reynolds L (2000) 5-HT$_{1A}$ agonist potential of pindolol: electrophysiologic studies in the dorsal raphe nucleus and hippocampus. *Biol Psychiatry* **47**: 1050–1055.

Sprouse JS, Reynolds L, Rollema H (1997) Do 5-HT$_{1B/1D}$ autoreceptors modulate dorsal raphe cell firing – in vivo electrophysiological studies in guinea pigs with GR127935. *Neuropharmacology* **36**: 559–567.

Stout SC, Owens MJ, Nemeroff CB (2001) Neurokinin$_1$ receptor antagonists as potential anti-depressants. *Ann Rev Pharmacol Toxicol* **41**: 877–906.

Zobel AW, Nickel T, Kunzel HE, Ackl N, Sonntag A, Ising M, Holsboer F (2000) Effect of the high affinity corticotropin-releasing hormone receptor I antagonist R121919 in major depression: the first 20 patients treated. *J Psychiatry Res* 34: 171–181.

15

Sleep Research and Affective Disorders

Sue J. Wilson and David J. Nutt

University of Bristol, Bristol, UK

There is a very strong association between sleep and major depression (see Table 15.1). Sleep disturbance is one of the key symptoms of the disease and may be the reason that depressed patients first seek help (Thase, 2000; Agargun et al., 1997a). Up to 95% of patients with major depressive episode have at least one complaint of sleep, either difficulty in initiating or maintaining sleep or early wakening (Hamilton, 1989; Thase, 1999) and depression-related insomnia seems to be a high risk factor for suicide (Agargun et al., 1997b). As well as subjective symptoms, there are changes in sleep architecture in major depression, and in those patients with recurrent depression who have sleep abnormalities the long-term efficacy of cognitive therapy is reduced (Thase et al., 1998). Antidepressants in general change sleep architecture in the opposite direction to the changes in depression. This alteration in sleep is one of the few consistent and measurable biological effects in this disease, and therefore it is important to study it and the effects of treatment.

HOW SLEEP IS MEASURED

Information about sleep may be obtained in the simplest way by asking the subject about sleep, either informally or in a structured way using a questionnaire. These methods will give information about the subject's perception of the ease of going to sleep, quality of sleep and timing. Subjective perceptions are very important in the study of sleep disturbance in patients, but the insights into neurochemical processes

TABLE 15.1 Associations between depression and sleep

• sleep architecture abnormal – REM latency shortened	• sleep disturbance common in depression – may be presenting complaint
• antidepressants change sleep architecture – REM latency lengthened	• may predict treatment outcome
• sleep deprivation improves mood in major depression	

Mood Disorders: Clinical Management and Research Issues. Edited by E. J. L. Griez, C. Faravelli, D. J. Nutt and J. Zohar.
©2005 John Wiley & Sons Ltd. ISBN 0 470 09426 5.

in the brain have been gained by recording brain electrical activity during the night using polysomnography. This has traditionally been carried out in sleep laboratories, but more recently, particularly in Europe, there is increasing use of home polysomnography using ambulatory equipment. This is effective and relatively cheap and allows the study of sleep in the real world and unconstrained by strange environment. In the study of depression in outpatients it has proved acceptable to patients who would be unwilling to volunteer to come into hospital for sleep studies. There is a wide choice of small digital recorders for home use and PC-based replay systems are available.

Recording sleep in order to analyse sleep stages requires the use of electroencephalography (EEG), electromyography (EMG) and electrooculography (EOG) and minimum requirements were laid down formally in a manual produced by a committee of experienced sleep researchers in the 1960s and published by the American Government Health Office (Rechtschaffen and Kales, 1968). There are five universally recognized stages of sleep in normal subjects; criteria for identifying these are known universally as the Rechtschaffen and Kales (R&K) criteria after the authors of the committee's report and are used worldwide by most sleep researchers.

Stages 1–4 of R&K are non-rapid eye movement or non-REM sleep. Sleep gradually increases in depth with 1 as the lightest and 4 as the deepest stage. EMG activity gradually diminishes from stage 1 to stage 4, but muscle tone does not entirely disappear. Stage 1 sleep is drowsiness during which normal alpha (8–13 Hz) and mixed fast (14–30 Hz) rhythms of the waking EEG are replaced by theta activity (4–7 Hz) and there are slow rolling lateral movements of the eyes picked up on the EOG. Stage 2 sleep contains sleep spindles (widespread lentiform runs of 12 or 14 Hz activity) and K complexes (large biphasic slow transients) in the EEG, and normally eye movements are absent. Stages 3 and 4 or slow wave sleep (SWS) may be considered as continuing from stage 2 but with more delta, or slow activity (0–4 Hz), such that activity at below 2 Hz and of amplitude greater than 75 μV occupies between 20% and 50% of the epoch for stage 3 sleep, and greater than 50% for stage 4. In contrast stage REM, or rapid eye movement sleep, has an EEG pattern of low amplitude mixed frequencies similar to waking or stage 1 sleep, with occasional sharper transients interspersed (these may be surface manifestations of the ponto-geniculate-occipital (PGO) waves recorded from these deeper structures in animals during REM sleep and associated strongly with saccadic eye movements). There is a total lack of tonic activity recorded on the EMG but phasic muscle twitches are often seen. There are frequent jerky conjugate eye movements, usually lateral but sometimes vertical, during this stage. Figure 15.1 illustrates some of these patterns.

Behaviourally, stage 1 sleep is the stage of drowsiness when subjects will usually deny being asleep when aroused. Stage 2 is peaceful light sleep from which it is fairly easy to wake subjects – about 50% of the night is spent in this stage, during which myoclonic jerks and 'falling' arousals occur. During stages 3 and 4, or slow wave sleep, subjects are pale and still, with slow regular heart rate and breathing. It is

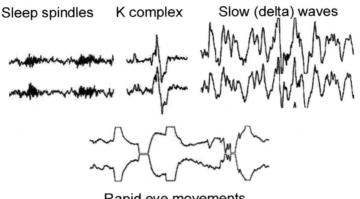

Figure 15.1 Some waveforms used to distinguish the various stages of sleep

difficult to wake someone from slow wave sleep, and the subject will feel 'groggy' and confused on waking. Most dreaming takes place during REM sleep.

During the course of a normal night's sleep a healthy subject will pass through the five stages of sleep several times, each episode of non-REM/REM sleep being termed a sleep cycle. This progression through the various stages may be plotted against time and is called a hypnogram (see Figure 15.2). From this normal hypnogram it may be seen that most of the SWS occurs in the first half of the night and most of the REM sleep in the second half. Various measures of amounts, timing and

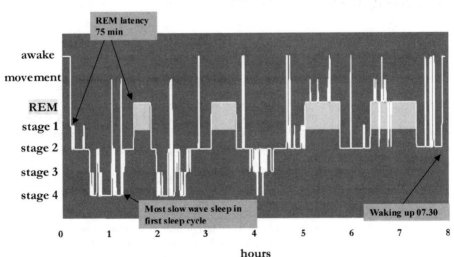

Figure 15.2 Hypnogram from a normal subject

proportions of the stages are derived from the hypnogram, and the structure of sleep as demonstrated in the hypnogram is called sleep architecture, supposedly from the hypnogram's similarity to a depiction of a city skyline. The maintenance of sleep, number of interruptions and stage changes etc., is called sleep continuity, and a widely used measure of sleep fragmentation is sleep efficiency, being the percentage of the time in bed which is actually spent asleep.

The amounts of time spent in each sleep stage, the number of cycles and the amount of interruption by waking is very variable from subject to subject, but less so within subjects. In general there are definite age effects in adulthood, with less slow wave sleep and lower sleep efficiency the older the subject.

The measurement of sleep structure is a useful tool which may be used to help elucidate various aspects of depressive illness.

STUDYING SLEEP ABNORMALITIES IN DEPRESSION

The most consistent sleep anomalies have been described for many years and briefly, consist of:

(1) REM advance, the most robust finding – onset of REM is earlier than in normal subjects and there is disruption of the normal preponderance of REM in the latter part of the night.
(2) Disruption of sleep continuity with early and middle insomnia and early morning wakening.
(3) Reduction of slow wave sleep, particularly in the first cycle.

An example of a depressed patient's sleep from our own studies is given in Figure 15.3.

REM Alterations in Depression

REM alterations have been found in depressed patients to varying degrees since originally described by Gresham et al. (1965) and later confirmed not only during a depressive episode but during remission by Kupfer and Foster (1972). A review of sleep studies by Benca et al. (1992) confirmed that this is a robust finding in depression. Many measures of REM such as total duration in minutes over the night, length of each episode, number of episodes and eye movement during REM (REM activity or density) have been studied. However, the most consistent abnormality has been the time taken to enter the first episode of REM (REM onset latency, ROL). This is widely reported as being shortened in depression (see Hicks et al., 2002; Wilson et al., 2000) particularly in endogenous subgroups (Hubain et al., 1995) and this abnormality increases with age and disease severity (Lauer et al., 1991). Indeed some of the findings of the earlier studies of depressed patients were disputed later because age and illness severity were not taken into

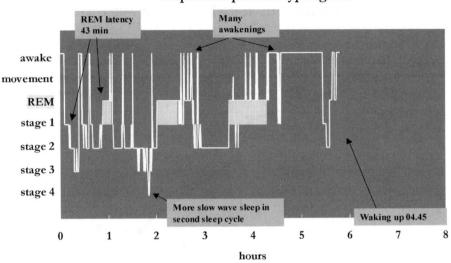

Figure 15.3 Hypnogram from a depressed patient

account (Berger and Riemann, 1993), but studies of young patients (Emslie et al., 1994) have confirmed the finding.

Lengthening of the first REM period, or general imbalance of REM so that a greater than normal amount occurs in the first half of the night, and increased number of eye movements (REM density) have also been described by many authors (for review see Reynolds and Kupfer, 1987). REM sleep abnormalities have been claimed to be not only a state marker for depression but also a trait marker, as they have been found during remission in patients with recurrent depression (Giles et al., 1987) and have been proposed as a predictor of recurrence. REM abnormalities in first-degree relatives of depressed patients have led to the proposal that these could be useful as vulnerability markers (Lauer et al., 1995).

A recent example of the use of sleep research in the study of the evolution of depression is the work by Thase et al. (1998) on recurrent depression. They evaluated sleep architecture and clinical parameters before, during and for two years after long-term successful cognitive treatment in patients with recurrent depression. They were able to prove that those patients with abnormal sleep architecture before treatment had a higher risk of recurrence within the two-year follow-up than those with a normal sleep pattern (Figure 15.4). This finding has huge clinical significance in the selection of treatment modality.

Slow Wave Sleep Abnormalities in Depression

The presence of SWS abnormalities is much less consistent in depression, but there does seem to be a robust finding of reduced SWS in the first sleep cycle, implying a

Effect of sleep abnormality at baseline on recurrence rate in depressed patients successfully treated with CBT

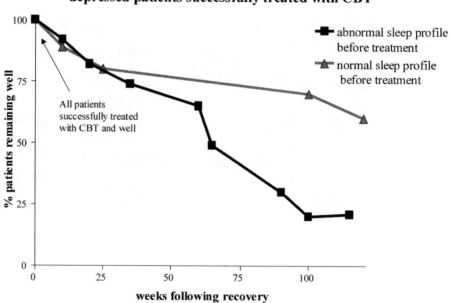

Figure 15.4 Difference in outcome between patients with recurrent depression with and without objective sleep disturbance. All patients were treated with psychological therapy and were recovered at the zero point. Those patients with sleep disturbance during their illness were more likely to relapse. Data from Thase et al., 1998

reduced 'pressure' of SWS (Kupfer et al., 1984, 1990). However this is difficult to differentiate from an increased pressure of REM sleep, with shorter REM latency making the time available for the first SWS period very short. Ehlers et al. (1996) have described an alteration of the distribution of SWS over the night during successful treatment with clomipramine, using the ratio between slow wave activity in the first to the second sleep cycle (delta sleep ratio, DSR) and have postulated that increasing the DSR may be necessary for the therapeutic action of antidepressants.

Another somewhat paradoxical link is that sleep deprivation, and in particular REM deprivation, has been known for many years to improve mood in major depression, and in a study by Vogel et al. (1975) REM sleep deprivation was found to be equally efficacious with imipramine therapy. However, it is difficult to perform and once uninterrupted sleep is allowed its effect disappears. Recent research has refined the methods of manipulation of sleep and circadian rhythm to maximize its effects on mood and there have been several strategies proposed to prolong the effect (see Giedke and Schwarzler, 2002).

STUDYING EFFECTS OF ANTIDEPRESSANTS ON SLEEP IN DEPRESSION

In general, drugs which are known to affect central neurotransmission tend to alter sleep, either continuity or architecture or both, but those which affect primarily 5-hydroxytryptamine (5-HT) or noradrenaline (NA) have large effects.

Acute Effects on REM Sleep

Antidepressant (AD) drugs are known to have profound effects on sleep architecture and continuity acutely, both in volunteers and in depressed patients; these effects are greatest and most consistent on REM sleep, and tend to be in the opposite direction to the sleep abnormalities found in major depression, but are usually of greater degree (for review see Vogel et al., 1990).

REM sleep effects are twofold, consisting firstly of a delay in the onset of the first REM period, and secondly in a decrease in the total amount of REM sleep over the night (see Table 15.2). In addition in some studies REM density, that is the amount of eye movements per unit time of REM sleep, has been studied and found to be altered by antidepressants. The mechanism of this REM suppression is not entirely clear, but has been widely attributed to the effects of increased serotonergic and noradrenergic transmission induced by these drugs. Mechanisms of REM sleep generation have been studied extensively in both animals and humans and, through use of specific agents affecting neurotransmission, it is known that cholinergic neurons in the brainstem nuclei, responsible for generation of the REM state, are influenced by alterations in serotonin and noradrenaline; in particular serotonergic effects on REM are probably mediated via $5-HT_{1A}$ receptors on the REM initiating cholinergic cells in the brainstem (Monaca et al., 2003). Mechanisms of noradrenergic influences on REM are less clear but altering noradrenergic balance in the brain has large effects on REM. A simplified schematic diagram of these effects is given in Figure 15.5. The extent of REM suppression is a good non-invasive pharma-

TABLE 15.2 Acute effects on sleep of antidepressant drugs in depressed patients

	REM latency	REM amount	Sleep continuity	Examples
Tricyclics 1	↑	↓	↓	Clomipramine, imipramine
Tricyclics 2	↑	↓	↑	Amitriptyline, doxepin (trimipramine no effect on REM amount)
SSRIs	↓	↓	↓	All
MAOIs	↓↓	↓↓	↓	Phenelzine, (moclobemide only minor effects on REM)
$5-HT_2$ Receptor blocks	↓/no change	↓/no change	↑	Nefazodone, mirtazapine
SNRI	↓	↓	↓	Venlafaxine

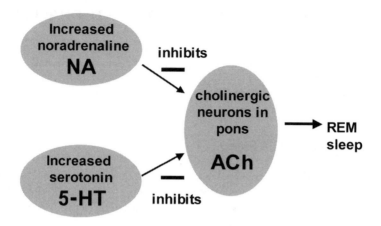

Brainstem control of REM sleep

Figure 15.5 Simplified diagram of neurotransmitter influences on REM sleep generation in the brainstem

codynamic measure of brain effects. Most antidepressants increase monoaminergic transmission either by preventing reuptake or by blocking autoreceptor mechanisms of homeostasis.

Other Acute Effects

REM suppression after antidepressants is very often accompanied by an increase in arousals during sleep, almost as if the transition to REM sleep is replaced by one to awakening. Vogel (1990) has postulated that this type of arousal REM suppression is characteristic of antidepressants. However, drugs affecting other neurotransmitter systems also have effects on arousal, and therefore some antidepressants improve sleep efficiency because of their effects to block, for example, histamine, alpha-1 adrenoceptors or serotonin receptors (see below). There are no consistent effects of antidepressants on non-REM sleep.

Chronic Effects

One of the most interesting uses of sleep studies of antidepressants is in the investigation of long-term effects. These effects are important, as most patients remain on treatment for many months, and also interesting in psychopharmacological terms given that our theories of antidepressant mechanisms are predicated on receptor adaptation over weeks.

Sleep laboratory studies of long-term administration of antidepressants in depressed patients have included work on the SSRIs fluoxetine, zimelidine, fluvoxamine and citalopram (Rush et al., 1998 8 weeks; Wilson et al., 2000 12 weeks; Hendrickse et al., 1994 >7 weeks; Shipley et al., 1985 4 weeks) the TCAs imipramine, clomipramine, nortriptyline and amitriptyline (Mendlewitz et al., 1991 3 weeks; Dunleavy et al., 1972; Kupfer et al., 1991 3 weeks; Ciapparrelli et al., 1994 4 weeks). Most have shown that the marked effects of increased REM latency and decreased REM time seen early in treatment are slightly diminished over the course of weeks, although they remain significantly changed from baseline. Effects on sleep efficiency have been less well studied chronically, and their relationship to subjective effects remains unclear.

In our studies we have used home recording with ambulatory equipment, which made patients more likely to volunteer, since they were not required to come into hospital, and some clinical assessments could be done at home. This procedure obviated the need for adaptation nights, as the 'first night effect' (the first night in a strange environment being different from a usual night's sleep) has been shown not to occur using home recordings (Sharpley et al., 1988). Subjective measures of sleep are also important, as we have shown that perception of sleep changes during treatment of depression, independently of objective measures (Wilson et al., 2000).

An example of one of these studies is our examination of sleep effects after during long-term treatment of depression with an SSRI, paroxetine, and the mixed SSRI and $5\text{-}HT_2$ receptor blocker nefazodone (Hicks et al., 2002). 40 depressed outpatients were studied for 8 weeks treatment, with sleep recordings and clinical measures at baseline and at three and ten days and eight weeks of treatment. As well as measuring objective sleep we studied subjective perception with questionnaires and diaries.

Depression ratings improved in both groups of patients, and we found that as expected REM sleep was immediately suppressed by paroxetine but not by nefazodone (Figure 15.6). REM latency remained lengthened throughout the eight weeks after paroxetine while amount of REM sleep recovered to baseline. Sleep disruption measures such as amount of time spent awake after sleep onset and number of awakenings were increased in the paroxetine group and decreased in the nefazodone group early in treatment.

The sleep profiles of the two antidepressants were very different, and this is interesting in the light of their different pharmacological profiles. Paroxetine, the selective 5-HT uptake blocker markedly suppressed REM sleep as expected, and also disrupted sleep continuity, whereas nefazodone, with its main action as a $5\text{-}HT_2$ receptor blocker, and without the anticholinergic and antihistaminic actions of the sleep-promoting TCAs, improved sleep continuity. Thus we can postulate that there is a sleep-promoting action of $5\text{-}HT_2$-blocking drugs, and this is interesting in the light of previous findings that ritanserin, a selective $5\text{-}HT_2$ antagonist increases slow wave sleep dose-dependently (Idzikowski et al.,

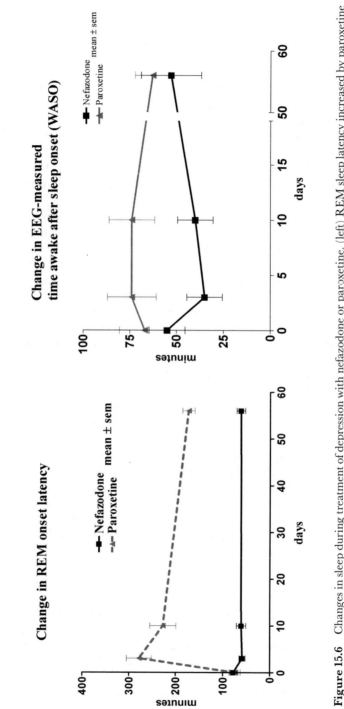
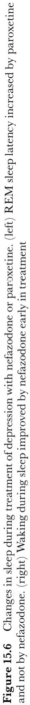

Figure 15.6 Changes in sleep during treatment of depression with nefazodone or paroxetine. (left) REM sleep latency increased by paroxetine and not by nefazodone. (right) Waking during sleep improved by nefazodone early in treatment

1991) and mCCP, an agonist at these receptors, reduces SWS and disrupts continuity (Lawlor et al., 1991).

It has been suggested that slow wave activity in non-REM sleep (SWA) and delta sleep ratio (DSR) are normalized by successful antidepressant treatment (Ehlers et al., 1996), that is that slow wave sleep and slow wave activity become greater in the first than the second and subsequent sleep cycles. In that study, the balance of SWA was shifted towards the beginning of the night in the responders to clomipramine, thus increasing the DSR. Since this index differentiated responders from non-responders, it was hypothesized that changes in SWA, rather than in REM sleep, may be associated with the clinical effect of antidepressants. If this were true, DSR could prove to be the elusive laboratory marker predicting response to treatment.

In the nefazodone and paroxetine study we used automatic frequency and period analysis of slow wave activity; we hoped to be able to separate the REM suppressant action from the action on slow wave sleep, because one antidepressant suppressed REM and the other did not. We found that the DSR changed significantly with treatment, the balance of SWA shifting towards the beginning of the night. This change was not associated with clinical improvement, but it was associated with the type of the medication used. While DSR increased in patients treated with paroxetine, it was largely unaffected in those treated with nefazodone, despite the fact that there was no drug group difference in the clinical outcome (see Figure 15.7). This contrasts with the previous report, where DSR changes predicted

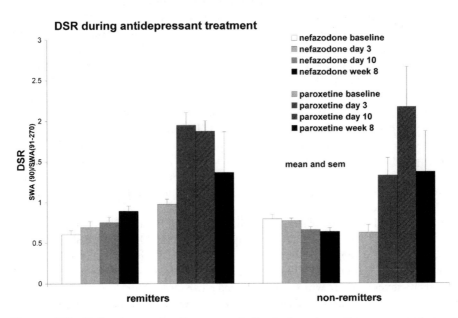

Figure 15.7 Delta sleep ratio changes markedly during paroxetine treatment but not during nefazodone treatment

response or non-response to clomipramine. The DSR was higher in remitted paroxetine patients than non-remitters only in night 3, but the difference did not reach significance.

MEASURING PHARMACODYNAMIC EFFECTS USING SLEEP

One of the most useful ways in which the study of sleep may contribute research is to use sleep to investigate psychopharmacological theories. One of these theories is the use of pindolol to speed up and augment therapeutic effects of SSRIs.

Animal studies have shown that after acute administration of an SSRI there is an immediate decrease in the firing rate of 5-HT neurons and only a small increase in the amount of 5-HT released into the synapse (Romero et al., 1996). After two weeks' treatment the firing rate of 5-HT neurons is found to recover and there is a marked increase in synaptic 5-HT (Bel and Artigas, 1993; Kreiss and Lucki, 1995). It is thought that this can be explained by the fact that serotonergic neurons in the raphe nucleus have autoreceptors on their cell bodies and dendrites which respond to increased 5-HT by switching off cell firing (Artigas, 1993). SSRIs produce increased levels of 5-HT around the cell body and dendrites of 5-HT neurons as well as at the synapse, and thus may activate the $5-HT_{1A}$ autoreceptors described above and cause inhibition of cell firing and a reduction in the amount of 5-HT released (Invernizzi et al., 1992). After chronic treatment with an SSRI there is a progressive desensitization of these $5-HT_{1A}$ autoreceptors in the raphe nuclei with a consequent recovery of cell firing and a rise in 5-HT levels in the terminal regions (e.g. frontal cortex), which is probably the site of antidepressant action in humans (Blier and de Montigny, 1994; see Figure 15.8). If this model does represent the onset of therapeutic action, then if the $5-HT_{1A}$ receptors were blocked and prevented from inhibiting cell firing early in SSRI treatment then release of 5-HT in the cortex might be accelerated. There is no selective $5-HT_{1A}$ antagonist available for human use, but pindolol, a beta-adrenoceptor antagonist, also has a high affinity for $5-HT_{1A}$ receptors where it also acts as an antagonist (Hamon et al., 1986). Pindolol has been shown in some studies to accelerate therapeutic effects of SSRIs when it is co-administered in depression (Artigas et al., 1994, Blier and Bergeron., 1995, Vinar et al., 1996, Bakish et al., 1997).

So how could the study of sleep contribute to the validation of the animal model? It is known that there is a dose-related suppression of REM sleep by SSRIs, and we hypothesized that the sleep effects of the combination of pindolol and SSRI would be much larger than the SSRI alone. We studied 12 healthy volunteers in a randomized crossover study in which they received paroxetine 20 mg/day (or its placebo) for nine days with a washout period of five days between (Bell et al., 2003). On day 7 and 9 of each treatment they also received pindolol 2.5 mg (or its placebo) three times a day. Sleep EEG recordings were made on each of the nights on pindolol (or

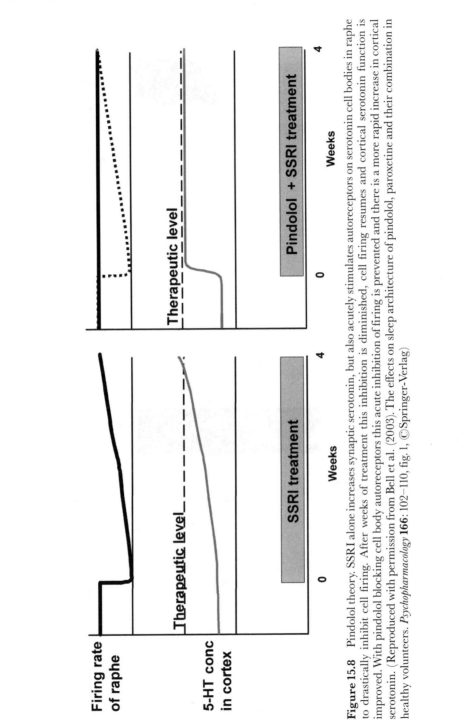

Figure 15.8 Pindolol theory. SSRI alone increases synaptic serotonin, but also acutely stimulates autoreceptors on serotonin cell bodies in raphe to drastically inhibit cell firing. After weeks of treatment this inhibition is diminished, cell firing resumes and cortical serotonin function is improved. With pindolol blocking cell body autoreceptors this acute inhibition of firing is prevented and there is a more rapid increase in cortical serotonin. (Reproduced with permission from Bell et al. (2003). The effects on sleep architecture of pindolol, paroxetine and their combination in healthy volunteers. *Psychopharmacology* **166**: 102–110, fig. 1, ©Springer-Verlag)

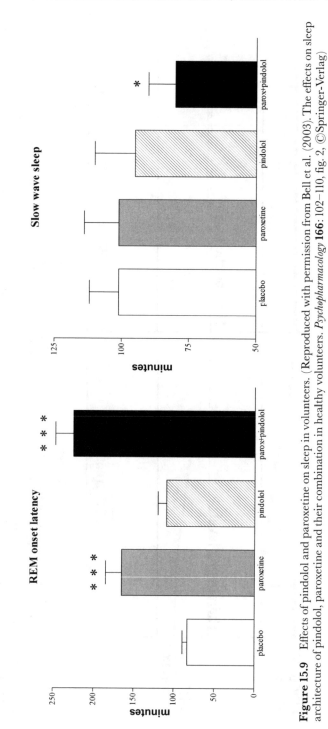

Figure 15.9 Effects of pindolol and paroxetine on sleep in volunteers. (Reproduced with permission from Bell et al. (2003). The effects on sleep architecture of pindolol, paroxetine and their combination in healthy volunteers. *Psychopharmacology* **166**: 102–110, fig. 2, ©Springer-Verlag)

its placebo) and thus four drug conditions were tested – placebo, pindolol alone, paroxetine alone and pindolol+paroxetine.

We found that both paroxetine and pindolol alone suppressed REM and that the REM effects of the combination were greater than either drug alone; however, the magnitude of the REM effects was approximately equal to the sum of individual drug effects (see Figure 15.9). However, there was a significant suppression of slow wave sleep only after the combination, which would fit with the hypothesis that pindolol and paroxetine in combination produce an increase in the net synaptic release of 5-HT in the synapse.

The examples above have shown how measurement of sleep can answer questions not only about depression and the effect of antidepressants but about the effects of drugs on neurotransmitter systems in the brain. For instance study of sleep structure in depression and after antidepressants may shed light on processes which are common to sleep and depression. We are also able to track effects of serotonin-modifying drugs by measuring their effects on sleep, and perhaps make assumptions about adaptive mechanisms in the brain which contribute to antidepressant action.

An interesting topic is slow wave sleep in depression. Slow wave sleep is very important for restoration/recovery processes and it may be that the build-up of pressure for slow wave sleep during the day is disturbed in depression, allowing REM sleep pressure to dominate. Studies of the REM and non-REM processes in depression, and how they are affected by antidepressants may shed light on underlying neurotransmitter and receptor processes, and could be particularly useful in the investigation of new agents affecting 5-HT$_2$ receptors.

REFERENCES

Agargun MY, Kara H, Solmaz M (1997a) Sleep disturbances and suicidal behavior in patients with major depression. *J Clin Psychiatry* **58**(6): 249–251.

Agargun MY, Kara H, Solmaz M (1997b) Subjective sleep quality and suicidality in patients with major depression. *J Psychiatr Res* **31**(3): 377–381.

Artigas F (1993) 5HT and antidepressants: new views from microdialysis studies. *Trends Pharmacol Sci* **14**: 262.

Artigas F, Perez V, Alvarez E (1994) Pindolol induces a rapid improvement of depressed patients treated with serotonin re-uptake inhibitors. *Arch Gen Psychiatry* **51**: 248–251.

Bakish D, Hooper CL, Thornton MD (1997) Fast onset: an open study of the treatment of major depressive disorder with nefazodone and pindolol combination therapy. *Int Clin Psychopharmacol* **12**: 91–97.

Bel N, Artigas F (1993) Chronic treatment with fluvoxamine increases extracellular serotonin in the frontal cortex but not in raphe nuclei. *Synapse* **15**: 243–245.

Bell C, Wilson S, Rich A, Bailey J, Nutt D (2003) The effects on sleep architecture of pindolol, paroxetine and their combination in healthy volunteers. *Psychopharmacology* **166**: 102–110.

Benca RM, Obermeyer WH, Thisted RA, Gillin JC (1992) Sleep and psychiatric disorders. A meta-analysis. *Arch Gen Psychiatry* **49**(8): 651–668.

Berger M, Riemann D (1993) REM sleep in depression – an overview. *J Sleep Res* **2**: 211–223.

Blier P, Bergeron R (1995) Effectiveness of pindolol with selected antidepressant drugs in the treatment of major depression. *J Clin Psychopharmacol* **15**: 217–222.

Blier P, de Montigny C (1994) Current advances and trends in the treatment of depression. *Trends Pharmacol Sci* **15**: 220–226.

Ciapparelli A, Gemignani A, Figura A, Guerrini I, Palagini L, Guazzelli M (1994) Effect of fluoxetine and clomipramine on EEG delta activity during sleep in major depression. *J Sleep Res* **3**: 415.

Dunleavy DLF, Brezinova V, Oswald I, Maclean AW, Tinker W (1972) Changes during weeks in effects of tricyclic drugs on the human sleeping brain. *Brit J Psychiat* **120**: 663–672.

Ehlers CL, Havstad JW, Kupfer DJ (1996) Estimation of the time course of slow-wave sleep over the night in depressed patients: effects of clomipramine and clinical response. *Biol Psychiatry* **39**(3): 171–181.

Emslie GJ, Rush AJ, Weinberg WA (1994) Sleep EEG features of adolescents with major depression. *Biol Psychiatry* **36**: 573–581.

Giedke H, Schwarzler F (2002) Therapeutic use of sleep deprivation in depression. *Sleep Med Rev* **6**(5): 361–377.

Giles D, Jarrett RB, Roffwarg HP, Rush AJ (1987) Reduced rapid eye movement latency: a predictor of recurrence in depression. *Neuropsychopharmacology* **1**: 33–39.

Gresham SC, Agnew HW, Williams RL (1965) The sleep of depressed patients. *Arch Gen Psychiatry* **13**: 503–507.

Hamilton M (1989) Frequency of symptoms in melancholia (depressive illness). *Br J Psychiatry* **154**: 201–206.

Hamon M, Cossery JM, Spampinato U, Gozlan H (1986) Are there selective ligands for 5HT1a and 5HT1b receptor binding sites in brain. *Trends Pharmacol Sci* **7**: 336–338.

Hendrickse WA, Roffwarg HP, Granneman BD, Orsulak PJ, Armitage R, Cain JW, Battaglia J, Debus JR, Rush AJ (1994) The effects of fluoxetine on the polysomnogram of depressed outpatients: a pilot study. *Neuropsychopharmacology* **10**: 85–91.

Hubain PP, Souery D, Jonck L, Staner L, Van Veeren C, Kerkhofs M, Mendlewitz J, Linkowski P (1995) Relationship between the Newcastle scale and sleep polysomnographic variables in major depression: a controlled study. *Eur Neuropsychopharmacol* **5**: 129–134.

Idzikowski C, Mills FJ, James RJ (1991) A dose–response study examining the effects of ritanserin on human slow wave sleep. *Br J Clin Pharmacol* **31**(2): 193–196.

Invernizzi R, Belli S, Samanin R (1992) Citalopram's ability to increase the extracellular concentration of serotonin in the dorsal raphe prevents the drug's effects in the frontal cortex. *Brain Res* **584**: 322–324.

Kreiss DS, Lucki I (1995) Effects of acute and repeated administration of antidepressant drugs on extracellular levels of 5HT measured in vivo. *J Pharmacol Exp Ther* **284**: 866–876.

Kupfer DJ, Foster DG (1972) Interval between onset of sleep and rapid eye movement sleep as an indicator of depression. *Lancet* **2**: 648–649.

Kupfer DJ, Franke E, McEachran AB, Grochocinski VJ (1990) Delta sleep ratio. A biological correlate of early recurrence in unipolar affective disorder. *Arch Gen Psychiatry* **47**(12): 1100–1105.

Kupfer DJ, Ulrich RF, Coble PA, Jarrett DB, Grochocinski V, Doman J, Matthews G, Borbely AA (1984) Application of automated REM and slow wave sleep analysis: II. Testing the assumptions of the two-process model of sleep regulation in normal and depressed subjects. *Psychiatry Res* **13**(4): 335–343.

Lauer CJ, Riemann D, Wiegand M, Berger M (1991) From early to late adulthood: changes in EEG sleep of depressed patients and healthy volunteers. *Biol Psychiatry* **29**: 979–993.

Lauer CJ, Schreiber W, Holsboer F, Krieg JC (1995) In quest of identifying vulnerability markers for psychiatric disorders by all-night polysomnography. *Arch Gen Psychiatry* **52**: 145–152.

Lawlor BA, Newhouse PA, Balkin TJ, Molchan SE, Mellow AM, Murphy DL, Sunderland T. A preliminary study of the effects of nighttime administration of the serotonin agonist, m-CPP, on sleep architecture and behavior in healthy volunteers. *Biol Psychiatry* **29**(3): 281–286.

Mendlewicz J, Kempenaers C, de Maertelaer V (1991) Sleep EEG and amitriptyline treatment in depressed inpatients. *Biol Psychiatry* **30**: 691–702.

Monaca C, Boutrel B, Hen R, Hamon M, Adrien J (2003) 5-HT 1A/1B receptor-mediated effects of the selective serotonin reuptake inhibitor, citalopram, on sleep: studies in 5-HT 1A and 5-HT 1B knockout mice. *Neuropsychopharmacology* **28**(5): 850–856.

Monti JM, Monti D (2000) Role of dorsal raphe nucleus serotonin 5HT1a receptor in the regulation of REM sleep. *Life Sciences* **66**: 1999–2012.

Rechtschaffen A, Kales A (1968) A manual of standardized terminology, techniques and scoring system for sleep stages in normal subjects. Washington, DC: US Dept of HEW.

Reynolds CF, Kupfer DJ (1987) Sleep research in affective illness. *Sleep* **10**: 199–215.

Romero L, Bel N, Casanovas JM, Artigas F (1996) Two actions are better than one: avoiding self-inhibition of serotonergic neurones enhances the effects of serotonin uptake inhibitors. *Int Clin Psychopharmacol* **11** (Suppl 4): 1–8.

Rush AJ, Armitage R, Gillin JC, et al. (1998) Comparative effects of nefazodone and fluoxetine in outpatients with major depressive disorder. *Biol Psychiatry* **44**: 3–14.

Sharpley AL, Solomon RA, Cowen PJ (1988) Evaluation of first night effect using ambulatory monitoring and automatic sleep stage analysis. *Sleep* **11**: 273–276.

Shipley JE, Kupfer DJ, Dealy RS, Griffin SJ, Coble PA, McEachran AB, Grochocinski VJ (1984) Differential effects of amitriptyline and of zimelidine on the sleep electroencephalogram of depressed patients. *Clin Pharmacol Ther* **36**: 253–259.

Shipley JE, Kupfer DJ, Griffin SJ, Dealy RS, Coble PA, McEachran AB, Grochocinski VJ (1985) Comparison of effects of desipramine and amitriptyline on EEG sleep of depressed patients. *Psychopharmacology* **85**: 14–22.

Thase ME (1999) Antidepressant treatment of the depressed patient with insomnia. *J Clin Psychiatry* **60**(Suppl 17): 28–31.

Thase ME (2000) Treatment issues related to sleep and depression. *J Clin Psychiatry* **61**(Suppl 11): 46–50.

Thase ME, Simons AD, Reynolds CF III (1998) Psychobiology correlates of poor response to cognitive behavior therapy: potential indications for antidepressant pharmacotherapy. *Psychopharmacol Bull* **29**(2): 293–301.

Vinar O, Vinarova E, Horacek J (1996) Pindolol accelerates the therapeutic action of SSRIs in depression. *Homeostasis* **37**: 93–95.

Vogel GW, Buffenstein A, Minter K, Hennessey A (1990) Drug effects on REM sleep and on endogenous depression. *Neurosci Biobehav Res* **14**: 49–63.

Vogel GW, Thurmond A, Gibbons P, Sloan K, Walker M (1975) REM sleep reduction effects on depression syndromes. *Arch Gen Psychiatry* **32**(6): 765–777.

Wilson SJ, Bell CJ, Coupland NJ, Nutt DJ (2000) Sleep changes during long-term treatment of depression with fluvoxamine – a home based study. *Psychopharmacology* **149**(4): 360–365.

16

Implementing Clinical Trials

Fiammetta Cosci and Carlo Faravelli

University of Florence, Florence, Italy

Clinical trials are now the most common procedure for testing new psychotropic compounds to be used in medicine and psychiatry. Almost all the principles of present therapeutics are based upon the results obtained (and published) by means of clinical trial methodology. All national regulatory agencies consider a new drug suitable for the market only if its efficacy and safety are sustained by the evidence derived from randomized trials.

The methods of clinical trials derive from a clearly stated epistemological framework, where the principles of scientific empiricism demand well-established rules in order to control for validity, reliability (reproducibility) and control of the various sources of bias.

Unfortunately, a potentially unaccounted bias is that all the newer compounds are developed by private industry, whose ultimate goal is neither new discoveries nor benefit to public health, but profit. Thus, the ethical standards for evaluating scientific research are not entirely respected.

Consequently, clinical trials have been, on more than one occasion, a means of twisting the methodological rules and empirical principles to drive the results toward a specific end.

For this reason, it is the intention of the authors to set the record straight concerning the critical analysis of the results of clinical trials, which, when published, are considered part of the training and education of clinicians.

HISTORY AND DEVELOPMENT OF CLINICAL TRIALS

The history of clinical trials in psychiatry began with Linford Rees. As early as 1949, while working in Cardiff, Rees conducted a study where electronarcosis, which had been introduced as a new method for treating schizophrenia, was compared with electroconvulsive therapy and insulin coma. In that study, the three treatment groups were selected for comparability of age, sex, and clinical features. Although the study was not fully randomized, nothing like this had

Mood Disorders: Clinical Management and Research Issues. Edited by E. J. L. Griez, C. Faravelli, D. J. Nutt and J. Zohar.
©2005 John Wiley & Sons Ltd. ISBN 0 470 09426 5.

been done in this area of psychiatry before. Subsequently, in 1950 and 1952, Rees ran placebo-controlled, double-blind studies looking at desoxycortisone acetate and later cortisone in the treatment of schizophrenia. The fact that the outcomes were negative in all these comparisons perhaps obscured the dramatic break-through that had occurred.

Beginning in 1953, Joel Elkes studied 27 patients with schizophrenia, giving them either a placebo followed by chlorpromazine or vice versa, and found that the active drug made a difference. In 1954, Rees randomized 100 anxious patients to either a placebo or chlorpromazine, and found that the drug was anxiolytic. In 1952–54, David Davies and Michael Shepherd studied the effect of reserpine in anxious depressives, while Mogens Schou and Eric Stromgren ran a placebo-controlled study of lithium in mania, finding it to be of benefit in 1954.

The Conference on the Evaluation of Psychotropic Drugs in 1956 was an important landmark for the future development of randomized clinical trials (RCTs) in psychiatry. The development of the use of clinical trials presented basilar issues of methodology. There was a general belief that it was not possible to measure subjective changes of the kind as those involved in psychiatric illness. Stemming from this, one of the key issues at the Conference was the use of rating scales for the mapping of clinical change. The most frequent question was 'How could a process that was so subtle and nuanced involving interactions between the subject and his friends, family and co-workers be captured by an instru-ment?' Nathan Kline, in particular, strongly argued against the use of rating scales. He contended that outcome measures, other than discharge from the hospital, risked producing a variation of the rabbit out of the hat effect. Rating scales were a means of putting the rabbit into the hat. When it was subsequently pulled out, it would fool the investigator as much as anyone else into thinking that something wonderful had happened.

Kline lost the argument and a strict process of standardization of psychiatry was born. Since the early 1960s, no proof of efficacy of a new drug was accepted unless substantiated by the use of rating scales (interestingly, no really innovative thera-peutic agent has been discovered since). After 1962, the standardization of diagnostic practice was all but inevitable. All research was first based on the use of 'quantitative' assessment measures, and then was accompanied by operational criteria.

The big change, when it came, was symbolized by the publication of the third edition of the *Diagnostic and Statistical Manual of Mental Disorders* (DSM III) in 1980 (APA, 1980).

Currently, the clinical experimentation for new drugs follows precise and standardized rules, initially dictated by the major American regulatory agency (the Food and Drug Administration, FDA) and later generalized internation-ally with the adoption of the Good Clinical Practices. The curious change that occurred during these years is that agencies existing to regulate the indus-tries have now become the standard to arbitrate on science (Healy, 2000a, 2000b).

CLINICAL TRIALS AS A STEP IN PHARMACOLOGICAL EXPERIMENTATION

Clinical trials are conducted when preclinical studies on animals have already produced sufficient knowledge about a compound's potential therapeutic activity, safety and toxicity. Pharmacokinetic and pharmacodynamic studies are the basis for identifying dosage, rate of administration per day and scheme of titration that will be applied to human beings who will take part in subsequent clinical trials.

The process of clinical experimentation is represented by:

- Phase 1 study: aimed to define the drug tolerability profile;
- Phase 2 study: aimed to quantify drug activity;
- Phase 3 study: aimed to compare the drug's efficacy and effectiveness;
- Phase 4 study: aimed to assess the drugs already on the market and used in everyday practice.

This is a precise programme of research which may proceed both in series and in parallel; it is also possible to go back to previous steps and repeat the same process *iter*.

From a practical point of view, these phases follow strict rules:

Phase 1: study on healthy volunteers, and sometimes on a small sample of patients. This phase provides initial indications on the clinical toxicity of the drug, and in particular, on the maximum dose which can be reasonably well tolerated. Moreover, it demonstrates the basic pharmacokinetics of the drug, the relationship between pharmacokinetics and pharmacodynamics, especially referring to long-term effects, and the relationship between dose-plasmatic concentrations and outcome. In addition, these studies must give information about significant pharmacokinetic variations in specific subgroups of subjects (elderly, patients with diseases interfering with hepatic metabolism or decreasing urinary clearance, etc.) and/or pharmacokinetic and pharmacodynamic interactions between the new compound and other drugs eventually associated in poly-therapy. Finally, Phase 1 studies should identify pharmacokinetic and pharmacodynamic characteristics of a new formulation compared to the ones already studied.

Phase 1 studies are usually conducted on 20–80 healthy subjects, and sometimes, on small samples of patients.

When the information on pharmacokinetics and clinical toxicity collected are clear and clinically and ethically acceptable, the drug can be investigated by means of a Phase 2 study.

Phase 2 is a larger and more consistent sample of patients usually exposed to the new drug to identify more detailed evidence of the therapeutic efficacy and to define the optimum dose range (minimal effective dose, maximum effective dose, therapeutic range related to safety and tolerability). During this phase the following information should be collected: optimum scheme of administration, titration and withdrawal symptoms. The last two points can be better defined during Phase 3 trials, even if information coming from Phase 2 studies allow for better design of subsequent protocol.

Briefly, Phase 2 is clinical research on the initial effects of the treatment, conducted on samples of around 100–200 patients. Rarely, it can also identify a secondary positive effect of the drug that indicates a probable new therapeutic indication. In this case, the drug will run the first phase again and be tested for the supposed new therapeutic indication.

Phase 3 evaluates a larger number of subjects. For drugs with psychotropic effect, around 2000–3000 subjects are usually included. During this phase, data previously collected are verified referring to a larger sample and using less strict inclusion/exclusion criteria. The aim of Phase 3 studies is to confirm and fortify the data on efficacy and effectiveness, and to give a precise description of the tolerability and safety of the compound in a wide range of patient groups and settings, and identify specific symptoms and patient groups in which the drug is especially effective. The comparative studies should confirm the drug's hypothesized psychotropic activity in a population for which clinical use is proposed, and should provide specific information about symptoms and the types for which the drug is especially effective. The studies should be conducted under conditions which resemble those of actual therapeutic use to establish optimal dosage in those populations for which the drug is intended. Moreover, these trials should establish the safety of the new psychotropic agent when given daily for three to six months and assess the nature and significance of any side effects with regard to incidence and control.

METHODOLOGY OF CLINICAL TRIALS

The Sample

In general, in Phase 3 clinical trials, it is important to sample the varieties of patient material for which the drug is intended. This objective may be served by one or both of two alternative strategies: (1) the population's differing age, sex, diagnostic categories, treatment setting, previous treatment and other qualities may be studied independently but, within each study, patients should be selected to be as homogeneous as possible. In this way, the diverse intended uses are tested by separate studies and each study has the advantage of a homogeneous sample; (2) since the identification of the pertinent qualities of the intended sample are often discovered both late and serendipitously, an alternative approach to sampling may be preferable. Large, heterogeneous samples are selected for each study with the aim of identifying the most responsive subgroup and providing precision in estimations of drug effects per se. Because of the post hoc nature of such findings, mutually comparable results must be apparent in comparable studies.

As far as sample size is concerned, experience with psychotropic drugs would suggest that in comparative trials fewer than 20 patients in any treatment group is disappointing, but treatment groups of 25 to 30 patients can be satisfactory. More than 30 patients in a treatment group (30 to 50) is strongly recommended, particularly for anxiolytic and antidepressant drugs.

Females of childbearing potential may be included if results from animal reproductive and teratology studies and from previous clinical studies are satisfactory.

After comparative studies have indicated the drug's basic therapeutic activity, later studies in this phase may explore its efficacy and safety in patients with organic illnesses requiring concomitant medications.

Children may be studied in separate trials provided the clinical picture warrants drug administration and safety is assured to the fullest extent possible. Geriatric samples should be studied separately as responsiveness in different age groups is unpredictable.

Different treatment environments may be used by the independent investigators, and the different intended uses will require different treatment settings: inpatients, outpatients, private practice, psychiatric, non-psychiatric, with or without concurrent psychotherapy, or any other practice where there is an intended use.

Design

Phase 1, 2 and 3 studies can be conducted in a single group or in two or more groups of randomly included subjects. In any case, they refer to an open, single- or double-blind scheme, respectively, if both subject and researcher know who is receiving the drug, if only the researcher knows or if neither subject nor researcher knows who is receiving the drug or the placebo.

Unless features of ethics, safety and feasibility are contraindicated, each subject should have a drug-free washout period prior to receiving the study medication. If after washout the patients' symptom severity has dropped below the selection threshold, the patient should be dropped.

Phase 3 studies are sometimes conducted in single groups to evaluate the long-term outcome in a large number of subjects. In these cases, biological and laboratory parameters are monitored to collect clear data about the safety of the molecule. These kinds of studies are necessary to register a new drug in Europe since the European Committee for the development of new drugs expects exposure of at least 100 subjects to the therapeutic dose of the new compound for at least 12 months. It is obviously easier and faster to conduct such studies according to an open scheme rather than a single- or double-blind one.

A property typical of the open Phase 3 studies is that the dose can be flexible in order to adjust it to side effects and efficacy.

They can be conducted under controlled or uncontrolled conditions. The uncontrolled model refers to the assignment of a particular drug to a number of the eligible patients subsequently observed (usually around 50% of them). The other patients are included as controls and receive a different treatment. The choice of the group to treat with the new drug is absolutely random and casual. The control group is used to eliminate the bias linked to the natural variability of the disease; correct randomization should produce the same variability between the patients and the control group.

When the studies are conducted in two or more groups, they usually follow two different designs: the parallel group and the crossover design. In the first study group, patients are randomized in double-blind studies into two or more groups, each subject receives only one treatment (placebo or active compound). Instead, in the crossover design, each subject receives both treatments in two different phases according to a randomized order.

The parallel group design has the advantage of eliminating biases due to dropout and the data obtained can be easily analysed. The most important limitation is linked to the risk of inadequate randomization that makes the groups not perfectly comparable for variables that could interfere with treatment response. The parallel group design is widely used in Phase 3 clinical trials of psychotropic drugs. The new molecule can be compared to an 'old' active one (in the case of an anxiolytic, an antidepressant or an antipsychotic) and to both the placebo and the active drug (in case of an anxiolytic or an antidepressant), or only to the placebo (if the corresponding active drug has not already been marketed). The use of the placebo is necessary to collect information about efficacy and tolerability. Moreover, the placebo is ethically acceptable when an active comparable drug for the control group is not available (Hill, 1963).

The parallel group design is usually characterized by an initial period under placebo treatment according to a single-blind study, with the aim of conducting laboratory tests, collecting data for subjects inclusion in the 'active' part of the experimentation, washing out, if necessary, and excluding people with a high response rate to the placebo. The parallel group design can also be used to test a specific hypothesis, for instance, to evaluate withdrawal symptoms after the sudden termination of chronic treatment. In this case, one group stops the treatment, while the parallel group continues as a control. This scheme is particularly useful in evaluating the long-term response to a drug, especially when it is used in chronic or highly recurrent disorders, such as chronic depression. Moreover, the parallel group design can be flexible and, in this sense, adequately modulated to test specific hypotheses.

The crossover design has some important advantages similar to the parallel group scheme. It has a limited variability of response to the treatment because two drugs are tested on the same subjects. This brings a significant increase to the statistical efficiency of the comparison between the two compounds. Moreover, given that each subject receives both treatments, the researcher needs a smaller sample, or half the number of subjects required in a parallel group design, to test the hypothesis. On the other hand, there are also some important disadvantages: (1) due to the variable, episodic course of most psychiatric disorders, any advantages of the crossover design to clinical psychopharmacology may be more apparent than real. Due to either treatment effects or spontaneous changes, the patient may be significantly different in his requirements during each of the successive medication periods. In addition, experience with the first medication may significantly influence the attitude of the patient's family toward his illness, as well as the attitude of the therapist or of the patient himself; (2) subjects under study should present with a chronic disorder that lasts for the entire trial period; (3) subjects should be evaluated only after a complete washout to avoid any residual pharmacological or pharmaco-kinetic effects of the treatment received during the first half of the trial (the so-called 'carry over' effect).

Considering these strict rules, the crossover design can be used only rarely. In fact, some acutely psychotic patients, as well as many anxious and depressed patients, can become virtually asymptomatic after relatively brief exposure to effective medication and may present important symptomatological fluctuations during that time. Thus, a therapeutic response to the first effective medication can lead to the withdrawal of the most responsive patients and leave a smaller and perhaps more treatment-resistant sample for subsequent treatments in the crossover design. It is even more difficult to use such a design in clinical trials studying antidepressants if we consider that a long period of washout is sometimes necessary to eliminate any 'carry over' effects (Uhlenhuth et al., 1979) and that antidepressants have a two–three week latency of action. For this reason, clinical trials for antidepressants rarely use the crossover design.

Moreover, in depressive syndromes, spontaneous remissions and response to aspecific care may occur (FDA, 1979). On the other hand, the crossover design can be properly applied in studies on obsessive-compulsive disorders.

To support a claim of efficacy, it is scientifically desirable that from three to five studies in Phase 3 compare the new compound with both a placebo and an estab-lished efficacious drug of a pharmacological class similar to that of the drug under investigation. These studies should be double-blind and utilize standard methods of assessment of change. When it is concluded that the drug's basic therapeutic efficacy has been clearly established by comparative studies, consideration may be given to undertake further studies on an open trial basis with new populations. Due to the lack of a control group for comparison, these types of studies carry with them the inherent risk of encountering difficulties in interpretation of unexpected findings. Such findings need further comparison study or other studies that can provide corroborative support of efficacy and valuable data regarding safety of the new drug, especially when researchers working separately obtain similar findings.

In addition, patients may be selected to evaluate claims of efficacy other than the major ones. Three double-blind studies should be sufficient to assess efficacy in each of these other areas. Prior to double-blind comparative studies, it may be necessary to conduct several open studies to familiarize the researchers with the drug's activity in a particular therapeutic situation or special population and to establish an appro-priate dosage range.

Long-term safety studies may be done on an open trial basis or in a parallel comparison group design. The dosage should be at least the level expected for even-tual general therapeutic use. The data may also be obtained from studies of samples where continued medication may be anticipated, as well as from a formally struc-tured, long-term study. Provision may be made for patients in therapeutic trials to continue on the drug if it is indicated. A concurrent comparison group receiving no treatment or placebo is highly desirable here. In the latter case, a related problem deals with attrition. The longer a trial continues, the greater the likelihood that patients will drop out; the sample finishing the trial will not be identical to that beginning the trial. Life-table methods and other statistical techniques derived from public health morbidity and mortality studies may be applicable in this area (FDA, 1979).

Long-term studies of safety and efficacy are increasing in importance as they present an opportunity to look for indications of tolerance and dependence. The goals of the studies correspond to the evaluation of the reduction in mortality, especially from suicide, prevention or reduction of re-hospitalization, reduction in risk of recurrence or relapse, social functioning, relief from minor symptoms and life satisfaction. Nevertheless, there are many unsolved problems. First, on the basis of presenting clinical symptoms, it is difficult to predict which patients are likely to have recurrences. The frequency of recurrences and the duration of the interval between relapses or recurrences are highly variable.

Nowadays, the majority of clinical trials use double-blind, randomized, two-arm studies, where a new compound is compared to a standard drug and placebo. They usually include an initial 'run in' phase in which the subjects receive the placebo, this allows a washout period and the individuation of placebo responders who will be excluded from further stages of experimentation.

The use of two arms implies the simultaneous comparison of the new compound with both the placebo and an active, standard drug. With this procedure it is possible to complete the *iter* quickly so as to market a new product in a shorter amount of time.

Duration

The duration of therapeutic trials may vary. The recommended duration of the treatment period should vary according to the nature of the drug, the treatment requirements of the patient sample, and the setting in which the treatment is conducted. From two to four weeks is usually sufficient to show anxiolytic effects among anxious patients, and for depressed patients from three to four weeks is usually sufficient to show antidepressant action. For psychotic patients a treatment period of approximately four weeks is usually sufficient to show a therapeutic effect, but trials of six to eight weeks are preferable.

Weekly post-treatment evaluations for two to four weeks are needed when the rapidity of relapse is to be determined.

For tests of indications other than the major efficacy claims, the sample using the drug should be followed for a period comparable to that employed in normal clinical usage.

The duration of long-term safety studies is usually three to six months.

Assessment

Baseline observations should be carried out in all patients immediately before initiation into the treatment programme. The baseline evaluation should include all tests and assessments anticipated for later use in documenting the sample, inferring therapeutic change or monitoring safety considerations.

Since some disorders may remit rapidly, the second evaluation should generally take place within one week. The frequency of successive evaluations may vary from days to weeks.

For most cases of acute anxiety and many cases of depression, the episodes are relatively short-lived and within three or four weeks substantial spontaneous remission may occur among many patients. A placebo group, as well as a group receiving an inactive drug, may show at four weeks a level of remission comparable with that obtained after one or two weeks of effective treatment. This especially depends on the fact that at the beginning antidepressant drugs have a latency of action of around two–three weeks. During this period, patients do not reap any benefit from the active treatment but, in the majority of the cases, only side effects and a possible increase in the initial symptoms due to the biphasic action of antidepressants (especially selective serotonin reuptake inhibitors, SSRIs).

Thus it is possible that assessments conducted on a monthly basis will fail to reveal evidence of immediate therapeutic effect, i.e. during the first or second week of treatment. Since the speed with which a clinically significant effect is attained is of practical interest, most, if not all, assessment programmes should be repeated at frequent intervals during, at least, the first four weeks subsequent to the pretreatment baseline determination.

The criteria for evaluating the treatment response is crucial. Pertinent areas for assessment are necessary, as well as specific tests and procedures for observing or identifying untoward changes.

Classes of assessments specifically identified as criteria for evaluating psychotropic agents include: (1) global rating scales; (2) symptom rating scales (even if, unfortunately, their ad hoc nature makes most such scales unreliable and the mixed dissimilar symptoms found in a group of similarly diagnosed patients present problems in data summary, analysis and interpretation); (3) self-descriptive inventories; (4) mood adjective checklists (providing quantitative assessments of various mood dimensions, including anxiety/tension and depression); (5) ratings of social adjustment; (6) behavioural measures; (7) physiological measures; (8) evaluation of side effects (including their duration, onset, severity, likelihood of association with the study medication and action taken).

Drug-effect criteria in clinical trials of psychotropic agents should include a global rating, a standardized symptoms ratings by the clinicians, and, if possible, an independent standardized self-rating by the patient. An assessment of adverse events is essential as well.

In selecting the specific measures, the following properties of each measure should be considered: (1) reliability, i.e. consistency of the measurements obtained from a standard, unchanging selection; (2) validity, i.e. the ability of the measure to reflect the intended aspects of the problem of interest; (3) normative data, i.e. data allowing the investigators to set the minimum level of pathology for including patients in the study, to set the maximum level of other pathologies acceptable and to interpret the effectiveness of the treatment in reducing the pathology; (4) ease of administration (ECDEU, 1978).

Clinical trials aimed to study antidepressants evaluate both severity of the symptoms and side effects induced by the compounds under study. Symptom severity is usually measured by means of rating scales. The Hamilton Rating Scale for Depression (HAM-D) (Hamilton, 1960) and the Montgomery–Asberg Depression Rating Scale (MADRS) (Montgomery and Asberg, 1979) are the most widely used. Symptom severity is evaluated at regular intervals during the trial and the difference between the final and initial scores is a measure of treatment response. A 50% reduction in the initial score is commonly considered the cut-off point establishing efficacy. Such a reduction does not necessarily mean recovery or improvement for the patients, as the scale measures only the severity of a limited number of symptoms and not what the patients actually feel.

Side effects are usually measured by means of rating scales, such as the Dosage Record and Treatment Emergent Symptom Scale (DOTES) (Guy, 1976) and the Systematic Assessment for Treatment Emergent Events (SAFTEE) (SysteMetrics). These scales were properly realized after the discovery of tricyclic antidepressants (TCAs) with the objective of underlining the presence/absence of the most common secondary side effects of TCA treatment. Unfortunately, after the discovery of SSRIs and the newer compounds, which have a side-effect profile completely different from TCAs, the scales have not been modified. Consequently, although it is now possible to know if, for instance, an SSRI produces xerostomia, it is not possible to demonstrate if it induces a modification in the pattern of coagulation, as no rating scales include parameters like the INR. In fact, these types of side effects have been discovered by means of post-marketing surveillance and not by means of clinical trials.

ETHICS

Studies should be conducted in accordance with the Declaration of Helsinki and the laws of the country in which the research is conducted. This means, first of all, that voluntary consent is always required. Second, it is frequently necessary to exclude from drug research studies female patients who are, or may become, pregnant to eliminate the possibility of foetal damage. The first trimester is particularly at risk to the foetus. Sexually active women should be included only if they do not plan on becoming pregnant and are taking appropriate measures to avoid conception. On the other hand, the use of contraceptive drugs of established efficacy may pose a risk of adverse interaction with the investigational drug. Only after the results of reproductive and teratologic studies in animals have been reviewed and judged satisfactory may sexually active women be included.

Studies involving children should not be initiated until safety and efficacy studies in adults are well advanced.

The clinical use of placebo comparisons poses a true moral dilemma. Is it ethical to treat countless patients with a marketed but inadequately tested substance not proven to be more effective than an inert placebo? Is it ethical, for the sake of proof of efficacy based on placebo comparisons, to make deliberate investigational use of inert medication in a limited number of patients requiring treatment? The urgency of this dilemma varies from situation to situation as investigators weigh the alternatives. Although specific circumstances of prevailing ethics may contraindicate the use of placebo comparisons, claims for efficacy must provide an acceptable alternative, i.e. comparisons of dosage–response curves. In psychopharmacology, masses of data are not regarded as an acceptable alternative for studies involving unambiguous comparisons.

In conditions such as depression and anxiety, many investigators believe that the superiority of standard existing drugs over placebo is sufficiently modest to make the administration of placebo to some patients entirely justifiable, particularly if there are specific provisions to remove from the study those patients whose clinical condition worsens or fails to improve over a limited period of time. There is, however, a large body of opinion in some countries which questions the ethics of the use of a placebo, especially in depressed outpatients for whom even a modest level of superiority of drug over placebo might be sufficient to avert a suicide.

On the other hand, nowadays there is a wide opinion supporting the use of placebo-controlled studies on the basis that the comparison between a new drug and the placebo is necessary because the new drug must be at least superior to the placebo in terms of efficacy. In fact, the results of controlled clinical studies without comparison with a placebo usually show an efficacy of the drug four to five times higher than the one demonstrated by clinically controlled studies with a placebo comparison. Moreover, the ethical use of a placebo is supported also by the fact that about 25% of patients improve without drug treatment (the so-called placebo effect).

Considering these issues and assuming the substantial superiority of available standard psychotropic drugs over the placebo, it seems reasonable to first determine whether the drug under investigation has the same general efficacy as a standard drug. If it is not inferior to the standard drug, placebo-controlled studies should be initiated. If patient condition worsens, however, provisions should be made for removing them from the study.

Depending on the nature of the disorder, the type of drug under investigation and the safety and reliability of drugs available, placebo comparisons may be regarded as unethical or unsuitable. Where the placebo controls are not to be used, the drug under investigation is compared to a standard active drug, amytriptiline or imipramine, according to past procedures, and fluoxetine, according to the present procedure. The past use of TCAs as comparison drugs imposed the exclusion of patients with organic illnesses, such as cardiac disorder, glaucoma, urinary disorders, that could worsen due to the TCA. However, such exclusion criteria remained when fluoxetine was introduced, even though it did not have the same contraindications as TCAs. This is a strong paradox because the comparison drug should stimulate the discovery of new, more effective and tolerable compounds instead of restricting the field of research with an over-selected sample.

On the other hand, the superiority of a new compound is usually shown by comparing it with another compound of a certain class of antidepressants, usually imipramine for TCAs and fluoxetine for SSRIs. This introduces a strong bias linked to the specific characteristics of each antidepressant that cannot be applied to all drugs of the same class. In practice, in a sample of depressed patients with a high anxiety level, a new antidepressant which induces sedation as a side effect may provide better results when compared with fluoxetine, but not with fluvoxamine. There is the risk of applying the properties of a specific compound to all the other drugs of the same class, even if clinical practice demonstrates how different the effects of the drugs may be.

Moreover, when a placebo is not used, the investigation must provide for other procedures to protect against type II errors (i.e. an acceptance of the null hypothesis when it is wrong). Large sample size, use of stringent selection criteria, use of well-validated rating scales, evidence of inter- and intra-rater reliability and avoidance of all confounding therapeutic influences will help to reduce the hazard of error. Moreover, as alternatives to placebo-controlled studies, dose–response curves for the experimental and standard drug can be compared, or at least two dosage levels of the experimental drug may be compared under double-blind conditions to demonstrate dosage effect on efficacy. It may be desirable in some situations to consider a design where a group receiving the experimental drug is compared with a group receiving placebo in terms of the amount of standard drug supplementation required to maintain patients at a specific level (ECDEU, 1978).

Concerning the comparison of a drug versus placebo to study tolerability, Phase 3 studies are only partially useful and satisfactory. They should be completed by post-marketing surveillance, represented by Phase 4 studies. These studies focus on effectiveness and primarily on tolerability of the marketed drug, administered to a large sample of subjects during the daily clinical practice. The aim is to improve knowledge concerning the use of the drug, the risk/benefit ratio, the correlation between epidemiology of the disorder and the use of the corresponding drugs, the interactions between efficacy and tolerability of drugs used off-label, as well as the long-term positive and adverse effects.

This phase is particularly important for drugs previously studied through experimental designs or for drugs showing toxicity in specific populations (e.g. pregnant women, genetically selected subjects, chronically treated populations). A paradigmatic example in this case are the studies concerning clozapine (Healy, 2000a).

Although surveillance is fundamental for obtaining adequate knowledge of drugs and their use in daily clinical practice, it is not so common and widely practised. A good example of this is represented by the IFPMA Compendium on Regulation of Pharmaceuticals for Human use, formulated by the World Health Organization (WHO), which describes (section 6) the post-marketing procedures for 58 countries. Among the 58 included, 27 countries have specific legislation about drug surveillance, while seven countries do not have any legislation, but only recommendations for pharmacological industries and/or for general practitioners. 24 countries, on the other hand, do not have any kind of regulation.

LIMITATIONS OF CLINICAL TRIALS

The general methodology of clinical trials should be based on the principles of empirical science: (a) reliability, that is the principle for which the same result must be reproduced by different researchers (inter-rater reliability), or by the same researcher on different occasions; (b) control of biases (the systematic mistakes); and (c) use of inferential statistics to generalize on the entire patient population with a specific diagnosis the results of data collected in a small, but representative sample. The effort to respect these three aspects has often been the cause of a disregard for validity or the inadequacy of the experimental design to solve the scientific problem and the transposition of the results in situations different from the experimental ones.

Moreover, one of the most important principles of the scientific procedure is to look for and find the truth, respecting the ethical rules for which the only required reward is the discovery itself.

As mentioned above, in reality, the pharmaceutical industry's aim is usually to finance clinical trials in order to increase profit, independent of the possibility of discovering the truth. Therefore, research is driven by economic interests, rendering the ethical context of clinical trials markedly different from that envisaged by the epistemological principles of scientific research.

The fact that the majority of clinical pharmacological research is ordered and supported by the pharmaceutical industry perpetuates the suspicion that in controlled clinical trials there is a bigger and more dangerous bias than in the case of a complete absence of clinical evaluation. It is noteworthy, for instance, that negative results are not published and emphasized as well as positive results.

Considering these points, it seems necessary to critically evaluate clinical trials, as they are the most important step toward endorsement of new experimental drugs.

INCLUSION AND EXCLUSION CRITERIA

The selection of patients to participate in a clinical trial is of paramount importance (Endicott et al., 1994). Generally, five to ten patients are screened out for every one or two patients enrolled in the clinical trial for an antidepressant. Indeed, the average depressed patient in a psychiatrist's practice would probably be ineligible to participate in a Phase 3 clinical trial, often because of comorbid medical or psychiatric illness. High-volume sites may even operate on a 'don't ask/don't tell' strategy. If the exclusion criterion is questionable, it is in the best interest of the research entrepreneur to enrol the patient without clarifying the presence or absence of the ambiguous exclusion criterion (Thase, 1999), especially when the researcher must complete the trial in a short time. This means that subjects can be over-included using softer exclusion criteria.

Fortunately, young women can now participate in industry-sponsored clinical trials except when they are pregnant, breast-feeding, or – if sexually active – unwilling to use an acceptable form of birth control (Merkatz et al., 1993). Unfortunately, inclusion criteria are still strict and exclude from clinical trials the elderly (the FDA now requires representative samples of subjects including men and women aged 18 to 60 years from various regions of country for Phase 3 studies) (*New Drug Development in the United States*, 1976) (Endicott et al., 1994), non-responders and non-compliant people. This selection is even more evident and strict considering that a large part of clinical trials are conducted in highly regarded institutions (Simon et al., 1996; Thase, 1999), which usually treat subjects with extremely severe symptoms and poor response to treatments. Although antidepressants are effective in psychotic depression compared to the placebo, depressed patients manifesting hallucinations or delusions (and in particular those with suicidal tendencies) are usually excluded from trials conducted in the United States because the standard of care for psychotic depression is a combined therapy with an antidepressant and an antipsychotic, or electroconvulsive therapy. Similarly, cases with comorbidity with psychiatric disorders 'not better accounted for' or organic diseases are usually excluded, even if they include a large majority of patients observed in clinical practice.

In substance, clinical trials usually refer to tightly controlled conditions that may prevent detection of differences in real-world effectiveness (Feinstein, 1983). Moreover, in clinical trials for antidepressants, it is worse still that these tightly controlled conditions have been determined by a wider necessity to protect the researchers from a legal point of view and not protect the subjects under study from iatrogenic diseases, as in the past. It seems that this kind of research has been gradually modified in favour of bureaucratic requirements instead of scientific ones.

MEASUREMENT OF OUTCOME AND ANALYSIS OF THE RESULTS

The outcome is usually assessed as a good response to the drug if there is a 50% reduction in symptoms. Considering that the golden zone to detect efficacy of most antidepressants is probably in the moderate to moderately severe range of depression, a 50% reduction in symptoms cannot really identify a good response to treatment and does not match at all with patients' opinion of recovery (Perry, 1996; Nurnberg et al., 1999; Walters et al., 1999; Panteleeva et al., 2000), as the patient evaluates not only the mere reduction of symptoms but principally his functional impairment and quality of life. Therefore, a well-conducted clinical trial should include rating scales and questionnaires measuring the quoted parameters of functional impairment and quality of life.

On the other hand, placebo response rates of 50% to 70% are not uncommon in mild depression. Since this cut-off is not able to discriminate between a placebo and drug response, a ceiling effect sometimes compromises interpretation of studies of mild depression because of the lack of design power to show improvement when placebo response rates are high (Thase, 1999).

A further consideration refers to the statistical analysis of the results. Controlled clinical studies usually compare new drugs with traditional ones (typically the tricyclic antidepressants amitriptyline and imipramine) and lack of a significant difference between the two is taken as evidence that the new drug worked just as well as the older one. This kind of study indicates that given the numbers involved in a traditional antidepressant trial, the lack of difference between old and new treatments is not convincing evidence that the new treatment works. This is strictly linked to the common presence of the so-called type II error because small numbers are often likely (Thompson and Pocock, 1991; Greenberg et al., 1994; Hotopf et al., 1997). In reality, if drug 'A' is not statistically more effective than drug 'B', it does not mean that 'A' is as effective as 'B'. The bias is usually eliminated using a statistical design aimed to contradict hypothesis I (i.e. the two treatments are different) rather than not to contradict hypothesis I (i.e. the two treatments are equal). Briefly, when the results of a study do not show a significant superiority of one drug over the other, the only reasonable and correct conclusion is that the initial hypothesis cannot be confirmed (Faravelli 1994). Moreover, in theory, good clinical trials should analyse all the data collected in the sample observed, including dropout subjects.

DURATION OF CLINICAL TRIALS

For many patients, psychiatric disorder is a recurrent and potentially chronic illness that warrants long-term, preventive treatment. An acute phase response to a new agent thus will often lead to an indefinite course of maintenance phase therapy. At present, the vast majority of controlled clinical trials last less than one year. There are only a few published studies with a trial duration of greater than one year involving antidepressants introduced since 1988 (Montgomery et al., 1988; Stewart, 1998; Keller et al., 1998). Moreover, trial design adopted for registration purposes only calls for a six-week trial exposure. Ordinarily, six weeks is sufficient to show changes in Hamilton Rating Scale scores and significant differences from placebo administration. Thus, regulatory agencies such as the FDA accept evidence from such a trial sustaining a claim of antidepressant efficacy. Arguably, the relatively brief period of treatment involved in this design, or the widespread confusion between regulatory and scientific studies, or both factors combined, create an impression of therapeutic specificity; depression is rather similar to a bacterial infection, something that can be knocked out by a short, sharp course of treatment – an impression that is quite misleading. Thus far, there have been no major surprises, but issues such as loss of efficacy over time, late-emerging weight gain, and untoward antidepressant discontinuation syndromes, continue to be topical concerns.

An implication in favour of long-term evaluation of the results comes from studies showing that treatment with a placebo never maintains the Clinical Global Impression (CGI) score above 1–2 for a period of at least one to two months (Quitkin et al., 1984; Goodnick et al., 1987).

In reality, clinical trials are usually too short and there is no interest in deciding the criteria to stop a treatment. The controlled studies usually last for four, six or twelve weeks of treatment; follow-up periods are rare and their results are usually not published.

Moreover, antidepressants have a characteristic period of latency before producing a real therapeutic effect, and this time varies from subject to subject. The profile of improvement usually reported by controlled clinical trials, as a rapid reduction in symptoms in the first two weeks and a subsequent slower improvement, is far from what can be observed in clinical practice, where patients do not present an initial modification of symptom severity and have subsequent rapid improvement. In reality, what clinical trials show is a mean pattern of response, influenced by the initial rapid improvement typical of some patients. The direct consequence is that the mean pattern of response cannot be generalized and applied to all subjects. Therefore, it is necessary to have a follow-up period to clarify treatment response and the corresponding outcome.

THE MATTER OF GRANT

Phase 3 studies are tightly linked to regulatory agency rules that may favour pharmaceutical industries, which provide economic support of research but, above all, the use and widespread marketing of their new products (Stewart, 1998; Nurnberg et al., 1999; Thase, 1999). Moreover, they have access to all data on a specific product. Several authors have provided direct evidence of publication bias by investigating the publication status protocols submitted to ethics committees or research organizations (Dickersin and Min, 1993; Stern and Simes, 1997).

In this regard, it is interesting to notice that antidepressants, such as Prozac, have been licensed on the basis of demonstrated superiority over a placebo in patients with moderate rather than severe depression. But this superiority over the placebo says nothing about how good the compound is. Superiority over a placebo legitimizes a marketing claim that the compound has antidepressant efficacy, but is it as good as older compounds? A number of studies that have been done by independent groups, notably the Danish University Antidepressant Study Group (DUAG) have compared some of the newer compounds with clomipramine in more severely depressed populations. In most cases to date, clomipramine has been found to be superior (DUAG, 1986, 1990). The question of how an antidepressant acts against the more severe forms of depression is of no small importance, likewise, the question of what an antidepressant is and indeed what depressive disease might be is also important. Another ambiguity that the SSRIs are beneficial in moderate depression is consistent with an assumption that they will also be useful for milder depressions, but strictly speaking, this has not been shown to date. On the other hand, any anti-depressants, prior to the first of the SSRIs, have been shown to be antidepressant, at least to the FDA's satisfaction. The fact that the older compounds have not been withdrawn from the market, however, tacitly indicates that everyone 'knows' that they are antidepressants. There is a sense, then, that in the real (non-regulated) world, randomized placebo-controlled trials are not necessary to prove that a compound is an antidepressant.

Pharmaceutical industries, however, should not be considered uniquely evil in this regard. The trials that the industry has sponsored have established that certain compounds with particular biochemical profiles are at the very least antidepressant principles, if not specific magic bullets for depression. The various psychotherapies, in contrast, have conspicuously avoided testing the different therapeutic components contained in the treatment packages they offer to see which contributes what to the resolution of depressive or other nervous disorders. In short, a great deal of what a study reveals depends on who sponsors it, and the community at large has not, for the most part, been involved in sponsoring independent studies in the therapeutics of nervous disorders.

PUBLICATION OF RESULTS

As a consequence of the strict relationship between scientific research and economic interests, it is noteworthy that Phase 3 clinical trials, principally used to test new compounds before marketing, are easily published and largely represented in the literature. Moreover, the majority of the published results show the superiority, in terms of effectiveness, of the new compounds versus the old ones. This unfortunate phenomenon can explain the pharmaceutical industry's pressure to modify the presentation of results of clinical trials, or leave them unpublished. In other words, many negative trials are not published because of pressure or criticism exerted by drug firms upon authors, or as a result of a conflict of interest in the editorial processing of manuscripts (Fava, 1998). A striking example of this is the case of calcium channel blockers compared to a diuretic published in the *Journal of the American Medical Association* (Zalewski, 1997), but it is also the case with antidepressants. Only a small number of published results of randomized clinical trials show unfavourable results of the new antidepressants (DUAG, 1986, 1990; Peselow et al., 1989; Faravelli et al., 2003), while there are a myriad of clinical trials in favour of the new compounds. This could be explained by the true superiority of new antidepressants; however, in reality, meta-analyses of the trials comparing TCAs vs. SSRIs usually fail to demonstrate a clear advantage of the SSRIs (Anderson, 1998, 2000; Bech et al., 2000; Hotopf et al., 1996; Mitchell et al., 1997; Montgomery, 2001; Ottevanger, 1991; Pande and Sayler, 1993; Song et al., 1993; Steffens et al., 1997).

However, meta-analyses can be biased as well as clinical trials because they may include or exclude clinical trials and they usually refer to published data and not to all the available data for all randomized patients, since there is a large number of unpublished reports.

Concerning the inclusion of unpublished results, Bech and co-workers in 2000 used the Eli Lilly and Company (Lilly) fluoxetine database referring to patients from published and unpublished randomized clinical short-term trials of fluoxetine, aiming at obtaining quantitative estimates of the fluoxetine treatment effect compared with placebo and TCAs. The results were striking since fluoxetine was superior to placebo in all the trials while in trials comparing fluoxetine versus TCA, the results for all trials and for the USA trials showed a trend in favour of fluoxetine. Those for the non-USA trials showed a trend in favour of TCA. The authors concluded that fluoxetine was superior to placebo whereas the results obtained versus TCA depended on the approach used. In fact, in 65% of the USA trials compared with the 47% of the non-USA trials, old TCAs (imipramine and amitriptyline) were used as comparison compounds instead of the newer (nortriptyline, clomipramine, etc.). The choice of the comparison compound is fundamental as the results from meta-analyses can differ depending on how many patients are withdrawn from treatment early and how they are counted in the analysis.

Such manipulation of results is relevant as it is generally recognized that the standard basis for treatment guidelines is meta-analyses of all randomized controlled trials or systematic literature reviews.

Concerning the choice of clinical trials in a meta-analysis, different biases must be considered: multiple publications, selective publication, selective reporting in studies sponsored by the pharmaceutical industry. Melander et al. (2003) studied 38 publications presenting data from the 42 studies submitted to the Swedish drug regulatory agency to secure marketing approval for five SSRIs for the treatment of major depression. They found: (1) multiple publications: 21 studies contributed to at least two publications each, and three studies contributed to five publications; (2) selective publications: studies showing significant effects of drug were published as stand-alone publications more often than studies with non-significant results; (3) selective reporting: only 24% of the stand-alone publications reported the usually less favourable intention to treat results while many publications reported the more favourable per protocol analyses only.

On the basis of these findings, it is evident that without access to all studies (positive as well as negative, published as well as unpublished) and without access to alternative analyses (intention to treat as well as per protocol), any attempt to recommend a specific drug is likely to be based on biased evidence. In this sense, the authors talk about evidence-b(i)ased medicine.

FROM CLINICAL TRIALS' RESULTS TO CLINICAL PRACTICE: THE OFF-LABEL USE OF PSYCHOACTIVE DRUGS

Major biological treatments in psychiatry have been discovered by accident or serendipity, that is by means of chance as a necessary and/or sufficient condition. Good examples of serendipitous discovery are electroshock therapy, lithium, chlorpromazine, iproniazid and imipramine (Jeste et al., 1979). Since strict methodological rules have been introduced in research, the possibility of serendipitously discovering new psychoactive drugs have largely decreased. The only exception is due to the 'off-label' use of the new compounds. That is, some drugs have been found to be effective in psychiatric disorder different from those for which they initially had indications.

Actually, the only real improvement in clinical pharmacology during the last 40 years is due to the unexpected, off-label use of drugs developed for different purposes: antiepileptics as mood stabilizers, SSRIs for anxiety disorders, novel antipsychotics for bipolar disorders.

CONCLUSIONS

Considering all these issues, there are some doubts that Phase 3 studies do allow an extrapolation to the wider patient population which it is intended to treat.

This suggests that: (1) the simple transposition of the findings to the real world clinical reality is particularly difficult because the population samples of clinical trials have different characteristics from the patients of everyday clinical experience; (2) research conducted on a sample with a high rate of probable non-responders yields misleading results. The problem is even more complex if we consider that psychiatric samples are intrinsically heterogeneous, and this phenomenon is not mitigated by operational diagnoses.

On the basis of limitations described above, it is evident that the majority of the studies should be subjected to some form of criticism. For instance, it is now commonly accepted that SSRIs should be, together with other newer compounds, the first-choice treatment for mood and anxiety disorders (Keller, 2000; Zohar and Westenberg, 2000). However, this is far from being well established. Some studies still report greater efficacy of the TCAs (DUAG, 1990; Barbui and Hotopf, 2001; Faravelli et al., 2003) and the meta-analyses carried out on the trials comparing TCAs versus SSRIs failed to show a clear advantage of the SSRIs (Anderson, 2000; Bech et al., 2000; Montgomery, 2001).

There is a large gap between clinical trial findings and clinical practice. Clinical trials seem to serve the purpose of advocating new compounds (Fava, 2002) and to favour their registration with regulatory agencies, even when they are not in accordance with the requirements of every day clinical practice.

It is obvious that the new antidepressants have a lower risk of inducing rapid cycling and are safer in case of overdose, but it does not mean that they have high tolerability, especially if the tolerability is supported by the scores of inadequate rating scales. In fact, in everyday clinical practice, it is common to hear complaints after the very first oral administration of an SSRI. SSRIs are not lacking in subjective side effects, especially in those with a diagnosis of anxiety or mood disorders who have a low tolerance to any unpleasant effect induced by the therapy.

For this reason, even if it is speculated that Phase 4 studies could help solve the dilemma as they consider a naturalistic environment representing the real, everyday psychiatric practice, they also present with certain disadvantages. They require the enrolment of a large number of subjects to evaluate efficacy and/or tolerability, which involves important logistic and economic matters (Hollister et al., 1994; Thase, 1999); and they are not controlled; the prescription is based on subjective grounds and this may seriously bias the findings (Thase, 1999).

Therefore, it is the authors' opinion that the treatment of a patient still depends significantly on his relationship with the psychiatrist. The capacity of the clinician to communicate with the patient, to be understood, to mitigate his fears, doubts and complaints are basic to making a treatment effective. Besides guidelines and strong standardization in psychiatry, the prescription still continues to be an 'art' linked to science.

REFERENCES

APA (1980) *Diagnostic and statistical manual* (3rd edition). Washington, DC: American Psychiatric Association.

Anderson IM (1998) SSRIs versus tricyclic antidepressants in depressed inpatients: a meta-analysis of efficacy and tolerability. *Depress Anxiety* **7**(1): 11–17.

Anderson IM (2000) Selective serotonin reuptake inhibitors versus tricyclic antidepressants: a meta-analysis of efficacy and tolerability. *J Affect Disord* **58**(1): 19–36.

Barbui C, Hotopf M (2001) Amitriptyline v. the rest: still the leading antidepressant after 40 years of randomized controlled trials. *Br J Psychiatry* **178**: 129–144.

Bech P, Cialdella P, Haigh MC, Birkett MA, Hours A, Boissel JP, et al. (2000) Meta-analysis of randomized controlled trials of fluoxetine versus placebo and tricyclic antidepressants in the short-term treatment of major depression. *Br J Psychiatry* **176**: 421–428.

Calabrese JR, Shelton MD, Rapport DJ, Kimmel SE, Elhaj O (2002) Long-term treatment of bipolar disorder with lamotrigine. *J Clin Psychiatry* **63**(10): 18–22.

Dickersin K, Min YL (1993) NIH clinical trials and publication bias. *Online J Curr Clin Trials* **28**: Doc No. 50.

DUAG (Danish University Antidepressant Group) (1986) Citalopram: clinical effect profile in comparison with clomipramine. A controlled multicenter study. *Psychopharmacology* **90**(1): 131–138.

DUAG (Danish University Antidepressant Group) (1990) Paroxetine: a selective serotonin reuptake inhibitor showing better tolerance, but weaker antidepressant effect than clomipramine in a controlled multicenter study. *J Affect Disord* **18**(4): 289–299.

ECDEU (Early Continuous Drug Evaluation Unit) (1978) International guidelines for clinical trials of psychotropic drugs. *Psychopharmacol Bull* **14**(1): 47–65.

Endicott J, Schwartz GE, Lee JH (1994) Classification issues in patient selection and description. In Prien RF, Robinson DS (eds) *Clinical Evaluation of Psychotropic Drugs*. New York: Raven Press, pp. 69–83.

Evans L, Moore G (1981) The treatment of phobic anxiety by zimelidine. *Acta Psychiatr Scand Suppl* **290**: 342–345.

Faravelli C (1994) Che cosa non funziona nelle sperimentazioni cliniche controllate. In Maj M, Racagni G (eds) *La Sperimentazione dei Nuovi Farmaci in Psichiatria*. Milan: Masson, pp. 81–89.

Faravelli C, Cosci F, Ciampelli M, Scarpato MA, Spiti R, Ricca V (2003) A self-controlled, naturalistic study of selective serotonin reuptake inhibitors versus tricyclic antidepressants. *Psychother Psychisom* **72**: 95–101.

Fava GA (1998) All our dreams are sold. *Psychother Psychosom* **67**: 191–193.

Fava GA (2002) Long-term treatment with antidepressant drugs: the spectacular achievement of propaganda. *Psychother Psychosom* **71**: 127–132.

FDA (Food and Drug Administration) (1979) FDA guidelines for the clinical evaluation of psychotropic drugs – antidepressants and antianxiety drugs. *Psychopharmacol Bull* **14**(2): 45–63.

Feinstein A (1983) An additional basic science for clinical medicine, II: The limitations of randomized trials. *Ann Intern Med* **99**: 544–550.

Goodnick PJ, Fieve RR, Peselow ED, et al. (1987) Double blind treatment of major depression with fluoxetine: use of pattern analysis and relation of HAM-D score to CGI changes. *Psychopharmacol Bull* **23**: 162.

Greenberg RP, Bornstein RF, Zborowski MJ, Fisher S, Greenberg MD (1994) A meta-analysis of fluoxetine outcome in the treatment of depression. *J Nerv Ment Dis* **182**: 547–551.

Guy W (1976) ECDEU *Assessment Manual for Psychopharmacology* (revised, 1976). DHEW Publication No. (ADM) 76-338.

Hamilton M (1960) A rating scale for depression. *J Neurol Neurosurg Psychiatr* **23**: 56.

Healy D (2000a) *The Antidepressant Era*. Cambridge, MA: Harvard University Press, pp. 111–142.

Healy D (2000b) *The Antidepressant Era*. Cambridge, MA: Harvard University Press, pp. 78–110.

Hill AB (1963) Medical ethics and controlled trials. *BMJ* **1**: 1043–1049.

Hollister LE, Jones JK, Fisher S (1994) Post-marketing surveillance of drug. In Prien RF, Robinson DS (eds) *Clinical Evaluation of Psychotropic Drugs*. New York: Raven Press, pp. 217–235.

Hotopf M, Lewis G, Normand C (1996) Are SSRIs a cost-effective alternative to tricyclics? *Br J Psychiatry* **168**: 404–409.

Hotopf M, Hardy R, Lewis G (1997) Discontinuation rates of SSRIs and tricyclic antidepressants: a meta-analysis and investigation of heterogeneity. *Br J Psychiatry* **170**: 120–127.

Jeste DV, Gillin JC, Wyatt RJ (1979) Serendipity in biological psychiatry – a myth? *Arch Gen Psychiatry* **36**(11): 1173–1178.

Keller MB (2000) Citalopram therapy for depression: a review of 10 years of European experience and data from U.S. clinical trials. *J Clin Psychiatry* **61**(12): 896–908.

Keller MB, Kocsis JH, Thase ME, Gelenberg AJ, Rush AJ, Koran LM, Schatzberg AF, Russell JM, Hirschfeld RMA, Klein DN, McCullough JP, Fawcett JA, Kornstein SG, LaVange L, Harrison WM (1998) Maintenance phase efficacy of sertraline for chronic depression. A randomized controlled trial. *JAMA* **280**: 1665–1672.

Melander H, Ahlqvist-Rastad J, Meijer G, Beermann B (2003) Evidence b(i)ased medicine-selective reporting from studies sponsored by pharmaceutical industry: review of studies in new drug applications. *BMJ* **326**(7400): 1171–1173.

Merkatz RB, Temple R, Sobel S, et al. (1993) Women in clinical trials of new drugs. *N Engl J Med* **329**: 292–296.

Mitchell J, Greenberg J, Finch K, Kovach J, Kipp L, Shainline M, et al. (1997) Effectiveness and economic impact of antidepressant medication: a review. *Am J Manag Care* **3**(2): 323–330; quiz 331.

Montgomery SA (2001) A meta-analysis of the efficacy and tolerability of paroxetine versus tricyclic antidepressants in the treatment of major depression. *Int Clin Psychopharmacol* **16**(3): 169–178.

Montgomery SA, Asberg M (1979) A new depression scale designed to the sensitive to change. *Br J Psychiatry* **134**: 382.

Montgomery SA, Dufour H, Brion S, Gailledreau J, Laqueille X, Ferrey G, Moron P, Parant-Lucena N, Singer L, Danion JM, et al. (1988) The prophylactic efficacy of fluoxetine in unipolar depression. *Br J Psychiatry* Suppl (3): 69–76.

New Drug Development in the United States (1976) HHS publication. Rockville, MD: Department of Health Human Services, Food and Drug Administration.

Nurnberg HG, Thompson PM, Hensley PL (1999) Antidepressants medication change in a clinical treatment setting: a comparison of the effectiveness of selective serotonin reuptake inhibitors. *J Clin Psychiatry* **60**(9): 574–579.

Ottevanger EA (1991) The efficacy of fluvoxamine in patients with severe depression. *Br J Clin Res* **2**: 125–132.

Pande AC, Sayler ME (1993) Fluoxetine – a clinical and research update: severity of depression and response to fluoxetine. *Int Clin Psychopharmacol* **8**: 243–245.

Panteleeva GP, Abramova LI, Korenev AN (2000) Selective serotonin reuptake inhibitors in the therapy of various types of endogenous depression. *Zh Nevrol Psikhiatr Im S S Korsakova* **100**(3): 36–41.

Perry PJ (1996) Pharmacotherapy for major depression with melancholic features: relative efficacy of tricyclic vs selective serotonin reuptake inhibitor antidepressants. *J Affect Disord* **39** (1): 1–6.

Peselow ED, Filippi AM, Goodnick P, Barouche F, Fieve RR (1989) The short- and long-term efficacy of paroxetine HCl. A. Data from a 6-week double-blind parallel design trial vs imipramine and placebo. *Psychopharmacol Bull* **25**: 267–271.

Quitkin FM, Rabkin JG, Ross D, et al. (1984) Identification of true drug response to anti-depressants. *Arch Gen Psychiatry* **41**: 782.

Simon GE, VonKorff M, Heilingenstein JH, Revicki DA, Grothaus L, Katon W, Wagner EH (1996) Initial antidepressant choice in primary care. Effectiveness and cost of fluoxetine vs tricyclic antidepressants. *JAMA* **275** (24): 1897–1902.

SysteMetrics, Inc. Pharmacological and Somatic Treatment Research Branch, 5600 Fishers Lane, Rockville, MD, 20857, USA.

Song F, Freemantle N, Sheldon TA, House A, Watson P, Long A, et al. (1993) Selective serotonin reuptake inhibitors: meta-analysis of efficacy and acceptability. *BMJ* **306**(6879): 683–687.

Steffens DC, Krishnan KR, Helms MJ (1997) Are SSRIs better than TCAs? Comparison of SSRIs and TCAs: a meta-analysis. *Depress Anxiety* **6**(1): 10–18.

Stern JM, Simes RJ (1997) Publication bias: evidence of delayed publication in a cohort study of clinical research projects. *BMJ* **315**: 40–45.

Stewart A (1998) Choosing an antidepressant: effectiveness based pharmacoeconomics. *J Affect Disord* **48**(2–3): 125–133.

Thase ME (1999) How should efficacy be evaluated in randomized clinical trials of treatments for depression? *J Clin Psychiatry* **60**(Suppl 4): 23–31.

Thompson SG, Pocock SJ (1991) Can a meta-analysis be trusted? *Lancet* **338**: 1127–1130.

Uhlenhuth EH, Glass RM, Fischman MW (1979) Multiple cross-over designs with an anti-anxiety agent and an antidepressant. *Psychopharmacol Bull* **15**(3): 37–40.

Walters G, Reynolds III CF, Mulsant BH, Pollock SG (1999) Continuation and maintenance pharmacotherapy in geriatric depression: an open-trial comparison of paroxetine and nortrptyline in patients older than 70 years. *J Clin Psychiatry* **60**(Suppl 20): 21–25.

Zalewski D (1997) Ties that bind: do corporate dollars strangle scientific research? *Lingua-franca* **7**: 51–59.

Zohar J, Westenberg HG (2000) Anxiety disorders: a review of tricyclic antidepressants and selective serotonin reuptake inhibitors. *Acta Psychiatr Scand* **403**: 39–49.

17

Mood and Anxiety Disorders – a Diagnostic Pleonasm?

Herman M. van Praag

Academic Hospital, University of Maastricht, Maastricht, The Netherlands

THE BOND THAT TURNED OUT TO BE INEXTRICABLE

The border between depression and anxiety is befogged, if discernible at all. The two groups of psychic dysfunctions constitute a true Gordian knot. That is true on two levels: the level of disorders and that of symptoms (Table 17.1). In other words: anxiety and mood *disorders* often co-exist (Table 17.2), while anxiety disorders are often accompanied by depressive *symptoms* and, vice versa, mood disorders frequently by anxiety *symptoms* (DiNardo and Barlow, 1990).

Moreover, one distinguishes presently the so-called subthreshold anxiety disorders and subthreshold mood disorders, being anxiety and mood states that do not fulfil the DSM criteria for a true disorder but yet cause substantial discomfort. Those subthreshold conditions also occur frequently together (Judd et al., 1997). Finally, in an attempt to resolve the diagnostic problems posed by the overlap of mood and anxiety disorders, the constructs of atypical depression and mixed anxiety–depression disorder were introduced, hybrid constructs composed of elements known from the anxiety and affective disorders (West and Dally, 1959; Zinbarg et al., 1994). Diagnostically, all this makes for a pretty messy situation.

How come? What could be the reason for this curious overlap? It is not known for sure, but I will discuss four possible explanations.

(1) Anxiety and mood disorders are independent categories, each with their own symptomatology and pathophysiology, that happen to occur often simultaneously.
(2) Mood and anxiety disorders share a common pathophysiology.
(3) Anxiety disorders (or disturbances in anxiety regulation) may trigger depression (or disturbances in mood regulation) or vice versa.

Mood Disorders: Clinical Management and Research Issues. Edited by E. J. L. Griez, C. Faravelli, D. J. Nutt and J. Zohar.
©2005 John Wiley & Sons Ltd. ISBN 0 470 09426 5.

TABLE 17.1   Comorbidity of anxiety and depression exist on various levels

- Mood and anxiety disorders often occur together
- Anxiety symptoms often accompany a mood disorder
- Depressive symptoms often accompany an anxiety disorder
- Subthreshold mood and anxiety disorders often go hand-in-hand
- Mixed anxiety–depression disorder

TABLE 17.2   Comorbidity mood and anxiety disorders, both lifetime and cross-sectionally (From Wittchen et al. (2001). John Wiley & Sons Limited. Reproduced with permission)

• Community samples • Primary care samples	} approximately 33%
• Clinical samples	approximately 65%

(4)   The nosological disease model is invalid and thus it is futile to try to separate a variety of discrete anxiety and mood disorders.

THE POSSIBLE REASONS WHY

Mere Coincidence

For a number of reasons coincidental intertwining of mood and anxiety disorders is not a likely explanation (Table 17.3).

First, affective and anxiety disorders tend to respond to the same treatments. Antidepressants are effective in mood disorders and in most anxiety disorders, whereas certain anxiolytics are effective in depression as well (Henn et al., 2001). Mood and anxiety disorders have, in the second place, several biological features in common, for instance disturbances in 5-hydroxytryptamine (5-HT; serotonin)-mediated systems, particularly those served by 5-HT_{1A} and 5-HT_{2C} receptors; corticotropin-releasing hormone (CRH) overdrive and disinhibition of the noradrenergic (NA-ergic) system (Nemeroff, 1996; Anand and Charney, 1997; Van Praag et al., 2004).

TABLE 17.3   Comorbidity anxiety/depression

Hypothesis 1: *Independent categories that often occur together*

• Respond to the same drugs • Share biological disturbances • Share many symptoms • Early adversities increase vulnerability for mood *and* anxiety disorders • High parental rates of anxiety/depression comorbidity	} Makes this assumption unlikely

TABLE 17.4 Symptomatological overlap between dysthymia and generalized anxiety disorder (GAD)

Dysthymia	GAD
Depressed mood (in adolescents: irritability) (≥2 years)	Excessive anxiety or worry (≥6 months)
2/6 of the following symptoms:	3/6 of the following symptoms:
Poor appetite or overeating	Restlessness
Insomnia or hypersomnia	Fatigue
Fatigue	Poor concentration
Low self-esteem	Irritability
Poor concentration	Muscle tension
Hopelessness	Sleep disturbances

Third, both groups of disorders share many symptoms. Generalized anxiety disorder, for instance, overlaps to a substantial degree with dysthymia (Table 17.4), and co-occurs very often together with major depression. In a majority of patients with an affective or an anxiety disorder mood and anxiety symptoms are thoroughly mixed and shade off one into the other.

A fourth argument against coincidence is that early developmental adversity, such as sexual and/or physical abuse and emotional deprivation, increases the risk of both anxiety and mood disorders later in life (Wittchen et al., 2001) (Table 17.5).

A final argument against coincidence is the observation that parents of patients suffering from a combination of mood and anxiety disorders also show high rates of the two types of disorder combined (Wittchen et al., 2001).

TABLE 17.5 Prevalence and risk factors of anxiety and mood disorders (in %). (From Wittchen et al. (2001). © John Wiley & Sons Limited. Reproduced with permission)

	Anxiety disorder	Mood disorder	Both
Prevalence	18.9	7.1	7.4
Parental history of:			
any anxiety disorder	32.1	27.8	34.2
any mood disorder	43.2	54.0	62.5
mood+anxiety disorder	17.7	19.4	25.6
Early development risks			
parental separation	22.5	18.2	23.4
traumatic events	22.8	28.4	38.6

TABLE 17.6   Comorbidity anxiety/depression

Hypothesis 2: *Anxiety (disorder) triggers mood disturbances/depression or vice versa*

Plausible possibility
    Exemplified by the novel diagnostic construct: anxiety/aggression-driven depression

TABLE 17.7   Psychopathological evidence supporting the construct of anxiety/aggression-driven depression

- Precursor symptoms: anxiety and increased outward-directed aggression
- Some episodes are characterized by anxiety and increased aggression, only
- Anxiety and aggression are highly intercorrelated, across diagnoses

Anxiety Disorders May Trigger Mood Disorders (or Vice Versa)

Anxiety serving as a pacemaker of depression seems to be an arguable possibility, at least in a subgroup of depression (Table 17.6). Whether the reverse is also true is not known.

Recently we postulated a new diagnostic construct named: anxiety/aggression-driven depression (Van Praag, 1992b, 1994, 1996, 2001). It refers to a subtype of depression in which the core disturbance lies not in mood regulation but in anxiety- and aggression-regulation; mood lowering is hypothesized to be a subsidiary. Paradoxically thus, this depression type is considered not to be a (primary) mood disorder. Briefly summarized, this hypothesis is based on the following observations.

- In a subgroup of depression the first symptoms to appear are anxiety and signs of disturbed aggression regulation, manifesting itself in such symptoms as irritability, short-temperedness, anger outbursts with no or little provocation, and the like. Mood lowering comes later, if it appears at all. In some episodes psychopathology remains restricted to symptoms of anxiety and hostility towards others (Table 17.7). Anxiety and aggression apparently, *may* serve as pacemakers for depression, but act not necessarily as such (Van Praag, 1996). Anxiety and aggression, moreover, do not occur independently but appear to be psychopathological features firmly linked. They occur highly intercorrelated across diagnoses (Apter et al., 1990).
- In depressed patients in whom increased anxiety and aggression are precursor symptoms and possibly pacemaker symptoms, anxiety and aggression are the first symptoms to respond to successful antidepressant treatment. Mood elevation follows after some delay (Katz et al., 1987; Van Praag, 1996) (Table 17.8).

TABLE 17.8 Psychopharmacological evidence supporting the construct of anxiety/aggression-driven depression

---

• Anxiety and aggression are the first symptoms to respond to antidepressant treatment

---

TABLE 17.9 Biological evidence supporting the construct of anxiety/aggression-driven depression

---

• 5-HT disturbances are observed in a subgroup of depression
• Both 5-HT metabolism and 5-HT receptors (amongst others the 5-HT$_{1a}$ receptor) are involved
• 5-HT$_{1a}$ receptor system involved in both anxiety- and agression-regulation
• 5-HT disturbances accumulate in depression heralded by anxiety and aggression

---

• Finally some biological data seem to validate the proposed diagnostic construct. In a subgroup of depression 5-HT-ergic disturbances have been established, i.e. diminished 5-HT metabolism and signs of diminished 5-HT receptor function in which the 5-HT$_{1A}$ receptor is involved (Sargent et al., 2000) (Table 17.9). These disturbances are not specific for (a particular subtype of) depression but have also been found in some patients with other diagnoses such as schizophrenia and certain anxiety states. This was explained by the observation that the pertinent 5-HT disturbances are correlated not with a particular, discrete categorical diagnosis but with disturbances in the regulation of anxiety and aggression, both inward- and outward-directed aggression – irrespective of the diagnostic category in which these phenomena occurred (Van Praag et al., 1987; Coccaro, 1992).

Moreover it was ascertained that both the metabolic and the receptor disturbances of the 5-HT system are trait-related (Van Praag et al., 1987; Golden et al., 2002). This gave rise to the hypothesis that they might be vulnerability factors, increasing the risk of disturbances in anxiety- and aggression-regulation in times of mounting stress (Van Praag and De Haan, 1980).

5-HT disturbances were shown to accumulate in anxiety/aggression-driven depression, i.e. depression in which anxiety and aggression are hypothesized to lie at the root of the depressive syndrome.

All in all, anxiety/aggression-driven depression, though still a hypothetical construct, demonstrates that anxiety (and aggression) may, in some cases, indeed trigger a mood disorder.

Anxiety and Depression Share a Common Pathophysiology

It is conceivable that the pathophysiological variables underlying anxiety and depression partly overlap or that pathophysiological disturbances underlying one state trigger pathophysiological changes generating the other (Table 17.10). In that

TABLE 17.10   Comorbidity anxiety/depression

Hypothesis 3: *Anxiety and depression share common pathophysiology*

For two systems data are available:
- 5-HT system
- CRH system

TABLE 17.11   Anxiety/depression comorbidity: 5-HT system as a common denominator

- In a subgroup of depression 5-HT receptor hyposensitivity
- 5-HT_{1a} receptor system involved in down-regulation $\Rightarrow$ mood disturbances
- Secondarily up-regulation 5-HT_{2c} system $\Rightarrow$ anxiety

TABLE 17.12   Anxiety/depression comorbidity: CRH system as a common denominator

- In subtype of depression CRH overdrive
- CRH overdrive in PVN $\Rightarrow$ hyperactivity of HPA axis
- CRH overdrive in regions beyond PVN $\Rightarrow$ behavioural symptoms:
  — anxiety
  — depression-like

case one would expect it to be next to impossible to unravel signs of disturbed anxiety regulation and those of disturbed mood regulation.

The 5-HT (Table 17.11) and CRH systems (Table 17.12) provide possible examples of pathophysiological blending.

5-HT as a Common Denominator

As was discussed in the previous subsection, 5-HT disturbances do occur in a subgroup of depression – both metabolic disturbances and disturbances in receptor function. Challenge tests with 5-HT_{1A} receptor agonists (Klaassen et al., 2002) and direct receptor measurements with PET technology (Sargent et al., 2000) point towards hypofunction of the 5-HT_{1A} receptor system. Whether other 5-HT receptors are likewise deranged is unknown. The fact that several types of antidepressants increase the responsivity of the postsynaptic 5-HT_{1A} receptors (Blier and De Montigny, 1994) supports the hypothesis that lowered 5-HT_{1A} receptor reactivity is associated with certain types of depression.

It has been demonstrated in animal experiments that the 5-HT_{1A} and 5-HT_{2C} receptor are reciprocally related, in that down-regulation of the 5-HT_{1A} receptor leads to up-regulation of the 5HT_{2C} receptor (Takao et al., 1997). The 5-HT_{2C} receptor is involved in anxiety regulation. Its activation with the relatively selective

5-HT$_{2C}$ receptor agonist *m*-chlorophenylpiperazine (mCPP), for instance, leads to increased anxiety, in particular in sensitive individuals such as those suffering from panic disorder (Kahn et al., 1988). 5-HT$_{1A}$ down-regulation, followed by 5-HT$_{2C}$ up-regulation would thus induce a mixture of symptoms known from the anxiety and mood disorders.

CRH as a Common Denominator

Dysregulation of the CRH system would likewise be a mechanism leading to a clew of anxiety and depressive symptoms.

In a subgroup of depression CRH is overproduced as is apparent from increased CRH concentrations in the brain and in cerebrospinal fluid, increased plasma levels of ACTH and cortisol and decreased suppression of plasma cortisol by dexamethasone (Nemeroff, 1996).

From a functional point of view the CRH system comprises two components. One innervating the paraventricular nucleus (PVN) and responsible for activation of the hypothalamic–pituitary–adrenal (HPA) axis and as such for the autonomic and endocrine responses to stress.

The second group of CRH neurons is located extrahypothalamically, in the hippocampus and some other locations and is held responsible for the behavioural responses to stress. If CRH is administered directly into the brain the animal develops two symptom clusters, a group considered to represent anxiety, such as increased sensitivity to the anxiogenic nature of novel environments, and a group that might be analogous to human depression, with phenomena like decreased food intake, reduced sexual behaviour, sleep disturbances and psychomotor agitation.

CRH overdrive, as has been observed in subtypes of depression, as well as in certain anxiety disorders, then, would produce a cluster of anxiety and depressive symptoms in variable combinations, dependent on the vulnerability/plasticity of the CRH systems.

Non Applicability of the Nosological Disease Model

The Nosological Disease Model

The nosological disease model has dominated psychiatry ever since Kraepelin used it to systematize mental disorders (Table 17.13). The model considers mental disorders as discrete entities, separable one from the other, and each characterized by a particular symptomatology, course, outcome and response to treatment. In principle such an entity is thought to be 'carried' by a particular pathophysiology – in principle, because as yet we know little about the neurobiological determinants of mental disorders. It is this latter supposition that has driven biological psychiatric

TABLE 17.13   Comorbidity anxiety/depression

Hypothesis 4: *The nosological disease model is flawed. Consequently it is futile to distinguish discrete anxiety and mood disorders*

Alternative disease model: reaction-form model

research over the past 40 years, searching as it had been for the neurobiological roots of categorical entities like schizophrenia, major depression and panic disorder.

The nosological disease model has been accepted in psychiatry almost axiomatically, though it is of questionable validity (Van Praag, 1992a, 1997, 2000). Take, as one example out of many, the construct of major depression. It predicts little as to symptomatology, course, outcome and response to biological and psychological treatment. Biological variables, such as disturbances in the 5-HT and/or CRH system, may or may not be demonstrable. Specific drug treatment is lacking: antidepressants are helpful in depression but in a multitude of non-depressed conditions as well, and other psychotropic drugs, such as particular benzodiazepines may be useful in combating depression. Finally biological research has failed to find biological markers indicative of this condition. One has to wear blinkers to call a disorder of that nature a discrete entity.

The Reaction-form Disease Model

An alternative disease model exists, though it has been reviled in psychiatry, and rejected without having been seriously studied (Table 17.14). It is the reaction-form model (Van Praag, 1992a). It conceives mental disorders not as discrete entities with more or less fixed boundaries, but as conglomerates of psychic dysfunctions that vary in composition both inter-individually and over time intra-individually.

Consequently, the term depression, is not used as a collective term for a series of discrete mood disorders but rather as an indication for a group of psychiatric conditions characterized primarily by disturbances in mood-, anxiety- and

TABLE 17.14   Nosological and reaction-form disease model of mental disorders

Nosological model	Reaction-form model
Fixed boundaries	Variable, foggy boundaries
Particular symptomatology	Clusters of psychic dysfunctions of varying composition
Particular and predictable course and outcome	Course and outcome variable and unpredictable
Quite stable intra- and inter-individually	Variable inter-individually and over time intra-individually

aggression-regulation of varying intensity. The same is thought to be true for the group of anxiety disorders. The reason for this fluidity is thought to be the following. Mental disorders are conceived as responses to noxious stimuli, biological or psychological in nature, originating in the outside world or from within, genetically determined or acquired. They have in common that the individual cannot cope with them, neither biologically nor psychologically.

Stimuli of this nature will disrupt a number of neuronal circuits in the brain either via a direct action or via the evoked stress response. The degree of disruption in the various circuits differs individually, the reason being variability in plasticity. Due to pre-existing imperfections, certain circuits may function marginally, just undisturbed under normal conditions, but failing under taxing circumstances. Hence the psychiatric conditions associated with those disruptions will be lacking in symptomatological consistency. Mood lowering, for instance, will be mixed with varying amounts of anger, irritability, anxiety, cognitive disturbances and a variety of somatic disturbances.

Anxiety and Depression in the Light of the Reaction-form Model

With the reaction-form model as a starting point it would be futile to try to separate mood disorders from anxiety disorders and to divide each grouping into discrete 'packages'. Instead the proper approach would be to chart carefully in each individual patient the mood- and anxiety-related symptoms and to study the psychic dysfunctions underlying these psychopathological symptoms. Only in that way one would gain a proper insight into the structure of the psychopathological condition.

A categorical diagnosis of a given patient would therefore not be the endpoint of the diagnostic process, as it is today, but just the beginning: a first diagnostic step to be followed by a refined analysis of the syndromal and symptomatological composition of the disorder and, most importantly, by an analysis of the psychic dysfunctions underlying the psychopathological symptoms.

Within the context of this disease model it would be inappropriate to speak of high comorbidity of mood and anxiety disorders. The appropriate phrasing would be: disturbances in mood- and anxiety-regulation often go hand in hand, resulting in mixtures of depressive and anxiety symptoms, the composition of which is highly varied and variable and to be assessed dimensionally and individually. Biological research would not be directed towards the biological roots of a particular mood or anxiety disorder, but at elucidation of the biological determinates of disturbed regulation of mood and anxiety.

CONCLUSIONS

Depression and anxiety, taken as discrete disorders or as symptoms, are tightly intertwined. It seems improbable that this is a matter of coincidence. Much more likely are the following two propositions. First, anxiety may trigger depression or vice versa. The first pathway has been shown to be a likely one. In a subgroup of depression, anxiety (together with dysregulation aggression) seems to be a pacemaker for depression, leading to what has been named: anxiety/aggression-driven depression.

The second conceivable possibility is that anxiety and depression share a common pathophysiology. The 5-HT and the CRH system are likely candidates for such a commonality.

As a final explanation it was proposed that the nosological disease model is not applicable in the realm of affective disorders, that it is futile to try to single out discrete mood and anxiety disorders – that, in other words, disturbances in mood- and anxiety-regulation present themselves clinically in highly variable and varying clusters of anxiety- and mood-related symptoms. Diagnosing them should be individualized and dimensional. In that case the reaction-form model would be more appropriate than the nosological disease model to characterize the conglomerate of mood and anxiety disorders.

Whichever explanation is the proper one, the knot of mood and anxiety disorders seems to be truly Gordian in nature.

SUMMARY

Depression and anxiety are tightly intertwined, both on a categorical and on a symptomatological level. Four possible explanations are discussed: coincidence, considered to be unlikely; anxiety precipitating depression or vice versa, a plausible explanation in certain cases; anxiety and depression sharing certain pathophysiological mechanisms, no more than a possibility yet, but several neuronal systems can be put forward as possible candidates.

Finally it is possible that the nosological disease model is not valid in this realm and that proper diagnosing of mood and anxiety disorders requires application of the reaction-form disease model.

REFERENCES

Anand A, Charney DS (1997) Catecholamines in depression. In Honig A, Van Praag HM (eds) *Depression: Neurobiological, Psychopathological and Therapeutic Advances.* Chicester, UK: John Wiley.

Apter A, Van Praag HM, Plutchik R, Sevy S, Korn M, Brown SL (1990) Interrelationships among anxiety, agression, impulsivity, and mood: a serotonergically linked cluster. *Psychiatry Res* **32**: 191–199.

Blier P, de Montigny C (1994) Current advances and trends in the treatment of depression. *Trends Pharm Sci* **15**: 220–226.

Coccaro EF (1992) Impulsive aggression and central serotonergic system function in humans: an example of a dimensional brain–behavior relationship. *Int Clin Psychopharm* **7**: 3–12.

Di Nardo PA, Barlow RD.(1990) Syndrome and symptom co-morbidity in the anxiety disorders. In Maser JD, Cloninger CR (eds) *Comorbidity in Anxiety and Mood Disorders*. Washington, DC: American Psychiatric Press.

Garbutt JC (2002) A longitudinal study of serotonergic function in depression. *Neuropsychopharmacology* **26**: 643–659.

Golden RN, Heine AD, Ekstrom RD, Bebchuk JM, Leatherman ME, Garbutt JC (2002) A longitudinal study of serotonergic function in depression. *Neuropsychopharmacology* **26**: 653–659.

Henn F, Sartorius N, Helmchen H, Lauter H (eds) (2001) *Contemporary Psychiatry.* Vol 3. *Specific Psychiatric Disorders*. Berlin: Springer.

Judd LL, Akiskal HS, Paulus MP (1997) The role and clinical significance of subsyndromal depressive symptoms (SSD) in unipolar, major depressive disorder. *J Affect Disord* **45**: 5–18.

Kahn R, Wetzler S, Van Praag HM, Asnis GM (1988) Behavioral indications for serotonin receptor hypersensitivity in panic disorder. *Psychiatry Res* **25**: 101–104.

Katz MM, Koslov S, Maas JW, Frazer A, Rowden C, Casper RC, Croughan J, Kocsis J, Redmond E (1987) The timing and specificity and clinical prediction of tricyclic drug effects in depression. *Psych Med* **17**: 297–309.

Klaassen T, Riedel WJ, Van Praag HM, Menheere PPCA, Griez E (2002) Neuroendocrine response to mCPP and ipsaperone in relation to anxiety and aggression. *Psychiatr Res* **113**: 29–40.

Nemeroff CB (1996) The corticotropin-releasing factor hypothesis of depression: new findings and directions. *Mol Psychiatry* **1**: 336–342.

Sargent PA, Husted Kjear K, Bench CJ, Rabiner EA, Messa C, Meyer J, Gunn RN, Grasby PM, Cowen PJ (2000) Brain serotonin 1_A receptor binding measured by positron emission tomography with (^{11}C) WAY-100635. Effects of depression and antidepressant treatment. *Arch Gen Psychiatry* **57**: 174–180.

Takao K, Nagatani T, Kitamura Y, Yamawaki S (1997) Effects of corticosterone on 5-HT_{1A} and 5-HT_2 receptor binding and on the receptor-mediated behavioral responses of rats. *Europ J Pharmacol* **333**: 123–128.

Van Praag HM, De Haan S (1980) Depression vulnerability and 5-hydroxytryptophan prophylaxis. *Psychiatry Res* **3**: 75–83.

Van Praag HM, Kahn R, Asnis GM, Wetzler S, Brown S, Bleich A, Korn M (1987) Denosologization of biological psychiatry or the specificity of 5-HT disturbances in psychiatric disorders. *J Affect Disord* **13**: 1–8.

Van Praag HM (1992a) *Make Believes in Psychiatry or the Perils of Progress*. New York: Brunner Mazel.

Van Praag HM (1992b) About the centrality of mood lowering in mood disorders. *Europ Neuropsychopharm* **2**: 393–402.

Van Praag HM (1994) 5-HT related, anxiety- and/or aggression driven depression. *Inter Clin Psychopharm* **9**: 5–6.

Van Praag HM (1996) Faulty cortisol/serotonin interplay. Psychological and biological characterisation of a new hypothetical depression subtype (SeCa depression). *Psychiatry Res* **65**: 143–157.

Van Praag HM (1997) Over the mainstream: diagnostic requirements for biological psychiatric research. *Psychiatry Res* **72**: 201–212.

Van Praag HM (2000) Nosologomania: a disorder of psychiatry. *World J Biol Psychiatry* **1**: 151–158.

Van Praag HM (2001) Anxiety/aggression-driven depression. A paradigm of functionalization and verticalization of psychiatric diagnosis. *Progress Neuro-Psychopharm Biol Psychiat* **25**: 893–924.

Van Praag HM, De Kloet R, Van Os (2004) *Stress, the Brain and Depression*. Cambridge, UK: Cambridge University Press.

West ED, Dally PJ (1959) Effects of iproniazid in depressive syndroms. *Br Med J* **1**: 1491–1494.

Wittchen HU, Schuster P, Lieb R (2001) Comorbidity and mixed anxiety–depressive disorder: clinical curiosity or pathophysiological need? *Hum Psychopharm* **16**: S21–S30.

Zinbarg RE, Barlow DH, Liebowitz M, Street L, Broadhead E, Keaton W, Roy-Byrne P, Lepine JP, Theherani M, Richards J (1994) The DSM-IV field trial for mixed anxiety depression. *Am J Psychiatry* **151**: 1153–1162.

At the Interface of Depression and Anxiety: Comorbidity and Concepts

Thea Overbeek and Eric J. L. Griez

University of Maastricht, Maastricht, The Netherlands

INTRODUCTION

The debate on comorbidity between anxiety and depression leans heavily on current nosography. The vast majority, if not all studies describe the co-occurrence of different disorders along the lines of the two main classificatory systems, the successive versions of the *Diagnostic and Statistical Manual of Mental Disorders* (DSM, American Psychiatric Association), and the *International Classification of Diseases and Related Health Problems* (ICD, World Health Organization).

As they are defined in the DSM and ICD, depressive and anxiety disorders obviously share a number of clinical features, as well as, most probably, the explanatory pathways to these features. However, for all the accumulated knowledge on the epidemiology and neurobiology of affective disorders, the issue of splitting or lumping together remains largely unresolved. The co-occurrence of anxiety and depressive disorders has led to hypotheses about a common aetiology, and several models have been suggested to explain associations between anxiety and depression (Frances et al., 1992). Roughly summarized, these models represent either a unitarian view (lumping the disorders together into one 'affective' spectrum) or a separatist view (splitting the spectrum), with various variants in between (Nemeroff, 2002). Another possibility that deserves attention is the 'artifactual' argument, which states that the problem of comorbidity is inherent to our imperfect current classification systems, which are based on rather arbitrarily defined criteria and thresholds, using strange combinations of various symptoms and featuring a considerable amount of definitional overlap. In consideration hereof, it may be improper to speak of 'comorbidity' in its true sense, the diagnostic framework itself having a deficient validity. Obviously, the way we conceive of psychiatric illnesses, and the constructs we use to describe and classify them,

Mood Disorders: Clinical Management and Research Issues. Edited by E. J. L. Griez, C. Faravelli, D. J. Nutt and J. Zohar.
©2005 John Wiley & Sons Ltd. ISBN 0 470 09426 5.

determine the way we explain associations between them. Some of these problems and the nosological challenge they create, are elaborated upon by Van Praag (this volume).

The present chapter represents quite a different approach of the relationship between depressive and anxiety disorders. It departs from the traditional appraisal of comorbidity in the current psychiatric literature and leaves largely aside the debate about whether or not DSM/ICD diagnoses are valid. A brief look at the assessment methods, and a review of the disparate results they have yielded so far in the study of co-existing depression and anxiety has led us to reflect on the concepts themselves, and the logical relationships that may follow from their meaning. Accordingly, we first discuss a range of clinical scales relevant to our subject: they illustrate the various ways in which depression and anxiety have been conceived of before the introduction of current classifications. Sadly, as a rule, the use of standardized depression and anxiety scales has been limited to assess progress in treatment studies. Despite their potential usefulness in collecting information on features of emotions like anxiety/fear and depression/sadness, they remain under-exploited to this effect. To our knowledge, no major comorbidity study has yet been conducted using classical depression and anxiety scales as a main assessment tool. Thus, while emphasizing the potential interest of assessing depression and anxiety at a very symptomatic level, we are left with comorbidity data from traditional epidemiology. As a result the next part of this chapter summarizes a number of major epidemiological surveys, taking for granted the DSM/ICD framework. After all, for communicative purposes we need a descriptive instrument to provide an overview of the evidence. The last part goes beyond the empirics and attempts to reflect on the link between anxiety and depression from a different perspective, conducting a concise inquiry into the concepts of emotions, sadness and anxiety in particular.

CLINICAL CONCEPTS OF DEPRESSION AND ANXIETY

The way we assess and classify a condition reflects the way we conceive of it.

Many quantitative instruments have been developed to assess depression and anxiety, and they cover a broad range of symptoms. It has been assumed that they do not represent diagnostic instruments, but add a quantifiable description of illness severity and profile of symptoms to an existing diagnosis. Because scales themselves cannot do anything but assessing (the severity of) symptoms, they can be considered as a more sensitive tool to evaluate the details of a clinical condition than the diagnostic interviews, which are aimed by definition at solving a dichotomy (diagnosis versus no diagnosis) on basis of some – rather arbitrarily – predefined criteria. Despite the claim that classification systems are atheoretical, they cannot be such, simply because behind each description some form of a priori framework is present. Paying attention to rating scales represents a plea for a return to the basics of descriptive psychopathology. Such a return could make sense in further studies on the meaning of such basic concepts as depression and anxiety. It is unfortunate that clinical scales have hardly been used in large population surveys. Although they serve no classificatory purpose, their analysis might add worthwhile information on the relative weight of individual symptoms in different conditions of depression and anxiety, on their co-occurrence and on the total profile of symptoms in distinct disorders.

It is not our intention to enter into a detailed methodological discussion on rating scales, or to discuss or comment on all individual scales. It will suffice to mention some representatives of the depression and anxiety scales, and to discuss some general aspects relevant to the subject.

The Assessment of Depression

Amongst the most widely used instruments for assessing depressive states at a symptomatic level are the Hamilton Rating Scale for Depression (HRSD, also abbreviated as HAM-D, Hamilton, 1960, 1967); the Beck Depression Inventory (BDI, Beck et al., 1961); the Montgomery–Åsberg Depression Rating Scale (MADRS, Montgomery and Åsberg, 1979) and the Zung Self-rating Depression Scale (SDS, Zung, 1965). With many other scales, they differ in various aspects as number of items, nature of items covered, and time needed for completion. Of course, there are also differences between them in validity, reliability and sensitivity. Scales are usually divided into two main categories, the self-rating ('subjective') scales and the clinician-rated ('objective') scales, each category having its own advantages and disadvantages. Faravelli et al. (1986) compared a number of depression rating scales, and showed that one difference between self-rating and observer-rated scales was that the self-rating scales showed more rightward asymmetry (higher severity) and observer-rated depression scales tended towards a leftward asymmetry (lesser severity). Moreover, the internal structure of the depression scales, as tested by means of factor analysis, showed considerable differences. Also, the reciprocal correlations between the rating scales are reasonably homogeneous, but not particularly high. In the various scales only a subset of items is dedicated to the core symptoms of depression, the other items being apparently dedicated to a variety of accessory symptoms concerning somatic issues, anxiety, or sleep.

In a more recent study Faravelli et al. (1996) analysed the merits of clinical scales in measuring the severity of depression. They showed that it is not so much the number of symptoms that determines the severity, but rather the presence of certain symptoms, especially those in the melancholic cluster. Different symptoms had different weights in establishing the gradient of severity. In passing, we note that Faravelli and co-workers' observations may be of relevance to our subject. If severity of depression is reflected more in the presence of some core (especially melancholic) symptoms, than in the number of symptoms present, we might infer that at some point there is a change in the quality of the affective state when severity increases.

However, which symptoms exactly are concerned, and at which degree of severity is difficult to determine. Scales greatly differ in the number of items devoted to particular core symptoms. Future studies addressing this issue should therefore take into account that information should only be inferred from the appraisal of individual items on these scales. The issue remains largely under-explored.

Another problem worth noting is that, particularly for a descriptive purpose, the total score on a scale does not give any indication as to what specific kind of items or clusters of items are important for an individual case. It should be kept in mind that when a broad range of symptoms is covered by a scale (Snaith, 1993), many patterns of response may lead to the same score.

The Assessment of Anxiety

Anxiety scales share the same pitfalls as depression scales, as emphasized in Keedwell and Snaith's review (1996). Even more than is the case with depression, the construct of 'anxiety' is far from unitary, with its repercussion on the validity of the concept as designating a single or complex affective state. Also, the term anxiety covers a different range of phenomena that is bound to language and culture. Constructs such as depression and anxiety refer to states that may fluctuate over time, displaying broad variations in severity from day to day, even within hours.

The Hamilton Anxiety Scale (HAS, also abbreviated as HAM-A, Hamilton, 1959), the State–Trait Anxiety Scale (STAI, Spielberger et al., 1977), and the Clinical Anxiety Scale (CAS, Snaith et al., 1982) are some of the frequently used scales that measure nonspecific anxiety.

Large differences have been shown in the emphasis on the various symptom-categories that items can be divided into, like features of anxious mood, anxious cognition, anxiety-bound behaviour (avoidance), over-arousal, somatic signs, and others (Himmelhoch et al., 2001).

It is worth noting that there are many more scales for anxiety than for depression. Traditional psychiatric nosography clearly distinguishes different types of anxiety disorders. Accordingly, besides 'general' scales covering anxiety as one single concept, other scales are specifically directed at the assessment of particular types of anxiety such as panic/agoraphobia (e.g. the Panic and Agoraphobia Scale, PAS, Bandelow, 1995), social anxiety (Liebowitz's social anxiety scale, Liebowitz, 1987) and obsessive-compulsive anxiety (e.g. Maudsley Obsessional Compulsive Inventory, MOCI, Hodgson and Rachman, 1977). This again underscores the complex reality that underlies the term anxiety.

Differentiating Depression and Anxiety

Special mention should be made of the Hospital Anxiety and Depression Scale (Zigmond and Snaith, 1983, HADS). This instrument has been constructed for use in general (somatic) hospital settings. The authors took special care to diminish the interference of physical symptoms, which was an important objection against the HRSD. Additionally, they tried to disentangle the constructs of depression and anxiety. Another focus was upon anhedonia, which was considered to be the most reliable clinical marker of likely response to antidepressant drugs. The HADS has been widely used in clinical settings in various countries, is quite easy to complete (containing 14 items) and well accepted by patients. It has been shown to have acceptable validity and reliability (Herrmann, 1997).

It is remarkable that most scales, that are meant to assess either depressive or anxiety states, contain items obviously related to symptoms of both anxiety and depression. As a consequence, it is risky to differentiate states of anxiety and depression by comparing total scores, even though the scales are supposed to be specific. Bramley et al. (1988) correlated several self-rating scales for either depression or anxiety with two criterion observer-rated scales (the CAS for anxiety and the MADRS-Modified – this is the MADRS without the items on inner tension and reduced sleep – for depression). Their results showed that self-rating scales for depression could discriminate between depressive and anxiety states, but anxiety scales did not. This conclusion also applied to the criterion scales of anxiety (CAS) and depression (MADRS-Modified). An earlier comparative study by Snaith and Taylor (1985) had reached the same conclusion.

A provisory comment on the issue of clinical rating scales is that caution should be exercised when using them in differentiating depression from anxiety on basis of the global quantification they yield as an end score. On the other hand, scales offer an interesting approach of clinical psychopathology, which, if used in conjunction with current classification systems, may add useful information at a descriptive level and challenge some taken-for-granted aspects of our present views.

Classification of Depression and Anxiety

The history of anxiety and depression throughout the development of the DSM and ICD systems is complicated. For an extensive historical overview of the relationship between anxiety disorders and mood disorders we refer to Himmelhoch et al. (2001), and Glas (2003). In DSM-I and DSM-II (APA, 1952, 1968) clear distinctions between anxiety and depression were not yet made (Levine et al., 2001). The disorders were more drawn apart from DSM-III (APA, 1980) onwards, especially where DSM-III was designed to be an atheoretical, symptom-oriented classification. It stated explicit criteria for inclusion and exclusion, and set thresholds for the various disorders. Diagnosing any anxiety disorder in the presence of a comorbid mood disorder was not allowed, major depression always took precedence. This position is actually very interesting from the conceptual point of view, as it attributes a more central role to the emotion of depression than anxiety. We will revisit this point in the final section of our chapter. Many authors challenged the validity of the hierarchical and exclusionary relationship between anxiety and mood disorders, and in the later DSM-III-R (APA, 1987) and DSM-IV (APA, 1994) this restriction on axis I was lifted, tolerating diagnosing separate co-existing disorders on axis I. From then on, many epidemiological studies showed the frequent comorbidity of separately predefined disorders. The clinical reality that did not tally with the categorical views on mental pathology was again 'explained' (Van Praag, 1996).

Clinical interviews have been developed within the framework of these systems, to reach diagnoses on basis of predefined criteria. Frequently used standardized instruments are for example the Structured Clinical Interview for DSM-disorders (SCID; Spitzer et al., 1992); the Diagnostic Interview Schedule (DIS; Robins et al., 1981); the Composite International Diagnostic Interview (CIDI; Robins et al., 1988) and the Schedules for Clinical Assessment in Neuropsychiatry (SCAN; Wing et al., 1990). The Mini International Neuropsychiatric Interview (MINI, Sheehan et al., 1998) is a more recently developed tool for both DSM and ICD diagnoses, and is relatively easy to administer as it takes about 15 minutes to complete. The MINI is increasingly accepted and used for the assessment of psychiatric disorders or screening purposes in epidemiological studies. All have been described in detail elsewhere (Burke et al., 1990; Arbabzadeh-Bouchez and Lepine, 2003). These (semi-)structured interviews often are used in addition to an unstructured interview, to assure that a broad spectrum of disorders has been covered. Not only do the above instruments vary in diagnostic coverage and classification framework they depart from, the timeframe considered also differs.

The above summary of the tools at our disposal, whether they are rating scales or sophisticated standardized interviews, illustrates the arbitrary way we currently conceive of depression and anxiety. The collection of the empirical data that appear below is inevitably endowed with the deficient validity of the existing frameworks. Therefore they should be cautiously interpreted with the exact amount of critical judgement they are calling for.

AT THE INTERFACE: PREVALENCE OF COMORBID CONDITIONS

Prevalence figures of comorbidity vary, partly due to a lack of clear conceptualization and definition of the term comorbidity (Wittchen, 1996). Also methodological differences regarding assessment instruments, time frame covered (lifetime or concurrent, past month, 6 or 12 months), case definition (diagnostic criteria or subthreshold conditions included), use of expert or lay interviewers contribute to uncertainty and confusion (Wittchen et al., 2001). Different types of anxiety disorder show different comorbidity figures with depression, and different types of mood disorders show different comorbidity figures with the separate anxiety disorders. Comorbidity-prevalence rates from population-based, primary care or clinical samples also differ according to the setting that the figures are derived from.

Population Surveys

The two largest epidemiological surveys are from the USA, and are frequently cited. The Epidemiologic Catchment Area (ECA) study was performed among 20 291 subjects from five sites within the US, aged 18 years and up (Regier et al., 1990). The ECA used the DIS for DSM-III diagnoses, and worked with lay interviewers. The National Comorbidity Survey (NCS) was developed as the continuation of the ECA and especially addressed the comorbidity of psychiatric disorders. This survey comprised 8098 subjects from age 15 to 54 years (Kessler et al., 1994). The NCS used an adapted version of the CIDI for screening, and lay interviewers. It also used a more intensive memory enhancement strategy, and found a considerably higher rate of lifetime disorders. The NCS unfortunately did not include diagnosis of OCD. A rough overview of estimated comorbidity figures is given in Table 18.1.

Data from the ECA study on anxiety disorders and comorbidity with mood (and addictive) disorders are reported by Regier et al. (1998). Lifetime prevalence of (any) anxiety disorder was 14.6% and prevalence of mood disorders was 8.3% of respondents. A comorbid anxiety disorder was present in 47.2% of people with lifetime depression. NCS data were reported by Kessler et al. (1994, 1996), and revealed on the individual diagnostic categories that 24.9% of respondents had one or more anxiety disorder lifetime, a lifetime (any) mood disorder was prevalent in 19.3%, and major depression (MDD) in 14.9% of the population. One-year prevalence rate for anxiety disorder was 17% and for depression 10%. Comorbidity figures from the NCS report that 51.2% of subjects with MDD had an anxiety disorder in the same 12-month period. Of the subjects with lifetime depression, 58% had any anxiety disorder lifetime, and 74% had at least one comorbid 'any' psychiatric disorder. The prevalence of MDD figures from the ECA are lower than the NCS figures; according to Kessler this is due to sampling and ascertainment problems in ECA that led to underestimation of prevalence. Whereas mostly anxiety disorders are shown to be the primary disorder and the MDD secondary, it is an important result from the analysis of the NCS data that this specific association also gives rise to a more persistent course of the depression, and more interference with activities of daily life, suicide and hospitalization for depression (Kessler et al., 1996). An overview by Kaufman and Charney (2000) showed that about 30–40% of anxiety disorder patients (OCD not included) had a comorbid MDD, with different figures for the individual disorders. Panic disorder and generalized anxiety disorder have a

TABLE 18.1. Estimates of lifetime comorbidity between anxiety disorders and MDD. Adapted from Kaufman and Charney (2000) and Levine et al. (2001)

Diagnosis	Anxiety disorder comorbid with MDD	MDD comorbid with anxiety disorder
Panic disorder	40–60%	10–30%
Social phobia	20–35%	30%
Generalized anxiety disorder	60%	20%
Post-traumatic stress disorder	30–40%	20%
Obsessive-compulsive disorder	30–60%	
Any anxiety disorder	40%	60%

comorbidity rate of about 65%, post-traumatic stress disorder 40%, and social phobia about 20%. With MDD as the index disorder, a mean comorbidity rate with anxiety disorders is 20%, the highest figure for social phobia 27%, the lowest for panic disorder 10%. Most frequently the anxiety disorder (social phobia, GAD and PTSD) precedes the MDD; PD equally frequently precedes, follows, or starts simultaneously with the MDD episode.

Levine et al. (2001) summarized that the whole group of anxiety disorders (including OCD) show comorbid lifetime major depression in about 40%. The individual anxiety disorders show some variation around this figure. GAD is in about 60% of cases seen with comorbid lifetime depression, PD in 40% to 50%, 30% of the OCD patients have a lifetime comorbid major depression, PTSD patients are in 30–40% of cases seen with depression, and 35% of social phobia also suffer from a major lifetime depression.

Starting from the other side, of the patients with major depression, on a lifetime basis about 60% suffer from any additional anxiety disorder. 20% of these have a GAD, 30% PD, 30% social phobia.

For GAD extraordinarily high comorbidity figures have been reported (Wittchen et al., 1994). Up to 90% of GAD patients have a lifetime comorbid psychiatric disorder, mainly mood disorders like MDD, 60%, and dysthymia, 40%.

Another review by Merikangas et al. (1996) computed data from a set of epidemiological population-based surveys, and concluded that there was a strong and consistent association between the mood disorders and anxiety disorders (and substance abuse); magnitude of comorbidity between mood disorders and anxiety disorders was greater than comorbidity between the affective disorders and substance abuse.

Epidemiological data on a newly proposed DSM-IV diagnosis of mixed anxiety depression (MAD), a syndrome combining features of both anxiety and depression (subthreshold conditions) where neither would qualify as a predominant, standalone diagnosis (Zinbarg et al., 1994; Rapaport, 2001; Barlow and Campbell, 2000), interestingly showed an unexpectedly low prevalence rate of about 1% (Wittchen et al., 2001).

Primary Care Studies

A large-scale study by the World Health Organization has investigated the prevalence of mental disorders in primary health care, a total of 25 916 subjects were screened across 15 different countries (Sartorius et al., 1996; Wittchen et al., 1999; Lecrubier and Ustun, 1998). In the second-stage assessment of 5438 subjects the CIDI was applied. From this study it was shown that 62% of all depressive cases also suffer from another mental health problem, most commonly anxiety disorders. Of the patients with anxiety disorders, 45% had a comorbid depression; of patients with a depression about 40% had an anxiety disorder as well. It was shown that an advantage of comorbidity was that the likelihood of recognition of mental disorders increased, and also the likelihood of receiving treatment was highly increased by the presence of comorbid disorders.

Clinical Comorbidity

Many clinical studies have reported on comorbidity between anxiety and mood disorders (Breier et al., 1984; Starcevic et al., 1992; Ball et al., 1995; Davies et al., 1995). Due to space limitations, we focus on some recently published studies.

Diagnostic comorbidity rates vary between clinical studies because they are influenced by several methodological factors, amongst others the number and nature of disorders assessed, the method of assessment (semi-structured interview versus clinical evaluation), and time period covered (current versus lifetime).

In a clinical population (Zimmerman et al., 2002) with major depressive disorder (N = 479), 64.1% of patients also met criteria for at least one comorbid axis I disorder, and 36.7% of depressed patients had two or more comorbid disorders. The most frequent comorbid diagnoses belonged to the group of anxiety disorders (56.8%), with social phobia being the most frequent individual disorder. This study also showed that 14% of patients had a current (any) comorbid disorder that was in partial remission. Also, not-otherwise-specified (NOS) categories were rather frequent: 14.6% had any NOS anxiety disorder, especially subthreshold PTSD and subthreshold PD.

Another clinical study from Finland, the Vantaa Depression Study, investigated 269 patients with MDD (Melartin et al., 2002). From this sample, 73% were female, 83% were outpatients. This study covered all DSM-IV axis I and axis II disorders when looking for comorbidity, and used the semi-structured SCAN. Most of the patients (79%) had at least one current comorbid diagnosis, and 52% even had two or more comorbid diagnoses. Anxiety disorders were present in 57%; 25% of patients had alcohol abuse or dependence; and 44% had a personality disorder. The last figure, on comorbid personality disorder, however, could be distorted by the fact that the SCID II was done while the patients were depressed. Nonetheless, the conclusion must be that comorbidity among psychiatric patients with MDD is very common, and often multiple.

Finally, let us mention that these recent results are in line with earlier reports that found high comorbidity rates among MDD patients, like Sanderson et al. (1990) who reported 60% of comorbid axis I disorders, most commonly anxiety disorders. The review by Wetzler and Sanderson (1995) reports that a range of 7–61% (mean 24%) of PD patients have a current comorbid depressive disorder; lifetime depression is reported in about 65% of PD patients. Of patients with primary depressive disorder, about 14% (range 9–69%) have a comorbid panic disorder; for this group no lifetime data were available.

The above prevalence figures apply to the various anxiety disorders and (unipolar) major depression. Several studies have suggested that comorbidity rates for the affective disorder subgroups differ. As was concluded in a review by Freeman et al. (2002), epidemiological studies as well as clinical studies have found a high co-occurrence of anxiety disorders with bipolar disorder. OCD has been suggested to show a high comorbidity rate with bipolar disorder (Chen and Dilsaver, 1995a), but results from different studies are not unequivocal (Kruger et al., 1995; Perugi et al., 1997). For the specific relationship of bipolar disorder and panic disorder, there seems to be more evidence, from an epidemiological study (Chen and Dilsaver, (1995b) and from several genetic studies (MacKinnon et al., 2002; Rotondo et al., 2002). Likewise, social phobia and PTSD have been associated with bipolar disorder (Freeman et al., 2002).

REFRAMING CONCEPTS

The bulk of the above surveys notwithstanding, ICD and DSM frameworks offer no explanation for the link they suggest between anxiety and mood disorders. This is something of a surprise. Both systems largely rely on a surface descriptive approach of clinical constructs, and a good proportion of these constructs suffer from a suspicious validity. A closer analysis of our basic concepts can make sense here. The definition of concepts determines the logical relationships between them. Clarifying the concepts of depression and anxiety may illuminate their interface.

The remainder of the present chapter is an attempt to pay attention to these issues. Which emotions, which behaviours, which functions of an organism do the constructs of depression and anxiety exactly refer to? Pathology will be subsumed and clinical categories somewhat de-emphasized. We will consider disturbed emotions, endorsing affectivity as the key feature of anxiety and depressive disorders. We will address the nature of emotions, focusing on sadness and fear. We assume that there is a close conceptual relationship between sadness and fear and that the logical link between depression and anxiety can be inferred from this proximity. We expect the following considerations to help shed light on the aggregation of anxiety and depression in the lifespan of some individuals.

ON THE NATURE OF EMOTIONS

The Force to Exist

In the *Ethics* (1677), a masterpiece of deductive inference, the Dutch philosopher Benedict de Spinoza, questions the nature of human affectivity. Apparently, Spinoza observes, everything in nature tends to persevere into existence. Inanimate objects simply persist. Living organisms survive: they grow, develop and reproduce. Life appears to be endowed with an appetite for life.

In their striving to be, organisms are driven towards everything that fosters their development, and they refrain from anything that thwarts their force to be. This we observe in unicellular beings approaching the nutriments they need to stay alive and consistently fleeing a drop of acid which threatens their existence. At the other end of complexity, humans' struggle for life is more sophisticated. The *Ethics* (III, prop. 9) posits that in humans, striving for life is conscious and appetite becomes desire. Beside food, water and warmth, humans tend to pursue such other goods as knowledge, wealth, honours and social recognition, to name a few. In contrast, they seek to avoid such things as illness, poverty and humiliation. They feel the former category to boost their quality of life, in other words their power to be, and the latter to endanger it. Accordingly, items belonging to the former category are called 'goods', while things in the second category are labelled 'evils' or 'adversity'.

Consciousness of the Ability to Be

Thus, in humans, appetite for life is a conscious desire which rests both in the body and in the mind. As a consequence, for each change in an individuals' capacity to be there is a concomitant change in his mind. These transitions we call emotions (*Ethics*, III, prop. 11). Therefore, emotions are the consciousness of the organisms' own capacity of existence.

This may be either a pleasant or a painful consciousness*, depending on whether the 'power to be' is going stronger or weaker. Each change in the organism that strengthens life is sensed as pleasure, and each change that weakens life, as pain. Pleasure is excellence of the mind to the same extent as fitness is excellence of the body. Pain in contrast, is a shrinking of the mind.

It follows that, basically, there are only two emotions, pain and pleasure. Sadness is the prototype of pain and joy the prototype of pleasure. However, humans do experience a great diversity of emotions because they tend to associate pain and pleasure with different ideas in various contexts.[†]

Thus emotions essentially are the conscious side of the organism's fitness for survival. Spinoza's fascinating suggestion is consonant with current evolutionary views in affective neuroscience (McGuire et al., 1992; Nesse, 1990, 1999; Damasio, 1995). Emotions are believed to have emerged from ancient brain processes that we, humans have inherited from ancestral species. The function of these homologous brain systems is to energize organisms, helping them to cope with their environment and to maximize their chances of survival. Panksepp (1998) posits that emotional systems 'generate an animal's egocentric sense of well-being with regard to the most important natural dimensions of life'. Throughout the ages, the primal issues of maintaining one's physical integrity, finding goods and protecting them, breeding, rearing and securing social support for oneself and the young progressively generated specific coordinated responses. In higher vertebrates, mammals in particular, these capacities turned out to encompass powerful internal feelings sensed as emotions. Panksepp argues that there is reasonable experimental evidence to iden-

---

[*] Psychologists nowadays refer to the positive or negative valence of emotions.

[†] 'Love is nothing else but pleasure accompanied by the idea of an external cause; hatred is nothing else but pain accompanied by the idea of an external cause. We further see that he who loves necessarily endeavours to have and keep present to him the object of his love, while he who hates endeavours to remote and destroy the object of his hatred' (*Ethics*, III, prop 13).

TABLE 18.2   Three main emotional systems corresponding to three major evolutionary challenges as suggested by Panksepp (1998)

	Seeking system	Fear system	Panic – loss system
Evolutionary challenge	Finding resources (e.g. food, water, sex)	Avoiding harm and destruction	Maintaining social bonds and cohesion
Emotive state			
Positive valence (fitness)	Desire, strive	*(absence of fear)*	Attachment, love, trust
Negative valence (unfitness)	*(absence of desire)*	Fear, anxiety	Separation, distress, grief, sorrow
Putative brain structures involved	Mesolimbic and mesocortical dopaminergic pathways	Central and lateral, amygdala, anterior and medial hypothalamus, periventricular grey	Midbrain periaqueductal grey, ventral septum, dorsomedial thalamus, stria terminalis, cingulate gyrus[a]

[a] Structures implicated in the distress vocalizations

tify a number of such 'basic emotional systems' in the brain. Panksepp's SEEKING, FEAR and PANIC/LOSS systems are of particular interest for the sake of our enquiry (see Table 18.2). Let us quote Panksepp describing the SEEKING system.

> This emotional system is a coherently operating neuronal network that promotes a certain class of survival abilities. This system makes animals intensely interested in exploring their world and leads them to become excited when they are about to get what they desire. It eventually allows animals to find and eagerly anticipate the things they need for survival, including, of course, food, water, warmth and their ultimate evolutionary survival need, sex [. . .] it helps fill the mind with interest and motivates organisms to move their bodies effortlessly in search of the things they need, crave, and desire. In humans, this may be one of the main brain systems that generate and sustain curiosity, even for intellectual pursuits.

Arguably, there is a conceptual analogy between seeking, *sensu* Panksepp, and striving to be, *sensu* Spinoza. But what further about pain, pleasure, and, for the sake of our inquiry, sadness and joy?

SADNESS

Sadness is the painful awareness of a decay in the capacity to keep oneself into existence. Therefore sadness is the consciousness of a loss relative to a previous state. The essence of sadness is the collapse from a higher to a lesser degree of fitness.

There is no emotion in having a particular degree of fitness. The way I am is not a matter of pain or pleasure. The way I am makes me neither happy nor miserable. Pain and pleasure only proceed from a *difference* in the way I am, compared to the way I was. Emotions are driven by desire, and desire constantly compares. Thus, pleasure and pain are not linked to a specific level of abilities: they are a function of passing to a higher or a lesser degree in the power of existence. Transitions, and transitions only trigger emotions.*

This explains why emotions are similar in all individuals, regardless of their level of success in coping, survival and self-fulfilment. Pain affects the successful, and the poor feel pleasure. This explains the sad person feeling deprived with no apparent appreciation of the success and the wealth that he or she may still have. The intimate relationship between the concepts of sadness and loss, has been commandingly conceptualized in Bowlby's attachment theory (1980), and to a lesser extend in Seligman's notion of learned helplessness (1975).

Bowlby's separation–loss theory points to the role of the primal bond between the mother and her offspring, and emphasizes the dramatic consequences of its disruption on the survival abilities of the infant. Abandonment of the vulnerable infant through loss of maternal care bears a relationship to prototypal sadness. One of the most fascinating experimental findings in this regard is the phenomenon of the so-called distress vocalizations (DVs). Animals, rat pups or young chickens separated from their mother and left alone in a strange place, start emitting very specific, usually ultrasonic vocalizations, seemingly to solicit the parent's attention. Following separation, the response often is biphasic, with an early phase attended by many vocalizations, intense motor activity and an active search for the caregiver; this is followed by a phase of despair-like behaviour, with progressive extinction of the DVs, prostration and immobility. In line with Bowlby, Panksepp (1998) refers to a single PANIC/LOSS/SORROW system. Laboratory studies have shown structures of this system to control DVs. Apparently, emotions linked to the PANIC/LOSS system provide safeguards for infant–mother attachment and social bonding. It is noteworthy that the PANIC/LOSS system reaches its highest development in the mammals, which are social beings par excellence; separation and abandonment have dramatic, life-threatening consequence for newborn mammals (Panksepp, 1998). Seligman (1975) developed the concept of learned helplessness, which he related to depressive behaviours. In Seligman's experimental paradigm, animals, most often dogs, were submitted to a series of electric shocks they could neither avoid nor escape. When later presented with similar aversive stimuli, most animals helplessly underwent the events despite having regained the opportunity to escape, in an apparently passive attitude towards forthcoming adversity. Seligman's experiments can be reinterpreted as instances of loss of ability in mastering one's environment. Seligman's dogs had lost the ability to exercise control over environmental parameters that profoundly affected them. Such a loss represents a definite shrinking of the organisms' ability to live and survive.

---

* 'For if man were born with the perfection to which he passes, he would possess the same, without the emotion of pleasure' (*Ethics*, III, Definition of the Emotions, iii, note).

FEAR

Fear is Pain in the Future

Throughout the Middle Ages scholars used to represent the principal emotions in a 2×2 table (Table 18.3), which scheme actually relied on the doctrine of the ancient Stoics. Humans' appraisal basically distinguishes between good and bad events. Pleasure is the present experience of good things, pain the experience of evils. Regarding the future, humans tend to desire things they believe to be good, and to fear those they believe to be bad. Thus fear is the emotion with a negative valence, pertaining to the future. Fear obviously belongs to the negative emotions, related to evils and associated with pain. Contemporary evolutionary views emphasize this negative valence of fear as a functionality that helps in keeping the organism away from adversity. Indeed, avoidance is constitutive of fear. It is worth noting that avoidance as a coping strategy dictated by fear makes sense as long as no irremediable damage has occurred to the organism. Once damage has occurred, it is too late to avoid: there is loss, and actual loss is sadness. Thus fear refers to unaccomplished pain, in other words, pain in the future.

TABLE 18.3   Basic emotions according to the Stoics

	In the present	In the future
Good	Pleasure	Desire
Evil	Sadness	Fear

Fear is diverse and the evils a particular organism seeks to avoid are numerous. Accordingly, naming fears has been a much appreciated pastime of earlier psychopathologists (Campbell, 1981). Yet a closer look at the content of highly prevalent fears is more interesting. Phobias typically represent fears of concrete, circumscribed external objects. Evolutionary views on phobias hold that phobic fears are related to innate mechanisms shaped by nature as safeguard for life in a hostile environment (Ohman and Mineka, 2001; Poulton and Menzies, 2002). Animals have been prepared via natural selection to avoid things that may more or less endanger their survival. Against the background of human psychopathology, Nesse (1990) lists a number of subtypes of anxiety, each of which he tentatively relates to a particular kind of primal danger (Table 18.4)

All fears have pain in common, and pain is the subjective side of a loss in the power to be. Therefore, experiencing pain is facing a loss in one's capacity of survival. For a living being, the ultimate loss is death. Thus, the ultimate fear is a fear of dying, and Epicurus rightly pointed to the fear of death as the core of all

TABLE 18.4   Putative primal dangers related to different types of anxiety according to Nesse (after Nesse, 1990)

Anxiety	Primal danger
Panic	Present vital threat (e.g. attack by predator)
Agoraphobia	Highly unsafe environment (attack likely)
Social anxiety	Rejection from group membership
Separation anxiety	Social loss and disruption of protective bond
Blood injury phobia	Blood loss
Hoarding compulsions	Lack of food and other goods
Washing compulsion	Infection
Animal phobias	(Vital) threat by dangerous animals

human misery (Diogenes Laertius (1999), book IX).* Thus all instances of fear are instances where possibly the organism's very existence is endangered. The case is clear for the prey—predator paradigm, as it is for specific phobias such as fear of heights, enclosed spaces, fire, natural disasters such as thunder and storms, sharp objects and animals. In all these situations, the animals' existence is at risk, either acutely (prey—predator) or remotely. Social fears represent a distinct category: they typically apply to higher vertebrates, mammals in particular. Mammals need social support to survive, should it only be for the immaturity of their young. For social animals, including humans, the loss of social integrity may be of vital importance; it is loss of life. This explains social fears in the perspective of an ultimate fear of death.[†]

In sum, there is nothing else in fear but pain, pain being conceived of as a deficit in the ability to survive.

Fear is Uncertain and Therefore Inconstant

In the *Ethics*, Spinoza conceptualizes fear as being an inconstant pain. This pain arises from the image of something concerning which we are in doubt. More precisely, the emotion of fear, he further writes, arises from the idea of something past or future, whereof we to a certain extent doubt the issue. Fear pertains to the

---

[*] However, Epicurus further reasoned that we should not fear death because in fact we never have knowledge of death: as long as we are, death is not, and once death is, we are not any more. In this he may have missed that the painful essence of fear lies in *waiting now* for the future evil, not the evil itself. Even though the object of the fear never materializes, fear hurts.

[†] From a conceptual point of view, one may argue that social fears occupy a specific place amongst fears. They are more recent in the history of evolution and, compared to archaic safeguards such as other phobias, they may be a more pertinent feature for well organized animals, such as humans. To a social beings such as mammals are, the threat of storm or of a small animal may have become less salient than the threat of separation and abandonment. To this extent social fears may have evolved very close to the image of acute loss, death, sadness and depression.

future, possibly to the past.* Insofar as the object of fear is in the future, to some extent the causality of fear is in the future. Now, the future is not certain. Therefore, uncertainty is constitutive of fear.

Uncertainty relates to unpredictability.† There has been quite a lot of experimental work on the link between unpredictability and anxiety (Mineka and Kihlstrom, 1978). Typically, an environment that goes unpredictable becomes anxiogenic. In an unpredictable environment cues are not reliable. A typical example in a learning paradigm of classical conditioning occurs when, given the occurrence of the UCS (the signalling event), the probability of occurrence of the CS (the signalled event), equates or approaches the probability of non-occurrence of the CS. In such an environment, the danger of losing control is great. And losing control of its environment entails a loss in the organism's ability to face the challenge of survival.

The view of fear as uncertainty may provide a first hint to illuminate its relationship to sadness. Fear is a foretokened loss of control over one's environment. Such a loss of control affects the organism's power to be. Thus fear is a threat of sadness.

Fear is not only uncertain. Fear is also inconstant. Fear is variable and changing over time. Why should we logically expect fear to be an inconstant emotion? The argument may run as follows. The future exists in the subject's mind as an image only. The same applies to the past. Past and future are kept in existence through images in the mind (Damasio, 1994). However, while facts are irrevocable, images are prone to change. When the subject has in mind an image of doom and loss, he feels pained and tends to substitute that image by a different one. The mind endeavours to repel images of doom and replace them by images of happiness. The individual naturally seeks a glimpse of success rather than failure, a glimpse of joy rather than pain.‡ Thus there is an inherent instability of fear. The inconstant pain of fear always mixes to some extent with the inconstant pleasure of hope. There is neither fear without hope, nor hope without fear, Spinoza insists.

The view of fear as inconstant emotion may provide us with a second hint concerning the relationship between fear and sadness. Take uncertainty away, and hope becomes pleasure. Take uncertainty away, and fear becomes despair (*Ethics*, III, prop. 17). We might expect fear to become sadness when images of doom overtake images of hope in the mind, making fear less inconstant. Fear closes down to sadness as a function of its constancy, in other words to the degree it is turning chronic.

---

* Fear related to a past event is typically obsessive fear. The obsessive subject has doubts about past as much as about future events. To this extent, obsessions are merely a particular case of anxiety. However, we will not further discuss the concept of obsessions in the present demonstration.

† Not each instance of uncertainty can be explained by unpredictability. Unpredictability may explain uncertainty only as far as future events are concerned. Unpredictability does not encompass uncertainty pertaining to past events.

‡ 'he who fears, in other words doubts, concerning the issue of something which he hates also conceives something which excludes the existence of the thing in question: to this extent he feels pleasure, and consequently to this extent he hopes that it will turn out as he desires' (*Ethics* III, Definitions of the Emotions, xiii).

FROM FEAR TO SADNESS

When Uncertain Sadness Turns Certain

At first, the mind of the fearful oscillates, expecting the worst but wishing the best. The subject with fear anticipates doom, but endeavours to keep in account that the threat may not materialize.

Then comes exhaustion, and images of doom start dragging on in the mind. Ups and downs in the subject's mood flatten, giving way to generalized negative expectations in face of adversity.* The fluctuating fear eventually freezes into a static state with a steady negative valence. The fleeting glimpses of disaster, originally mixed up with hope, merge into the protracted contemplation of a looming pain. Loss is now taken for granted. The *Ethics* emphasizes that if the elements of uncertainty are removed, fear turns into despair (*Ethics*, III, proposition 18). Despair encompasses the certainty of damage.

Painful Expectations, Lasting Injuries that Hurt, and a Place for Panic

In the flow of time, the mind continuously anticipates the future, considers the present and remembers the past. This incessant sequence is the measure of the subject's expectations. The time passing by is the ultimate evidence.

Fear looks forward to an uncertain harm. Sadness reflects on lost excellence. There is an evident temporal relationship between fear and sadness. The object of fear is the future; the object of sadness is the past. Fear and sadness are lasting emotions, extending of their essence beyond the time present. Fear waits for the future to materialize; sadness preserves the memory of the past.

In contrast panic is the immediate emotion linked to the assault of unfolding adversity. Panic is the internal experience of the acute threat to the organism's survival, when its very existence is at stake. It ensues that conceptually, not only are fear and sadness different, but between them there is a logically designated place for the distinct state of panic. This all is consonant with the view that putatively 'anxiety prepares the system for an anticipated trauma whereas panic deals with one that is already in progress' (Bouton et al., 2001).

Fear as Unfulfilled Sadness

The argument developed in the previous paragraphs suggests a number of ideas about the definition of emotions, and, regarding our original concerns, about the nature of sadness and fear. Emotions in general have been related to the drive of life

* Generalized apprehensive expectation: the link between fear and sadness?

and the striving for survival. They should be regarded as the 'contentment', or the absence thereof, of the organism sensing an increase or a decrease in its chances of coping with life. This satisfaction must be conceived of as an evolutionary concept, having grown from the reflex-like approach and avoidance reactions in single-cell organisms, to conscious desire and complex, cognitively loaded emotions in humans. At least in higher mammals, fear and sadness are essentially the painful perception of a threat to, or an actual loss in, the 'power to be'. Fear, leaning forward to the uncertain future, is intermittent sadness being mixed up with the hope of escaping danger. Sometimes the fearful subject forebodes a loss; sometimes he hopes for the best. Thus, fear is incipient sadness, which reaches completion when time consumes the anticipated loss. It ensues that there is continuity between fear and sadness in the flow of time. In order to become sadness, fear requires that time passes.

The process unfolds in the direction of the arrow of time, and this tells us that fear will eventually become sadness, but that sadness is not likely to change into fear.

Anxiety as Incomplete Depression?

Several arguments arguably illustrate the idea that anxiety is a putative state of unfulfilled depression.

When assessed on the independent dimensions of positive and negative affectivity, patients with anxiety states present increased ratings on both negative and positive affectivity. In contrast, subjects with depression yield high scores on negative affectivity only, having seemingly lost any significant profile of positive affectivity. This shows anxiety and depression to share a common profile, depression representing one further degree yet in psychological pathology (Tellegen, 1985; Clark and Watson, 1991). Van Praag discusses as plausible the possibility that anxiety induces depression, or at least a subtype of depression. He observes that anxiety symptoms, and anxiety-related irritability often precede the development of depression. He refers to this type of depression as being 'anxiety/aggression-driven' and links this construct to serotonergic disturbance (Van Praag, Chapter 17 in this volume).

Our analysis presents the passage from anxiety to depression as mediated by a phase of constant and chronic fear. As we have reported earlier in the present chapter, GAD, the anxiety disorder which arguably yields the highest degree of chronicity, strikingly shows one of the highest degrees of depressive comorbidity. The close proximity between GAD and depression has even led some authors to speculate on a common diathesis between the two disorders (Kendler, 1996; Mineka et al., 1998).

Addressing the cognitive correlates of anxiety and depression, Alloy and co-workers (1990) hypothesize that depression, compared to anxiety, is characterized by a sense of certainty encompassing hopelessness. This idea is perfectly consistent with our above analysis. Waikar and Craske (1997) investigated 329 patients with affective pathology and found support for Alloy and co-workers' suggestion.

We further infer that time is an essential dimension in the transformation of fear into sadness. We some years ago examined whether chronicity is a factor towards depression in a population of panic disorder (PD) patients. The results not only support the idea, but suggest as well a direct relationship between the severity of PD and the development of subsequent depression (Griez and Overbeek, 1997).

If fear 'prepares' for sadness, one should logically expect anxiety with subsequent (lifetime) depression to be more prevalent than depression alone. This is the case (Mineka et al., 1998). Pure depression nevertheless occurs independently, for instance as a result of acute unforeseen loss events, such as sudden grief.

In sum, it appears plausible that fear is a logical itinerary to sadness, and that there may be a continuum between clinical conditions of anxiety and depression.

A Note on the Concepts of Fear and Sadness in an Evolutionary Perspective

The above account of emotions broadly refers to evolutionary views. There is an extensive literature on evolutionary biology, while evolutionary views in psychiatry and clinical psychology are spreading fast. Yet investigators do not all agree in their interpretations. A number of authors tend to consider emotions in general, regardless of their valence, as being in themselves instances of adaptations. Following their view, anxiety and depression have supposedly been 'invented' by nature as adaptive responses to the challenges of ancient environments (see, for instance, Nesse, 1999; Troisi and McGuire, 2002). Accordingly, they deploy a lot of heuristic efforts to explain the potential virtues of painful conditions as depression and other psychiatric illnesses (Nesse, 2000). Others have challenged these 'adaptationist' positions. Criticism has been voiced on some methods used in evolutionary psychiatry (McLoughlin, 2002; Lane and Luchin, 1988; Dubrovsky, 2002).

The conceptual analysis in the present chapter is consistent with modern neuroscience (Panksepp, 1998, Damasio, 1994). However, it should be noted that our analysis does not present each emotion as being a blessing of nature in itself. Emotions are the internal sense of well-being that corresponds to the capacity for life, or the fitness of the organism. For each increase in fitness there is an emotion with a positive valence, for each decrease, an emotion with a negative valence. Fear and depression are the emotional side of a loss of power for life. Consequently, they express a decrease in fitness. From this point of view, the analogy drawn between anxiety and depression on one hand, cough and fever on the other hand (Nesse, 1999) may be conceptually wrong. Fear and sadness are not the consequence of a loss of life, let alone an adaptive reaction to it; they *are* loss of life and express a lack of fitness. Depressive individuals present hormonal and immunological disturbances, a sign that they are at increased vulnerability (vanWest et al., Chapter 8 in this volume). Another striking case is the increased prevalence of affective disorders in physically ill subjects, amongst others, cardiac patients (Griez et al., 2000;

Fleet et al., 2000; Frasure-Smith et al., 1993); in cardiac patients in particular, the occurrence of affective pathology has been associated with a poorer vital prognosis.

EPILOGUE

From a conceptual point of view, there is continuity between fear and sadness but no overlap. The continuity may be consistent with the idea that anxiety and depressive disorders belong to a same spectrum. The absence of overlap, however, argues against the idea of a diagnostic pleonasm (Van Praag, Chapter 17 in this volume). To the extent that fear is not merely sadness, anxiety is not depression.

Fear is sadness foreseen, moderated by uncertainty. From this point of view, one might argue that anxiety disorders are conceptually less severe than depression. Our analysis intends to clarify concepts. It does not come in the place of empirical research.

REFERENCES

Alloy LB, Kelly KA, Mineka S, Clements CM (1990) Comorbidity of anxiety and depressive disorders: a helplessness–hopelessness perspective. In Maser JD, Cloninger CR (eds) *Comorbidity of Mood and Anxiety Disorders.* Washington, DC: American Psychiatric Press.

APA (American Psychiatric Association) (1952) *Diagnostic and Statistical Manual of Mental Disorders* (1st edition). Washington, DC: American Psychiatric Press.

APA (American Psychiatric Association) (1968) *Diagnostic and Statistical Manual of Mental Disorders* (2nd edition). Washington, DC: American Psychiatric Press.

APA (American Psychiatric Association) (1980) *Diagnostic and Statistical Manual of Mental Disorders* (3rd edition). Washington, DC: American Psychiatric Press.

APA (American Psychiatric Association) (1987) *Diagnostic and Statistical Manual of Mental Disorders* (3rd revised edition). Washington, DC: American Psychiatric Press.

APA (American Psychiatric Association) (1994) *Diagnostic and Statistical Manual of Mental Disorders* (4th edition). Washington, DC: American Psychiatric Press.

Arbabzadeh-Bouchez S, Lepine JP (2003) Measurements of depression and anxiety disorders. In Kasper S, Den Boer J, Sitsen J (eds) *Handbook of Depression and Anxiety.* New York: Marcel Dekker.

Ball S, Buchwald A, Waddell M, Shekhar A (1995) Depression and generalized anxiety symptoms in panic disorder. Implications for comorbidity. *J Nerv Ment Disease* **183**: 304–308.

Bandelow B (1995) The assessment of efficacy of treatments for panic disorder and agoraphobia. II. The Panic and Agoraphobia Scale. *Int Clin Psychopharmacol* **10**: 73–82.

Barlow DH, Campbell LA (2000) Mixed anxiety–depression and its implications for models of mood and anxiety disorders. *Compr Psychiatry* **41**: 55–60.

Beck AT, Ward CH, Mendelson M, Mock JE, Erbaugh JK (1961) An inventory for measuring depression. *Arch Gen Psychiatry* **4**: 561–571.

Beck A, Clark D (1988) Anxiety and depression: an information processing perspective. *Anxiety Res*, **1**: 23–36.

Bouton ME, Mineka S, Barlow DH (2001) A modern learning theory perspective on the etiology of panic disorder. *Psychol Rev* **108**(1): 4–32.

Bowlby J (1980) *Attachment and Loss.* New York: Basic Books.

Bramley PN, Easton AM, Morley S, Snaith RP (1988) The differentiation of anxiety and depression by rating scales. *Acta Psychiatr Scand* **77**: 133–138.

Breier A, Charney D, Heninger G (1984) Major depression in patients with agoraphobia and panic disorder. *Arch Gen Psychiatry* **41**: 1129–1135.

Burke JD, Wittchen HU, Regier DA, Sartorius N (1990) Extracting information from diagnostic interviews on co-occurrence of symptoms of anxiety and depression. In Maser JD, Cloninger CR (eds) *Comorbidity of Mood and Anxiety Disorders.* Washington, DC: American Psychiatric Press.

Campbell RJ (1981) *Psychiatric Dictionary.* Oxford: Oxford University Press.

Chen YW, Dilsaver SC (1995a) Comorbidity for obsessive-compulsive disorder in bipolar and unipolar disorders. *Psychiatry Res* **59**: 57–64.

Chen YW, Dilsaver SC (1995b) Comorbidity of panic disorder in bipolar illness: evidence from the Epidemiologic Catchment Area Survey. *Am J Psychiatry* **152**: 280–282.

Clark LA, Watson D (1991) Tripartite model of anxiety and depression: psychometric evidence and taxonomic implications. *J Abnorm Psycho* **100**: 316–336.

Damasio AR (1994) *Descartes' Error.* New York: Penguin Putnam.

Damasio AR (1995) On some functions of the human prefrontal cortex. *Ann NY Acad Sci.* **15**: **769**: 241–251

Davies F, Norman R, Cortese L, Malla A (1995) The relationship between types of anxiety and depression. *J Nerv Ment Disease* **183**: 31–35.

Diogenes Laertius (1999) *Vies et Doctrines des Philosophes Illustres.* French translation MO Goulet-Caze. Paris: Le Livre de Poche.

Dubrovsky B (2002) Evolutionary psychiatry. Adaptationist and nonadaptationist conceptualizations. *Progr Neuropsychopharmacol Biol Psychiatry.* **26**: 1–19.

Faravelli C, Albanesi G, Poli E (1986) Assessment of depression: a comparison of rating scales. *J Affect Disord* **11**: 245–253.

Faravelli, C, Servi, P, Arends, JA, Strik, WK (1996) Number of symptoms, quantification, and qualification of depression. *Compr Psychiatry* **37**: 307–315.

Fleet R, Lavoie K, Beitman BD (2000) Is panic disorder associated with coronary artery disease? A critical review of the literature. *J Psychosom Res* **48**: 347–356.

Frances A, Manning D, Marin D, Kocsis J, McKinney K, Hall W, Kline M. (1992) Relationship of anxiety and depression. *Psychopharmacology (Berl)* **106**(Suppl): S82–S86.

Frasure-Smith N, Lesperance F, Talajic M (1993) Depression following myocardial infarction. Impact on 6-month survival. *JAMA* **270**(15): 1819–1825.

Freeman MP, Freeman SA, McElroy SL (2002) The comorbidity of bipolar and anxiety disorders: prevalence, psychobiology, and treatment issues. *J Affect Disord* **68**: 1–23.

Glas G (2003) A conceptual history of anxiety and depression. In Kasper S, Den Boer J, Sitsen J (eds) *Handbook of Depression and Anxiety.* New York: Marcel Dekker.

Griez EJ, Mammar N, Loirat JC, Djega N, Trochut JN, Bouhour JB (2000) Panic disorder and idiopathic cardiomyopathy. *J Psychosom Res* **48**: 585–587.

Griez E, Overbeek T (1997) Comorbidity of depression and anxiety. In Honig A, Anseau M, van Praag HM (eds) *Depression: Neurobiological, Psychopathological and Therapeutic Advances.* Chichester, UK: John Wiley.

Hamilton M. (1959) The assessment of anxiety states by rating. *Br J Med Psychol,* **32**, 50–55.

Hamilton M (1960) A rating scale for depression. *J Neurol Neurosurg Psychiatry* **23**: 56–62.

Hamilton M (1967) Development of a rating scale for primary depressive illness. *Br J Soc Clin Psychol* **6**: 278–296.

Herrmann C (1997) International experiences with the Hospital Anxiety and Depression Scale – a review of validation data and clinical results. *J Psychosom Res* **42**: 17–41.

Himmelhoch J, Levine J, Gershon S (2001) Historical overview of the relationship between anxiety disorders and affective disorders. *Depress Anxiety* **14**: 53–66.

Hodgson RJ, Rachman S (1977) Obsessional-compulsive complaints. *Behavioural Research and Therapy* **15**, 389–395.

Kaufman J, Charney D (2000) Comorbidity of mood and anxiety disorders. *Depress Anxiety* **12**(Suppl 1): 69–76.

Keedwell P, Snaith RP (1996) What do anxiety scales measure? *Acta Psychiatr Scand* **93**: 177–180.

Kendler KS (1996) Major depression and generalised anxiety disorder. Same genes, (partly) different environments: revisited. *Br J Psychiatry* **30**(Suppl): 68–75.

Kessler RC, McGonagle KA, Zhao S, Nelson CB, Hughes M, Eshleman S, Wittchen HU, Kendler KS (1994) Lifetime and 12-month prevalence of DSM-III-R psychiatric disorders in the United States: results from the National Comorbidity Survey. *Arch Gen Psychiatry* **51**: 8–19.

Kessler RC, Nelson CB, McGonagle KA, Liu J, Swartz M, Blazer DG (1996) Comorbidity of DSM-III-R major depressive disorder in the general population: results from the US National Comorbidity Survey. *Br J Psychiatry* **30**(Suppl) : 17–30.

Kruger S, Cooke RG, Hasey GM, Jorna T, Persad E (1995) Comorbidity of obsessive compulsive disorder in bipolar disorder. *J Affect Disord* **34**: 117–120.

Lane LW, Luchin D (1988) Evolutionary approaches to psychiatry and problems of method, *Comprehensive Psychiatry* **29**(6): 598–603

Lecrubier Y, Ustun TB (1998) Panic and depression: a worldwide primary care perspective. *Int Clin Psychopharmacol* **13**(Suppl 4): S7–S11.

Levine J, Cole DP, Chengappa KN, Gershon S (2001) Anxiety disorders and major depression, together or apart. *Depress Anxiety* **14**: 94–104.

Liebowitz MR (1987) Social phobia. *Mod Probl Pharmacopsychiatry* **22**: 141–173.

MacKinnon DF, Zandi PP, Cooper J, Potash JB, Simpson SG, Gershon E, et al. (2002) Comorbid bipolar disorder and panic disorder in families with a high prevalence of bipolar disorder. *Am J Psychiatry* **159**: 30–35.

Marks IM, Nesse RM (1994) Fear and fitness:an evolutionary analysis of anxiety disorders. *Ethol Sociobiol* **15**: 247–261.

McGuire MT, Marks I, Nesse RM, Troisi A (1992) Evolutionary biology: a basic science for psychiatry? *Acta Psychiatr Scand* **86**(2): 89–96.

McLoughlin G (2002) Is depression normal in human beings? A critique of the evolutionary perspective. *Int J Ment Health Nurs* **11**: 170–173.

Melartin TK, Rytsala HJ, Leskela US, Lestela-Mielonen PS, Sokero TP, Isometsa ET (2002) Current comorbidity of psychiatric disorders among DSM-IV major depressive disorder patients in psychiatric care in the Vantaa Depression Study. *J Clin Psychiatry* **63**: 126–134.

Merikangas KR, Angst J, Eaton W, Canino G, Rubio-Stipec M, Wacker H, et al. (1996) Comorbidity and boundaries of affective disorders with anxiety disorders and substance misuse: results of an international task force. *Br J Psychiatry* **30**(Suppl): 58–67.

Mineka S, Kihlstrom J (1978) Unpredictable and uncontrollable events: a new perspective on experimental neurosis. *J Abnorm Psychol*, **87**(2): 256–271.

Mineka S, Watson D, Clark LA (1998) Comorbidity of anxiety and unipolar mood disorders. *Ann Rev Psychol*, **49**: 377–412.

Montgomery SA, Åsberg M (1979) A new depression scale designed to be sensitive to change. *Br J Psychiatry* **134**: 382–389.

Nemeroff CB (2002) Comorbidity of mood and anxiety disorders: the rule, not the exception? *Am J Psychiatry* **159**: 3–4.

Nesse RM (1990) Evolutionary explanations of emotions. *Human Nature* **1**(3): 261–289.

Nesse RM (1999) Proximate and evolutionary studies of anxiety, stress and depression: synergy at the interface. *Neurosci Biobehav Rev* **23**(7): 895–903.

Nesse RM (2000) Is depression an adaptation? *Arch Gen Psychiatry* **57**: 14–20.

Ohman A, Mineka S (2001) Fears, phobias, and preparedness: toward an evolved module of fear and fear learning. *Psychol Rev* **108**(3): 483–522.

Panksepp J (1998) *Affective Neuroscience: The Foundation of Human and Animal Emotions*. New York: Oxford University Press.

Perugi G, Akiskal HS, Pfanner C, Presta S, Gemignani A, Milanfranchi A, et al. (1997) The clinical impact of bipolar and unipolar affective comorbidity on obsessive-compulsive disorder. *J Affect Disord* **46**: 15–23.

Poulton R, Menzies RG (2002) Fears born and bred: toward a more inclusive theory of fear acquisition. *Behav Res Ther* **40**(2): 197–208.

Rapaport MH (2001) Prevalence, recognition, and treatment of comorbid depression and anxiety. *J Clin Psychiatry* **62**(Suppl 24): 6–10.

Regier DA, Narrow WE, Rae DS (1990) The epidemiology of anxiety disorders: the Epidemiologic Catchment Area (ECA) experience. *J Psychiatr Res* **24**(Suppl 2): 3–14.

Regier DA, Rae DS, Narrow WE, Kaelber CT, Schatzberg AF (1998) Prevalence of anxiety disorders and their comorbidity with mood and addictive disorders. *Br J Psychiatry* **34**(Suppl): 24–28.

Robins LN, Helzer JE, Croughan J, Ratcliff KS (1981) National Institute of Mental Health Diagnostic Interview Schedule: its history, characteristics, and validity. *Arch Gen Psychiatry* **38**: 381–389.

Robins LN, Wing J, Wittchen HU, Helzer JE, Babor TF, Burke JD, Farmer A, Jablensky A, Pickens R, Regier DA, Sartorius N, Towle LH (1988) The Composite International Diagnostic Interview: an epidemiologic instrument suitable for use in conjunction with different diagnostic systems and in different cultures. *Arch Gen Psychiatry* **45**: 656–664

Rotondo A, Mazzanti C, Dell'Osso L, Rucci P, Sullivan P, Bouanani S, et al. (2002) Catechol o-methyltransferase, serotonin transporter, and tryptophan hydroxylase gene polymorphisms in bipolar disorder patients with and without comorbid panic disorder. *Am J Psychiatry* **159**: 23–29.

Sanderson WC, Beck AT, Beck J (1990) Syndrome comorbidity in patients with major depression or dysthymia: prevalence and temporal relationships. *Am J Psychiatry* **147**: 1025–1028.

Sartorius N, Ustun TB, Lecrubier Y, Wittchen HU (1996) Depression comorbid with anxiety: results from the WHO study on psychological disorders in primary health care. *Br J Psychiatry* **30**(Suppl): 38–43.

Seligman MEP (1975) *Helplessness*. San Francisco: WH Freeman.

Sheehan DV, Lecrubier Y, Sheehan KH, Amorim P, Janavs J, Weiller E, et al. (1998) The Mini-International Neuropsychiatric Interview (M.I.N.I.): the development and validation of a structured diagnostic psychiatric interview for DSM-IV and ICD-10. *J Clin Psychiatry* **59**(Suppl 20): 22–33.

Snaith P (1993) What do depression rating scales measure? *Br J Psychiatry* **163**: 293–298.

Snaith RP, Baugh SJ, Clayden AD, Husain A, Sipple MA (1982) The Clinical Anxiety Scale: an instrument derived from the Hamilton Anxiety Scale. *Br J Psychiatry* **141**: 518–523.

Snaith RP, Taylor CM (1985) Rating scales for depression and anxiety: a current perspective. *Br J Clin Pharmacol* **19**(Suppl 1): 17S–20S.

Spielberger CD, Gorsuch R, Lushene RE (1977) *The State–Trait Anxiety Inventory – Y Form*. Palo Alto: Consultant Psychologists Press.

Spinoza Benedict de (1677) *Ethics*. Translated from the Latin by RHM Elwes (1883). Middle Tennessee State University Philosophy Webworks, Hypertext Edition.

Spitzer RL, Williams JB, Gibbon M, First MB (1992) The Structured Clinical Interview for DSM-III-R (SCID). I: History, rationale, and description. *Arch Gen Psychiatry* **49**: 624–629.

Starcevic V, Uhlenhuth E, Kellner R, Pathak D (1992) Patterns of comorbidity in panic disorder and agoraphobia. *Psychiatry Res* **42**: 171–183.

Tellegen A (1985) Structures of mood and personality and their relevance to assessing anxiety, with an emphasis on self-report. In Tuma AH, Maser JD (eds) *Anxiety and the Anxiety Disorders*. Hillsdale NJ: Lawrence Erlbaum.

Troisi A, McGuire M (2002) Darwinian psychiatry and the concept of mental disorder. *Neuroendocrinol Lett* Special issue, **23**Suppl 4): 31–37.

Van Praag HM (1996) Comorbidity (psycho) analysed. *Br J Psychiatry* (Suppl): 129–134.

Van Praag HM (2000) Nosologomania: a disorder of psychiatry. *World J Biol Psychiatry* **1**: 151–158.

Waikar SV, Craske MG (1997) Cognitive correlates of anxious and depressive symptomatology: an examination of the helplessness/hopelessness model. *J Anx Disord* **11** (1): 1–16.

Wetzler S, Sanderson W (1995) Comorbidity of panic disorder. In Asnis G, van Praag H (eds) *Panic Disorder. Clinical, Biological and Treatment Aspects*. New York: John Wiley pp. 80–98.

Wing J, Babor T, Brugha T, Burke J, Cooper JE, Giel R, Jablensky A, Regier D, Sartorius N (1990) SCAN: Schedules for Clinical Assessment in Neuropsychiatry. *Arch Gen Psychiatry* **47**; 589–593.

Wittchen HU (1996) Critical issues in the evaluation of comorbidity of psychiatric disorders. *Br J Psychiatry* (Suppl): 9–16.

Wittchen HU, Lieb R, Wunderlich U, Schuster P (1999) Comorbidity in primary care: presentation and consequences. *J Clin Psychiatry* **60**(Suppl 7): 29–36; discussion 37–38.

Wittchen HU, Schuster P, Lieb R (2001) Comorbidity and mixed anxiety–depressive disorder: clinical curiosity or pathophysiological need? *Hum Psychopharmacol* **16**: S21–S30.

Wittchen HU, Zhao S, Kessler RC, Eaton WW (1994) DSM-III-R generalized anxiety disorder in the National Comorbidity Survey. *Arch Gen Psychiatry* **51**; 355–364.

World Health Organization (1992) *The ICD-10 Classification of Mental and Behavioural Diseases*. Geneva: WHO.

Yerevanian BI, Koek RJ, Ramdev S (2001) Anxiety disorders comorbidity in mood disorder subgroups: data from a mood disorders clinic. *J Affect Disord* **67**: 167–173.

Zigmond AS, Snaith RP (1983) The hospital anxiety and depression scale. *Acta Psychiatr Scand* **67**: 361–370.

Zimmerman M, Chelminski I, McDermut W (2002) Major depressive disorder and axis 1 diagnostic comorbidity. *J Clin Psychiatry* **63**: 187–193.

Zinbarg RE, Barlow DH, Liebowitz M, Street L, Broadhead E, Katon W, et al. (1994) The DSM-IV field trial for mixed anxiety–depression. *Am J Psychiatry* **151**: 1153–1162.

Zung WW (1965) Self-rating depression scale. *Arch Gen Psychiatry* **12**: 63–70.

Index

Note: Page numbers in *italics* refer to tables or figures. Abbreviations used in the index are: BPD = bipolar disorder; CBT = cognitive-behavioural therapy; CRF₁ = corticotropin-releasing factor1; IRS = inflammatory response system; SSRIs = selective serotonin reuptake inhibitors; TMS = transcranial magnetic stimulation; VNS = vagus nerve stimulation.

diagnostic *see* diagnostic assessment;
standardized scales
association studies 49–52
attachment theory 362–363, 515
attention deficit hyperactivity disorder (ADHD)
107
attributional style 360
atypical depression 297, 311, 312, 319, 375
atypical features, mood-spectrum 136–137
automatic thoughts 361, 362

B lymphocytes 211, 212, 213, 222
behaviour therapy 352–357, 366, 368
effectiveness 367
neuroimaging studies 240, *241*
suicide prevention 171
being, force for 512–514, 520
benzodiazepine receptor binding, neuroimaging
233
generalized anxiety disorder 257
panic disorder 247, 248
post-traumatic stress disorder 253
benzodiazepines 257
bereavement
complicated 298
suicide risk 164, 173
biological factors
suicide *155*, 162, 163, 198, 200
treatment resistance 385–389
see also biological theories
biological markers
antidepressant response 318
depression 96–97, 203–204
biological rhythms
bipolar disorder 108–109
depression 58–59, 83, 409
sleep deprivation therapy 454
biological symptoms of depression, ICD-10
89–90, *89*
see also somatic symptoms/signs
biological theories
bipolar disorder 105
depression 19
inflammatory hypothesis 211–224, 388
neurobiology *see* neurobiology of depression
see also biological factors
bipolar disorder 103–112
adolescents 14, 108
biology 105
children 14, 108
classification 106

bipolar–unipolar dichotomy 86, 92,
124–126, 138–139
BPI 106
BPII 106
and genetic studies 37
historical background 85–86, 103–104,
124–125
problems with 92, 124–126, 127, 138–139
rapid-cycling BPD 106
spectrum concept 92, 126, 127–128, 138
clinical management 109–110
comorbidity 12, 15–16, 107, 512
course of 17, 107–109
definition 103
drug treatment 110–111, 261, 326–330, *332*, 333
bipolar–unipolar dichotomy 125–126
and genetics 43–44, 54, *56*, *57*
and mood-spectrum approach 126–127
neuroimaging studies 268
resistance to 375, 382–385
suicide prevention 170
tolerance 307
triggering mania 312–313, 327, *329*, 384
electroconvulsive therapy 110, 329
epidemiology 104
age of onset 16, *19*, 38–39, 104
bipolar–unipolar dichotomy 125
comorbidity data 12, 15–17, 512
correlates 20
course 17
gender differences 18, 38, 104
prevalence rates 9, *13*, 14, 39, 104, 125
genetic factors 104
adoption studies 42, 104
anticipation 52
association studies 50, 51
classification and 37
family studies 39–40, *41*, 104
linkage studies 44, 45–48, *46–47*, 49
mode of inheritance 43
pharmacogenetics 54, *56*, *57*
twin studies 41–42, 104
historical background 85–86, 103–104,
124–125
mixed episodes 106
mood-spectrum approach 126–137, 138–139
mortality 109
neuroimaging studies 261–262, 268, 269
onset of 16, *19*, 38–39, 104
outcomes 109
post-episodic maladjustment 132–134
psychology of 107